W0018648

MEDICAL RADIOLOGY

Diagnostic Imaging and Radiation Oncology

Springer
Berlin
Heidelberg
New York
Barcelona
Budapest
Hong Kong
London
Milan
Paris
Tokyo

Thermoradiotherapy and Thermochemotherapy

Volume 1: Biology, Physiology, Physics

Contributors

J.C. Bolomey · P. Burgman · I.B. Choi · J. Crezee · O. Dahl · M.W. Dewhirst
C.J. Diederich · R. Felix · K. Hynynen · D.K. Kelleher · A.W.T. Konings
J.J.W. Lagendijk · D. Le Bihan · E.R. Lee · G.C. Li · S. Mizushina
J. Mooibroek · J. Nadobny · B. S. Nah · A. Nussenzweig · R. Olmi
J.L. Osborn · K.D. Paulsen · D.M. Prescott · D.I. Roos · S.K. Sahu
C.J. Schneider · M. Seebass · M.H. Seegenschmiedt · C.W. Song · B. Sorbe
P.R. Stauffer · C. Streffer · J.D.P. van Dijk · G.C. van Rhoon P.W. Vaupel
C.C. Vernon · A.G. Visser · F.M. Waterman · P. Wust

Edited by

M.H. Seegenschmiedt, P. Fessenden, and C.C. Vernon

Foreword by

L.W. Brady and H.-P. Heilmann

With 266 Figures, 6 of Them in Color and 45 Tables

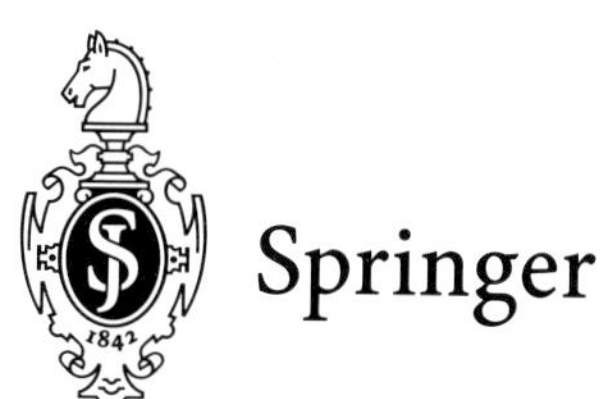

Springer

Priv.-Doz. Dr. M. HEINRICH SEEGENSCHMIEDT
Strahlentherapeutische Klinik
Universität Erlangen-Nürnberg
Universitätsstraße 27
91054 Erlangen, Germany

PETER FESSENDEN, PhD
Professor Emeritus, Radiation Oncology
Radiation Oncology
Physics Division
Stanford University Medical Center
SUMC Room S-044
Stanford, CA 94305, USA

CLARE C. VERNON, MA, FRCR
Department of Clinical Oncology
Hammersmith Hospital
Ducane Road
London W12 OHS, UK

MEDICAL RADIOLOGY. Diagnostic Imaging and Radiation Oncology
Continuation of
Handbuch der medizinischen Radiologie
Encyclopedia of Medical Radiology

ISSN 0942-5373
ISBN 3-540-57229-5 Springer-Verlag Berlin Heidelberg New York

Library of Congress Cataloging-in-Publication Data. Thermoradiotherapy and thermochemotherapy/contributors, J.C. Bolomey . . . [et al.]; edited by M.H. Seegenschmiedt, P. Fessenden, and C.C. Vernon; foreword by L.W. Brady and H.-P. Heilmann. p. cm. – (Medical radiology) Includes bibliographical references and index. Contents: v. 1. Biology, physiology, and physics. ISBN 3-540-57229-5 1. Cancer – Thermotherapy. 2. Cancer – Chemotherapy. 3. Cancer – Radiotherapy. 4. Cancer – Adjuvant treatment. I. Bolomey, J.C. (Jean-Charles) II. Seegenschmiedt, M.H. (Michael Heinrich), 1955– . III. Fessenden, P. (Peter) IV. Vernon, C.C (Clare C.) V. Series. [DNLM: 1. Neoplasms – therapy. 2. Hypothermia, Induced. 3. Radiotherapy, Adjuvant. 4. Chemotherapy, Adjuvant. QZ 266 T412 1995] RC271.T5T44 1995 616.99'406—dc20 DNLM/DLC for Library of Congress 95-11653

Printed in Germany

Cover design: Springer-Verlag, Design & Production

Typesetting: Best-set Typesetter Ltd., Hong Kong

SPIN: 10089909 21/3135/SPS – 5 4 3 2 1 0 – Printed on acid-free paper

Foreword

Hyperthermia has been found to be of great benefit in combination with radiation therapy or chemotherapy in the management of patients with difficult and complicated tumor problems. It has been demonstrated to increase the efficacy of ionising radiation when used locally but also has been of help in combination with systemic chemotherapy where hyperthermia is carried out to the total body.

Problems remain with regard to maximizing the effects of hyperthermia as influenced by blood flow, heat loss, etc.

The present volume defines the current knowledge relative to hyperthermia with radiation therapy and/or chemotherapy, giving a comprehensive overview of its use in cancer management.

Philadelphia/Hamburg, June 1995

L.W. Brady
H.-P. Heilmann

Preface

In an attempt to overcome tumor resistance, hypoxia, or unfavorable tumor conditions, oncological research has come to focus on gene therapy, immunotherapy, new cytotoxic agents, and increasingly sophisticated radiotherapy. Radiation research has been directed towards heavy particle therapy and modification of the radiation response by either protecting or sensitizing agents. Improved dose localization using rotational or conformal strategies has also been implemented. Recently, changes in radiation fractionation schedules have shown promise of better results. *Hyperthermia in cancer therapy* can be viewed similarly as another means to increase the sensitivity of tumors to radio- and chemotherapy.

Hyperthermia (i.e., the application of heat to attain elevated tumor temperatures, usually in the range of 41°–44°C) as an *adjuvant* to chemo- and radiotherapy is primarily employed to improve local control, while its combination with systemic chemotherapy and sometimes even whole-body radiotherapy obviously aims at the control of systemic metastases as well. It is in *local control of the primary lesion* that hyperthermia will have the greatest impact, and it is *in combination with radiotherapy* that hyperthermia appears to have its greatest potential at present. Therefore it should be implemented in patients in whom the percentage of local failure is high, such as those with the common tumors of the brain, breast, lung, oropharynx, upper gastrointestinal tract, and pelvis including the prostate, uterus, cervix, ovary, and bladder. Even if the impact on survival from improved local control were to be as low as 5%, this increase would still represent a very significant number of patients saved from a cancer death.

In cases where no hope for better survival can be expected from improved local control, many patients could still benefit from alleviation of the extremely unpleasant effects of uncontrolled local disease (bleeding, pain, infection, etc.). This is particularly true for breast cancer patients who experience a local failure at the operated breast or chest wall, such failure often being associated with a variety of very distressing symptoms and circumstances. Thus, *palliation of uncontrolled local disease* is another important indication for hyperthermia.

A general rationale for the use of hyperthermia began to evolve from the laboratory in the early 1960s, but the actual task of inducing and monitoring the heat application clinically proved to be much more technically difficult than was anticipated. Nevertheless, even early clinical trials using crude technical heating equipment sometimes achieved encouraging results when hyperthermia and appropriate radiotherapy where combined.

More recently we have seen some very positive clinical results emerging from well-controlled phase III randomized trials (including malignant brain tumors, melanomas, head and neck and breast tumors) where good quality assurance has been assured. Most of these trials were of multi-institutional design to recruit sufficient numbers of patients within a reasonable period. Studies involving heat in combination with chemotherapy and even triple-modality therapy are now underway for tumors with a high tumor growth fraction or high metastatic potential. Innovative and invasive techniques, such as interstitial and intracavitary hyperthermia, have become available to strengthen our oncological armamentarium. Presently unresolved questions point to the following areas of research:

1. *Biologists* may deepen or even complete our insight into the development of thermotolerance, and specific assays of heat shock proteins may provide us with information about the optimal treatment schedule.
2. *Physiologists and pharmacologists* may induce artificial alterations of the cellular environment by means of specific thermosensitizers, vasodilators, or the infusion of glucose to alter the pH. Using positron emission tomography or magnetic resonance spectroscopy, the induced changes might easily be monitored and used for the prediction of tumor response.
3. *Physicists or engineers* may improve present heating systems: applicators are now being designed to provide broader field sizes, improved control of power deposition, thermal homogeneity and heat delivery to areas of limited access, better shielding of sensitive adjacent normal tissues, better conformity to curved body surfaces, improvement of overall treatment comfort for patients and improved equipment and computer operation for staff.
4. There is a further need for useful noninvasive thermometry techniques, e.g., microwave or ultrasound radiometry, applied potential tomography, or particularly magnetic resonance imaging; however, clinical applications are likely to be some years off.
5. *Clinical oncologists* (surgeons, radiotherapists, and medical oncologists) must cooperate to an even greater extent in multicenter trials and quality control, and design appropriate controlled clinical studies for suitable tumors and body sites.

Despite this "work-in-progress situation," there is no doubt that the addition of hyperthermia to chemo- and radiotherapy provides a significant and worthwhile improvement in cancer control, and that it holds good promise as a cancer treatment for selected body sites. In the two volumes of *Thermoradiotherapy and Thermochemotherapy* we have aimed to bring together a group of experts of international reknown to present up-to-date knowledge and future perspectives in the fields of hyperthermic biology, physiology, and physics (volume 1) and clinical options for combined hyperthermia and ionizing radiation or chemotherapy (volume 2). The two volumes include 45 contributions (21 chapters in volume 1 and 24 chapters in volume 2) which demonstrate the advanced state of this multidisciplinary field. We have structured the contents of the book into six sections: historical review, biological principles, pathophysiological mechanisms, physical principles and engineering, clinical applications, and multicenter trials and future research.

The logical order of the chapters, the many figures and tables, the concise tabulation of parameters for hyperthermia data evaluation, and the comprehensive subject index provide a clear orientation in the field. The reader will find the important aspects summarized and highlighted at the end of each chapter. The two volumes are designed to allow the specialist as well as the interested newcomer to start with any desired topic or preferred area of research and then easily to proceed to any other topic of interest.

In publishing these two volumes we hope to promote further scientific exchange among the countries of Europe, America, Asia and other areas in order to stimulate the diffusion of knowledge of thermoradio- and thermochemotherapy in all specialized oncological fields. Biological research, technical improvements, and new clinical concepts and therapeutic ideas may pave the way for a broad spectrum of oncological and even nononcological applications. We hope that you will find this book interesting, informative, and stimulating: it certainly was for all three of us as we participated in the writing and editing of it.

Erlangen/London/Stanford

M. Heinrich Seegenschmiedt
Clare C. Vernon
Peter Fessenden

Contents

Contents of Volume 2

Clinical Applications of Hyperthermia

Historical Review

1 A Historical Perspective on Hyperthermia in Oncology

M.H. SEEGENSCHMIEDT and C.C. VERNON

CONTENTS

1.1 Introduction

"*Cancer*" today means a "*malignant growing tumor*" which nearly always threatens life if it has reached its advanced form, but may be "curable" if detected in any early stage of development. One special section of medicine called "oncology" deals with these malignant diseases. Despite extensive research in the past, the etiology, possible preventive measures, and the diagnostic assessment are still incompletely understood; similarly, the therapeutic management of cancer is still not too well established in our present health care system. By the public, cancer is mostly perceived as a fatal disease which is often associated with pain or other dreadful symptoms, malnutrition, severe individual discomfort, and many psychosocial problems.

Throughout medical history, the diagnostic and therapeutic management of cancer have been a matter of controversy and never regarded as a truly rewarding task. Even now, the early detection, refined diagnosis, and description of the clinical development of various tumors along with their specific clinical symptoms are emphasized more in the medical curricula and practical training, continuous medical education, and medical research than in the complicated and empirical therapeutic practice of surgical, medical, and radiation oncology.

Due to the overt lack of success with the more conventional oncological methods, i.e., surgery, radiotherapy, and chemotherapy, improved cancer treatments are desperately sought. They are often wholeheartedly and quickly embraced if they offer hope of even a small improvement in cancer management. However, if the methods in question fail to prove their therapeutic potential within a certain period, they also may be too quickly condemned, without careful assessment. Thus, historical, political, economic, and even intrinsically medical aspects may not be disregarded if new oncological treatment modalities like "hyperthermia" are to occupy their appropriate place in oncology.

This introductory chapter to the two volumes on "Thermoradiotherapy and Thermochemotherapy" briefly reviews the developing field of oncology and tries to address the specific role of hyperthermia in this field from a more historical perspective. This historical review is intended to point out only the most interesting areas of hyperthermic research, which have come under intensive investigation in recent years. We rely in this chapter on several excellent summaries of the same issue as well as some historical comments on hyperthermia (LICHT 1965; DIETZEL 1975; HORNBACK 1984; MEYER 1984; OVERGAARD 1985; STORM 1983; SUGAHARA 1989). We are aware that the presented selection of historical details and their specific interpretation is a somewhat subjec-

M.H. SEEGENSCHMIEDT, MD, Department of Radiation Oncology, University of Erlangen-Nürnberg, Universitätsstraße 27, D-91054 Erlangen, FRG
C.C. VERNON, M.A., FRCR, MRC Hyperthermia Clinic, Hammersmith Hospital, Du Cane Road, London W12 OHS, UK

tive view and certainly does not represent a complete assessment of the available historical sources.

1.2 Historical Perspective on Cancer Therapy

1.2.1 Ancient Times

It is almost certain that some of the "swellings" and "ulcers" of the skin, breast, and female genitalia exactly described in different Egyptian papyri (Papyrus Ebers, Papyrus Edwin Smith, and Papyrus Kahoun) were true malignant tumors. On account of their easy accessibility they were the best-known and best-described "cancers" of antiquity. Similar descriptions of malignant tumors are also encountered in the available ancient medical writings of the Mesopotamian, Indian, and Persian cultures. The Greek priests of Asklepios (about 1260 B.C.), the Asklepiades, who were known for their medical skills, already knew of and differentiated the continuously progressing "swellings" with or without ulceration. Because of the rather similar appearance of a protruding and locally infiltrating tumor of the breast and the crayfish, they called this disease "*καρκινος*" (*karkinos*) (Fig. 1.1).

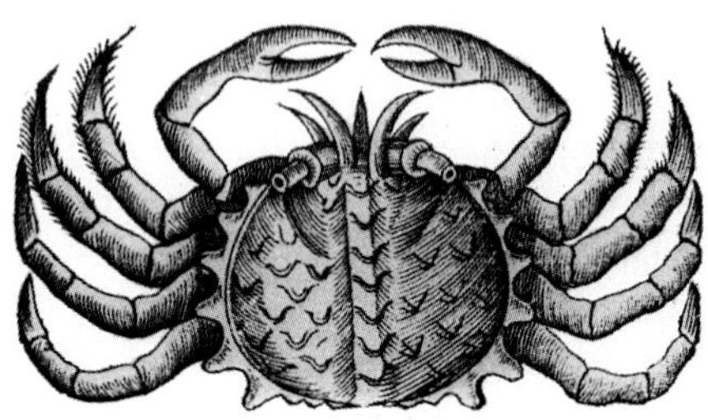

Fig. 1.1. "*Le chancre.*" Copperplate engraving from the medical book *Œuvres d'Ambroise Pare, 10th edition*, Lyon 1641. This engraving illustrates the animal, a crayfish or crab, which gave the name to our modern disease "cancer." The writers at the time of Hippocrates (500–400 B.C.) used the words "*karkinos*" and "*karkinoma*" to describe indiscriminately chronic ulcerations and swellings that appear to have been malignant tumours. The Roman Celsus (25 B.C.–50 A.D.) translated the Greek word "*karkinos*" into the Latin "cancer," a term which was used for open and deeply penetrating types of ulcers, while he used "carcinoma" for closed lesions corresponding to our premalignant and malignant tumors. As late as the nineteenth century both terms were used as synonyms to describe malignant tumors

For noninflammatory tumors, hard swellings, and ulcers of the skin, female breast, and genitalia with a tendency to generalization, locoregional relapse, and a fatal outcome, the *Hippocratic aphorisms* derived from the famous Greek physician Hippocrates of Kos (460–370 B.C.; Fig. 1.2) used the expressions "*karkinos*" (in an early tumor stage) or "*karkinoma*" (in an advanced tumor stage). These expressions were later translated into the Latin language as the term "*cancer.*" Occasionally another term, "*σκιρρος*" (Latin: *scirrhus*), was used; however, in later times this expression was applied in a more or less confusing manner even for noncancerous hard tumors,

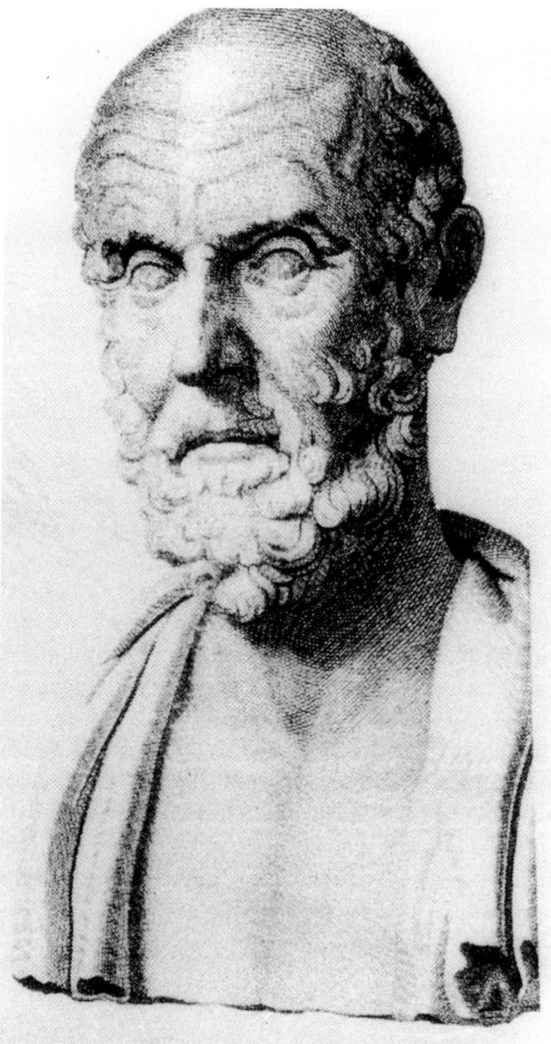

Fig. 1.2. Hippokrates of Kos (460–370 B.C.), the famous Greek physician who became famous for his so-called *Hippocratic aphorisms*, which comprised a collection of items of practical advice for the physicians of the time

precancerous tumor lesions, and some particular types of cancer.

The ancient physicians were often reluctant to treat these malignant diseases, which they regarded as cancers. In many instances, cancer therapy was considered useless or even disastrous for the patient, and also potentially damaging to the reputation of the physician, especially when the prescribed treatment was failing. Thus, a "prudent" physician with wide clinical experience had to learn through theoretical studies and clinical practice to "touch" only the easily curable small tumors (i.e., those in their early stages), and to leave untreated those patients who displayed large protruding, ulcerated, or generalized tumors (i.e., those in their more advanced stages). Thus, a broad *therapeutic pessimism* governed oncological practice in antiquity. One of the Hippocratic aphorisms even specifically warns against the treatment of the "*nonulcerated cancers*," which were then already regarded as a more advanced form of cancer, by saying (JONES and HENRY 1959): "It is better to give no treatment in the cases of hidden cancer, as the treatment causes speedy death, while to omit treatment is to prolong life."

Also the term "*μεταστασις*" (metastasis) was coined from the Hippocratian medicine meaning "to change" or "to transform".

The Roman encyclopedist Aulus Cornelius Celsus (25 B.C.–50 A.D.) included in his famous encyclopedia a chapter on "*De Medicina*," which added to the diagnostic but not to the therapeutic knowledge of cancer. It was the most renowned physician of antiquity, Clarissimus Claudius Galen from Pergamon (130–120 A.D.), who wrote a special volume on "*tumors*"; however, among the 61 presented "tumors" he also described several nontumorous diseases like "*edema*," "*erysipelas*," and "*lipomas*." More importantly, Galen codified the "humoral theory" of disease which arose about 400–500 B.C. in analogy to the theory of the four elements and was explained in the treatise "*On the Nature of Man*," written by Hippocrates or his son-in-law Polybos.

This humoral theory, although not undisputed in antiquity, became established for the next 1500 years and handed down to the scholastic school of medicine in the Middle Ages. This fundamental theory of physiology explained that the physical condition is due to the relative balance among its four "humors" – the liquids blood, yellow bile, black bile, and phlegm. If the mixture (*krasis*) of these four humors is in good balance (*eukrasia*), the human being enjoys a state of health, while the imbalance (*dyskrasia*) of the humors is the cause of diseases, including cancer. This conceptual idea of disease as an imbalance of the four natural "forces," so-called humoralistic medicine, became very popular among physicians and scientists and convinced almost everybody of antiquity and thereafter.

With regard to the development of malignant tumors, Galen held one of the four humors responsible, the "*melan cholos*" – the nonexistent black bile. As long as such an interpretation of cancer was accepted as the truth, it was bound to discourage a more "logical" approach to the treatment of cancers, including the surgical excision of tumors. Instead, general treatments such as diets or drugs or bleedings prevailed as common therapeutic strategies far into the nineteenth century. Even nowadays, plenty of quacks still thrive on this "alternative treatment" of cancer.

1.2.2 The Middle Ages

Arabian medicine helped to pass on several ideas of ancient medicine to the "dark" Middle Ages. Of itself, this period added little to the knowledge of cancer, although a few aspects, especially in respect of the internal tumors, were developed and broadened. For example, the Arab physician Rhazes (900 A.D.) differentiated nasal polyps and cancer, and Avenzoar (about 1150 A.D.) suggested external feeding and nutritional support by means of clysters and sounds for patients suffering from slowly growing esophageal and gastric cancers. The medieval physicians were as sceptical about the performance of surgical procedures for cancers as were those of antiquity, and the nascent separation of the two practical medical fields of surgery and medicine clearly hampered progress in oncology.

1.2.3 The Sixteenth, Seventeenth, and Eighteenth Centuries

In the sixteenth century, the physicians of the Renaissance provided little new information and developed no new clinical strategies for the treatment of cancer. For example, the German anatomist Andreas Vesalius (1514–1564), who published his famous anatomical book "*De humani corporis fabrica libri septem*" in 1543, helped to improve the clinical understanding and the differentiation of malignant tumors, but again, his studies were far more targeted at diagnostic rather than therapeutic progress in oncology. As a representative example, one of the most famous surgeons of that time, the Frenchman Ambroise Paré, still interpreted the occurrence of metastases in the traditional humoralistic fashion, namely as a local manifestation of the "melancholic diathesis."

In the seventeenth century and the period of the Enlightenment, the French genius René Descartes (1596–1650) – who was a philosopher, mathematician, and physician at the same time – was one of the first to challenge the popular humoralistic "black bile theory" of Galen through a widely acclaimed *mechanistic lymph theory* which was in accordance with the then newly discovered lymphatic system. In a long historical perspective, his "mechanistic" concept encouraged later surgeons to take a logical approach to treating cancer by removing all involved cancerous lymph nodes together with the primary tumor. In that century, which was sorely troubled by plague epidemic throughout Europe, the view of cancer as a "contagious disease" was adopted by many physicians and the public. This opinion derived from analogies with other tumor-like diseases including leprosy and elephantiasis. As a fatal consequence, all sufferers from cancer were rigorously barred from most hospitals at that time, a policy which was retained even up to the middle of the nineteenth century. This is well reflected in a dramatic conflict in 1874 between James Marion Sims (1813–1883), who is regarded as the father of surgical gynecology in North America, and the managers of the first gynecological hospital in New York, the famous "Women's Hospital of the State of New York", who intended to bar all patients with malignant tumors from the hospital. Finally, patients with tumors were also treated.

Due to major advances in anatomy and general pathology, the eighteenth century witnessed the first great scientific debate in medicine between the declared proponents of the "humoralistic diathesis" and those of "solidistic localism," which was then being newly applied to oncological diseases. The most important promoter of *localism*, the Italian Giovanni Battista Morgagni (1682–1771), taught anatomy in Bologna and Padua; he precisely described and characterized numerous cancers which he saw at autopsies from this new perspective. An important contribution to the clarification of the etiology of malignancies was also made by the Dutch clinician Herman Boerhaave (1668–1738), who regarded cancer as a consequence of *local irritation*, an important clinical observation which was later confirmed in respect of many types of occupational cancer, such as scrotal cancer in chimney sweeps, pulmonary cancer among the Schneeberg miners, bladder cancer in aniline workers, and bone tumors among dial-makers. It was not until this time, in 1740, that the first specialized hospital for cancer patients was opened; this hospital, in Rheims (France), remained open for almost a hundred years.

1.2.4 The Nineteenth Century

It was not until the nineteenth century that oncology made a more decisive step forward through further progress in pathological anatomy and detailed histological studies on the various tissues composing different organs rather than mere macroscopic observation and description of organ changes. The founder and promoter of histopathology, the young French physician Marie François Xavier Bichat (1771–1802), was able to differentiate between the stroma and parenchyma of cancers and precisely observed their lobular structure. He rejected the ancient differentiation between open (ulcerated) and nonulcerated cancers.

The ingenious inventor of the stethoscope, the precise diagnostician, observant clinician, and brilliant pathological anatomist, René Théophile Hyacinthe Laennec (1781–1826), divided the malignant tumors into a "homologous" (i.e., analogous to existing tissues) and a "heterologous" group (i.e., without any parallelism to normal tissues). He was already convinced of the *local origin of cancer*, whereas several of his collaborators still believed in the "dyscrasic cancerous diathesis." Even 30 years later, the Austrian pathologist Karl von Rokitansky (1804–1878) upheld the old humoralistic idea in his early years and was much supported by the French physician Jean Cruveilhier (1791–1874), who emphasized the existence of a "cancer juice." Many other cancer theories originated in the nineteenth century which tried to overcome the traditional hypotheses. However, this was still a scientific debate on the origin, development, and diagnosis of cancer rather than on the appropriate treatment.

In the nineteenth century, new concepts and ideas were transferred from the autopsy to the operation room. With the introduction of anesthesia more aggressive surgeons developed new treatment concepts. Thus, the field of "surgical oncology" started to develop and slowly helped to improve the therapeutic standards achieved with drugs and diets. This is reflected in the famous book by the American surgeon John Collins Warren (1778–1856), "*Surgical Observations on Tumours with Cases and Operations*," which was published in 1837 (Pollay 1955). Warren also stressed the importance of complete surgical removal of "precancerous lesions."

A completely new oncological understanding arose from microscopy and the interpretation of pathological findings according to the Schleiden-Schwann "cell theory" (Matthias Jakob Schleiden, 1804–1881; Theodor Schwann, 1810–1880) and the Remak-Virchow cell theory, which is reflected by the hypothesis "*omnis cellula e cellula*" (Robert Remak, 1815–1865; Rudolf Virchow, 1821–1902). It was the German anatomist and physiologist Johannes Peter Müller (1801–1858) and his remarkable book entitled "*Über den feineren Bau und die Formen der krankhaften Geschwülste*" (published in 1838) who finally paved the way for a revolutionary interpretation which still influences our allopathic medical thinking and current oncological concepts. Müller's work stimulated the fundamental studies of his famous disciple Rudolf Virchow, who successfully applied his "cellular pathology" (i.e., pathology of various diseases from the perspective of their cellular changes) to the various malignant diseases. He was the first to completely define and describe the "cancerous cell," the tumor structure, and the various stages of tumor formation. Virchow was a very strong proponent of the *local origin of cancer*, an interpretation which subsequently stimulated all the modern therapeutic approaches of surgical oncology.

Despite some errors in Virchow's oncological concept (e.g., that *all* tumors originate from connective tissue), his basic ideas have prevailed until today. Based on the dramatic input of bacteriology around 1870–1900 and the rapid technical progress made in various medical disciplines, including the discovery of x-rays in 1895 by Wilhelm Conrad Röntgen (1845–1923) and their immediate use in diagnostic and therapeutic radiology, as well as the increasing sophistication of surgery as a whole and of radical operations in particular, the treatment of cancer has experienced considerable progress in the twentieth century. Due to the aforementioned progress and the development of anesthesiological techniques, some remarkable new oncological operations were performed at the end of the nineteenth and the beginning of the twentieth century, including the *Halstedt operation* on the breast (William Stewart Halstedt, 1852–1922), the *Wertheim operation* on the uterus (Ernst Wertheim, 1864–1920), and the renowned *Billroth operation* on the larynx, esophagus, and stomach (Theodor Billroth, 1829–1894).

1.2.5 The Modern Ages

During the twentieth century our basic understanding of cancer has exploded, resulting in an immense specialization and subspecialization of oncological research. The most remarkable contributions during this century have come from biology, biochemistry, pathophysiology, pharmacology, microbiology, virology, immunology, and human genetics, but there have also been contributions from environmental medicine, epidemiology, biomedical statistics, and many other related disciplines. Nowadays experimental research is booming and clinical practice still diversifying. There is far greater awareness of individual and general preventive measures, external and internal diagnostic procedures have improved dramatically, and for many malignancies single-modality therapy has been abandoned and replaced by a multimodality approach.

Nevertheless, not only the patients and the public but also most physicians and scientists are confused, frustated, and even intimidated by this immense diversification, as few are able to achieve a broad overview of this accumulated knowledge. Another observation is troublesome: It is not known whether there has been an actual increase in cancer in our times or whether the increased prevalence is attributable to improved cancer registration, better diagnostic tools, or increased life expectancy; however, cancer is the *symbolic disease of our modern era*, as leprosy was during the Middle Ages or cholera during the nineteenth century.

Despite scientific conquests and advances in clinical practice, many old questions are still unanswered and with any new answer even more questions seem to arise. Unfortunately, this is also reflected in the persistent lack of successful management for most solid tumors, at least when they have progressed beyond a merely local stage. Thus, we must ask ourselves of the field of oncology:

1. Where have we arrived with our present scientific knowledge?
2. Is Hippocrates' pessimistic view on cancer treatment still valid?
3. Are we now experiencing a new battle between "humoralists" (represented by laboratory medicine, medical oncology, and immunology) on the one hand and "solidists" (represented by diagnostic imaging or surgical and radiation oncology) on the other?
4. Will the imminent economic constraints on our health care systems allow us to pursue new therapeutic avenues while we continue in the frustrated therapeutic efforts of the past, or will we be forced to abandon costly treatments?
5. Can we define better prognostic parameters to allow more strict selection of patients?

Certainly it will be the task of the next century to synthesize the multifaceted research efforts, to improve interdisciplinary cooperation, to introduce stringent quality assurance and control in diagnostic and therapeutic practice, and to conduct controlled multidisciplinary and multicenter trials where there is a clear indication of any therapeutic progress from various single institutions. When we reflect on this arduous and still on-going development of oncology, it should be evident that the development of hyperthermia in oncology should be given a fair chance and that a similar patient attitude should be adopted with regard to other new treatment concepts and ideas as tentative steps are taken to define their role in oncology.

1.3 Historical Perspective on Hyperthermia

1.3.1 General Definitions

The term "*hyperthermia*," which is derived from the Greek "*hyper*" (i.e., beyond, above, over, or excessive) and "*therme*" (i.e., heat), has to be clearly distinguished from the term "*fever*," which derives from the Latin word "*febris*." While the former term refers to the artificial, either external or internal induction of localized or systemic heat deposition in the human body, the latter term describes an internally induced pathophysiological phenomenon which may be caused by abnormalities of the brain or triggered by toxic agents that affect the temperature-regulating centers in the hypothalamus and lead to a systemic increase in the body temperature. Viruses, bacterial toxins, drugs, tissue breakdown, and foreign proteins can act as so-called pyrogens. While under the former condition, the normal thermoregulatory forces react with vasodilatation and increasing perfusion to maintain the normal body temperature, under the latter condition the central thermoregulatory system and the thermal feedback control mechanisms are still functioning, but are switched and regulated at a higher than normal body temperature level.

In contrast, the term "*malignant hyperthermia*" is used to describe the sudden and often fatal rise in body temperature which is mostly associated with the induction of general anesthesia by means of halothane, methoxyflurane, cyclopropane, and diethylether. It occurs preferentially in young people and in specific families. It is characterized by the sudden onset of extremely high body temperatures and by tachycardia, cardiac arrhythmia, and rigidity of muscles. Succinylcholine may be one triggering agent, and the underlying defect in susceptible patients seems to be a faulty calcium metabolism in muscles which results in the typical tetany symptoms. The burst of muscular activity produces tremendous quantities of heat which overwhelm the normal compensation mechanisms of the human body, and the central temperature and feedback control mechanisms may be damaged as well. Systemic temperatures may reach far beyond 42°C.

"*Environmental heat illness*" is another scenario in which the body temperature is elevated above the normal level. This temperature elevation can derive from two sources. First, heat can be transferred from the environment to the human body by radiation (i.e., via electromagnetic waves) and by conduction and convection from warm air, hot water, or other hot media. For example, when exposed to direct sunlight, the human body can accumulate up to 150 kcal/h. Secondly, heat can be produced metabolically by the body itself, especially by intense muscular activity. During maximal physical exercise the metabolic heat production reaches 600–900 kcal/h, which raises the core body temperature to as high as 40°C

(Bard 1961). All individuals suffering from "heat stroke" have an intact thermoregulatory center.

Today "hyperthermia" in oncology is used as a sensitizing agent for ionizing radiation (radiosensitization) or chemotherapy (chemosensitization). Generally this can be achieved with heat treatments in the range of 41°–43°C, while temperatures above 43°C induce direct thermal cytotoxicity depending upon the duration of heating. Other means of inducing "hyperthermia" like photocoagulation or laser therapy work at considerably higher temperatures beyond 50°–60°C or even 100°C or higher. Thus, the present meaning of "hyperthermia" is rather diverse and strongly related to the applied technique and the purpose of its application.

1.3.2 General Historical Considerations

The obvious ignorance and confusion about the exact diagnosis and treatment of "cancer" may well explain many of the remarkable case reports of "cancer cure" by exposure to heat which have been handed down in medical history. In ancient times most cancers (some of which may not have been of a truly malignant nature) were treated by local excision (surgery), diets or drugs (medicine), and/or bleedings. Another oncological treatment termed "cauterization" was also commonplace in various ancient cultures. This treatment consisted in the local application of extreme heat either by the use of specific chemicals, such as "cauterizing salves," or by direct physical contact of the tumor with the so-called *ferrum candens*, which has been translated as "fire drill" or "red hot iron" (Fig. 1.3). Besides these rather local measures, the use of hot baths was another traditional means of treating various types of disease, though only sometimes cancer (Fig. 1.4).

If we accept that these widely applied caustic measures represent typical applications of "*local hyperthermia*" (at high temperatures for a short period of time) and the use of hot baths or the artificial induction of fever, applications of "*systemic hyperthermia*" (at relatively mild temperatures for a much longer treatment duration), then hyperthermia has a very longstanding tradition in the treatment of cancer. However, it was not until the beginning of the twentieth century that a much more scientific approach was taken to the application of heat as a means of cancer therapy, and this will be the focus of most of our remarks.

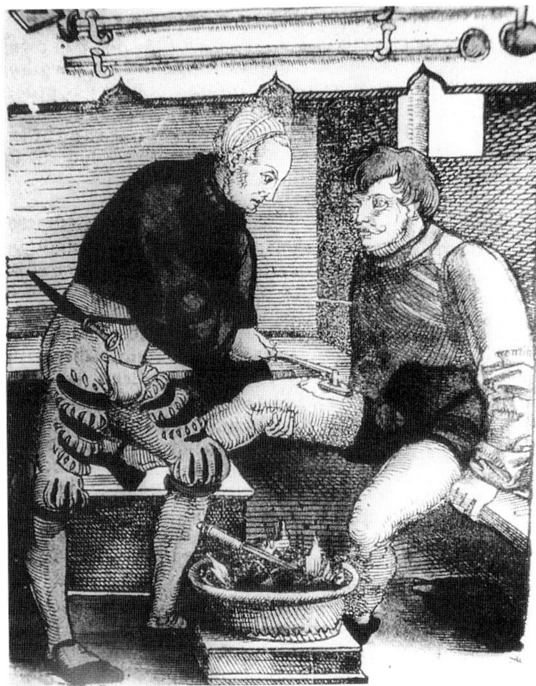

Fig. 1.3. Illustration of a typical cautery treatment in the Middle Ages with the "*ferrum candens*" (red hot iron). Copperplate engraving from the sixteenth century. (Philadelphia Museum of Art, Philadelphia. Purchased: SmithKline Beckman Corporation Foundation)

During this century and especially during recent decades new heating techniques and clinical applications have been developed and many types of tumors have been treated. For induction of *external local hyperthermia* a variety of methods have been applied, including radiofrequency, shortwave, microwave, ultrasound, and hot water perfusion techniques. In addition, *internal, intracavitary, and interventional heat treatments* have been carried out by means of galvanocautery, electromagnetic heating, and conductive hot water perfusion. *Systemic heating* has been induced by hot baths, artificial fever therapy, and external heating devices, e.g., heating cabinets. Technical progress and the growth of clinical expertise, especially during the last two decades, have helped us to stimulate the development and implementation of various heating methods. Thus, nowadays a broad spectrum of heating methods and techniques is available for clinical applications, as summarized in Table 1.1.

Dises puchlein sagt vns von allen paden die võ natur heiß sein

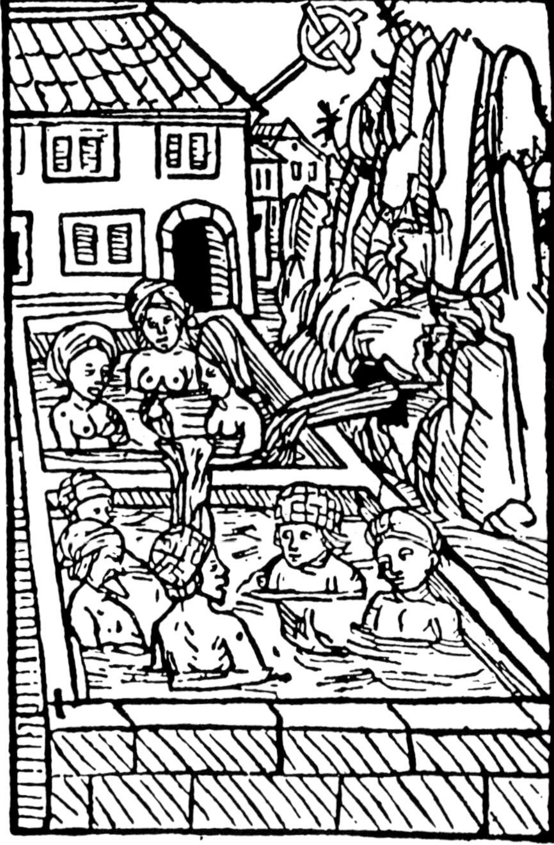

Fig. 1.4. Open thermal bath located at a hot spring illustrated on the title page of a book from the sixteenth century. The writing on top of the wood engraving gives the title of the book: "This booklet tells us about all natural hot baths." German wood engraving from around 1500 A.D. (Paris, Bibliothèque des arts decoratifs)

1.3.3 Localized Heating Methods

1.3.3.1 External Cautery

In ancient times heat was applied to various types of disease, including cancer. One of the oldest historical reports on the use of heat to treat tumors was handed down by the Indian "*Ramajana.*" Its use as an oncological treatment is also mentioned in the Egyptian *Edwin Smith Surgical Papyrus*, which dates back to about 3000 B.C. (BREASTED 1930). Therein a clinical report is presented of a woman suffering from a (malignant?) breast tumor. In this case it was recommended that the tumor be treated by means of the so-called fire drill, which was clearly meant to be a local caustic therapy. Subsequently, such local heat treatments were described in numerous other reports by Greek and Roman physicians. This ancient confidence in the application of local heat is underscored by one of the famous aphorisms of the Greek physician Hippocrates, who stated (translated in Latin words, according to OVERGAARD 1985):

Quae medicamenta non sanant, ferum sanat.
Quae ferum non sanat, ignis sanat.
Quae vero ignis non sanat, insanobilia reportari oportet.

which means:

Those who cannot be cured by medicine can be cured by surgery.
Those who cannot be cured by surgery can be cured by heat.
Those who cannot be cured by heat are to be considered incurable.

While in this specific Hippocratic aphorism (local) cautery was regarded as a very effective means of treating advanced malignant superficial tumors, Hippocrates warned against the use of (systemic) heat when he stated in another aphorism:

Heat produces the following harmful results in those who use it too frequently: softening of the flesh, impotence of the muscles, dullness of the intelligence, hemorrhages, fainting, and death ensuing in certain cases.

The broad application of "local heat" throughout antiquity is addressed in several ancient Roman scripts, for example in "*De medicina*," the famous encyclopedia of the Roman physician Celsus (CELSUS 1967), and in the writings of Galen, who also recommended the use of "*ferrum candens*" for accessible localized tumors.

However, this "solidistic" or "mechanistic" approach to cancer therapy stood somewhat in contrast to the otherwise "humoralistic concept" of disease which was commonplace at the time. Apparently the therapeutic success of local heat treatment spoke for itself. The records on local cautery usually state that the involved area was entirely burnt out, including a margin of surrounding healthy tissue, thereby destroying the tumor and coagulating the underlying bleeding vessles. The Greek physician Leonidas from

Table 1.1. Principal methods and special techniques of heating

Heating method	Specific technique	Clinical applications
Microwave heating methods (50–2450 MHz)		
Single external devices	Direct tissue contact at the body surface with use of bolus material	Small superficial tumors
Multiple external devices	Direct tissue contact with applicators placed around the lesion	Extensive superficial tumors
Phased array devices	Applicators surround the patient for regional deep heating	Deep-seated tumors of abdomen, pelvis, or extremities
Interstitial devices ("antennae")	Single antenna or antenna array directly inserted into the timor	Any accessible body site; tumors of the brain, head, and neck, chest wall, pelvis, extremities, and soft tissue
Intracavitary devices ("antennae")	Different antenna designs inserted into preformed body cavities	Accessible tumors of the pharynx, esophagus, bile duct, cervix, uterus, prostate, rectum, and anus
Radiofrequency heating methods (0.5–27 MHz)		
Inductive external device	Loops or coils positioned against the body surface or surrounding the patient	Large or deep-seated tumors in any body site
Capacitive external devices	Pairs of plate electrodes placed on opposite sites of the body	Various sites of the body (superficial or deep)
Inductive interstitial devices	Ferromagnetic material (wires, seeds) implanted directly into the tumor	Any accessible body site; as for microwave heating
Capacitive or inductive interstitial and intracavitary devices	Arrays of paired or unpaired needle electrodes implanted into the tumor	Any preformed body cavity; as for microwave heating
Ultrasound heating methods (0.5–5.0 MHz)		
Single external device	Direct tissue contact at body surface with use of bolus material	Small superficial or medium-depth tumors
Multiple external devices	Direct tissue contact with applicators placed around the lesion	Extensive superficial or medium-depth tumors
Focused array devices	Applicators are focused into the depth of the patient's body for deep heating	Superficial and deep-seated tumors of abdomen, pelvis, or extremities
Interstitial devices ("antennae")	Single- and multiple-element antennae or array inserted directly into the tumor	Any accessible body site; as for microwave heating (under development)
Intracavitary devices ("antennae")	Single- and multiple-element antenna inserted into preformed cavity	Any preformed body cavity; as for microwave heating
Local and regional perfusion methods		
Intravascular blood perfusion	Warmed blood into catheterized vessel	Tumors in regions with regional vessel network; liver, extremities, etc.
External saline perfusion	Warmed saline perfused across the mucosal surfaces	Superficial intracavitary tumors: bladder, cervical anorectal tumors
Interstitial hot water perfusion	Warmed water perfused with high pressure within implanted catheters	Any accessible body site; as for microwave heating
Systemic heating methods		
Induction of fever	Injection of pyrogenic material	Metastatic and advanced tumors
Intravascular blood perfusion	Extracorporeal blood heating	Metastatic and advanced tumors
External heating techniques	Hot bath and blankets, heat boxes, space suites, radiative devices	Metastatic and advanced tumors

Alexandria (about 200 A.D.) treated large or fixed tumors of the breast with local cautery. Similar reports are known from the "*Hypomnema*" of Paulos from Ägina (625–690 A.D.), who helped to transmit many of the ideas and concepts of Greek and Roman medicine to the Arabs when they conquered the ancient Egyptian metropolis of Alexandria (Paulos von Aegina 1914).

External cautery was also a very prominent treatment for many nononcological disorders and cancers from antiquity through to the nineteenth century (Fig. 1.5a,b). Moreover, in many other old cultures of the Middle East, Asia, and Middle and South America similar treatment techniques were handed down to us by various scripts and sketches. Fig. 1.6 depicts a typical medieval illustration from the medical script "*Armamentarium chirurgicum*" by Johann Schultes (Amsterdam, 1672) which demonstrates the typical cauterization of a female patient with a large ulcerated breast carcinoma. Similar caustic treatments of tumors are reported in other body sites and in different cultures. Most interestingly, in the Middle Ages and thereafter caustic treatments were usually performed by the "barbers," who were obviously responsible for the "solidistic" treatment methods, while the "physicians" tended to follow the traditional guidelines of "humoralistic" therapy. These two competing professions and medical concepts continued their dispute over diagnosis and the best means of treating diseases, including cancer, until the twentieth century. Interestingly, modern methods of "local heat" application for the treatment of tumors include the use of electrocoagulation and laser techniques, which are mostly applied in the operation room.

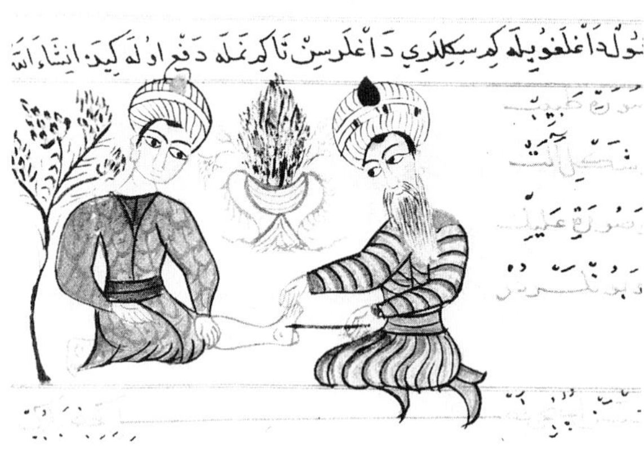
a

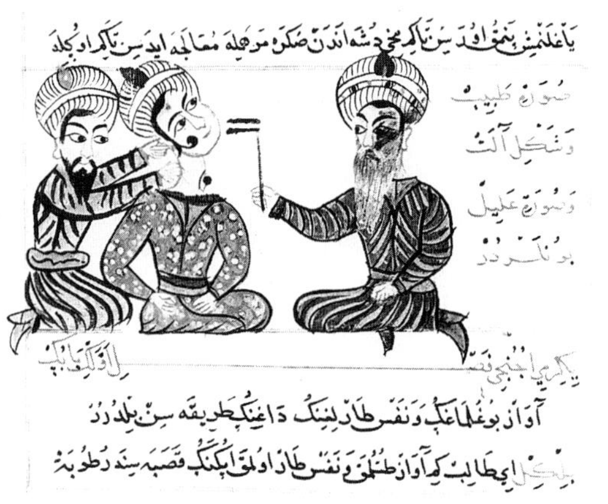
b

Fig. 1.5a,b. Cautery treatment of localized tumors, boils, and warts in medieval Arabian medicine. **a** Removal of a foot lesion. **b** Removal of a neck node lesion (*depicted in black*). Medieval Turkish Surgical Manuscript from Charaf ed-Din, 1465 (Paris, Bibliothèque Nationale)

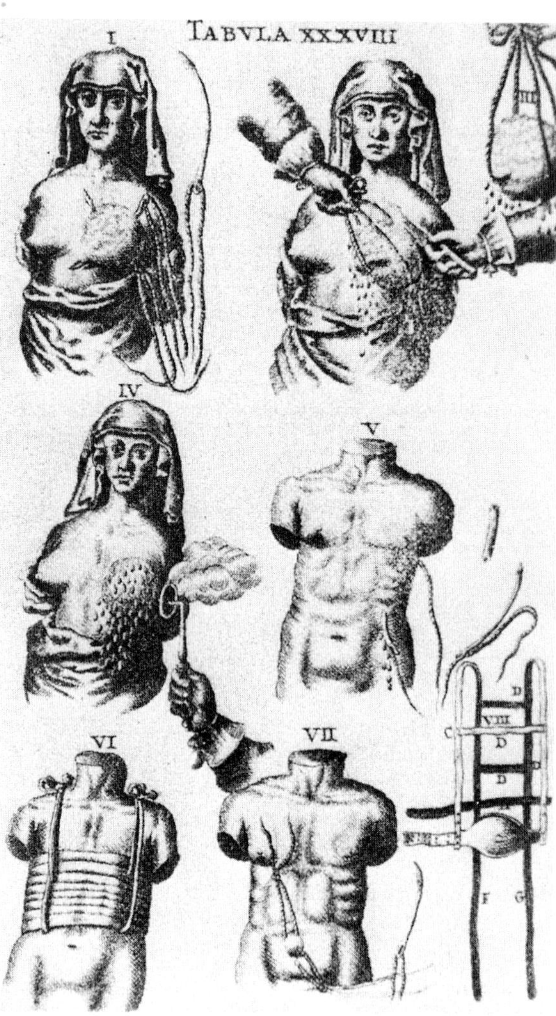

Fig. 1.6. Use of a ring-shaped hot iron to cauterize a tumorous lesion of the breast in the seventeenth century. The illustration explains the preoperative preparation, the performance of the surgical procedure, and the special bandage technique postoperatively. The author entitles this illustration "How to remove the breast with an apparent breast carcinoma and to bandage the site according to Sostratus." Illustration from the *Armamentarium chirurgicum* of Johann Schultes, Amsterdam 1672 (Paris, Bibliothèque de Faculté Médecine)

1.3.3.2 Internal and Interventional Cautery

Localized heating was not only applied externally but also used as an internal heating method for many diseases, especially gynecological disorders (Fig. 1.7), and some accessible tumors. About 1830 the French surgeon Joseph Claude Anthelme Récamier (1774–1856) began to use intracavitary electrical heating ("galvanocautery") for the treatment of uterine cancers. Subsequently in 1889, the American surgeon Byrne published his successful 20-year experience in 367 patients suffering from cancer of the cervix and/or corpus uteri. He reported an excellent long-term tumor response, a reduced or delayed relapse rate, reduced metastases in operable cases, and excellent palliative effects on pelvic and perineal pain in inoperable cases. He also stated what is now well known, namely that "*deeper lying cancer cells are destroyed by less heat than will destroy normal tissues*" (BYRNE 1889, 1892). Several devices and applicators were invented to apply galvanocautery to various organs (Fig. 1.8a,b).

The Swedish gynecologist F. Westermark (1898) implemented intracavitary heating without using the typical cauterizing approach. Instead, he induced localized conductive heating by means of hot water that was perfused through an intracavitary spiral metal tube which he placed in the vagina. The temperature of the circulating hot water was constantly controlled between 42° and 44°C over a 48-h treatment period. Although he applied this approach primarily for nononcological disorders and did not consider this method a typical cancer treatment, he observed excellent clinical responses in seven ulcerated and inoperable cervical carcinomas (WESTERMARK 1898). These beneficial clinical results in ulcerated or inoperable cervical tumors were confirmed by GOTTSCHALK (1899), who believed that higher temperatures and shorter treatment times would result in a similar tumor response. Interestingly, some recent clinical studies suggest that long-term mild hyperthermia at 41°–41.5°C appears to be equally as effective as a short-term high-temperature heat treatment (GARCIA et al. 1992).

Despite the rapid development of gynecological surgery in the late nineteenth and the early twentieth century, with Ries-Wertheim hysterectomy replacing the formerly popular "galvanocautery," the American gynecologist PERCY (1912, 1913, 1916) again reinforced the use of local cautery for inoperable uterine cancers. He performed galvanocautery during laparotomy and kept the temperatures of the vagina, rectum, and bladder well controlled between 43° and 46°C by means of invasively implanted thermometers. Thus, this could be regarded as the first report on the use of *intraoperative hyperthermia*. Percy noted some excellent palliative effects in inoperable cases and reported several long-term survivors.

These positive clinical findings were independently confirmed by two American surgeons from the Mayo Clinic: MAYO (1913, 1915) and

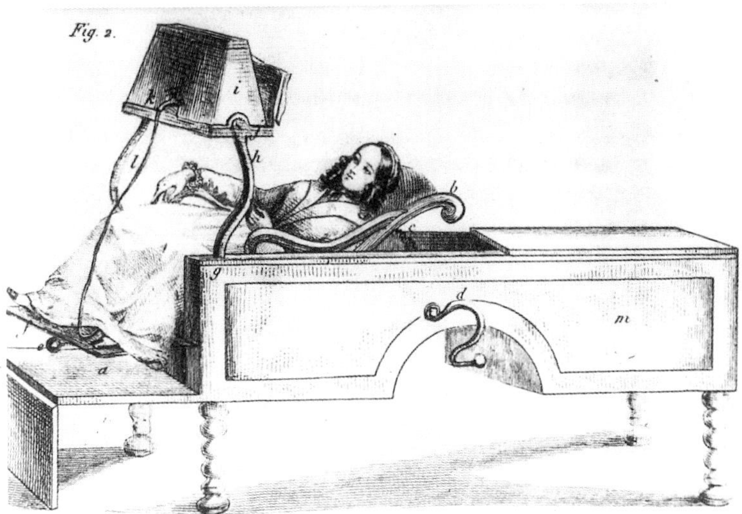

Fig. 1.7. Heating apparatus for treatment of various diseases of the uterus. Apparently the patient feels comfortable while reading a book during the treatment, the book being mounted on the apparatus. From: E. Matthieu, *Etudes cliniques sur les maladies des femmes.*, Paris, 1874 (Paris, Bibliothèque de Faculté Médecine)

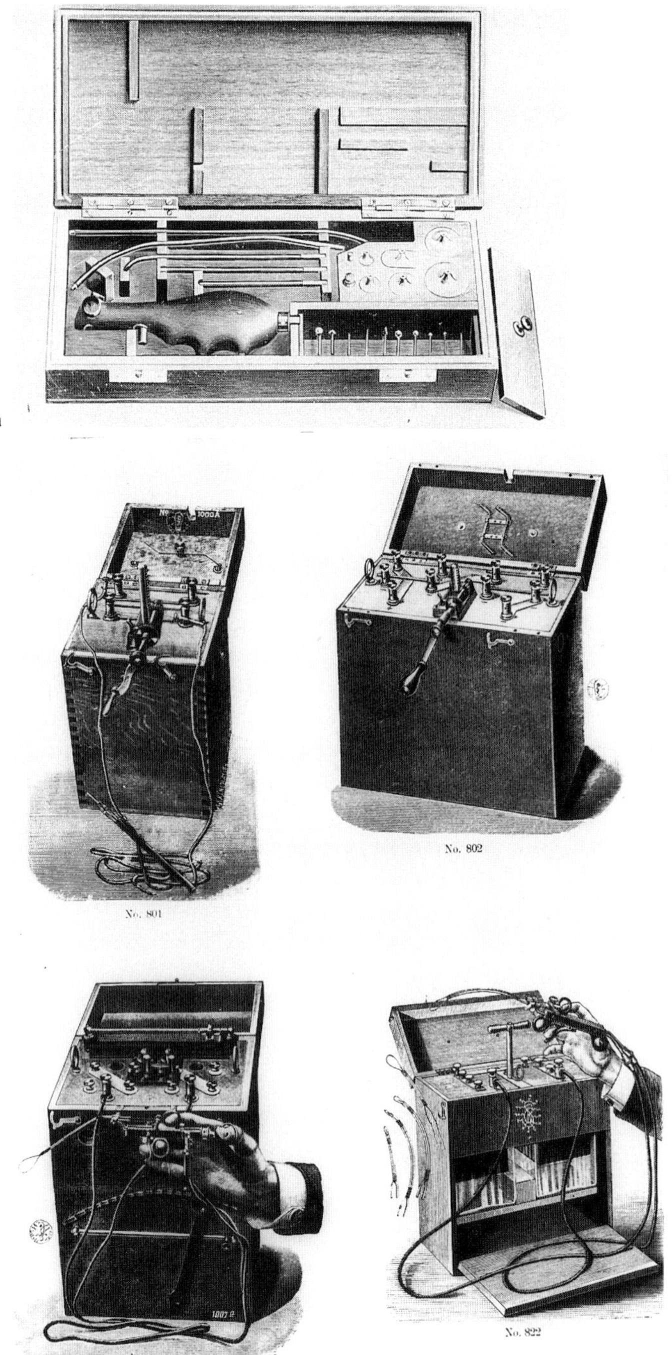

Fig. 1.8a–d. Galvanocautery. **a** Wooden box containing a complete tool set for surgical galvanocautery (according to Hirsch) around 1900. The box contains an insulated ceramic handle with connecting plugs (*lower left*), connecting tubes (*upper left*), and different electrodes (*lower right*). Catalogue offer from the electromedical company Reiniger, Gebbert, and Schall, Erlangen (Germany). (Courtesy of Siemens Medical Archives, Erlangen). **b** Various galvanocaustic devices including batteries for galvanocautery from around 1892. Catalogue offer from the electromedical company Reiniger Gebbert, and Schall, Erlangen (Germany). (Courtesy of Siemens Medical Archives, Erlangen). **c** Galvanocaustic instruments (according to Paquelin) around 1908 with a set of different electrode tips of various shapes. Catalogue offer from the electromedical company Reiniger, Gebbert, and Schall, Erlangen (Germany). (Courtesy of Siemens Medical Archives, Erlangen). **d** Various platin-ceramic tips of galvanocaustic instruments around 1908. The individual shapes are used for different types of surgery. Catalogue offer from the electromedical company Reiniger Gebbert, and Schall, Erlangen (Germany). (Courtesy of Siemens Medical Archives, Erlangen)

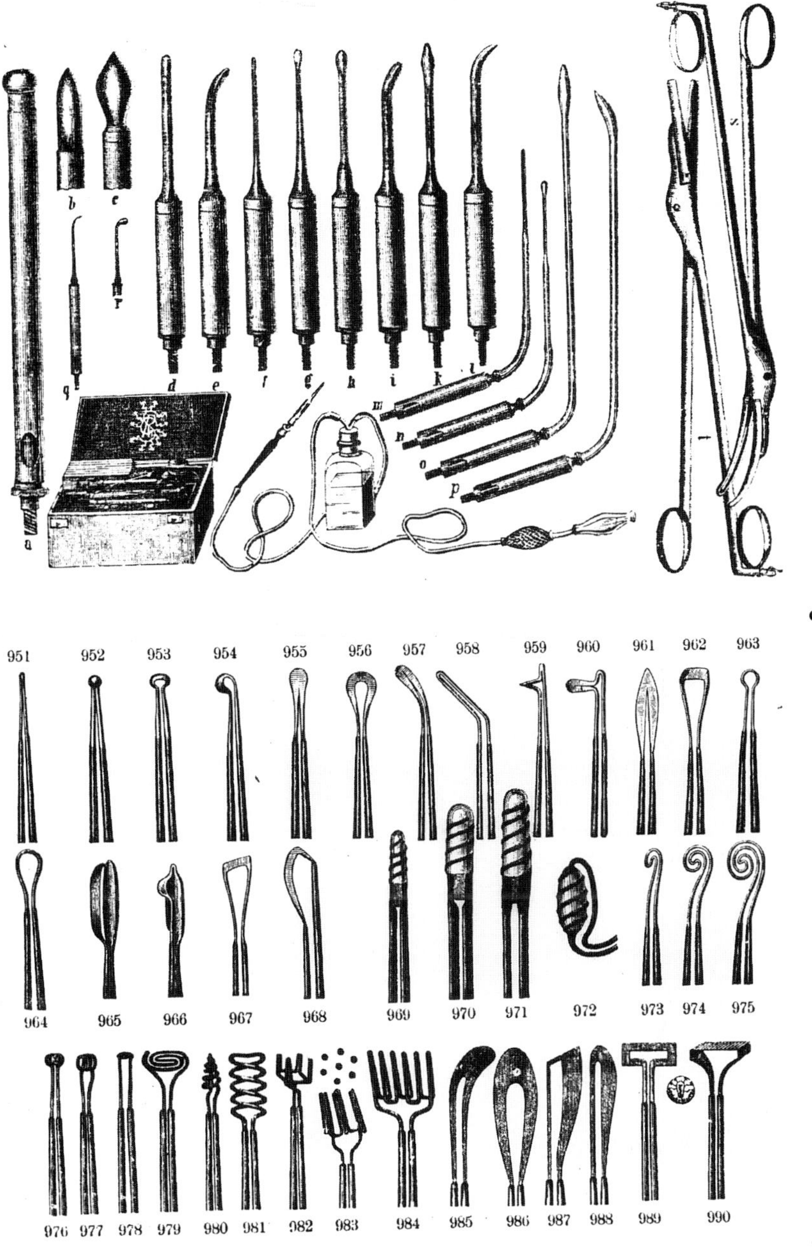

Fig. 1.8c,d

BALFOUR (1915) applied an "electrocautery" procedure for the treatment of cervical carcinomas. Mayo assumed that preoperative cautery could prevent the dissemination of malignant cells during the course of the surgical trauma. Stimulated by the encouraging results obtained, in 1923 the American surgeon Ochsner published his modified galvanocautery technique, which was used to treat advanced oral cancers involving the jaw. He reported on very favorable results in more than 100 patients suffering from various oral cancers (OCHSNER 1923).

1.3.3.3 Local Hot-Water Applications

Most historical reports dealing with the use of hot water for hyperthermia refer to systemic heat applications by means of hot baths. Only a few authors have reported on cancer treatment by means of localized hot water conductive heating. As mentioned previously, the earliest report came from F. WESTERMARK (1898), who used a circulating hot water device in the treatment of cervical cancer. However, hot water heating was also applied externally to treat finger and extremity tumors as well as penile carcinoma (GOETZE 1928, 1930; GOETZE and SCHMIDT 1932): for this purpose the whole extremity or penis was immersed in a hot water bath for several minutes. To avoid cooling effects due to heat convection, the tourniquet technique was applied, which required the additional use of general anesthesia. The temperatures were usually not measured, but probably did not exceed the skin pain threshold of 45°C, since all heat treatments were well tolerated and no late effects were observed. With this method good palliation was attained with remarkable tumor regression in several patients.

Only a few other authors have observed similar cures with external localized hot water applications: HOFFMAN (1957), HEYN and KURZ (1967), LAMPERT (1948, 1965, 1970), and CRILE (1962) reported on tumor cures in penile carcinomas, melanomas, and other malignancies. HOFFMANN (1957) achieved 14 cures among 64 pretreated melanoma metastases when tumor temperatures of 45°C were achieved in anesthesized patients, and CRILE (1962) observed the cure of neuroblastoma metastases using a local hot water bath exposure of 45°C for 1–2h.

1.3.3.4 Electromagnetic Heating Methods

In 1886, the German physicist Heinrich Hertz (1857–1894) demonstrated the physical nature of electromagnetic waves and described their characteristic features, thereby confirming the theories on electromagnetism formulated by the English physicist James C. Maxwell (1831–1879). Shortly afterwards in France, d'Arsonval reported that such currents could also affect physiological mechanisms in living tissues (d'ARSONVAL 1892, 1897), and around 1900 the famous Croatian physicist Tesla (1856–1943) recognized the heating capability of high-frequency currents in various biological tissues. In the following years "Arsonvalisation" became a very fashionable but controversial treatment method for various diseases which could be applied to the whole body or parts of it; however, with these devices only a slight increase in the temperature could be achieved (Fig. 1.9a–d).

In 1907, the German physicist Nagelschmidt was the first to demonstrate the possibility of deep heating ("thermopenetration") in the arm and chest of the human body and subsequently coined the expression "diathermy." With the design of appropriate powerful generators the medical applications of local diathermy developed rapidly in the following decades: while longwave diathermy (0.5–3.0 MHz) was already used by 1900, shortwave diathermy with frequencies of up to 100 MHz became the standard approach by 1920, and with frequencies of 100–3000 MHz by 1930. These heating techniques and HF currents were also introduced into the surgical practice of the time (Fig. 1.10a–d).

At this point it is worthwhile to reflect on the available technical means of impacting on human tissues from a physical perspective. Heat energy, in reality, is energy of molecular motion within a particular body. The potential energies include gravitational, elastic, chemical, and nuclear energy

Fig. 1.9a–d. Arsonvalisation. The technique of Arsonvalisation used high-frequency currents and large coils to induce current flow and warmth within human body or parts of it. Devices for systemic and local autoconduction could be distinguished. Arsonvalisation was used for disorders of (1) blood circulation, (2) metabolism, (3) central nervous system, and (4) skin. Other indications were tuberculosis, gastrointestinal disorders, and hemorrhoids. Arsonvalisation was also said to influence the central thermoregulation. **a** Photograph of whole-body autocondensation on the Apostoli condensator couch (around 1907–1912). The primary current, derived from accumulators, is distributed to switches, resistances, amperemeters, and voltmeters and brought to a large coil (above the table). From this coil the secondary currents pass into the high-frequency machine (below the table), which is a modified Oudin resonator, and from there to two conducting cables. One of the conducting cords is attached to the couch, whilst the other is led to a conducting handle. The couch itself consists of completely insulating beech-wood. (Courtesy of Siemens Medical Archives, Erlangen). **b** Whole-body autoconduction for treatment in horizontal position with a whole-body solenoid surrounding the patient positioned on the Apostoli couch (around 1908–1912). (Courtesy of Siemens Medical Archives, Erlangen). **c** Whole-body autoconduction cage for treatment in the vertical position of a standing or sitting person within the whole-body solenoid (around 1900). (Courtesy of Siemens Medical Archives, Erlangen). **d** Partial-body autoconduction with double resonating system; one of the electrodes is hand-held by the patient and connected to a large solenoid (*left*), while the other electrode is attached to a second solenoid and held by the therapist. (Courtesy of Siemens Medical Archives, Erlangen)

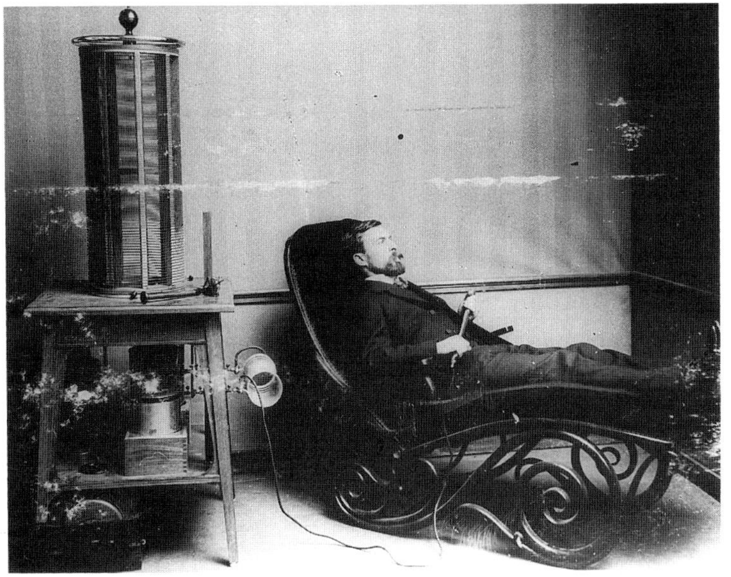

a

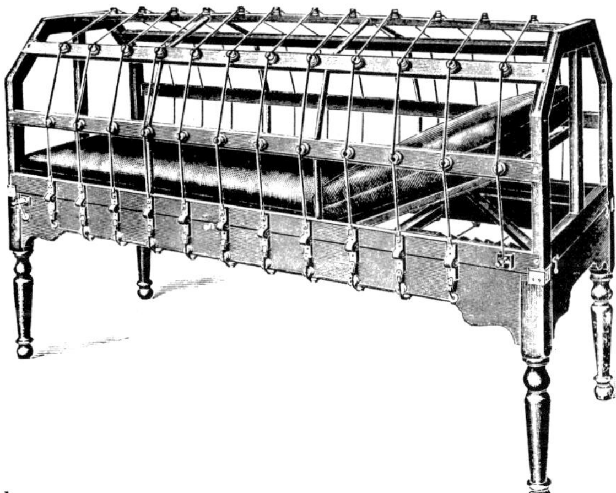

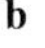

b

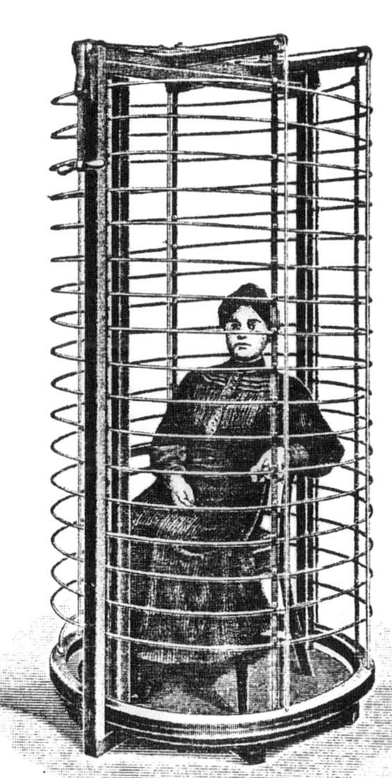

c

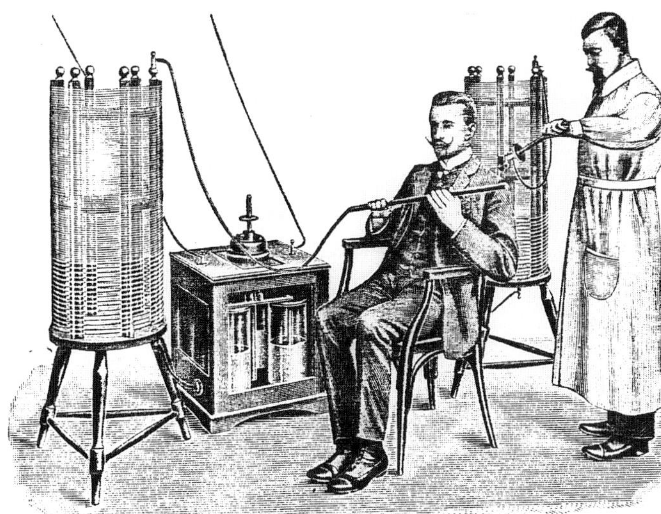

d

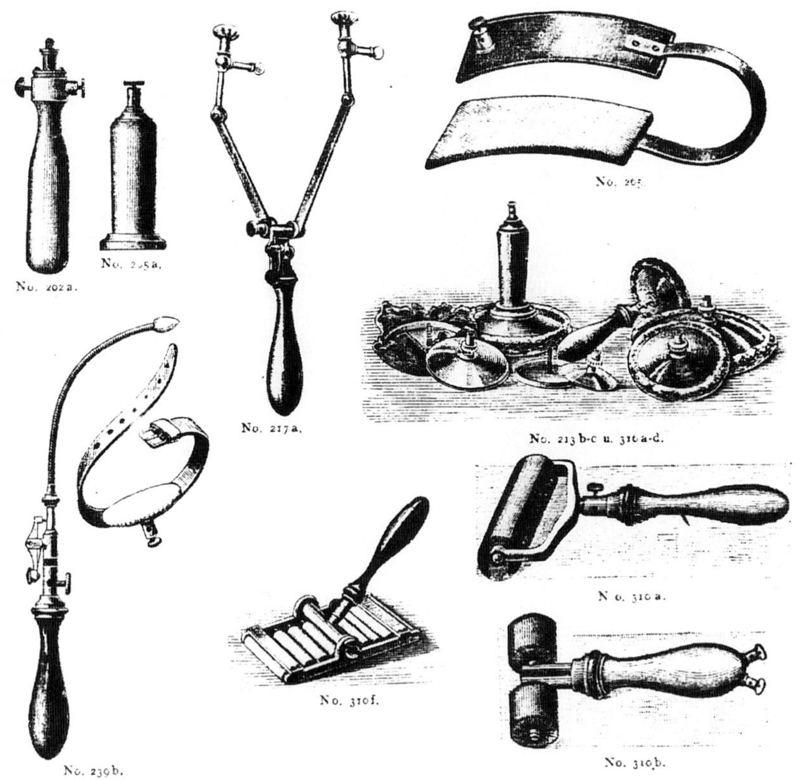

a

No. 152. Transportwagen für Elektrisier-Apparate

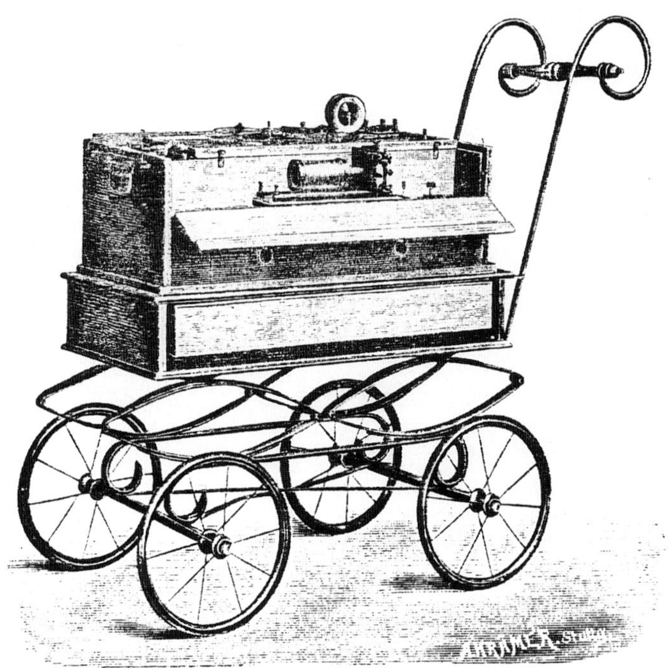

mit kräftigem Eisengestell, Eifedern, Rädern mit Gummireifen und tischförmigem Oberteil von Eichenholz zur leichteren Beförderung schwerer transportabler Apparate, z. B. unserer grösseren konstanten Leclanché-Batterieen und Leclanché - Doppel - Apparate, in Spitälern von einem Krankensaal zum andern und event. von Klinik zu Klinik M. 50.—,

152. **Derselbe Wagen mit zwei lenkbaren Rädern** M. 70 —.

b

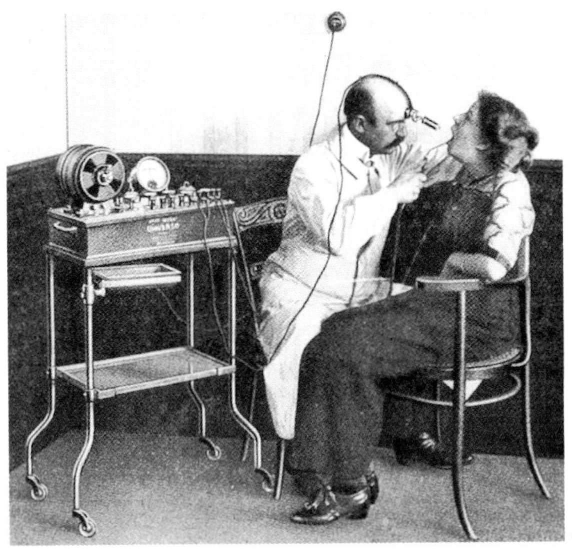

c

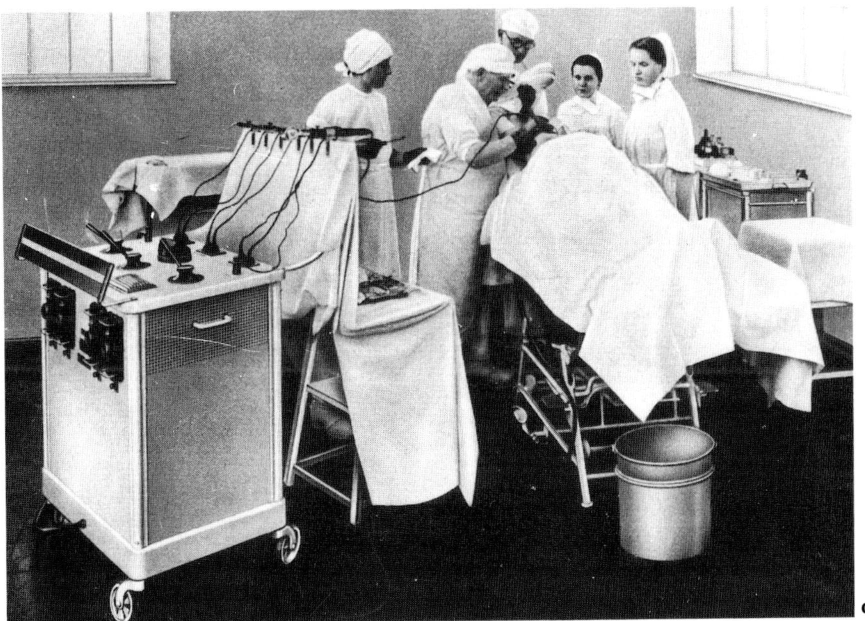

d

Fig. 1.10a–d. Surgical diathermy for localized lesions. **a** Different electrodes and holders for electrocautery around 1908. The holder (*upper left*) has an interrupter; one electrode (*lower left*) is designed to treat larynx lesions with a small transorally placed (active) electrode and a large external (passive) electrode which is incorporated in a cervical cuff. Catalogue offer from the electromedical company Reiniger, Gebbert, and Schall, Erlangen (Germany). (Courtesy of Siemens Medical Archives, Erlangen). **b** Vehicle for transportation of galvano- or electrocautery supplies around 1908. Catalogue offer from the electromedical company Reiniger, Gebbert, and Schall, Erlangen (Germany). (Courtesy of Siemens Medical Archives, Erlangen). **c** Surgical diathermy of a localized mouth lesion around 1910. The ENT surgeon uses a lamp on his forehead and a hand-held electrocautery which is attached to the power supply. (Courtesy of Siemens Medical Archives, Erlangen). **d** Surgical diathermy with the "Elchir-Thermoflux System" for large abdominal operations around 1933/1934. (Courtesy of Siemens Medical Archives, Erlangen).

and some electrical energies. Table 1.2 summarizes the complete spectrum of electromagnetic waves and their specific physical details (frequency, wavelength, photon energy). The theoretical concept of the electromagnetic (EM) wave spectrum was first developed by Maxwell in about 1860. The waves are defined as bundles of massless energy (photons) which travel through a vacuum at different frequencies and wavelengths at the speed of light (i.e., at 3×10^{10} cm/s).

Table 1.2. Spectrum of electromagnetic waves and photon beams

Properties of and use for thermo- or radiotherapy	Frequency (Hz)	Wavelength	Photon energy
Radiowaves			
Ranging from longwaves, broadcast band, and shortwaves to ultrashortwaves; produced by electrical oscillations; pass through nonconducting materials	$1 \cdot 10^5$ –	3 km –	413 peV –
Special hyperthermia implementations: Diathermy (30 m–50 m waves), shortwave therapy (50 m–3 m), microwaves (300 cm–10 cm waves)	$3 \cdot 10^{10}$	0.01 m	124 meV
Infrared radiation			
Typical heat waves which are produced by the molecular vibration and excitation of outer electrons in atoms	$3 \cdot 10^{12}$ –	100 μm –	12.4 meV –
Special hyperthermia implementations: Infrared lamps, radiators (0.3 mm–1 μm waves)	$3 \cdot 10^{14}$	1 μm	1.24 eV
Visible light			
From red through yellow, green, and blue to violet light; produced by excitation of the outer electrons in atoms; generated by electrical discharge in lamps and gas tubes No special hyperthermia implementations	$4.3 \cdot 10^{14}$ – $7.5 \cdot 10^{14}$	700 nm – 400 nm	1.77 eV – 3.1 eV
Ultraviolet light			
Produced by excitation of the outer electrons in atoms; causes erythema of the skin and kills bacteria No special implementations	$7.5 \cdot 10^{14}$ – $3 \cdot 10^{16}$	400 nm – 10 nm	3.1 eV – 124 eV
Soft x-rays			
Produced by excitation of the inner electrons in atoms; causes erythema of the skin and kills bacteria Radiotherapy implementations: grenz rays	$3 \cdot 10^{16}$ – $3 \cdot 10^{18}$	10 nm – 100 pm	124 eV – 12.4 keV
Diagnostic x-rays			
Produced by excitation of the inner electrons in atoms Radiotherapy implementations: superficial therapy	$3 \cdot 10^{18}$ – $3 \cdot 10^{19}$	100 pm – 10 pm	12.4 keV – 124 keV
Deep therapy x-rays, linac x-rays			
Produced by excitation of the inner electrons of an atom Radiotherapy implementations: orthovolt/linac therapy	$3 \cdot 10^{19}$ – $3 \cdot 10^{22}$	10 pm – 10 fm	124 keV – 124 MeV
Large linacs/proton synchrotron x-rays			
Produced by excitation of the protons in atoms Radiotherapy implementations: proton therapy	$3 \cdot 10^{22}$ – $3 \cdot 10^{23}$	10 fm – 1 fm	124 MeV – 1.24 GeV

Thereby the energy of EM waves is directly proportional to the frequency ν and the wavelength λ, i.e., as the frequency increases, the wavelength decreases and the energy of the photons increases. If heating methods are compared with the light photons and x-ray photon beams which have been simultaneously developed during this century, it is obvious that the useful "heating methods" have energies several orders of magnitude weaker than the "ionizing radiation methods" (Table 1.2).

In 1908, Freund reported on an electrical device to soften and eventually remove superficial tumor nodules, which he called "fulguration" (FREUND 1908) (Fig. 1.11a,b). At about the same time, KEATING-HART (1909) reported on a similar new treatment method which was applied in a total of 247 patients with various accessible tumors. The applied electromagnetic energy was sparked from a hand-held electrode through the cancerous lesion. Keating-Hart was also one of the very first clinical investigators to combine local heat and radiation therapy in cancer patients, and he thereby observed considerably improved results. Similarly, DOYEN (1910) was able to produce tumor necrosis by means of high-frequency currents; he called his treatment method "electrocoagulation."

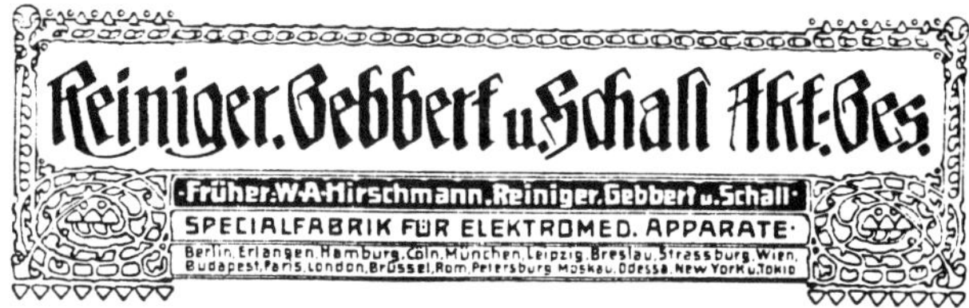

Eine neue elektro-chirurgische Methode!

Fulguration

Funkenbestrahlung bösartiger Geschwülste

mit Hochfrequenzströmen von grosser Spannung, in Kombination mit operativer Entfernung

nach Dr. de Keating-Hart (Marseille).

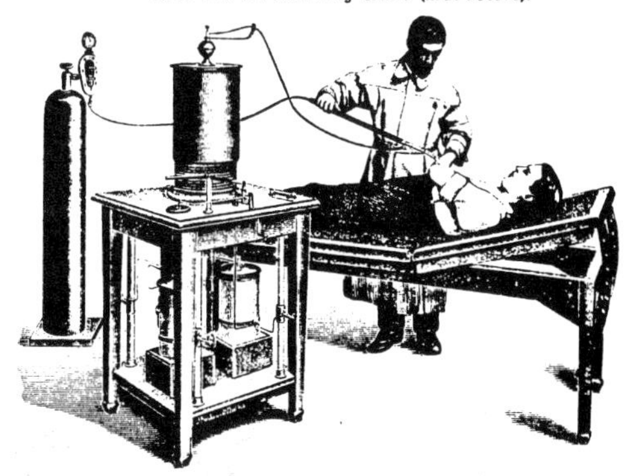

a

Empfohlen von:

Exzellenz Geh. Med.-Rat Professor Dr. **Czerny,** Heidelberg
(Münchener medizinische Wochenschrift, No. 10, 1908).

Geh. Hofrat Dr. **Benckiser,** Karlsruhe
(Deutsche medizinische Wochenschrift, No. 10, 1908).

Oberarzt Dr. **Krumm,** Karlsruhe
(Deutsche medizinische Wochenschrift, No. 10, 1908).

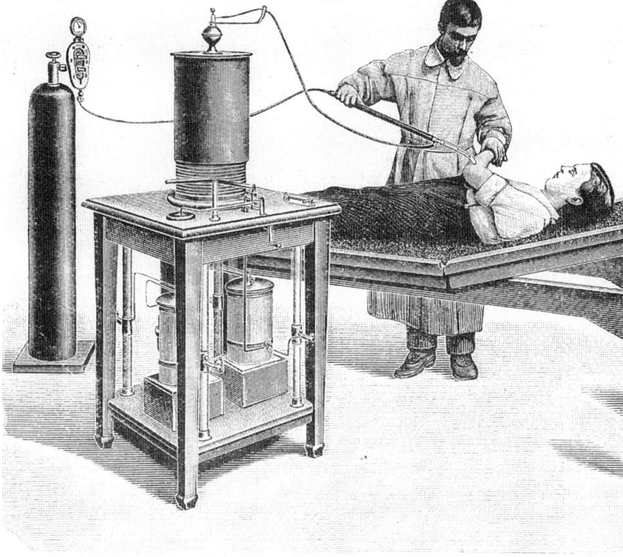

b

Fig. 1.11a,b. Fulguration. **a** Catalogue offer from Reiniger, Gebbert, and Schall Company, Erlangen (Germany): "Eine neue elektro-chirurgische Methode! Fulguration – Funkenbestrahlung bösartiger Geschwülste mit Hochfrequenzströmen von grosser Spannung, in Kombination mit operativer Emtfernung nach Dr. de Keating-Hart (Marseille)" (A new electrical surgery method! Fulguration! Sparking irradiation of malignant tumors with high-frequency currents in combination with surgical removal). (Courtesy of Siemens Medical Archives, Erlangen). **b** Details of the fulguration method. The handheld electrode is attached to the resonator (top of table) and positioned close to the lesion. The electrode is activated with the right thumb (interrupter). The undesired (!!) heat is counteracted with high-pressure nitrogen gas from a gas reservoir

Surgical diathermy was also applied in the treatment of cancers of the rectum and sigmoid colon by Strauss as early as 1913 (STRAUSS 1935). Later Strauss used this procedure in almost all cases of rectal cancer and applied up to four treatments depending on the extent of the tumor. He reported that in the majority of his patients an otherwise necessary colostomy was thereby avoided, and full rectal and sphincter function retained. Other positive findings in his patients included weight gain and improved laboratory findings (hemoglobin, red blood cell counts). Interestingly Strauss also noted that 75% of his patients developed periods of low fever (around 100°F = 37.7°C) after the tretment which sometimes lasted for several days—a mechanism which may indicate tumor necrosis and an early immunological response which in itself may have had therapeutic potential.

The German physician Müller was one of the first to report (in great detail) on the clinical effects of combined radiotherapy and heat by means of diathermy (MÜLLER 1912, 1913) (some technical devices were already available at that time to combine these treatments: Fig. 1.12). Of 100 patients with tumors of different body sites including the skin, breast, mediastinum, liver, rectum, uterus, and testis, about one-third showed a complete response with long-term tumor control and another third showed a substantial response though with subsequent tumor regrowth or metastases. He concluded that "the deeper the tumor location, the less the options are for treatment success" and strongly recommended this combined treatment because the tumor responses obtained were "definitely greater" than could have been expected by radiotherapy alone. Unfortunately, from a modern scientific perspective this study was not designed as a randomized clinical trial.

In 1919, the German gynecologist Theilhaber reported on a fractionated heating course of 10–20 heat sessions (15–20 min per session) for uterine and vaginal cancers which he applied by means of high-frequency currents (THEILHABER 1919, 1923). Considerable tumor regression and necrosis was noted, which histologically appeared to be "similar to that seen after X-irradiation." Despite these successful applications of heat, surgical diathermy for gynecological tumors was soon supplanted by other treatment strategies, including some improved surgical techniques and the use of radium. Nevertheless, MASSEY (1925) still stated:

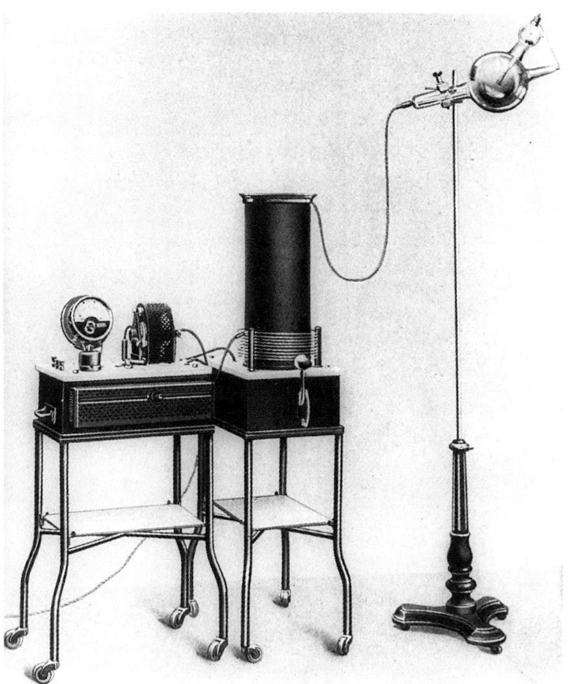

Fig. 1.12. Combination of diathermy and x-rays in one apparatus (ca. 1911). This is probably the first instrumentalization of combined "heat" and "ionizing radiation." Catalogue offer from Reiniger, Gebbert, and Schall Company, Erlangen (Germany). (Courtesy of Siemens Medical Archives, Erlangen)

"Electrocoagulation is now widely understood to be the method of choice in the removal of a carcinoma or sarcoma of the surface region or in an accessible cavity of the body."

TYLER (1926) published a quite remarkable case study on a patient with rapidly progressing breast cancer and extensive metastatic abdominal and liver involvement. After completion of 19 diathermy treatment sessions using opposing electrodes in the right upper quadrant of the abdomen, the involved liver decreased in size and the malignant ascites was markedly reduced for several months. At about the same time other radiofrequency heating methods were also implemented in various animal experiments (JOHNSON 1940; OVERGAARD 1940a; OVERGAARD 1940b; ROHDENBURG and PRIME 1921; WESTERMARK 1927), and it was believed that heat could induce a *selective* antitumor effect.

Other clinical reports confirmed the advantages of surgical diathermy when applied to tumors of the oral cavity, pharynx, larynx, esophagus, breast, genitalia, skin, bladder, rectum, prostate, and other sites (CLARK et al. 1925; CUMBERBATCH

1928), and thus *surgical diathermy* soon became a well-established method. In contrast, the rationale for nonnecrotizing applications of *medical diathermy* was much less clearly defined. Similar to Arsonvalisation, medical diathermy was applied for a rather diffuse spectrum of nononcological diseases including infections (e.g., pneumonia, angina, appendicitis), bone fractures, chronic disorders (e.g., hypertension), neurological diseases (e.g., epilepsy, migraine), and unspecific disorders such as obesity (Fig. 1.13). Interestingly, these medical diathermy treatments were not usually recommended in cancer therapy for fear of possible induction of tumor progression or distant metastases (BIERMANN 1942; SCOTT 1957). Instead, medical diathermy became an established method in physical therapy which underwent continuous improvement (Fig. 1.14a–c).

In 1929, the German Schliephake studied the biologic effects of shortwave treatment on various tissue types. Subsequently, he developed a set of *paired electrodes* to induce (capacitive) heating in locally advanced uterine cancers (SCHLIEPHAKE 1935). To heat these deeply located abdominal tumors, usually one of the two paired electrodes was placed anteriorly over the pelvis, while the other was posteriorly positioned over the sacrum. Schliephake used 20- to 50-MHz radiofrequencies with a wavelength between 6 and 15 m and applied several heating periods of up to 40 min. He observed marked destruction of the tumor tissue when the heat treatment was combined with x-rays; however, after several weeks all patients had experienced a relapse and no long-term survivors were observed. This method was subsequently modified and applied for various other pelvic tumors (Fig. 1.15a–c).

Shortly afterwards FUCHS (1936) reported on the clinical experience at the Vienna City Hospital with a combination of 20-MHz shortwave therapy (15 m wavelength) and ionizing radiation. The shortwave treatment lasted 20 min and was followed by radiotherapy a few hours later. The author concluded that there was an improved tumor response rate without increased radiation side-effects on the skin in the irradiated field. MEYER and MUTSCHELLER (1937) also demonstrated a large increase in the biological efficacy of ionizing radiation on tumors when heat was added. In six patients with superficial malignancies, only one-half of the radiation dose was sufficient to control the malignant skin lesions. All tumors regressed rapidly and without inflammatory reactions, while skin reactions were less pronounced than with the normal dose of radiotherapy.

The so-called synergistic effect between heat and radiation was also observed by KORB (1939, 1943, 1948) in patients with basal cell carcinoma of the skin. Korb applied a rather modern clinical study design, a matched-pair analysis of two identically sized lesions within the same patient, one of which was treated with radiation alone while the other received both treatment modalities. He demonstrated a clear advantage of the combined treatment. In contrast, BIRKNER and WACHSMANN (1949) treated several skin carcinomas using shortwave hyperthermia and observed a remarkable tumor growth inhibition, but were unable to achieve a complete tumor

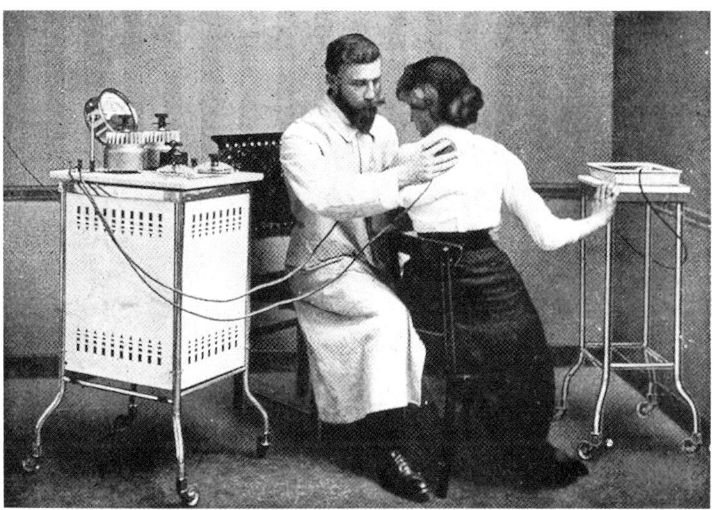

Fig. 1.13. "Universal Thermoflux" apparatus for localized heating of various body sites around 1910. The two opposing insulated electrodes are connected to the high-frequency generator and hand-held by the therapist. (Courtesy of Siemens Medical Archives, Erlangen)

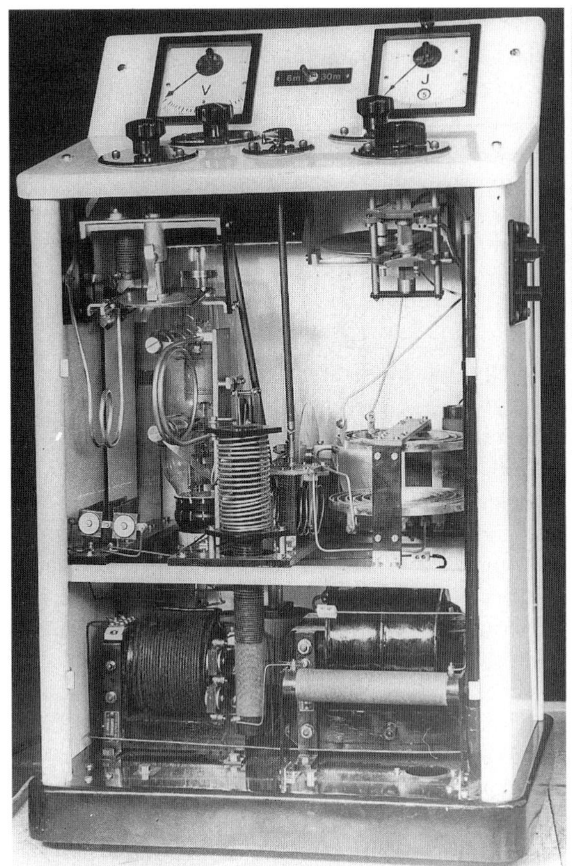
a

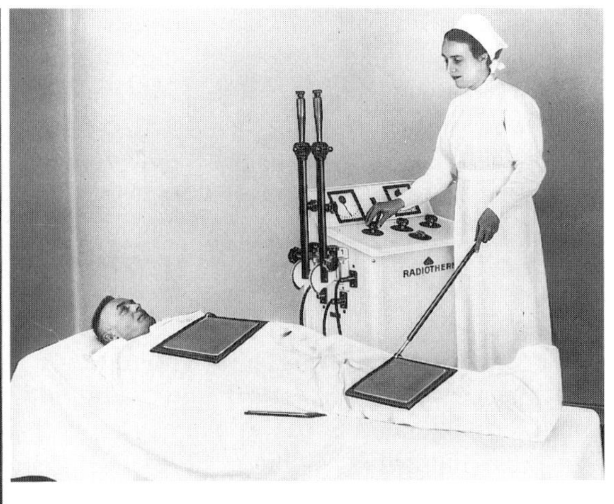
c

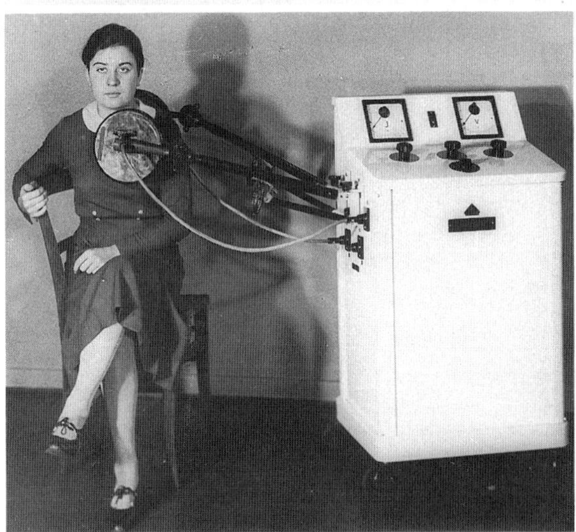
b

Fig. 1.14a–c. Medical diathermy in physical therapy. **a** The heating device "Radiotherm" from Siemens in 1933. The high-frequency generator offers two currents of 6 and 30 m wavelength and a maximum power output of 400 W. The heat treatment is applied with two electrodes on opposing sides of the medium, e.g., parts of the human body. (Courtesy of Siemens Medical Archives, Erlangen). **b** Local heating with "Radiotherm" around 1933–1938. Two 20-cm-diameter round electrodes are connected to the high-frequency generator and placed on opposite sides of the upper chest. (Courtesy of Siemens Medical Archives, Erlangen). **c** Regional heating with "Radiotherm" in 1947. The patient is wrapped into insulating blankets to avoid unnecessary heat loss. The therapist controls the power manually on the apparatus by turning a knob. She is holding the insulated active electrode against the upper portion of the patient's limbs, while the other active electrode is positioned over the upper abdomen and the passive electrode underneath the pelvis. (Courtesy of Siemens Medical Archives, Erlangen)

cure, although they applied long-term fractionated heat treatments (13 sessions of 2–4 h each) with tumor temperatures in the range of 42°–44°C.

1.3.3.5 Ultrasound Heating Methods

Ultrasound is characterized by its intensity (W/cm^2), which is the rate at which energy is transmitted by the wave. As the energy is absorbed, the temperature of the absorbing material rises. In 1920, the first patent was granted on the newly developed piezoelectric crystals and some related methods to induce ultrasound (Langevin 1920). Ten years later, ultrasonic research already focused on the different biological effects in normal and tumor tissue. In the

1930s, two Japanese research groups observed growth delay and complete regression of different animal tumors when they were exposed to several ultrasound treatments (NAKAHARA and KOBAYASHI 1934; NAMIKAWA 1938). Tumor inhibition by ultrasound was confirmed by KRANTZ and BECK (1939).

Similar to the implementation of x-rays at the time, the new ultrasound applications raised high expectations concerning their potential value in cancer treatment. Thus, in the 1940s technical development and clinical work were initiated to test the method in human tumors (Fig. 1.16). The first report of the use of ultrasound in human

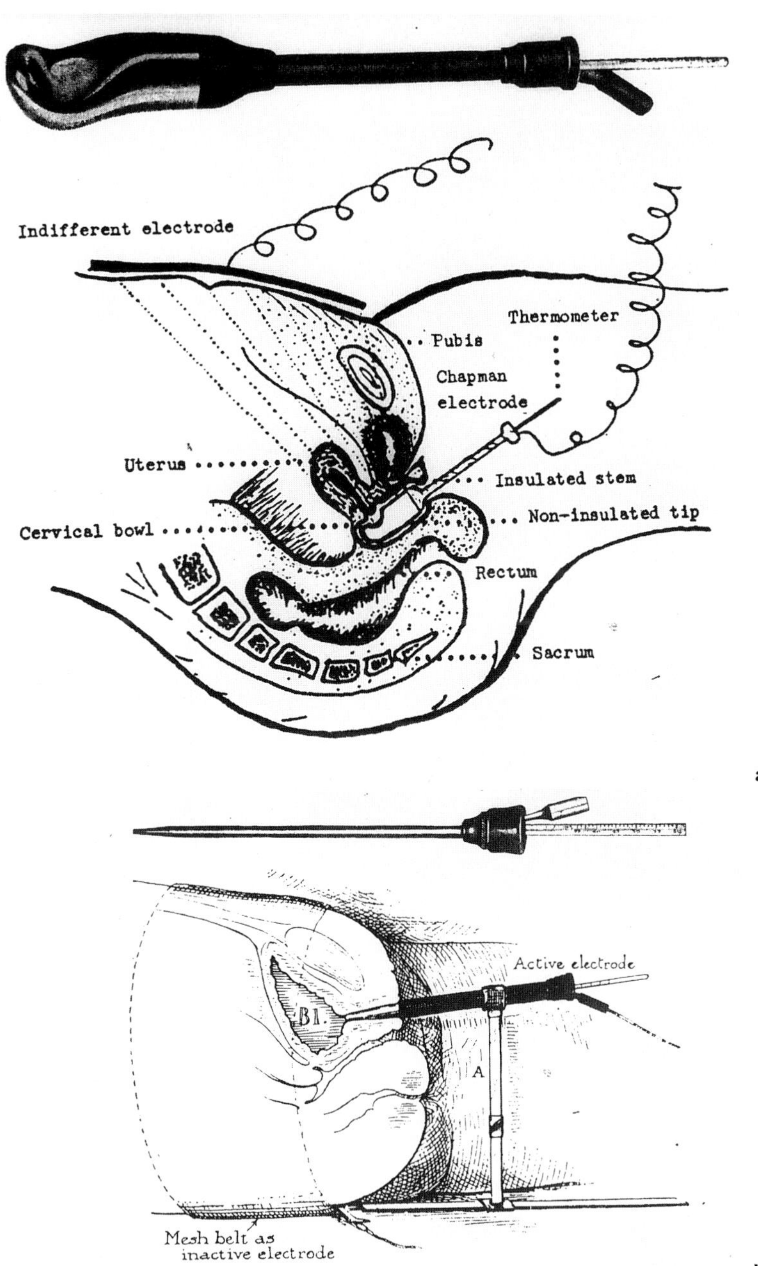

Fig. 1.15a–c. Deep (capacitive) diathermy. Combination of a small (active) intracavitary electrode and a large (passive) external electrode. **a** Abdominovaginal diathermy (for treatment of vaginal and cervical lesions) with the Chapman Vaginal Electrode. **b** Abdominourethral diathermy (for urethral and base of bladder lesions) with the Corbus Thermophore. **c** Abdominorectal diathermy (for prostate lesions) with the Corbus prostatic electrode

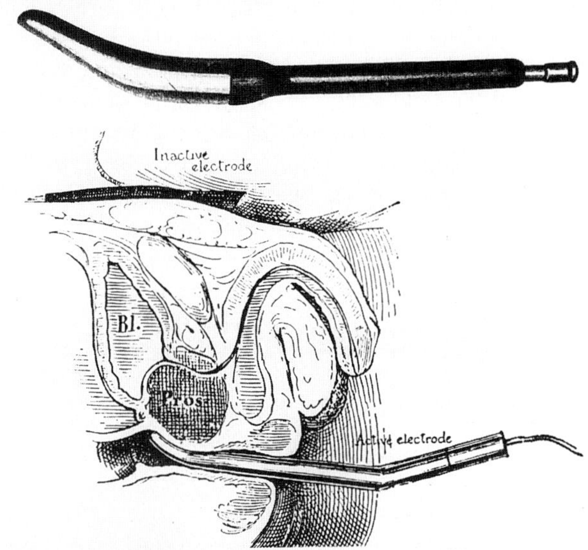

c

Fig. 1.15a–c. *Continued*

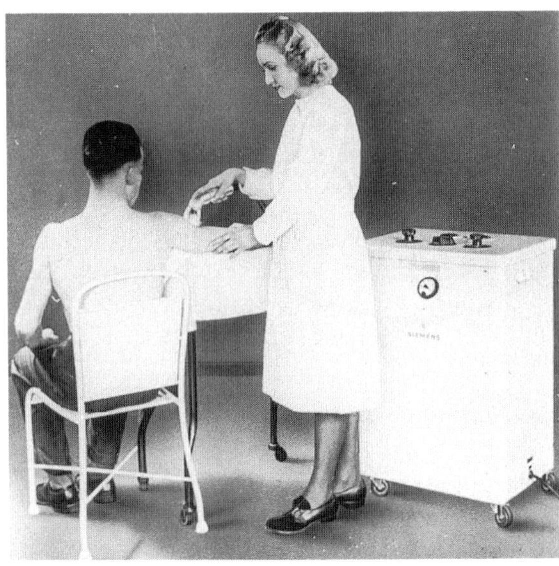

Fig. 1.16. Ultrasonic treatment of a soft tissue lesion with an 800-kHz device around 1949. (Courtesy of Siemens Medical Archives, Erlangen)

cancer therapy was published by the German investigator HORVATH (1946). He observed reduced tumor growth and some complete tumor regressions after ultrasound treatments in patients with skin cancers and one with lymphoma; however, the observed clinical effects were only transitory. Another early researcher in the field of ultrasound therapy was WOEBER (1949, 1955, 1956, 1965), who accumulated considerable clinical experience with combined ultrasound and radiation therapy in the treatment of skin cancers. Based on extensive animal experiments, WOEBER (1955, 1956, 1965) also treated 50 patients with skin cancers and observed that low-dose radiation therapy (30–40 Gy) combined with ultrasound heating achieved a response rate similar to that with high-dose radiotherapy alone (40–60 Gy), which clearly indicates a considerable thermal enhancement.

DEMMEL (1949) also achieved positive results and applied about three or four ultrasound sessions (20 min) in patients with basal cell skin cancer. DITTMAR (1949), while working with animal tumors, was one of the first investigators to state that the effects of ultrasound on tissue were exclusively thermal and involved no intrinsic anticancer effect. The Russian BUROV (1956) investigated the effects of pulsed ultrasound at very high intensity (150 W/cm^2) and at short time intervals (1.3 s) on animal tumors. When he applied this technique to human patients who suffered from malignant melanomas, he observed several complete tumor responses. Unfortunately, most early investigators working with ultrasound never realized or commented on the role of hyperthermia in their clinical results, nor did they document any temperatures.

Nevertheless, these and other positive findings (DMITRIEVA 1960; WIETHE 1949) were soon outweighted by other clinical studies which observed no impact of ultrasound on tumor growth (CLARKE et al. 1970; SOUTHAM et al. 1953). Moreover, it was even believed that ultrasound could trigger and stimulate tumor growth (POHLMANN 1951). The Congress on Ultrasound in Medicine, which was held in Erlangen (Germany) in 1949, presented a clear recommendation to avoid ultrasound therapy for the treatment of human tumors – a fatal error now completely reversed by modern technical developments in ultrasound (HYNYNEN 1990). It is assumed today that the rather negative impression derived from inappropriate or ineffective (i.e., insufficient heating) applications (CLARKE et al. 1970).

The current resurgence of interest in ultrasound in the treatment of human cancer is based entirely on its suitability as a modality for the induction of controlled localized hyperthermia, i.e., well-collimated beams, focusing abilities, and beneficial absorption characteristics in body tissues which are proportional to frequency and therefore lower in fatty tissue than in all soft tissues. In the early clinical studies at Stanford University (MARMOR et al. 1979) the investigators achieved 40% objective tumor responses to ultrasound hyperthermia alone, but most responses lasted less than 6 weeks. However, the clinical responses were clearly improved by the combination of ultrasound and x-rays (MARMOR et al. 1979; MARMOR and HAHN 1980). Ultrasound-induced hyperthermia for the treatment of human superficial tumors was also developed at the M.D. Anderson University Hospital (CORRY et al. 1982). Other research groups recognized that in experimental tumors the effect of x-rays could be enhanced by the application of ultrasound (LEHMANN and KRUSEN 1955; SPRING 1969; WOEBER 1955, 1956, 1965). LEHMANN and KRUSEN (1955) observed that ultrasound increased radiation-induced growth inhibition of a rodent tumor, this effect being prevented if the tumor was cooled during the ultrasound treatment.

1.3.4 Systemic Heating Methods

The Greek philosopher and scientist Parmenides from Elea (about 500 B.C.) claimed that he could cure all illness, including malignant tumors, if he could induce "sufficient fever" in the patient. This is probably the first historical note on the beneficial effects of systemic heating on cancer. The effects of exposure of the whole body to high temperatures have been widely recognized throughout medical history, whether achieved by hot bath or spa treatment, or (in the nineteenth century and later) by the artificial induction of fever by pyrogens, or (in modern times) by the use of special heating cabinets. Nowadays we assume that "fever" may directly affect malignant tumors, but also stimulates and reflects an immunological response of the human body.

1.3.4.1 Hot Bath Treatment

In all cultures and throughout the history of mankind, the use of "bath" has had not only a physical but also a mythological and religious significance (Fig. 1.17a–c). Some records dating back to the era of the Greek writer Homer (about 800 B.C.) describe the wonderful healing qualities of the hot steam bath in the treatment of many ailments. The Greeks and Romans are reported to have taken baths in various forms.

The ancient metropolis of Rome was very famous for its public baths, the so-called thermals (from the Greek word "*thermos*," meaning warmth). Many Roman emperors like the cruel militarist Caracalla (211–217 A.D.) tried to pacify and please the public by building new large public baths. Interestingly, these Roman baths usually included a "*frigidarium*" (for cold water) and a "*caldarium*" (for hot water). The highly developed spa culture of antiquity, with numerous types of hot baths, was practiced in various modifications including the hot steam bath, the hot bath in tubs, and the whole-body bath in hot springs. The latter is a habit specifically in countries with high geothermic and vulcanic activity like Iceland or Japan (SUGAHARA 1989).

Despite the use of hot baths being recommended for many ailments, there have to date been few reports on the treatment of cancer by hot baths in the literature. While in several older textbooks malignant neoplasms were regarded as a contraindication to spa therapy, recent researchers have suggested on the basis of experimental research that heat exposure has potential for the prevention of cancer (MITCHEL et al. 1986). Moreover, SUGAHARA (1989) indicated that hot baths may even serve this purpose, given the low incidence of breast cancer and the frequent use of hot baths in Japans. These speculations might find a more solid justification in modern immunologic research, which is providing increasing evidence

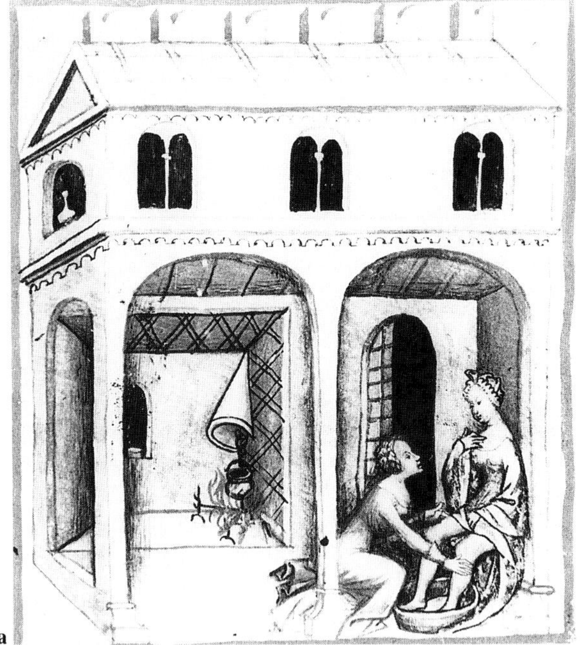

a

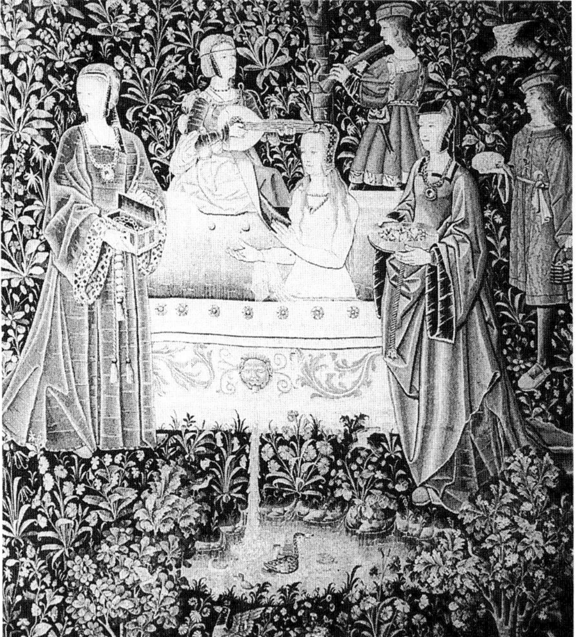

c

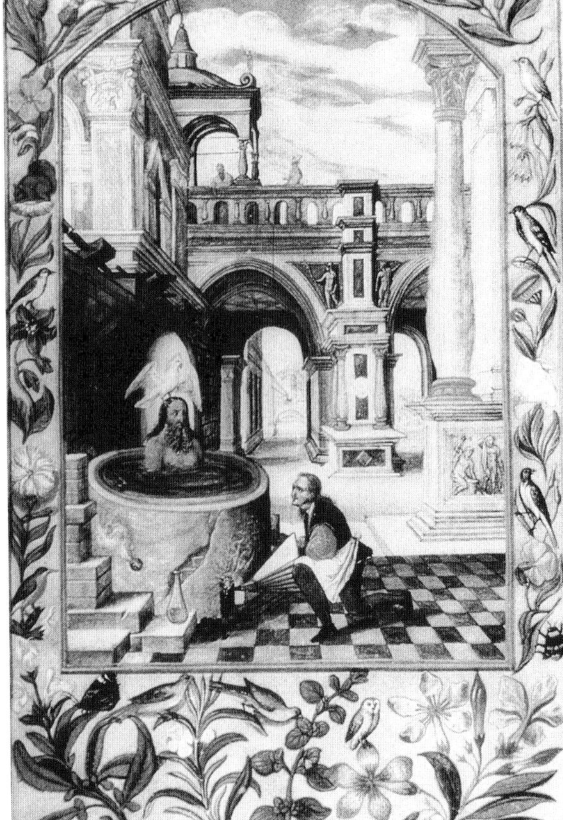

b

Fig. 1.17a–c. Hot bath treatment. **a** Old painting from *Tacuinum sanitatis* (The book of health) around 1500 A.D. The booklet gives medical advice in accordance with humoralistic medicine. The illustration explains the meaning and use of "hot water": it is strongly recommended for humans with a "cold complexion" (predisposition), for sick and weak persons, and for persons living in cold regions. (Courtesy of Heimeran Publishing Company). **b** Old medieval tapestry showing the hot bath of a person with a dove (symbol of the "Holy Spirit") above his head. The second person uses a bellow to increase the heat underneath the bath tub. **c** The hot bath – a typical scene from medieval aristocratic life around 1500. Old tapestry from around 1500 (Paris, Museum Cluny)

for a cascade of immunological reactions in humans after systemic heat exposure, which includes the synthesis of cytokines and interferons (Dewning et al. 1988).

Unfortunately many experimental and clinical studies on the use of systemic heating or induction of artificial fever fail to describe their basic treatment concept and their purpose. However, when reviewing the literature two rationales for systemic heating can be clearly distinguished: (a) to stimulate the immune sytem against the existing tumor cells by using moderate temperatures in the range of 39°–40.5°C (indirect thermal effects), and (b) to induce at least a tumor growth delay by use of higher temperatures in the range of 41°–43°C or to directly destroy the tumor cells at temperatures above 43°C (direct thermal effects).

1.3.4.2 Febrile Infections and Cancer Prevention

Epidemiological data assembled in the twentieth century indicate that in most countries the incidence of cancer is increasing at the same time as the incidence of infections is decreasing. Even at the beginning of this century, several studies noted that malignant tumors appeared to be less common in patients who had experienced several febrile infections during their life (Busch 1866a; Busch 1866b; Fehleisen 1883; Coley 1894; Eschweller 1898; Schmidt 1910; Wolffheim 1921; Braunstein 1929; Engel 1934; Sinek 1936; Schulz 1969). It was also assumed that acute productive tuberculosis could inhibit tumor growth (Fürth 1937). Others pointed out that a lower incidence of cancer occurs in geographical areas with endemic malaria (Levin 1910; Braunstein 1929, 1931; Schrumpf-Pierron 1932; Fürth 1937; Koller 1937).

The exact purpose and function of the febrile response which accompanies bacterial and viral infections are unknown, but generally it represents a "defense mechanism" of the body. It also remains unclear whether febrile infections have a direct cancer-preventive potential or whether the fever (or heat) stimulates preventive immunological reactions. According to Ashman (1979) the febrile response may act as a body defense in the following ways: (a) potentiation of interferons and cytokines; (b) promotion of the cell-mediated immune response; (c) potentiation of the cellular immune response; and (d) enhancement of nonspecific defense mechanisms.

1.3.4.3 Febrile Infections and Spontaneous Tumor Remission

In modern times, interest in systemic hyperthermia for cancer therapy arose from several remarkable case studies which reported spontaneous tumor remissions after exposure to febrile infections. The first clinical observations were published by two German physicians, Busch (1866a,b) and Bruns (1887): In 1866, Busch described a patient with a recurrent and histologically confirmed sarcoma of the face which had rapidly regressed after exposure to a prolonged erysipelas infection. Therefore Busch assumed that the long period of high fever ("whole-body hyperthermia") was responsible for this completely unexpected tumor regression. In 1887, Bruns observed complete regression of a widespread superficial malignant melanoma in a terminally ill patient who developed a high fever beyond 40°C for several days due to an erysipelas infection.

Subsequently many other investigators experienced similar spontaneous remissions of primary and metastatic cancers following a prolonged febrile episode due to bacterial infections (Fehleisen 1883; Gerster and Hartley 1892; Czerny 1895, 1907; Vidal 1907 Bolognino 1908; Rohdenburg 1918; Wolffheim 1921; DeCourcy 1933; Everson and Cole 1956; Selawry 1957; Selawry et al. 1958; Schulz 1969). Two opposing opinions were expressed about the mode of the anticancer action of febrile infections. While Fehleisen (1883) was convinced that the streptococcal bacteria themselves exerted an antagonistic influence upon malignant tumors, Vidal (1907) believed that the elevated body temperature alone was responsible for the induced tumor remission, since in his patients the fever had developed only as a result of a traumatic rather than an infectious event. Interestingly, DeCourcy (1933), in a review of the literature, found spontaneous tumor regression after febrile attacks of malaria, tuberculosis, and typhoid infections, and he believed that this was due to vasodilatation, hemorrhage, necrosis, thrombosis, and lymphatic infiltration of the tumor.

In a carefully documented review, Rohdenburg (1918) was able to locate a total of 302 case reports where spontaneous regression of histologically proven malignancies had occurred. In the search for common factors between these patients, he was able to detect a close relationship between tumor remission and the occurrence of fever due to infections. Those infections most commonly associated with high fever were smallpox, malaria, pneumonia, tuberculosis, and, particularly, erysipelas. These infections are typically characterized by continuous elevations of mild temperatures ranging from 39.4° to 40°C for several days.

Selawry (1957) reviewed 450 spontaneous tumor remissions in histologically proven cancers of which about one-third were related to previous febrile infections including erysipelas, malaria, typhus, scarlet fever, pneumonia, and many other diseases. Among these tumors, sarcomas were more frequently represented than carcinomas. In several other instances the spontaneous tumor remissions ultimately led to the complete cure of cancer (Selawry et al. 1958; Beeks 1966). Another but rather exotic case report was provided by Allison (1880), who described a patient with a lip carcinoma who experienced a complete tumor remission after being struck by lightning.

In 1971, Stephenson and co-workers carefully analyzed several clinical reports in the literature (2500 specific variables) on a total of 294 patients who had experienced spontaneous tumor regression. They noted that uncommon histological subtypes of tumors accounted for more than half of the cases, which included (a) hypernephroma, (b) malignant melanoma, (c) neuroblastoma, and (d) chorioncarcinoma. Unfortunately from a modern oncological perspective, these tumor types represent less than 4% of all cancers that develop in humans. While the gender was not important, younger age implied a more favorable prognosis. It was also noted that only a few patients survived beyond a period of 5 years after undergoing spontaneous tumor regression, and that most patients died of recurrent disease. The authors concluded that the spontaneous regression of cancer was most likely related to some alterations in the immune system. This is supported by evidence that lymphoid centers in humans are involved in tumor surveillance. Moreover, the higher incidence of neoplasms in patients with an impaired autoimmune system also suggests a direct relationship between spontaneous regression of tumors and the immune system.

1.3.4.4 Artifical Induction of Fever

The early case reports on the spontaneous regression of malignant tumors came to the attention of the New York surgeon William B. Coley, who assumed that the febrile response to bacteria causing erysipelas or other febrile infections would also be effective against cancer. In 1891 he initiated his own experimental studies after he had experienced and followed up a patient with an inoperable recurrent round-cell sarcoma for more than 7 years, who was surprisingly cured after an accidental erysipelas infection. In his clinical experiments Coley devised a heat treatment by deliberately producing fever through the administration of attenuated fluid cultures of *Streptococcus erysipelatis* containing *pyrogenic toxins* (Coley 1893). With this approach Coley was able to observe many tumor remissions and noted that a better response was achieved with the "more virulent bacterial strains" (Fig. 1.18). Most cancers regressed regardless of their histological subtype. Similar observations with viable and virulent bacteria strains were made by Czerny (1895, 1907, 1911) and Koch and Petruschky (1896).

Coley was the chief of the Bone Tumor Service at Sloan Kettering Memorial Hospital in New York at that time and therefore was able to teach and publish extensively on the usefulness of his new cancer treatment, which he called "*pyrogen therapy*" (Coley 1894, 1896, 1897). Certainly he was wrong in his belief that microparasitic organisms themselves were responsible for the development of cancer and that the streptococcal bacteria produced toxins which were able to destroy these cancer-causing organisms. However, his idea of the induction of fever as a means of whole-body hyperthermia and its obvious therapeutic effect on various tumors subsequently gave rise to considerable controversy about the

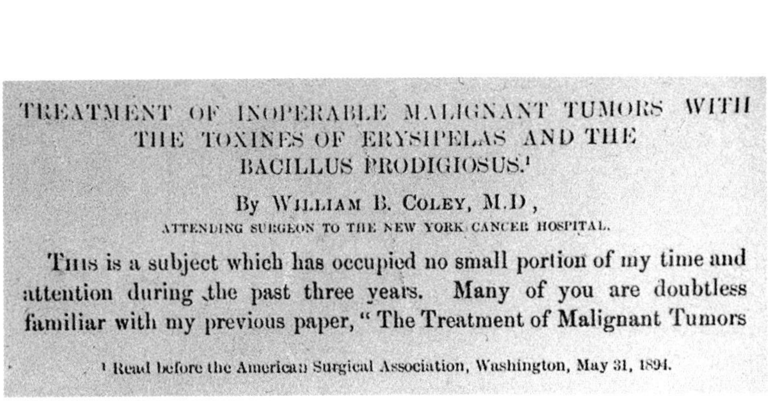

TREATMENT OF INOPERABLE MALIGNANT TUMORS WITH THE TOXINES OF ERYSIPELAS AND THE BACILLUS PRODIGIOSUS.[1]

By William B. Coley, M.D.,

ATTENDING SURGEON TO THE NEW YORK CANCER HOSPITAL.

This is a subject which has occupied no small portion of my time and attention during the past three years. Many of you are doubtless familiar with my previous paper, "The Treatment of Malignant Tumors

[1] Read before the American Surgical Association, Washington, May 31, 1894.

Fig. 1.18. Title page of one of the initial articles of William B. Coley's on his "pyrogen therapy method" in 1896, which was published in the American Journal of the Medical Sciences

treatment of cancer which has prevailed until now. Although Coley persisted in his experimental and clinical research for several decades in this century and finally had accumulated clinical experience in almost 1200 patients (Nauts et al. 1953, 1959), he was not able to achieve consistent clinical results and to produce a reliable strain of bacterial cultures as a standard pyrogen which he called "mixed bacterial vaccine" (MBV). Since few other investigators were able to duplicate his results (DeCourcy 1933), his work with toxin therapy rapidly fell into disrepute and was subsequently regarded by the American Cancer Society as an unproven and even "dubious" cancer treatment.

In 1918, Konteschweller reviewed most available pyrogens of the time which were used to induce fever, including typhoid vaccines, milk, colloidal selenium, tuberculin, various bacterial vaccines, antidiphtheria serum, peptones, pollens, and gelatin. He observed no difference between bacterial vaccines and colloidal preparations. The pyrogens usually induced a marked leukopenia which peaked at about 1 h but was soon followed by leukocytosis, which was maximal at about 6 h, while the white blood count ultimately reverted to pretreatment levels at 48 h. This indicates that fever and immune response both may be responsible for the antineoplastic effects of heat; however, even today the underlying mechanisms have not been fully uncovered and any clinical results which have been achieved with these methods are still speculative. In 1957, Huth reviewed the clinical results achieved with the application of Coley's toxins, i.e., special preparations of *Streptococcus erysipelatis* sera. Of the 484 tumor-bearing patients a total of 49% achieved a 5-year survival. The best results were achieved in operable cases and in soft tissue sarcomas and lymphoid sarcomas; unfortunately, however, an appropriate control grup was not presented.

Some decades later, Coley's daughter, Helen Coley Nauts, carefully reviewed her father's clinical work on "pyrogen therapy" (Nauts 1975, 1976). She meticulously followed the individual patients for up to 35 years and found a correlation between the survival rate and the thermal level of the induced fever therapy. The highest cure rate was obtained in patients who were exposed to fever therapy for as long as 4–6 months. She concluded that the "stimulation of the host's immunity" is the major anticancerous component of pyrogen therapy and especially linked it to the exposure to *Corynebacterium parvum*. She stated literally: "Fever alone is not the most important factor . . . and if it were, every (agent causing) fever should be equally effective. This is not the case."

Nauts also supported the relationship between hyperthermia and cancer prevention. She felt that this theory was confirmed by the low incidence of penile, skin, and breast cancer in the Japanese population, which was frequently exposed to hot baths (42°–48°C); as we know, such exposure can lead to rectal temperatures of up to 39°C. Later Nauts (1982) updated the review of Huth (1957) and reported that complete regression and 5-year survival occurred in 46% of the 523 inoperable cases and 51% of the operable cases treated with Coley's MBV (Table 1.3).

Miller and Nicholson (1971) reviewed the records of 52 patients with bone sarcoma who received Coley's toxin either alone or in conjunction with surgery and/or radiotherapy. In all but two patients, additional high doses of localized radiotherapy were administered. An overall 5-year survival rate of 64% was achieved. The authors reported on several prognostic factors influencing survival, including stage of disease, timing and dosage of radiotherapy, tumor site, and the dosage, frequency, and type of toxin injection. They also found that the temperature level (at least 38.3°–40°C) which was achieved during the febrile period was another important prognostic indicator. They concluded that Coley's toxins were effective in inducing fever and helped to improve survival as compared to the rate observed without the toxins. Among the many tested strains *Streptococcus pyogenes* and *Serratia marcescens* were the most effective.

1.3.4.5 Heating Cabinets and Systemic Heating Devices

As a reaction to the relatively inconsistent induction of fever by bacterial pyrogens (Coley's toxin), pyrogen therapy was quite soon replaced by externally applied systemic heating methods. For this purpose so-called heating cabinets were invented. They usually combined various radiant heating devices (radiators or light bulbs) with medical diathermy (Neymann and Osborne 1929). Carpenter and Page (1930) utilized a shortwave transmitter in combination with a non-heat-conducting box and produced systemic body

Table 1.3. Review of clinical results with Coley's toxins ("pyrogen therapy") (results summarized by NAUTS 1982)

Type of tumor	Number	Inoperable cases		Operable cases	
		No.	5-year survival	No.	5-year survival
Bone tumors (total)	*417*	*151*	*42 (28%)*	*266*	*109 (41%)*
Ewing's sarcoma	114	52	11 (21%)	62	18 (29%)
Osteogenic sarcoma	162	23	3 (13%)	139	43 (31%)
Reticular cell sarcoma	72	49	9 (18%)	23	13 (57%)
Multiple myeloma	12	8	4 (50%)	4	2 (50%)
Giant cell tumor	57	19	15 (79%)	38	33 (87%)
Soft tissue sarcomas (total)	*289*	*239*	*130 (54%)*	*50*	*36 (72%)*
Lymphosarcoma	86	86	42 (49%)	0	–
Hodgkin's lymphoma	15	15	10 (67%)	0	–
Other soft tissue sarcomas	188	138	78 (57%)	50	36 (72%)
Gynecologic tumors (total)	*63*	*49*	*33 (67%)*	*14*	*14 (100%)*
Breast cancer	33	20	13 (65%)	13	13 (100%)
Ovarian cancer	16	15	10 (67%)	1	1 (100%)
Cervical cancer	3	3	2 (67%)	0	–
Uterine sarcoma	11	11	8 (73%)	0	–
Other tumors (total)	*128*	*84*	*33 (39%)*	44	31 (70%)
Testicular cancer	64	43	14 (33%)	21	15 (71%)
Malignant melanoma	31	17	10 (59%)	14	10 (71%)
Colorectal cancer	13	11	5 (45%)	2	2 (100%)
Renal cancer (adults)	8	7	3 (43%)	1	1 (100%)
Renal cancer (children)	3	0	–	3	1 (33%)
Neuroblastoma	9	6	1 (17%)	3	2 (67%)
Total experience	897	523	238 (46%)	374	190 (51%)

temperatures in the range of 40°–40.5°C in a volunteer. This temperature level could be maintained for several hours without any severe side-effects (Fig. 1.19a–d).

A combination of systemic artificial heating and ionizing radiation was clinically studied and reported by WARREN (1935). In 29 of 32 patients with advanced malignant tumors an almost immediate improvement in general condition was noted which lasted as long as 6 months. Considerable shrinkage of the metastatic burden was observed in many patients, together with an improvement in general physical performance parameters, i.e., body weight and overall physical strength. A remarkable regression was observed in a patient with metastatic hypernephroma who was treated with five sessions of 41.5°C systemic (i.e., rectal) heating. Tumor remissions reached 1 to 6 months, but eventually all patients experienced tumor regrowth. Warren heated his patients with a heat cabinet by utilizing five radiating 200-W carbon filament light bulbs. The body temperature was elevated to 41.5°C for about 5 h without major toxicity. Warren concluded that "in cases previously treated by deep roentgen therapy, and in untreated cases, fever therapy seems to have a definite destructive effect upon the tumor cells."

At the same time, DOUB (1935) reported palliation in advanced malignancies, including osteogenic sarcoma. Systemic hyperthermia as high as 42° combined with modest doses of radiation achieved good palliative effects, but no permanent cures. Similar results were reported by SHOULDERS and TURNER (1942). By 1939 more than 500 scientific papers had been published on this type of externally induced systemic hyperthermia, which was then called "electropyrexia therapy" (NEYMAN 1939). Artificial fever as treatment for malignant tumors was just one of its many medical applications being investigated at the time, one further example being the inoculation of malaria for the treatment of tertiary syphilis. Clinical applications of systemic hyperthermia included gonorrhea, Sydenhan's chorea, rheumatic heart disease, rheumatoid arthritis, multiple sclerosis, and asthma. In this context, the various forms of heat applications in physical therapy are not addressed. They have been rapidly evolving since the beginning of the century. Most of these techniques have induced various types of currents or

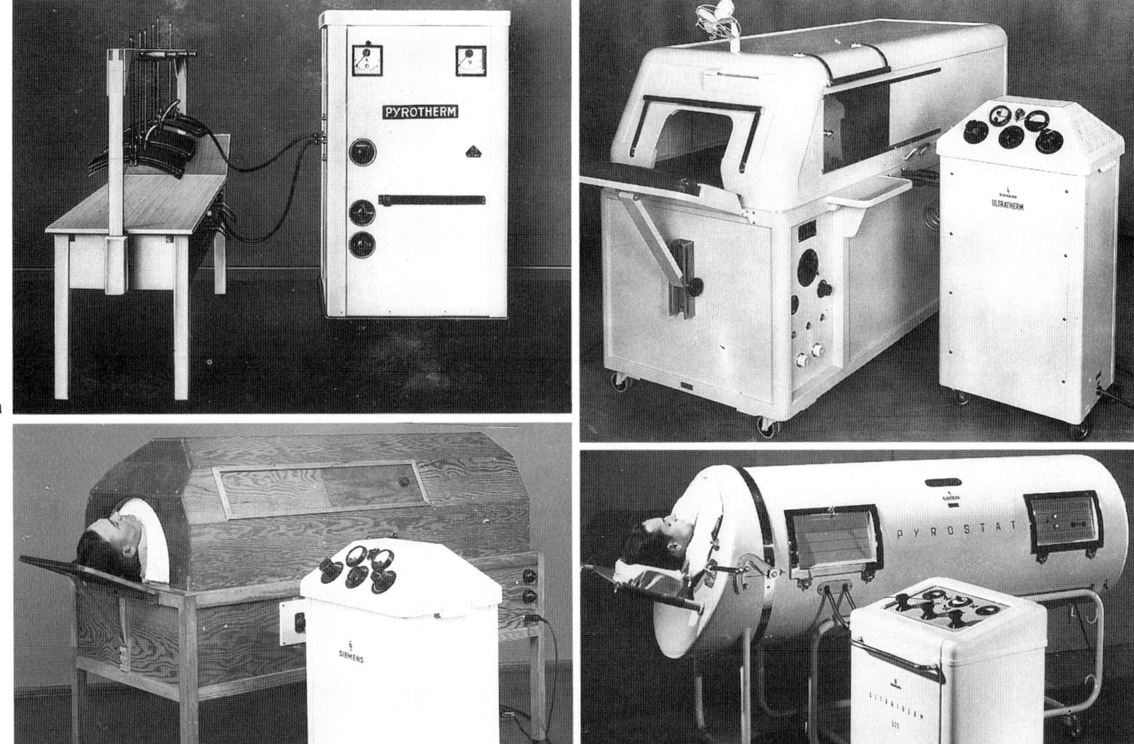

Fig. 1.19a–d. Systemic heating cabinets. **a** "Pyrotherm" apparatus combined with special electrode table for regional and whole-body heating around 1933: One large electrode is integrated within the wooden plate of the table, while three opposing concave-shaped electrodes are positioned above the table. The power deposition (400 W) is tuned manually with a turning knob. Amperemeter and voltmeter are implemented for treatment control. (Courtesy of Siemens Medical Archives, Erlangen). **b** Systemic heating box (fever cabinet) around 1940. The patient is positioned within the wooden box. The power is generated by the "Ultratherm" (400 W) apparatus from Siemens Company. (Courtesy of Siemens Medical Archives, Erlangen). **c** Systemic heating device (fever cabinet) which is attached to the power generator "Ultratherm" from Siemens Company around 1946. Note the small ventilator attached on the top of the heating box for cooling of the patient's face during therapy. (Courtesy of Siemens Medical Archives, Erlangen). **d** Systemic heating device "Pyrostat 601" (fever cabinet) which is attached to the power generator "Ultratherm 525" (700 W power supply) from Siemens Company around 1953/1954. (Courtesy of Siemens Medical Archives, Erlangen)

electrical fields within the human body and parts of it and thereby caused warmth and reactive hyperemia. Representative for these devices is a hydro-electric whole body bath tub, illustrated in Fig. 1.20.

These early efforts at artificial fever induction triggered all the later improved implementations of regional and systemic heating techniques. In the late 1960s and the early 1970s the first clinical efforts were made to implement hyperthermic perfusion of the extremities in patients with melanomas or soft tissue sarcomas (Cavaliere et al. 1967; Cavaliere 1970; Moricca 1970; Stehlin 1969, 1980). Also in the late 1960s modern techniques were implemented to induce systemic whole-body hyperthermia for advanced or metastatic tumors. The technical designs included hot blankets, hot wax baths, closed heating cabinets and radiating sources in combination with hot air exposure (Fig. 1.21).

Nowadays whole-body hyperthermia is usually applied in an adjuvant combination with either chemo- or radiotherapy for certain metastatic and advanced malignancies (Pettigrew et al. 1974; Bull et al. 1979; Larkin 1979; Parks et al. 1979). Several questions still remain with regard to the

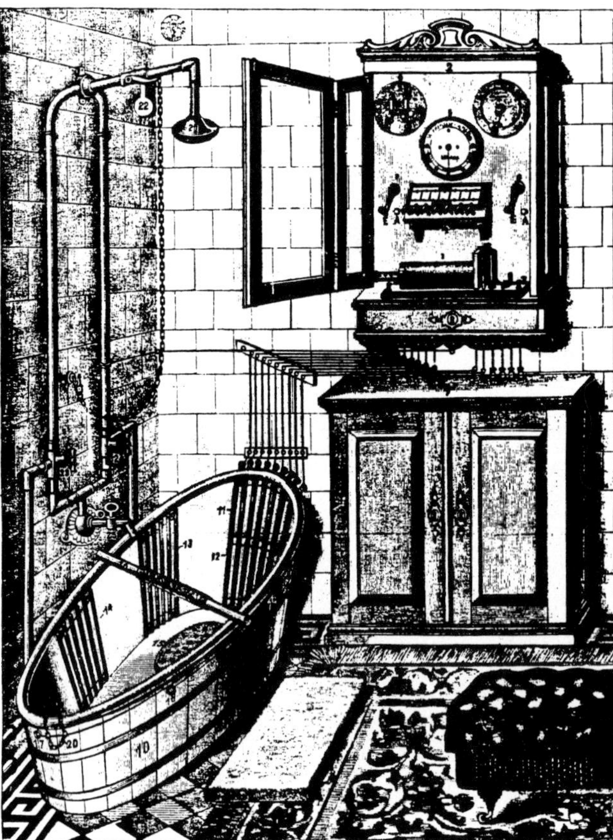

Fig. 1.20. Hydroelectric whole-body bath around 1900 with battery and induction coil for physical therapy. Catalogue page from the electromedical company Reiniger, Gebbert, and Schall, Erlangen (Germany). (Courtesy of Siemens Medical Archives, Erlangen)

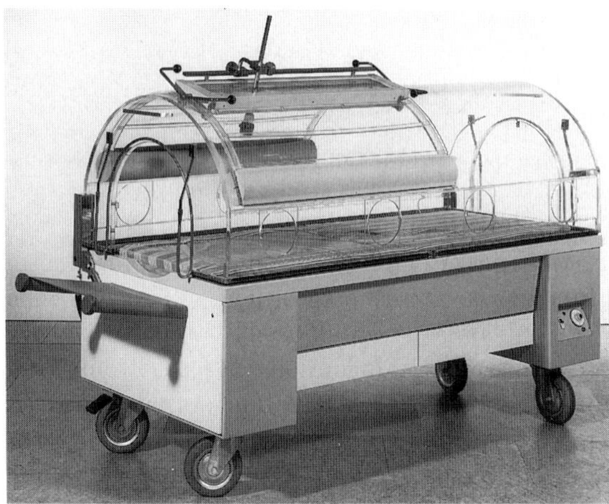

Fig. 1.21. Recent systemic heating device (fever cabinet) with transparent housing around 1969. (Courtesy of Siemens Medical Archives, Erlangen)

mechanisms involved in the potential antineoplastic activity of systemic heating, and these questions have been addressed in recent laboratory investigations.

1.3.5 Laboratory Hyperthermia Research

1.3.5.1 Heat Alone in Normal Tissues

Laboratory research on the effects of heat was initiated as long ago as the beginning of the twentieth century. Early investigators evaluated the tolerance of normal tissues to different degrees of thermal exposure. Cohnheim (1873) observed the response of rabbit ears following transient vascular ligation and immersion in hot water. While 45°C for 30 min produced no macroscopic effects, higher temperatures of 49°–50°C caused heavy inflammatory signs and severe tissue damage. With further research in this century (Burger and Fuhrmann 1964) it became evident that there is marked variation in the thermal response pattern among different mammalian tissues within the same species and also between the different mammalian species themselves. Moritz and Henriques (1947), however, established that the thermal tolerance of porcine and human skin is very similar. In their clinical experiments the lowest skin temperature responsible for inducing a cutaneous burn was 44°C for 360 min. They also found that at between 44°–51°C the heating time required to produce a thermal injury decreased by about one-half for each degree rise in temperature. Nowadays these dose-response findings are clearly reflected in the "thermal dose" equation proposed by SAPARETO and DEWEY (1984).

Until now the effects of heat on the various *normal tissues in humans* have not been systematically assessed. Autopsy examinations have been conducted with regard to fatal cases of artifically induced systemic heating (GORE and ISAACSON 1949) and fatal heat stroke (MALAMUD et al. 1946). These pathology studies suggested that individual organ susceptibility exists to different thermal exposures: myocardial damage (subendocardial hemorrhage and rupture of muscle fibers), brain damage (edema, diffuse petechial hemorrhage), renal, and liver damage have been described and related to different threshold temperatures. A review on the pathological effects of hyperthermia on the different organs of humans and animals was provided by FAJARDO (1984), who observed a clear time- and temperature-dependent dose-response relationship in the different organs.

1.3.5.2 Heat Alone in Tumors

In 1903, the thermal sensitivity of spontaneous or experimental malignant tumors was studied in vivo and in vitro by LOEB (1903) and JENSEN (1903). Loeb found that rat sarcoma cells were inactivated by 45°C for 30 min. Other investigators confirmed these observations in rodent tumors with different heat treatments ranging from 44°C for 30 min to 47°C for 5 min (HAALAND 1907, 1908; EHRLICH 1907), but no comparison was made between different tumor types or specific tumors and the surrounding normal tissues in these experiments.

HAALAND (1907, 1908) concluded from his animal experiments that malignant tumor cells have an individual susceptibility to heat. LAMBERT (1912) was probably the first to compare the heat sensitivity of different malignant and normal cells by using the special technique of cell cultures in hanging plasma drops. He applied heat treatments between 42°–47°C for various time intervals and showed that mouse sarcoma cells were able to survive an exposure of 43°C for 3 h, while the normal counterpart cells, proliferating connective tissue cells derived from the aorta, survived for twice as long. Thus, Lambert concluded from his study, that "the normal cells were more resistant to heat than malignant cells."

Several recent experimental in vitro studies have confirmed the rather individual thermal susceptibility of different tumors (BENDER and SCHRAMM 1966, 1968; GERICKE 1970, 1971). For example, in a large study BENDER and SCHRAMM (1966, 1968) tested 46 animal and human tumor cell lines under identical heating conditions and confirmed a *specific thermal sensitivity for each tumor cell line*, but their findings also suggested that tumors are not generally more sensitive to heat than normal tissues. They stated: "A thermal exposure which may induce complete tumor regression in some tumors, may still lead to rapid tumor growth stimulation in other tumors".

In transplantable murine tumors, ROHDENBURG and PRIME (1921) observed a rapid tumor regression after thermal exposures between 42° and 46°C. Careful histological studies 1–6 days after the hyperthermia exposure revealed complete tumor cell death, while no obvious side-effects were observed in normal tissues. This finding was another indication of the higher sensitivity of tumor cells as compared to normal cells, although the exact reasons were not known at that time. Similar observations were made by STEVENSON (1919) and LIEBESNY (1921).

A well-conducted study by N. WESTERMARK (1927) showed that rat Flexner-Jobling carcinoma or Jensen sarcoma regressed completely after radiofrequency heating. The temperature-time profiles which were required to obtain a tumor cure closely followed an Arrhenius relationship. For example, total tumor regression occurred to an equal extent after 180 min at 44°C and after 90 min at 45°C, while normal tissues were not damaged under similar temperature conditions. Westermark introduced the concepts of dose-time thermal effects and histopathological examination and he concluded from his study that "these tumors can be healed by heat treatment without destruction being cause to surrounding tissues."

Many other investigators confirmed the potential of heat to induce a tumor growth delay in vivo independently of the heating technique, i.e., by means of hot water bath heating (WESTERMARK 1927) or by implementation of electromagnetic high-frequency techniques (HAAS and LOB 1934; REITER 1933; BAUMEYER 1938; KORB 1939, 1943, 1948; OVERGAARD 1934, 1935, 1936l; OVERGAARD and OKKELS 1940a, 1940b; CHRONOWA 1948; SCHLIEPHAKE 1960). The Danish scientist K. OVERGAARD (1934, 1935) described cures of the Crooker sarcoma in mice by using diathermy yielding intratumoral temperatures of 42°–46°C. If lower temperatures were induced, a short-term tumor growth delay and inhibition was observed, but shortly thereafter regrowth occurred which was mostly located at the edge of the treated region.

Another study using high-frequency (8.3- to 135-MHz) currents in a transplanted mouse sarcoma resulted in tumor growth delay or inhibition and complete disappearance of some tumors (SCHERESCHEWSKY 1928a,b). The greatest effects were observed at a frequency range of 66–68 MHz – a frequency which is preferentially used in modern annular phased array heating systems. While in his original studies Scherescheswky felt that the lethal action of the shortwave diathermy was due to the specific wave frequency characteristics, he reversed his statement in a later study (SCHERESCHESWKY 1933), when he had additionally examined the body and tumor temperature of the heat-exposed mice. He stated in his conclusion that the "curative effects" of high-frequency fields were more related to the heating than to a specific frequency effect.

1.3.5.3 Heat Combined with Radiation

Although heat was used in cancer therapy at the beginning of the twentieth century, it was not until 1921 that studies emerged in the scientific journals concerning the effect of combined radiation and heat on malignant tumors. Besides their studies on the effects of heat alone, ROHDENBURG and PRIME (1921) were the first to analyze the combined effects of heat and radiation in the Crooker mouse sarcoma 180 and some spontaneously developing breast tumors using temperatures between 42° and 46°C. They revealed a definite *synergistic effect* above 42°C for the combined treatment. As was pointed out earlier, one of their observations was the "thermal dose-response relationship" between the heat-induced effects and treatment time and level of heating: low temperatures (41°C) were as effective as high temperatures (46°C) when the low temperatures were maintained for much longer treatment times. This finding was exactly confirmed by more recent thermobiology studies (DEWEY et al. 1982); it also forms the main rationale for the so-called "thermal dose concept" proposed by SAPARETO and DEWEY (1984).

ROHDENBURG and PRIME (1921) stated that "the combination of a given sublethal dose (of irradiation and heat) produces the same effect as four times the dose of heat alone, and as five times the dose of irradiation alone." The authors also noted no impact of the treatment sequence on the lethal effect of the combined therapy. In histological examinations they observed an intense congestion of small blood vessels between 24 and 72 h following the heat exposure. They observed that during this period the tumor cell contour became obscure and rapid karyorrhexis occurred. Massive coagulation necrosis and large areas of liquefaction developed between 72 and 144 h after the heat exposure. After the 7th day the necrotic tumor area was slowly replaced by fibrosis. This was the first observation of the induced physiological effects of heat which are thought to be responsible for the selective effects on tumor versus normal tissues.

Some years later, WESTERMARK (1927) investigated the localized effect of diathermy on two malignant rat tumors (Flexner-Jobling carcinoma, Jensen sarcoma). Tumor regression was observed after heat exposures of 44°C for 180 min and 45°C for 90 min, respectively, while skin and normal tissues were unaffected under thermal conditions which were lethal to the malignant tumor tissue. However, the author also pointed out that the differential heat sensitivity between tumor and normal cells diminished at a thermal level above 42°C, and he was concerned about the possible inhomogeneous heat distribution achieved by diathermy. This represents an instance of very early attention to the *quality assurance* issues which have recently been addressed in clinical hyperthermia trials (DEWHIRST et al. 1990).

Using chicken heart fibroblasts, BUCCIANTE (1928) was able to analyze differences in thermal susceptibility between the dividing and the resting cell populations – a phenomenon which is well known today and which forms one of the rationales for the combination of heat and radiotherapy. In addition, several decades later, SELAWRY et al. (1957) and HARRIS (1967) were able to clearly demonstrate increasing heat resistance after repeated thermal exposures. This phenomenon, which has been termed "*thermotolerance*," was also extensively studied by CRILE (1961), who stated: "Exposure of a tumor to heat for a period of time shorter than that required to destroy it makes the tumor temporarily resistant to subsequently applied heat."

Hill (1934) also observed rapid tumor regression of Jensen sarcomas transplanted to mice when the tumors were subjected to sublethal doses of radiation in combination with heat. The impact of different sequences of heat and radiation were studied in the murine Wood's sarcoma by Jares and Warren (1937, 1939). When the heat was applied prior to radiation therapy a much higher response rate was observed than when the heat followed radiation therapy. The authors also observed that the synergistic effect of combined radiation and heat was significantly reduced when an interval of 12–24 h was interposed between the two modalities. The impact of the timing and sequencing of the two modalities on tumor regression has subsequently, been studied by many research groups.

Despite these encouraging experimental studies, not all research groups agreed with the premise that heat potentiates ionizing radiation. In 1936, Taylor compared the effects of ultrashort radiowaves followed by radium therapy with the effects of radium alone in Jensen rat sarcoma and Walker rat carcinoma. He stated that heat alone did not alter the tumor growth rate unless tissue necrosis was produced, and he observed no synergistic effect of heat and radiation. Since no thermometry was performed, and details of the treatment schedule and the duration of heat exposure were not provided, it appears rather difficult to evaluate this study properly.

Modern hyperthermic research began with the remarkable experimental studies of Crile (1961, 1963), some of which still represent a real benchmark in experimental hyperthermia research. In the early 1960s, Crile took up the work of other researchers and performed a series of experiments on transplanted mouse tumors. He observed several fundamental biological reactions to heat which were later quantitatively assessed. The described biological phenomena included: (a) the time- and temperature-dependent cytotoxicity of heat; (b) the delayed in situ increased cytotoxicity in, and increased sensitivity of, large as compared with small transplanted tumors; (c) the thermotolerance of both normal and tumor tissue; and (d) the radiation sensitization by heat and its slow decay during heating.

1.3.4.4 Heat Combined with Chemotherapy

The combined use of heat and chemotherapeutic agents has been investigated only in the modern era of oncological research, ever since researchers realized that heat may alter the tumor cell membrane permeability and enhance uptake of cytotoxic agents (Field et al. 1964). First clinical observations on the combined application of heat and chemotherapy were reported by Woodhall et al. (1960) and Shingleton et al. (1962). Woodhall et al. observed some remarkable tumor responses in head and neck cancer patients. In 1970, Giovanella and co-workers found that L-1210 leukemia cells remained unaffected by temperatures in the range 37°–40°C; however, a lethal effect was suddenly induced at slightly higher temperatures in the range of 41°–42°C. A hundredfold enhancement of cell kill was induced when a specific alcoholic agent (dihydroxybutyl aldehyde) was added (Giovanella et al. 1970). Block and Zubrod (1973) also confirmed adjuvant effects of heat in cancer chemotherapy.

Other drugs, like D,L-glyceroaldehyde, melphalan, and oxamate, also proved to be more cytotoxic in combination with heat than alone. In vivo studies by Hahn and co-workers (Hahn 1979, 1982; Hahn and Strande 1976) suggested a possible benefit of using hyperthermia in combination with Adriamycin, bleomycin, nitrosoureas, cisplatin, and perhaps other drugs. Goss and Parsons (1976) tested different human fibroblast strains and melanoma cell lines in combination with various concentrations of melphalan alone or in combination with heat (42°C, 4 h) and found that the combined modality acted synergistically and increased the differential between fibroblast and melanoma cell lines.

Some of the first clinical applications of combined heat and chemotherapy were reported by Stehlin and co-workers, who found a 35%–80% increase in tumor response when heat of 40.5°–41.5°C was given in conjunction with melphalan chemotherapy perfusion for the treatment of regionally metastatic melanoma (Stehlin 1975).

1.4 Present and Future Role of Hyperthermia

When reviewing the early experimental and clinical studies on the possible benefits of localized or systemic heating, it becomes obvious that firm evidence for beneficial clinical effects is still limited. In most clinical studies the applied heating technique and the obtained clinical results were poorly described. Most clinical trials also failed to demonstrate a definite benefit of the additional heat by not using an appropriate control group. Even worse is the fact that no proof was provided that tumors were actually being heated, as appropriate invasive thermometry was lacking. In addition, histological evidence of tumor necrosis was rarely obtained and often the possibility of preexisting necrosis was simply neglected. More importantly, the heatability of a tumor may not only depend on the applied heating technique, but may in itself constitute an intrinsically favorable biological marker which predicts the tumor response.

Some historical circumstances have also reduced interest in hyperthermia research. The rapid development of oncology within the twentieth century, which is represented by the introduction of chemotherapy in the 1940s and 1950s and modern megavoltage radiotherapy equipment in the 1950s and 1960s, diverted scientific interest and enthusiasm away from further investigations in hyperthermia, and this diversion has continued until today, since new surgical techniques, immunotherapy, and gene therapy have entered the field. Nevertheless, in the 1960s new insights into the biological effects of heat became available and rekindled interest in the antineoplastic efficacy of heat and its potential in combination with radiotherapy and chemotherapy.

Nowadays, hyperthermia research is a rapidly evolving field, as is evident from the increasing development of various clinical HT applications as demonstrated by clinical studies presented at previous international hyperthermia meetings: Washington DC (USA) 1975, Essen (Germany) 1977, Fort Collins (USA) 1980, Aarhus (Denmark) 1984, Kyoto (Japan), 1988, and Tucson (USA) 1992 (Fig. 1.22). New clinical approaches have become more complex, including regional and interstitial heating. No area of the human body has been excluded from efforts to apply heat to localized tumors and organs (Fig. 1.23). Nevertheless, after the rather uncritical embracement of hyperthermia in the early 80s, there is now some frustration about its potential role, accompanied by stagnation in clinical research. However, it is too simple to categorize possible problems through questions and answers derived from a previous great debate on the theme: "The biology is with us, but the physics is against us." We need to solve interdisciplinary questions:

1. How does heat actually act at the molecular or cellular level and in certain tissue compositions?
2. How, when, and with what other therapies should hyperthermia be used to achieve its greatest potential?
3. Which methods will be the most efficacious for a particular tumor situation, and what is the optimal treatment regimen?
4. Will hyperthermia work consistently in *all* tumors and in *all* patients, if it is applied in its *optimal* way?

Answers to these questions will not be provided by individual achievements, but only by the *concerted efforts of all fields* contributing to cancer

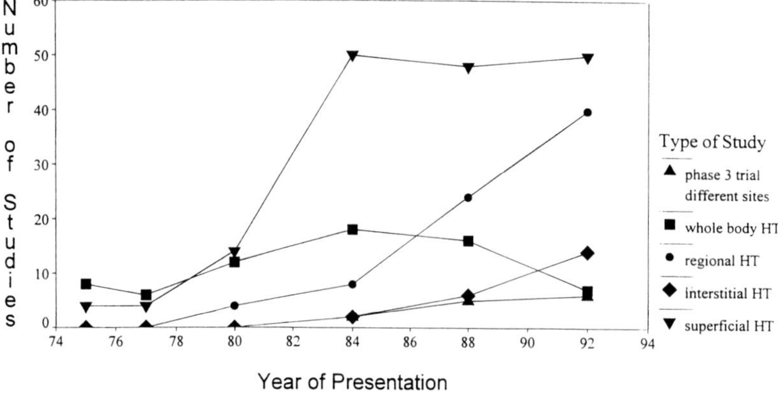

Fig. 1.22. Development of clinical hyperthermia research. Number of clinical studies presented at the International Hyperthermia Conferences in Washington (1975), Essen (1977), Fort Collins (1980); Aarhus (1984), Kyoto (1988), and Tucson (1992). The studies are grouped into the following categories: (1) superficial hyperthermia (HT), (2) interstitial HT, (3) regional HT, (4) whole-body HT and phase 3 HT studies in various body sites. (Modified from Overgaard 1993)

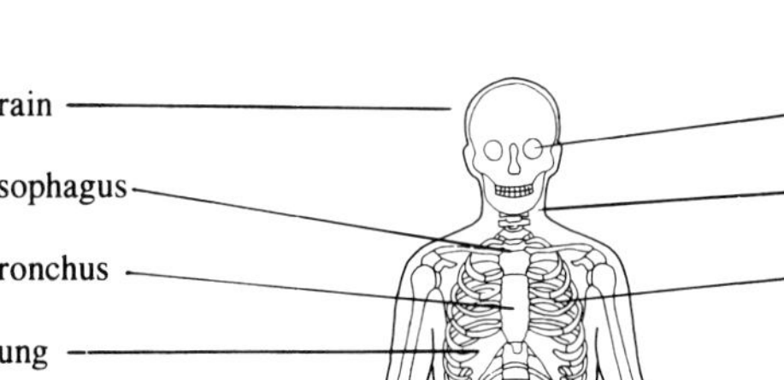

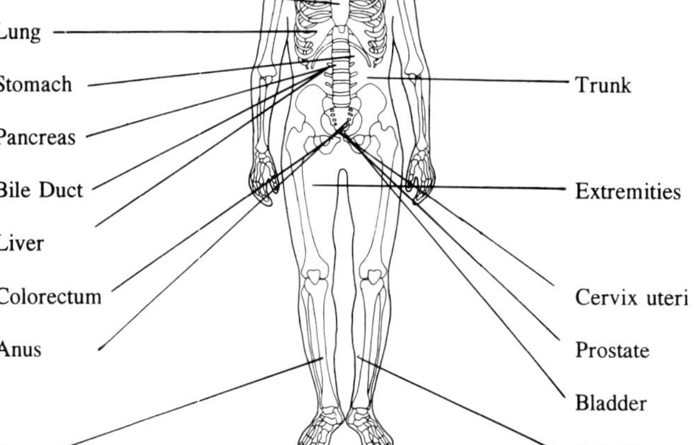

Fig. 1.23. Human body sites amenable to clinical hyperthermia research. Based on a survey on various human body sites approached with recent hyperthermia technology and clinical studies

therapy, including biology, physics, engineering, and clinical research. When we compare the present situation of hyperthermia with other oncological modalities from a scientific perspective, its situation is clearly no worse than that of chemotherapy, immunotherapy, and gene therapy: Despite immense experimental and clinical research efforts and enormous costs involved over several decades, cytotoxic agents have conquered only a small spectrum of clinical indications. Most trials using chemotherapy are still conducted as phase I–II trials, and phase III trials are often lacking "true" control groups. Immunotherapy and gene therapy, while being extremely expensive, have so far only theoretical promise, but have not achieved routine therapeutic efficacy. If only a small percentage of the financial resources, research funding, and staff devoted to chemotherapy were to be diverted to hyperthermia, this field would achieve a much broader spectrum of established clinical indications.

Moreover, the oversimplified criticism of early clinical hyperthermia studies should not result in condemnation of or a moratorium on further scientific investigations. Lack of success applies to many other fields in oncology and medicine today and is no argument against further funding of hyperthermia research. However, we believe that the development of hyperthermia as a useful tool in the oncological armamentarium must still depend on rigorously controlled scientific studies, and that presently hyperthermic therapy for human cancers must still be regarded as experimental. Therefore hyperthermia should not be used instead of established methods of cancer therapy.

We are just starting to apply new combinations of heat with cytotoxic agents or thermal sensitizers or with different radiation and chemotherapy schedules. We have obtained a better understanding of the complicated details of thermal cytotoxicity and thermal sensitization and we are rapidly developing more sophisticated technical tools to administer heat in a more predictable and controllable way. We are aware of the complex *quality assurance* issues, including appropriate selection of suitable patients, tumors, and heating techniques, and we have realized the necessity of appropriate treatment documentation and statistical analysis (Dewhirst et al. 1990). Furthermore, joint clinical efforts are being made in the form of better designed controlled multicenter studies (e.g., ESHO melanoma study, MRC breast study, and ongoing RTOG studies). Finally, we have a well-established scientific organization which offers the required scientific discussion and control.

Table 1.4. Rationale and aims for controlled clinical trials using thermoradiotherapy

1. *Better biological knowledge with regard to:*
   Thermal radiosensitization (inhibition of SLD/PLD repair)
   Effects of thermal cytotoxicity in normal and tumor tissue
   Sequencing of modalities and impact of thermotolerance
2. *Better physics and engineering support with regard to:*
   Homogeneity of the power deposition (heating distribution)
   Improved SAR coverage of the whole tumor volume
   Extensive invasive thermometry available
   Improved on-line treatment control during hyperthermia
   Improved power steering and feedback control
   Options for full treatment automatization
3. *Better selection of tumor sites and volumes with regard to:*
   Better diagnostic tumor extension assessment
   Improved methods of treatment planning
   Better ratio of power deposition to tumor volume
   Standardized documentation and treatment set-up
   Improved quality assurance conditions
4. *Future options and work-in-progress with regard to:*
   On-line treatment planning and thermal modeling
   Noninvasive thermometry control
   Physiological and pharmaceutical modification of heat effects

SLD, sublethal damage; PLD, potentially lethal damage

Thus, the rationale for the implementation of controlled clinical trials using hyperthermia in conjunction with radiotherapy has become even stronger in recent years, as can be seen from arguments listed in Table 1.4. If we continue our scientific research in this careful manner, we can conclude: "The past has not been with us, but the future will be with us." Despite previous shortcomings in research, pessimism about the potential role of hyperthermia in oncology is not justified.

References

Allison A (1880) Therapeutic effects of lightning upon cancer. Lancet 1: 77

Ashman RB (1979) The function of fever. Med J Aust 2: 532–539

Balfour DC (1915) The treatment by heat of advanced cancer of the cervix (Percy's method). Lancet, Minneapolis 35: 347–350

Bard P (1961) Medical physiology, 11th edn. Mosby, St. Louis, p 526

Baumeyer S (1938) Über die Wirkung der Kurzwellenbehandlung auf maligne Tumoren. Strahlentherapie 62: 373

Beck FF, Krantz JC (1940) Glycolysis in tumor tissue. III. The effect of ultrasonic vibrations on the growth and glycolysis of Walker sarcoma 319. Am J Cancer 39: 245

Beeks JW (1966) Hyperthermia as an adjunct to the treatment of neoplasms. J Kansas Med Soc 67: 527–543

Bender E, Schramm T (1966) Untersuchungen zur Thermosensibilität von Tumor- und Normalzellen in vitro. Acta Biol Med Germ 17: 527–543

Bender E, Schramm T (1968) Weitere Untersuchungen zur Frage der unterschiedlichen Thermosensibilität von Tumor- und Normalzellen in vitro und in vivo. Arch Geschwulstforsch 32: 215–230

Biermann W (1942) The medical applications of the short wave current. 2nd edn. Williams & Wilkins, Baltimore

Birkner R, Wachsmann F (1949) Über die Kombination von Röntgenstrahlen und Kurzwellen. Strahlentherapie 79: 93–102

Block JB, Zubrod CG (1973) Adjuvant temperature effects in cancer therapy. Cancer Chemother Rep 57: 373

Bolognino G (1908) Maligne Geschwülste und erysipelatöse Infektion. Z Krebsforsch 6: 261

Braunstein A (1929) Krebs und Malaria. Z Krebsforsch 29: 330, 486

Braunstein A (1931) Über durch Malaria bei Krebskranken hervorgerufene Reaktion en und ihre Beziehungen zum reticuloendothelialen System (RES). Z Krebsforsch 34: 230

Breasted JH (1930) The Edwin Smith surgical papyrus. In: Licht S (ed) Therapeutic heat and cold, 2nd edn. Waverly Press, Baltimore, p 196

Bruns P (1887) Die Heilwirkung des Erysipels auf Geschwulste. Beitr Klin Chir 3: 443–466

Bucciante L (1928) Ulteriori ricerche sulla velocita della mitosi nelle cellule coltivate in vitro in funzione della temperatura. Arch Exp Zellforsch 5: 1–23

Bull JM, Lees D, Schuette W et al. (1979) Whole body hyperthermia: a phase I trial of a potential adjuvant to chemotherapy. Ann Intern Med 90: 317–323

Burger FJ, Fuhrmann A (1964) Evidence of injury by heat in mammalian tissues. Am J Physiol 206: 1057–1061

Burov AK (1956) High intensity ultrasonic oscillation for treatment of malignant tumors in animals and man. Dokl Akad Nauk SSSR 106: 239

Busch W (1866a) Über den Einfluß, welchen heftigere Erysipeln zuweilen auf organisierte Neubildungen ausüben. Verhandlungen des Naturhistorischen Vereins der Preussischen Rheinlande und Westphalens 23: 28–30

Busch W (1866b) Verhandlungen ärztlicher Gesellschafter. Berl Klin Wochenschr 3: 245–246

Byrne J (1889) A digest of twenty years experience in the treatment of cancer of the uterus by galvano-cautery. Am J Obstet 22: 1052–1053

Byrne J (1892) Vaginal hysterectomy and high amputation, or partial exstirpation by galvanocautery in cancer of cervix uteri: an inquiry into their relative merits. Brooklyn Med J 6: 729

Carpenter CM, Page AB (1930) Production of fever in man by short radiowaves. Science 71: 450

Cavaliere R (1970) Hypertherme Perfusion erspart Extremitäten-Malignom Tumorrezidiv. Medical Tribune 9: 14

Cavaliere R, Ciocatto EC, Giovanella BC et al. (1967) Selective heat sensitivity of cancer cells. Biochemical and clinical studies. Cancer 20: 1351–1381

Celsus AC (1967) Über die Arzneimittelwissenschaft (de medicina) in 8 Büchern, vol V, G. Olms, Hildesheim, S. 288–289

Chronowa A (1948) Rezidivfreie Zerstörung von Carzinomzellen durch Ultrakurzwellen. Z Krebsforsch 56: 80–90
Clark WL, Morgan JD, Asnis EJ (1925) Electrothermic methods in the treatment of neoplasms and other lesions, with clinical and histological observations. Radiology 2: 233–246
Clarke PR, Hill CR, Adams K (1970) Synergism between ultrasound and X-rays in tumor therapy. Br J Radiol 43: 97
Cohnheim J (1873) Neue Untersuchungen über die Entzündung. Berlin
Coley W (1893) The treatment of malignant tumors by repeated inoculations of erysipelas: with a report of ten original cases. Am J Med Sci 105: 487–511
Coley W (1894) Treatment of inoperable malignant tumors with the toxines of erysipelas and the *Bacillus prodigiosus*: Trans Am Surg Assoc 12: 183
Coley W (1896) The therapeutic value of the mixed toxins of the *Streptococcus* of *erysipelas* and *Bacillus prodigiosus* in the treatment of inoperable malignant tumors. Am J Med Sci 112: 251
Coley W (1897) Inoperable sarcoma cured by mixed toxines of erysipelas. Ann Surg 25: 174
Coley W (1911) A report of recent cases of inoperable sarcoma successfully treated with mixed toxins of erysipelas and bacillus prodigiosus. Surg Gynecol Obstet 13: 174–190
Corry PM, Barlogie B, Tilchen EJ, Armour EP (1982) Ultrasound-induced hyperthermia for the treatment of human superficial tumors. Int J Radiat Oncol Biol Phys 8: 1225–1229
Crile G Jr (1961) Heat as an adjunct to the therapy of cancer – experimental studies. Cleve Clin Q 28: 75–89
Crile G Jr (1962) Selective destruction of cancers after exposure to heat. Ann Surg 156: 404–407
Crile G Jr (1963) The effects of heat and radiation on cancers implanted into the feet of mice. Cancer Res 23: 372–380
Cumberbatch EP (1928) Diathermy, its production and uses in medicine and surgery, 2nd edn. Mosby, St. Louis
Czerny V (1895) Über Heilversuche mit malignen Geschwülsten mit Erysipeltoxinen. Münch Med Wochenschr 36: 833
Czerny V (1907) Über unerwartete Krebsheilungen. Z Krebsforsch 4: 27
Czerny V (1911) Über die Therapie des Krebses. Münch Med Wochenschr 58: 1897–1900
d'Arsonval A (1892) Sur les effets physiologiques de l'état variable et des courants alternatifs. Conférence faite á la sociéte de physique. Bull Soc Int Electrol 20. April 1892
d' Arsonval A (1897) Action physiologique des courants alternatifs à grande fréquence. Arch Electrol Med 66: 133
DeCourcy JL (1933) The spontaneous regression of cancer. J Med 14: 141–146
Demmel F (1949) Ultraschallbehandlung von trauttumoren. Dtsch Med Wochenschr 3: 671
Dewey WC, Hopwood LE, Sapareto SA, Gerweck LD (1982) Cellular responses to combinations of hyperthermia and radiation. Radiology 123: 463–474
Dewhirst MW, Phillips TL, Samulski TV et al. (1990) RTOG quality assurance guidelines for clinical trials using hyperthermia. Int J Radiat Oncol Biol Phys 18: 1249–1259
Dewning JF, Martinez-Valdez H, Elizondo RS, Walker EB, Taylor MW (1988) Hyperthermia in humans enhances interferon-γ synthesis and alters the peripheral lymphocyte population. J Interferon Res 8: 143
Dietzel F (1975) Tumor und Temperatur. Aktuelle Probleme bei der Anwendung thermischer Verfahren in der Onkologie und Strahlentherapie. Urban & Schwarzenberg, München
Dittmar C (1949) Über die Wirkung von Ultraschallwellen auf tierische Tumoren. Strahlentherapie 78: 217–230
Dmitrieva NP (1960) The action of ultrasonics on spontaneous and transplantable tumours of animals and on malignant tumours of humans. Probl Oncol 6: 1379–1386
Doub HP (1935) Osteogenic sarcoma of the clavicle treated with radiation and fever therapy. Radiology 25: 355–356
Doyen E (1910) Traitement local des cancer accessibles par l'action de la chaleur au-dessus de 55°C. Rev Therap Med Chir 77: 551–577
Ehrlich P (1907) Experimentelle Studien an Mäusetumoren. Z Krebsforsch 5: 59–81
Engel P (1934) Über den Infektionsindex der Krebskranken. Wien Klin Wochenschr 47: 1118
Eschweiler R (1898) Die Erysipel, Erysipeltoxin- und Serumtherapie der bösartigen Geschwülste. Leipzig
Everson TC, Cole WE (1956) Spontaneous regression of cancer. Ann Surg 144: 366
Fajardo LF (1984) Pathological effects of hyperthermia in normal tissues. Cancer Res (Suppl) 44: 4826s–4835s
Fehleisen F (1883) Ätiologie des Erysipels. Verlag von Theodor Fischer's Medizinischer Buchhandlung, Berlin, p 21
Field M, Block JB, Oliverio VT, Rall DP (1964) Cellular accumulation of methyl-glyoxal-bis-guanylhydrazone in vitro. I. General characteristics of cellular uptake. Cancer Res 24: 1939–1942
Freund F (1908) Die elektrische Funkenbehandlung (fulguration) der Karzinome. Ferdinand Enke, Stuttgart
Fuchs G (1936) Über die Sensibilisierung röntgenrefraktärer Neoplasmen durch Kurzwellen. Strahlentherapie 55: 473–480
Fürth E (1937) Der Verlauf der Krebssterblichkeit in Europa. Z Krebsforsch 45: 310
Garcia DM, Nussbaum GH, Fathman AE et al. (1992) Concurrent iridium-192 brachytherapy and long-duration, conductive interstitial hyperthermia for the treatment of recurrent carcinoma of the prostate: a feasibility study. Endocurie Hypertherm Oncol 8: 151–158
Gericke D (1970) Studies on the thermosensitivity of experimental tumors in small animals. 10th International Cancer Congress, Houston (Texas), Abstract 572
Gericke D, Chandra P, Orii H, Wacker A (1971) In vitro thermosensibility of experimental tumors in small animals. Naturwissenschaften 58: 155–156
Gerster AG, Hartley F (1892) Sarcoma of the femur without recurrence five years after amputation through the trochanter minor. NY Med J 55: 641
Giovanella BC, Lohman WA, Heidelberger C (1970) Effects of elevated temperatures and drugs on the viability of L-1210 leukemia cells. Cancer Res 30: 1623–1631
Goetze O (1928) Lokale homogene Hyperthermierung der Gliedmaßen im Wasserbad, mit Hilfe der Blutleere. Langenbecks Arch Chir 152: 49–51
Goetze O (1930) Lokale Hyperthermisierung bei malignen Tumoren. Zentralbl Chir 36: 2258
Goetze O, Schmidt KH (1932) Örtliche homogene Überwärmung gesunder und kranker Gliedmassen. Dtsch Z Chir 234: 577–589

Gore I, Isaacson NH (1949) The pathology of hyperpyrexia. Am J Pathol 25: 1029–1060

Goss P, Parsons PG (1977) The effect of hyperthermia and melphalan on survival of human fibroblast strains and melanoma cell lines. Cancer Res 37: 152–156

Gottschalk S (1899) Zur Behandlung des ulcerierenden, inoperablen Cervixcarcinoms. Zentralbl Gynäkol 3: 79–80

Haaland M (1907) Die Metastasenbildung bei transplantierten Sarkomen der Maus. Z Krebsforsch 5: 122–125

Haaland M (1908) Contributions to the study of the development of sarcomas under experimental conditions. A.R. Imperial Cancer Research Fund, pp 175–261

Haas M, Lob A (1934) Die sogenannten spezifischen Effekte der Kurzwellen bei der Behandlung bösartiger Geschwülste. Strahlentherapie 50: 345

Hahn GM (1979) Potential for therapy of drugs and hyperthermia. Cancer Res 39: 2264–2268

Hahn GM (1982) Hyperthermia and Cancer. Plenum Press, New York, 1–285

Hahn GM, Strande DP (1976) Cytotoxic effects of hyperthermia and adriamycin on Chinese hamster cells. J Nat Cancer Inst 57: 1063–1067

Harris M (1967) Temperature-resistant variants in clonal populations of pig kidney cells. Exp Cell Res 46: 301–314

Heyn G, Kurz W (1967) Beitrag zur Behandlung des Peniscarcinoms. Z Urol 60: 103–105

Hill L (1934) Action of ultrashort waves on tumors. BMJ 2: 370

Hoffman M (1957) Erfahrungen bei der Behandlung Krebskranker mit Überwärmungsbädern. In: Lampert H, Selawry O (eds) Körpereigene Abwehr und bösartige Geschwülste. K.F. Haug, Ulm, 93–105

Hornback NB (1984) Historical aspects of hyperthermia. In: Hornback NB (ed) Hyperthermia in cancer, vol I. CRC Press, Boca Raton, Fl., pp 1–11

Horvath J (1946) Über die Wirkung der Ultraschallwellen auf das menschliche Karzinom. Klinik Praxis 1: 10–12

Huth E (1957) Die Rolle der bakteriellen Infektion bei Spontanremission maligner Tumoren und Leukosen. In: Lampert H, Selawry O (eds) Körpereigene Abwehr und bösartige Geschwülste. K.F. Haug, Ulm, 23–27

Hynynen K (1990) Biophysics and technology of ultrasound hyperthermia. In: Gautherie M (ed) Methods of external hyperthermic heating, Springer, Berlin Heidelberg New York, pp 61–115

Jares JJ Jr, Warren SL (1937): Combined effects of Roentgen radiation fever upon malignant tissue: preliminary summary. Cancer Probl Symposium: 225

Jares JJ Jr, Warren SL (1939) Physiological effects of radiation. I. A study of the in-vitro effect of high fever temperatures upon certain experimental tumors. Am J Roentgenol 41: 685

Jensen CO (1903) Experimentelle Untersuchungen über Krebs bei Mäusen. Z Bakt Parasit Infekt 34: 28–122

Johnson HJ (1940) The action of short radiowave, on tissues. III. A comparison of the thermal sensitivities of transplantable tumors in vivo and in vitro. Am J Cancer 38: 533–550

Jones S, Henry W (1959) Hippocrates, Harvard University Press, Cambridge, Mass

Keating-Hart W (1909) La fulguration et ses résultats dans traitement du cancer d'après une statistique personelle des 247 cas. J Med Intern (Paris) 13: 41

Koch R, Petruschky J (1896) Beobachtungen über Erysipelimpfungen am Menschen. Z Hyg Infekt 23: 477–489

Koller S (1937) Die Krebsverbreitung in Süd- und Westeuropa. Zugleich Darstellung der Vergleichsmethodik von Krebssterbeziffern unter Berücksichtigung der Fehlerquellen. Z Krebsforsch 45: 197–236

Konteschweller TC (1918) Pyretotherapy. A Maloine et Fils, Paris

Korb H (1939) Erhöhung der Wirkung von Röntgenstrahlen durch lokale Kurzwellenhyperthermie. Strahlentherapie 65: 649–656

Korb H (1943) Weitere Untersuchungen zur Frage der Erhöhung der Wirkung von Röntgenstrahlen durch lokale Kurzwellenhyperthermie. Strahlentherapie 72: 220–243

Korb H (1948) Über die Kombination der Röntgenbestrahlung mit der Kurzwellenbehandlung. Strahlentherapie 77: 301–303

Krantz JC, Beck FF (1939) Sound waves are tried as cancer treatment. Arch Phys Ther 20: 370

Lambert RA (1912) Demonstration of the greater susceptibility to heat of sarcoma cells as compared with actively proliferating connective-tissue cells. J Am Med Assoc 59: 2147–2148

Lampert H (1948) Überwärmung als Heilmittel. Hippokrates, Stuttgart

Lampert H (1965) Krebs und Überwärmung. Med Welt 49: 2721–2726

Lampert H (1970) Überwärmung und Krebs. Z Blut- und Geschwulstkrankheiten 2: 83–92

Langevin P (1920) British patent specifications. NS, 457, no. 145, 691

Larkin JM (1979) A clinical investigation of total body hyperthermia as cancer therapy. Cancer Res 39: 2252–2254

Lehman JF, Krusen FH (1955) Biophysical effects of ultrasonic energy on carcinoma and their possible significance. Archs Phys Med Rehabil 38: 452–459

Levin J (1910) Cancer among the American Indians, its bearing upon the thnological distribution of disease. Z Krebsforsch 9: 422–435

Licht S (1965) History of therapeutic heat. In: Licht S (ed) Therapeutic heat and cold. Waverly Press, Baltimore, pp 196–231

Liebesny P (1921) Experimentelle Untersuchungen über Diathermie. Wien Klin Wochenschr 34: 117

Loeb L (1903) Über Transplantation von Tumoren. Virch Arch Path Anat Physiol 172: 345–368

Malamud N, Haymaker W, Custer RP (1946) Heat stroke. A clinico-pathologic study of 125 fatal cases. Milit Surg 97: 397–449

Marmor JB, Hahn GM (1930) Combined radiation and hyperthermia in superficial human tumors. Cancer 46: 1986–1991

Marmor JB, Pounds D, Hahn GM (1979) Treatment of superficial human neoplasms by local hyperthermia induced by ultrasound. Cancer 43: 196–205

Massey GB (1925) Direct current electrocoagulation in the treatment of cancer. Lectures, clinics and discussions on electro-physiotherapy, Fischer, Chicago, p 73

Mayo WJ (1913) Grafting and traumatic dissemination of carcinoma in the course of operations for malignant disease. JAMA 60: 512

Mayo WJ (1915) The cancer problem. Lancet 35: 339

Meyer JL (1984) Hyperthermia as an anticancer modality – a historical perspective. In: Vaeth JM, Meyer JL (eds) Hyperthermia and radiation therapy / chemotherapy in the treatment of cancer. Frontiers of radiation therapy and oncology, vol 18. Karger, Basel, pp 1–22
Meyer WH, Mutscheller A (1937) Heat as a sensitizing agent in radiation therapy of neoplastic diseases. Radiology 28: 215
Miller RC, Connor WG, Heusinkveld RS, Boone MLM (1977) Prospects for hyperthermia in human cancer therapy. Radiology 123: 489–495
Miller TR, Nicholson JT (1971) End results in reticulum cell sarcoma of bone treated by bacterial toxin therapy alone or combined with surgery and/or radiotherapy (47 cases) or with concurrent infection (5 cases). Cancer 27: 524
Mitchel REJ, Merrison DP, Gragtmans NJ, Jeveak JJ (1986) Hyperthermia and phorbol ester tumor promotion in mouse skin. Carcinogenesis 7: 1505
Moricca G (1970) Applicazioni cliniche del trattamento ipertermico, dei tumori delig arti. Atti della Societa Italiana di Cancerologia (part 2), pp 77–89
Moritz AR, Henriques FC (1947) Studies of thermal injuries. II. The relative importance of time and surface temperature in the causation of cutaneous burns. Am J Path 23: 695–720
Müller C (1912) Therapeutische Erfahrungen an 100 Kombinationen von Röntgenstrahlen und Hochfrequenz, resp. Diathermie behandelten bösartigen Neubildungen. Münch Med Wochenschr 28: 1546–1549
Müller C (1913) Die Krebskrankheit und ihre Behandlung mit Röntgenstrahlen und hochfrequenter Elektrizität respektive Diathermie. Strahlentherapie 2: 170–191
Nakahara W, Kobayashi R (1934) Biological effects of short exposure to supersonic waves: local effects on the skin. Jap J Exp Med 12: 137–140
Nauts HC (1975) Pyrogen therapy of cancer: a historical review and current activities. In: Wizenberg MJ, Robinson JE (eds) Proceedings of the first international symposium on cancer therapy by hyperthermia and radiation. National Cancer Institute and American College of Radiology, Washington DC and Chicago, pp 239–244
Nauts HC (1976) Immunotherapy of cancer by bacterial vaccines. 3rd International symposium on detection and prevention of cancer, Plenum Press New York
Nauts HC (1982) Bacterial pyrogens: beneficial effects on cancer patients. In Gautherie M, Albert E (eds) Biomedical thermology. Liss, New York, pp 687–696
Nauts HC, Fowler GA, Bogatko FH (1953) A review of the influence of bacterial infections and bacterial products (Coley's toxins) on malignant tumors in men. Acta Med Scand 276: 1–103
Nauts HC, Pelner L, Fowler GA (1959) Sarcoma of the soft tissues, other than lymphosarcoma, treated by toxin therapy. New York Cancer Research Institute, Monograph no. 3, New York
Neyman CA (1939) Historical development of artificial fever in the treatment of disease. Med Rec 150: 89–92
Neyman CA, Osborne SL (1929) Artificial fever produced by high frequency currents. Ill Med J 56: 199
Ochsner AJ (1923) The treatment of cancer of the jaw with the actual cautery. JAMA 81: 1487
Overgaard J (1985) History and heritage – an introduction. In: Overgaard J (ed) Hyperthermic oncolgy 1984, vol 2. Taylor & Francis, London pp 3–8
Overgaard J (1993) The future of hyperthermic oncology. In: Gerner EW, Cetas TC (eds) Hyperthermic oncolgy 1992. Plenary and symposia lectures. Proceedings of the 6th International Congress on Hyperthermic Oncology. Arizona Board of Regents, Tucson, pp 87–92
Overgaard K (1934) Über Wärmetherapie bösartiger Tumoren. Acta Radiol 15: 89
Overgaard K (1935) Experimentelles über kombinierte Wärme-Röntgentherapie bösartiger Tumoren. Acta Radiol 16: 461–470
Overgaard K (1936) Experimentelles über Kurz- und Ultrakurzwellentherapie bösartiger Tumoren. Acta Radiol 17: 182
Overgaard K, Okkels H (1940a) Über den Einfluß der Wärmebehandlung auf das Woods Sarkom. Strahlentherapie 68: 587–619
Overgaard K, Okkels H (1940b) The action of dry heat on Wood's sarcoma. Acta Radiol 21: 577–582
Parks LD, Minaberry RN, Smith DP, Neely WA (1979) Treatment of far advanced bronchogenic carcinoma by extracorporally induced systemic hyperthermia. J Thorac Cardiovasc Surg 78: 883–892
Paulos von Aegina (1914) Die besten Artes Sieben Bücher (Epitomae medicae), vol VI, Verlagsbuchhandlung vormals E.J. Brill, Leiden, S. pp 511–512
Percy JF (1912) The results of the treatment of cancer of the uterus by the actual cautery, with a practical method for its application. JAMA 58: 696–699
Percy JF (1913) A method of applying heat both to inhibit and destroy inoperable carcinoma of the uterus and vagina. Surg Gynecol Obstet 17: 371–376
Percy JF (1916) Heat in the treatment of carcinoma of the uterus. Surg Gynecol Obstet 22: 77–79
Pettigrew RT, Galt JM, Ludgate CM, Smith AM (1974) Clinical effects of whole-body hyperthermia in advanced malignancy. Br Med J 4: 679–682
Pflomm E (1931) Experimentelle und klinische Untersuchungen über die Wirkung ultrakurzer elektrischer Wellen. Arch Klin Chir 166: 251
Pohlmann R (1951) Die Ultraschalltherapie, praktische Anwendung des Ultraschalls in der Medizin. Huber, Bern
Pollay M (1955) The first American book on tumours. Thesis, University of Madison, Wisconsin
Reiter T (1933) Tumorzerstörung durch Ultrakurzwellen. Dtsch Med Wochenschr 59: 160–166
Rohdenburg GL (1918) Fluctuations in the growth of malignant tumors in man, with special reference to spontaneous recession. J Cancer Res 3: 193–225
Rohdenburg GL, Prime F (1921) The effect of combined radiation and heat on neoplasms. Arch Surg 2: 116–129
Sapareto SA, Dewey WC (1984) Thermal dose determination in cancer therapy. Int J Radiat Oncol Biol Phys 10: 787–800
Schereschewsky JW (1928a) The action of currents of very high frequency upon tissue cells. A. Upon a transplantable mouse sarcoma. Public Health Rep (Wash) 43: 927
Schereschewsky JW (1928b) The action of currents of very high frequency upon tissue cells. B. Upon a transplantable fowl sarcoma. Public Health Rep (Wash) 43: 940
Schereschewsky JW (1933) Biological effects of very high frequency electromagnetic radiation. Radiology 20: 246
Schliephake E (1929) Tiefenwirkung im Organismus durch kurze elektrische Wellen. Teil II. Experimentelle Untersuchungen. Z Exp Med 66: 231–264

Schliephake E (1935) Short wave therapy. Actinic Press, London, p 181 ff.
Schliephake E (1960) Versuche zur Beeinflussung maligner Tumoren beim Menschen. Münch Med Wochenschr 102: 2020–2025
Schmidt R (1910) Krebs und Infektionskrankheiten. Med Klin 6: 1660–1693
Schulz G (1969) Verhütet Fieber Karzinome? Münch Med Wochenschr 111: 1051–1052
Schrumpf-Pierron P (1932) Die Seltenheit des Krebses in Ägypten und ihre wahrscheinlichen Gründe. (Ein Beitrag zur Ätiologie des Carcinoms). Z Krebsforsch 36: 145–163
Scott BO (1957) The principles and practice of diathermy. Heinemann, London
Selawry OS (1957) Zur Rolle erhöhter Körpertemperatur bei Spontanremissionen menschlicher Tumoren. Int Rundschau Phys Med 10: 162–164
Selawry OS, Goldstein MN, McCormick T (1957) Hyperthermia in tissue-cultured cells of malignant origin. Cancer Res 17: 785–791
Selawry OS, Carlson JC, Moore GE (1958) Tumor response to ionizing rays at elevated temperatures. A review and discussion. Am J Roentgenol 80: 833–839
Shingleton WW, Bryan FA, O'Quinn WL, Krueger LC (1962) Selective heating and cooling of tissue in cancer chemotherapy. Ann Surg 156: 408–416
Shoulders HS, Turner EL (1942) Observations on the results of combined fever and x-ray therapy in the treatment of malignancy. Strahlenther Med J 35: 966–970
Sinek F (1936) Versuch einer statistischen Erfassung endogener Faktoren bei Carcinomkranken. Z Krebsforsch 44: 492–527
Southam CM, Beyer H, Allen AC (1953) The effects of ultrasonic irradiation upon normal and neoplastic tissues in the intact mouse. Cancer 6: 390–396
Spring E (1969) Increased radiosensitivity following simultaneous ultrasonic and gamma-ray irradiation. Radiology 93: 175–176
Stehlin JS Jr (1969) Hyperthermic perfusion with chemotherapy for cancers of the extremities. Surg Gynecol Obstet 129: 305–308
Stehlin JS Jr (1975) Results of hyperthermic perfusion for melanoma of the extremities. Surg Gynecol Obstet 140: 339–348
Stehlin JS Jr (1980) Hyperthermic perfusion with chemotherapy for melanoma of the extremities: experience with 165 patients, 1967–1979. Ann NY Acad Sci 335: 352–355
Stephenson HE Jr, Delmy JA, Renden DI, et al. (1971) Host immunity and spontaneous regression of cancer evaluated by computerized data reduction study. Surg Gynecol Obstet 133: 649
Stevenson HN (1919) The effect of heat upon tumor tissues. J Cancer Res 4: 54
Storm FK (1983) Background, principles and practice. In: Storm FK (ed) Hyperthermia in cancer therapy. GK Hall, Boston, pp 1–8
Strauss AA (1935) Surgical diathermy of cancer of the rectum. Its clinical end results. JAMA 104: 1480
Sugahara T (1989) Hyperthermia and hot springs: scientific and cultural considerations. In: Sugahara T, Saito M (eds) Hyperthermic oncology 1988, vol 2. Taylor & Francis, London, pp 3–8
Taylor HJ (1936) The effect of ultra high-frequency currents (ultra short waves) combined with nonlethal doses of radium radiations upon experimental rat tumors. Br J Radiol 9: 467
Theilhaber A (1919) Der Einfluß der Diathermiebehandlung auf das Karzinomgewebe. Münch Med Wochenschr 71: 1260
Theilhaber A (1923) Der Einfluß der zellulären Immunität auf die Heilung der Carcinome (insbesondere der Mamma und des Uterus). Arch Gynäkol 18: 237–272
Vidal E (1907) Cancer et traumatism. In: Alcan F (ed) Assoc Franc de Chirurgie, Paris, p 1
Warren SL (1935) Preliminary study of the effect of artificial fever upon hopeless tumor cases. Am J Roentgenol 33: 75
Westermark F (1898) Über die Behandlung des ulcerierenden Cervixcarcinoms mittels konstanter Wärme. Zentralbl Gynäkol 22: 1335–1339
Westermark N (1927) The effect of heat upon rat tumors. Scand Arch Physiol 52: 257–322
Wiethe C (1949) Clinical experiences with ultrasonic waves. JAMA 140: 926
Woodhall B, Pickrill KL, Georgiades NG, Mahaley MS, Dukes HT (1960) Effect of hyperthermia upon cancer chemotherapy – application to external cancer of head and neck structures. Ann Surg 151: 750–759
Woeber K (1949) Über die Wirkung des Ultraschalls auf oberflächliche Tumoren. Arch Dermatol Syph 191: 400
Woeber K (1955) Combined x-ray and ultrasound treatment for dermatological conditions. Am J Phys Med 34: 376–378
Woeber K (1956) Biological basis and application of ultrasound in medicine. Ultrasonics Biol Med 1: 18
Woeber K (1965) The effect of ultrasound in the treatment of cancer. In: Kelly E (ed) Ultrasonic energy. University of Illinois Press, Urbana, Illinois, pp 137–149
Wolffheim W (1921) Über den heilenden Einfluß des Erysipels auf Gewebsneubildungen, insbesondere bösartige Tumoren. Z Klin Med 92: 507–526

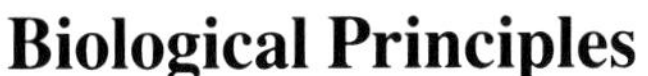

Biological Principles

2 Molecular and Cellular Mechanisms of Hyperthermia

C. STREFFER

CONTENTS

2.1 Introduction

The success of tumor therapy is determined by the efficiency with which the killing of tumor cells is achieved under conditions of no or only slight damage to the normal tissues. Cell killing in this sense means that the clonogenicity of stem cells is destroyed by agents such as ionizing radiation, cytotoxic chemicals, or heat. Hyperthermia, the heating of cells to 40°–45°C, can act as a cytotoxic agent by itself or as a sensitizing agent in combination with ionizing radiation or cytotoxic drugs (STREFFER 1990). The characteristics and mechanisms of sensitization by heat will be described in other chapters in the volume; therefore the focus of this chapter will be on the action of heat alone. During prolonged heating for several hours at temperatures of about 42°C and below or after a short heat shock, cells can become more thermoresistant. These phenomena of thermotolerance will also be described in a later chapter.

The application of hyperthermia has a long history in tumor therapy. However, the molecular and cellular mechanisms have been studied in depth only recently. Heat kills cells in a stochastic manner, as do other cell-killing agents. This means that a certain probability exists that a given cell will survive or die when a population of cells is subjected to a heat treatment. However, one of the outstanding features of heat treatment is that cellular effects can be observed very quickly after or even during treatment. Thus one can observe that structures of multimolecular complexes, like the cytoskeleton, are heavily damaged directly after heat treatment in the temperature range of 42°–45°C (DERMIETZEL and STREFFER 1992). In contrast to the rapid manifestation of these effects in the microscopic appearance of the treated cells, similar radiation-induced changes can be seen only days after a treatment with doses in a comparable therapeutic range. Furthermore, metabolic rates are increased during the heat treatment, which induces metabolic disturbances. These phenomena have mainly been studied with respect to energy and glucose metabolism and the biosynthesis of macromolecules (STREFFER 1985).

2.2 Molecular Effects

As stated above, during a hyperthermic treatment considerable molecular and metabolic changes occur. While after exposure to ionizing radiation DNA damage is the most important effect leading to reproductive cell death (ALPER 1979), the mechanism of cell killing by hyperthermia alone is less clear. It appears evident that events in the cytoplasm as distinct from the cell nucleus are important (HAHN 1982; STREFFER 1982, 1985). At the molecular and metabolic level heat predominantly induces two principal effects (STREFFER 1985): (a) conformational changes and

C. STREFFER, PhD, MD h.c., Professor, Department of Medical Radiobiology, Universitätsklinikum Essen, D-45122 Essen, FRG destabilization of macromolecules and multimolecular structures; (b) increased rates of metabolic reactions during the heat treatment followed by dysregulation of metabolism, mainly after hyperthermia.

2.2.1 Conformational Changes of Macromolecules

The conformation of biological macromolecules is mainly stabilized by covalent bonds between subunits of the macromolecules, by hydrogen bridges, by interactions of ionic groups within the macromolecules and with their environment, and by hydrophilic/hydrophobic interactions of groups within the macromolecules and their environment. The last three classes of bonds and interactions are comparatively weak; they can be altered easily, for instance, by an increase in temperature. For the biological activity of macromolecules specific conformational structures are usually a prerequisite. The conformation of DNA is irreversibly changed only at temperatures which lie far above the temperature range of cell killing (Lepock 1991). However, especially in proteins changes can be induced which lead to disturbances of the native protein conformation at temperature ranges which are near to or overlap with those that lead to cell killing (Privalov 1979; Lepock 1982; Lepock et al. 1983; Leeper 1985; Streffer 1985). A detailed study of protein denaturation in erythrocyte membranes by differential scanning calorimetry has shown that such processes begin in a temperature range of 40°–45°C (Brandts et al. 1977; Lepock 1991).

The range of temperatures at which structural transitions of proteins occur depends very much on the specific protein under consideration and differs over a wide range of proteins. For a number of proteins such transitions have also been demonstrated in more complex cells than erythrocytes, e.g., fibroblasts and hepatocytes, in the range 40°–45°C – a range at which killing of these cells also takes place and which is used for hyperthermic treatment in tumor therapy (Lepock 1991). The enthalpy calculated from Arrhenius plots for cell killing is in the same range as for protein denaturation (Lepock 1992; Streffer 1990). These phenomena will be discussed later (see p. 51). Furthermore, heat-induced structural changes in proteins are extremely dependent on the pH value (Privalow 1979). A similar pH dependence is found for the heat sensitivity of cells. The pH value determines whether the various ionic groups of amino acid residues exist in the protonated or deprotonated form (Streffer 1963). Quite a number of these groups, which stabilize protein conformation by ionic interactions, have pK values near the physiological pH. These pK values are dependent on temperature; therefore a change in temperature will also alter the protonation, and the ionic state of the amino acid residues and their interaction is thereby altered. Such alterations contribute to conformational changes of proteins during hyperthermia (Streffer 1963; Wallenfels and Streffer 1964, 1966).

Lepock et al. (1983) have reported that the fluorescence of proteins bound to membranes and its quenching by paranaric acid is altered when isolated cytoplasmic and mitochondrial membranes are heated. Lepock (1991) reported on Differential Scanning Calorimetry (DSC) scans of Chinese hamster lung V79 cells. Significant denaturation of proteins begins at 40°–41°C. In further investigation this author studied isolated cell nuclei, mitochondria, microsomes, and a cytosolic fraction of soluble proteins. Each cellular component contained proteins with an irreversible denaturation starting at 40°–41°C. It is concluded that these conformational changes of membrane proteins are responsible for the observed effects of heating on membranes. It has frequently been suggested that membranes are the main cellular targets for hyperthermia in bacteria as well as in mammalian cells (Wallach 1978; Hahn 1982; Konings 1987).

2.2.2 Membranes

The phospholipid bilayer is an essential part of biological membranes. The hydrophobic, nonpolar hydrocarbon chains of the fatty acids face each other in the middle of the membranes and the polar heads of the phospholipids are oriented to the aequous phase inside and outside the cells. Proteins which can be integrated into both phospholipid layers or only into one of the phospholipid layers are floating in the lipid bilayers. This represents a brief description of the fluid mosaic model of membranes which was proposed by Singer and Nicolson (1972) and is generally accepted today. The "fluidity" of these membranes greatly influences the function and stability of membranes. The lipid composition has a very marked influence on the fluidity. Unsaturated fatty acids increase fluidity, while cholesterol decreases it. Raising the temperature also increases the fluidity, and YATVIN (1977) proposed that this effect correlated with cell killing.

Much attention has therefore been paid to the lipids of membranes and their influence on membrane fluidity in relation to cell killing by heat (YATVIN et al. 1982). Such correlations have been observed for bacterial systems. YATVIN (1977) studied a mutant of *Escherichia coli* K12 which required unsaturated fatty acids for survival. With increasing incorporation of these unsaturated fatty acids (18:1 or 18:3) into the membrane, the fluidity of the membrane as well as cell killing by heating was enhanced. The thermosensitivity of the bacteria increased in proportion with microviscosity when cells were grown in unsaturated fatty acid at different temperatures (DENNIS and YATVIN 1981). These observations were confirmed to some extent with mammalian cells. Murine leukemia cells (L1210) were cultured with oleic acid (18:1) or docosahexanoic acid (22:6) and the heat sensitivity increased (GUFFY et al. 1982). KONINGS and RUIFROK (1985) studied heat-induced cell killing in mouse fibroblasts after increasing the polyunsaturated fatty acids (PUFA) in all cellular membranes. These cells showed a higher fluidity of the membranes and increased thermosensitivity. However, when thermotolerance was induced the fluidity of the membranes did not change. The authors conclude from these data that, "the lipid composition of cellular membranes is not the primary factor which determines heat sensitivity of mammalian cells."

The incubation of V79 Chinese hamster cells with cholesterol resulted in a higher microviscosity of membranes but the thermosensitivity of the cells was not changed (YATVIN et al. 1983). Similar results were observed by KONINGS and RUIFROK (1985). On the other hand, CRESS et al. (1982) observed a positive correlation between the cholesterol content of plasma membranes and cell killing in several cell lines. LI et al. (1980) found remarkable similarities between the action of hyperthermia and of ethanol on cell killing and interpreted these findings as representing a modification of membrane fluidity. However, in a further study cell killing by hyperthermia and its modification by ethanol apparently correlated more closely with protein denaturation in membranes than with lipid fluidity (MASSICOTTE-NOLAN et al. 1981).

Studies with electron spin resonance have demonstrated that lipid transitions occur in the temperature ranges around 7°–8°C and 23°–26°C in mitochondria as well as in whole cell homogenates, while conformational transitions in proteins were observed between 40° and 47°C (LEPOCK 1982; LEPOCK et al. 1983). Several studies on membrane-bound receptors have shown that they are inactivated or lost from the membranes. Epidermal growth factor (EGF) receptors of fibroblasts showed a decreased affinity for EGF after heating but the number of membrane-bound receptors remained unchanged (MAGUN and FENNIE 1981). Concanavalin A-induced capping and cell survival responded in a similar manner to hyperthermia (STEVENSON et al. 1981). CALDERWOOD and HAHN (1983) observed a heat-induced inhibition of insulin binding to the plasma membrane of CHO cells, which was apparently caused by a decrease in the number of available insulin receptors, and this effect correlated well with cell killing. Similar effects were found for the binding of monoclonal antibodies to murine lymphoma cells (MEHDI et al. 1984).

Studies with scanning electron microscopy have shown that proteins which go through both phospholipid layers of the membrane (intermembrane protein particles, IPPs) and which stabilize the membrane are removed by hyperthermia (Fig. 2.1) (STREFFER 1985). Such proteins have the function not only of stabilizing the membranes but also of performing enzymatic reactions. Such an enzyme is certainly Na^+/K^+-ATPase, which is involved in ion transport through membranes. BOWLER et al. (1973) observed an increase in membrane permeability and a loss of membrane-bound ATPase after heat treatment of cells. These effects correlated with the heat-induced cell killing. In HeLa cells a dramatic loss of Na^+/K^+-ATPase activity was observed after heating the cells at 45°C for 10 min. A partial restoration of the enzyme activity took place during subsequent incubation at 37°C. This recovery was impaired by actinomycin D and cycloheximide. Apparently RNA and protein synthesis is needed for these processes (BURDON and CUTMORE 1982), which were observed at the same time as maximal synthesis of heat shock proteins. After continuous heating at 42°C, which results in thermotolerant cells, the enzyme activity increased in HeLa cells. A further treatment at

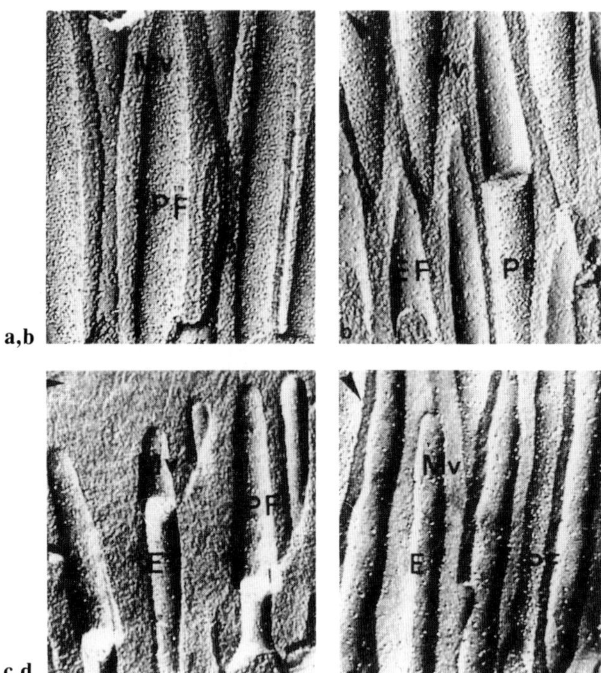

Fig. 2.1a–d. Electron micrograph of freeze-fractured small intestine mouse microvilli (*Mv*). *PF*, inner membrane; *EF*, external membrane. **a** Control, ×77 000; **b** nonexteriorized intestine after heating at 41°C for 30 min, ×98 000; **c** exteriorized intestine immediately after heating at 41°C for 30 min, ×77 000; **d** 3 h after heating at 41°C for 30 min, ×77 000. Note the reduction of IMP particles especially in **d**. (From Issa 1985)

45°C demonstrated that the thermosensitivity of Na^+/K^+-ATPase is not changed under these conditions; only the absolute levels are increased (Burdon et al. 1984).

In another study, by contrast, no decrease in Na^+/K^+-ATPase was observed after heating of mouse lung fibroblasts and HeLa cells (Ruifrok et al. 1986) as observed by Burdon and Cutmore (1982). Thus very contradictory results have been reported on this subject. In both cases (Burdon et al. 1984; Ruifrok et al. 1986) ouabain-sensitive ATPase was measured. By ouabain inhibition the Na^+/K^+-ATPase can be differentiated from other ATPase activities. However, the conditions of the assay differed. it certainly has to be elucidated whether these differences were responsible for the contradictory results. Ruifrok et al. (1986) also measured the ouabain-sensitive K^+ influx with $^{86}Rb^+$ as a tracer in mouse fibroblasts after incubation of the cells at 44°C. No decrease in K^+ influx was observed. This K^+ influx is driven by Na^+/K^+-ATPase and with a decrease in enzyme activity the K^+ influx should also decline. From these data it must be concluded that Na^+/K^+-ATPase and K^+ influx cannot be considered a general cause of cell death after hyperthermic treatments.

On the other hand the spontaneous loss of intracellular K^+ during and after severe hyperthermic treatments has frequently been related to cell death (Yi 1983). Ruifrok et al. (1985a,b) observed a dose-dependent decrease in K^+ in mouse fibroblasts after hyperthermia. This effect correlated well with cell killing. Other data which did not show an increased efflux were observed after nonlethal or less severe treatments (Boonstra et al. 1984). However, the K^+ efflux was modified by the addition of serum to the culture medium, while the clonogenic activity was not changed (Ruifrok et al. 1987). Furthermore, in other experiments a correspondence between cell killing and K^+ efflux was not observed (Vidair and Dewey 1986). Thus the loss of K^+ seems to be a consequence of heat-induced membrane damage but not a cause of cell death. When neuroblastoma cells were heated for 30 min at 45°C (survival 1%), the intracellular K^+, Na^+, and Cl^- concentrations were not changed directly after heating. However, 10–16 h after heating the ion gradients changed in some cells. At this time the cells underwent "metabolic" death (Borelli et al. 1986).

Hyperthermia may damage not only the cytoplasmic membrane but also the intracellular membranes; for instance, in the small intestine the latter show dramatic disturbances after heating (Breipohl et al. 1983). The loss of the receptor activities which are presented by membrane proteins, and other membrane proteins might be caused by conformational changes of the corresponding membrane proteins. However, a clear conclusion as to the role of lipids or proteins may be difficult. The cooperative state between the molecular species in membranes is dependent on both membrane fluidity and protein conformation (Wallach 1978). Studies with Raman spectroscopy on erythrocyte membranes show that temperature-dependent transitions involve concerted processes in which hydrophobic amino acid residues and lipids participate (Verma and Wallach 1976). Although the results obtained to date are not conclusive, many facts suggest that conformational changes of proteins and their cooperative effects with the lipid environment are very probably the main initiators of the observed effects on membranes. These membrane changes

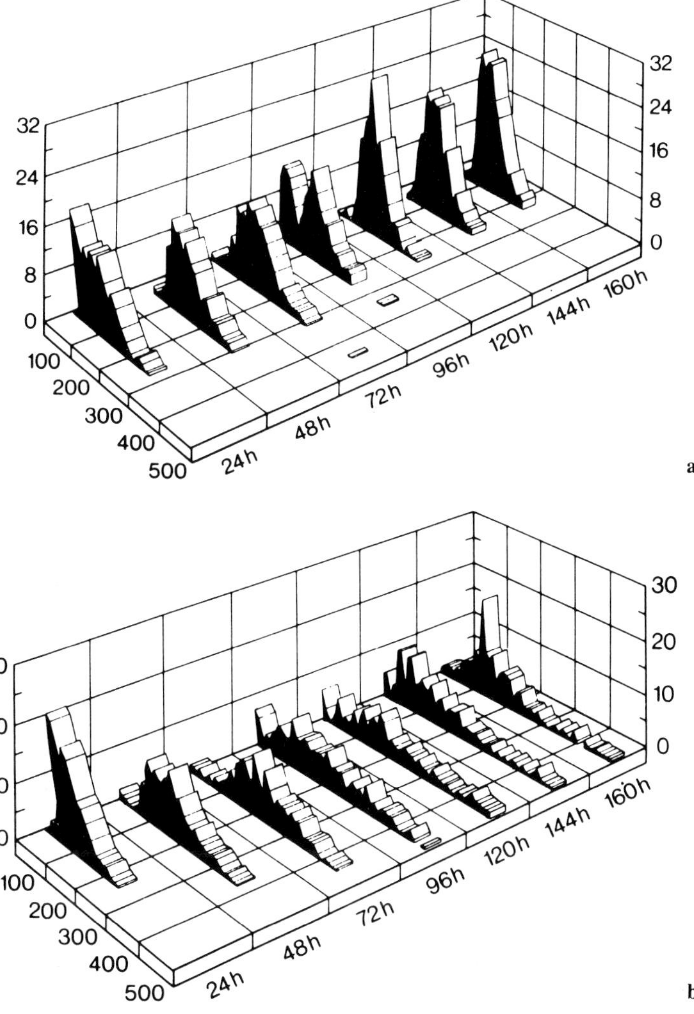

Fig. 2.2. **a** Nuclear size variation of MeWo cells (control sample, 37°C). Contours are expressed three-dimensionally. The *abscissa* indicates the entire period of cell cultivation, while the *ordinate* shows the mean of the absolute number of cells, and the z-axis ten classes of areas given in μm^2. For each nucleus or nuclear fragment the DAPI-stained areas were morphometrically measured and class differentiation computed. In the control samples the nuclei show a fairly well normal distribution of nuclear size over the entire period of cultivation. **b** Nuclear size distribution of MeMo cells (44°C, 1 h). The tendency in the disturbance of nuclear division is very pronounced. This is most apparent after 48 h of cultivation

also induce alterations of the ion permeabilities. As well as the above-described efflux of K^+, an increased influx of Ca^{2+} has frequently been reported (Leeper 1985; Vidair and Dewey 1986). A heat dose-response was observed for the intracellular increase in Ca^{2+}. Intracellular Ca^{2+} is bound to various cellular structures, e.g., smooth endoplasmic reticulum. After a heat treatment this Ca^{2+} is released and the concentration of free Ca^{2+} increases (Dewey 1989). These effects will be discussed further in connection with the mechanisms of cell killing.

2.2.3 Mitotic Spindles and Cytoskeleton

Mitotic cells have been found to be very heat sensitive. Hyperthermic treatment apparently prevents the aggregation of the globular proteins to the spindle apparatus or causes the disaggregation of spindles. As a consequence mitotic cells are unable to complete the mitotic division and cells with a tetraploid genome enter the G_1 phase (Coss et al. 1982). This observation is in agreement with the high thermosensitivity of mitotic cells. In fast-proliferating cell systems many tetraploid cells are seen (van Beuningen et al. 1978). The size of cell nuclei increases tremendously after heating of melanoma cells at 42° or 44°C in vitro. While the size of nuclei is quite uniform in untreated cells, the range becomes wider after heat treatment and this effect increases with increasing heat damage (Fig. 2.3) (Dermietzel and Streffer 1992).

In a similar way microtubules of the cytoskeleton disaggregate during hyperthermic treatment and reaggregate during subsequent incubation at 37°C (Lin et al. 1982). A correlation between cell killing and irreversible disturbances of the cytoskeleton has been observed in heated cells; no reassembly of the cytoskeleton occurs under these conditions (Cress et al. 1982). In heavily heat-damaged cells these structures have been completely lost. After heating at 42°C, and even more so at 44°C, the spindle-like melanoma cells rounded up, the tubulin structures became polymorph and concentrated in the perinuclear zone, and giant cells appeared with extreme pleomorphisms. Thus the structure of cytoskeletal organization was completely destroyed (Fig. 2.3) (Dermietzel and Streffer 1992). Again, it appears reasonable to assume that conformational changes of the proteins take place which lead to a disaggregation of the cytoskeletal structure. Under the same conditions DNA synthesis and the cytoskeleton were studied in melanoma cells after a hyperthermic treatment. It appeared that the damage to the cytoskeleton was more relevant for the heat-induced cell killing than the inhibition of DNA synthesis. The intermediate filaments which connect the microtubules to membranes seemed to be damaged more severely than the microtubules themselves (Dermietzel and Streffer 1992).

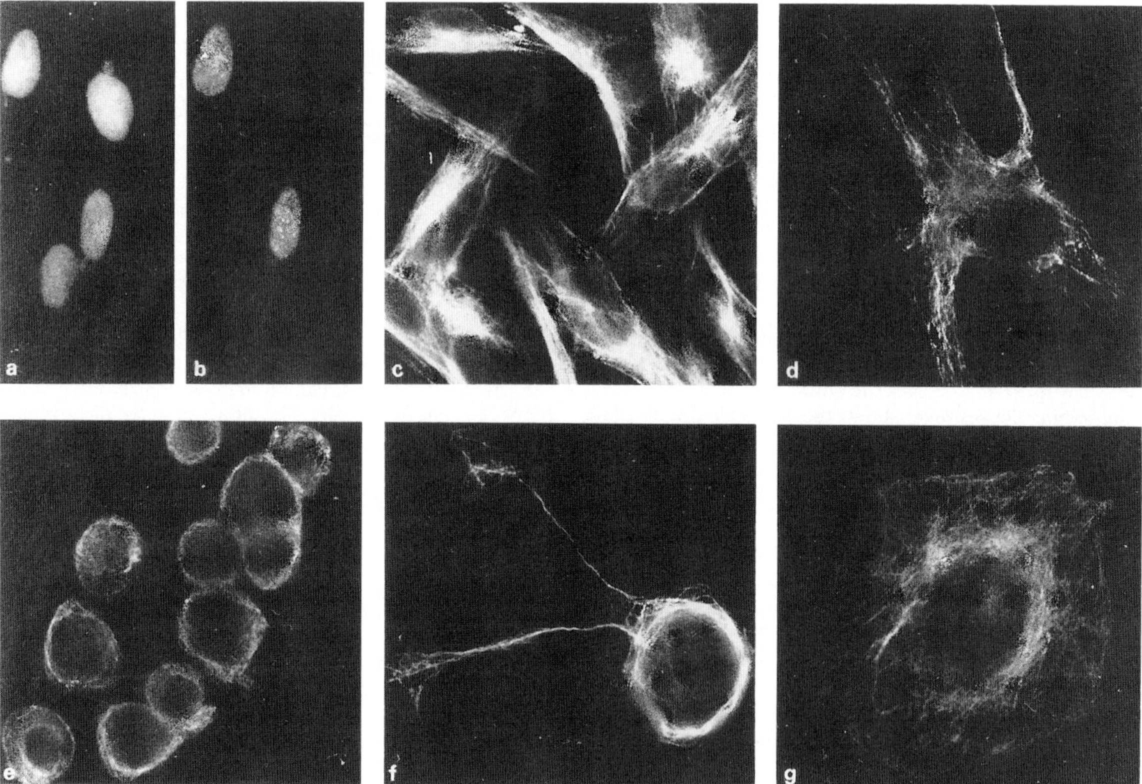

Fig. 2.3. Double labelling of MeWo cells with DAPI (**a**) and immunostaining with a monoclonal anti-BrdU antibody (**b**). This form of double staining served for quantification of MeWo cell survival and detection of proliferation kinetics. **c** Example of spindle-like cells (SPL cells) under control conditions, 48 h after plating. **d** Polymorph cell with intact microtubules (PM^- cells). **e** Round cells (RS cells) after heat treatment (1 h, 44°C), and prolonged cultivation (48 h). **f** Pleomorphic cell (PM^- cells) exhibiting rearrangement of microtubules. **g** Giant cell (G cell): a special class of cell which occurred after heat treatment

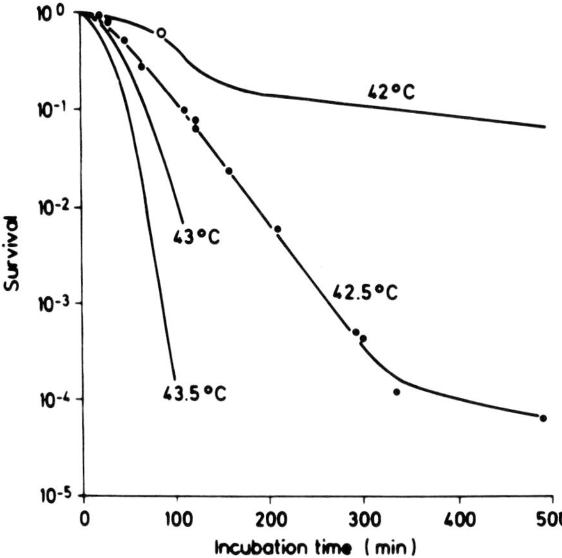

Fig. 2.4. Survival curves of asynchronous CHO cells heated at different temperatures for varying periods. (Redrawn from DEWEY et al. 1977)

2.2.4 Glucose and Energy Metabolism

Glucose metabolism is closely linked to the metabolism of lipids and a number of amino acids as well as to energy metabolism in general. These pathways are very dependent on the extra- and intracellular milieu. A number of differences exists between tumors and normal tissues with respect to glycolysis (WARBURG et al. 1926), pH (GERWECK 1982), and nutrients (HAHN 1982), which may be very important for hyperthermic treatment and cell killing by heat. However, it must be stressed that the variability of glucose metabolism between individual tumors even of the same entity and localization is extremely high (Table 2.1) (STREFFER et al. 1988). Nevertheless, some metabolic patterns may be characteristic in tumors. Thus in hepatomas the glycolytic pathway is increased and gluconeogenesis is reduced in comparison to normal liver tissue (WEBER 1983).

Glycolysis influences the intracellular milieu, and the rate of glycolysis is dependent on various factors, such as pH and oxygen tension. Glucose loading of rats decreases the pH in normal tissues and in tumors. This effect has been measured in the extracellular space (VON ARDENNE 1982; JÄHDE and RAJEWSKY 1982; VOLK et al. 1993). It is generally assumed that these processes lead to an accumulation of lactic acid in the heated tissues. In this connection it is of considerable importance that cell killing by hyperthermia is enhanced if cells are heated at low pH (GERWECK 1982).

A very remarkable increase in lactate levels was found by LEE et al. (1986) in the SCK tumor in mice. The authors also measured the lactate level under the same conditions in muscle. The heat-induced increase was much smaller in this normal tissue and the effect lasted only very briefly, whereas the lactate level in the SCK tumor was more than doubled after heating for 30 min at 43.5°C and the increase lasted longer than 24 h. The authors also observed an increase in β-hydroxybutyrate. However, as the level of lactate was much higher than that of β-hydroxybutyrate, the authors concluded that the lactate was responsible for a possible acidification of the tumor. Further studies demonstrated that the possible increase in lactate was very dependent on the characteristics of the tumour and differed in individual tumors under the same conditions (STREFFER 1987, 1988, 1990) (Table 2.1). However, in all tumors an increase in the lactate – pyruvate ratio was seen. These data demonstrate that glycolysis is apparently not inhibited during hyperthermic treatment as long as glucose is sufficiently available.

Burdon et al. (1984) have observed an increase (by 1%–40%) in lactate formation in HeLa cells, glioma cells, and some other cells directly after heating for 2–4 h at 42°C. The effect varied greatly

Table 2.1. Metabolites (μmol/g tissue) in three xenografts of melanoma after hyperthermia (Ht) at 43°C for 1 h (MIRTSCH and STREFFER, unpublished data)

	Bo		Mewo		Wi	
	Control	Ht	Control	Ht	Control	Ht
Glucose	1.8	1.1	1.9	1.9	1.6	–
Lactate	5.8	12.1	6.6	7.8	5.9	6.4
Pyruvate	0.19	0.17	0.25	0.20	0.15	0.14
Lactate/pyruvate	30.5	71.2	26.4	39.0	39.3	45.7

from cell line to cell line, however. No change was seen in normal human glial cells. During these studies BURDON et al. (1984) measured the lactate production from glucose and its release into the medium during the incubation of the cells in vitro. Such an effect was also obtained with melanoma cells (ISBRUCH 1986). However, when lactate levels were measured with very sensitive methods (bioluminescence) in melanoma cells directly, different results were obtained, the level being decreased by more than 30% after a severe heat treatment at 44°C for 1 h. Under the same conditions the pyruvate level was slightly increased. This led to a strong reduction in the lactate – pyruvate ratio (STREFFER 1988). It is interesting that this ratio increased after heating in tumors from the same melanoma cells which were grown on nude mice (Table 2.2).

Hyperthermic treatment speeds up metabolic reaction rates, including glycolysis (SCHUBERT et al. 1982; STREFFER 1982, 1985). More energy is needed by the heated cells in order to maintain ion gradients through membranes as well as the structural characteristics in the various cell compartments etc. Thus, investigations with ^{14}C-glucose (uniformly labelled) have demonstrated an enhanced turnover of glucose, as measured by expired labelled CO_2, during whole-body hyperthermia of mice at 40° and 41°C (STREFFER 1982; SCHUBERT et al. 1982). In addition, increased glucose degradation through the pentose phosphate pathway was observed during the first 55 h after heating cells in vitro (KONINGS and PENNINGA 1985). Under the same conditions of whole-body hyperthermia a strong decrease in liver glycogen has been observed in mice. The hepatic glycogen value remains low during the following 24 h and only a slow rise is induced by a glucose load after the hyperthermic treatment (SCHUBERT et al. 1982; STREFFER 1985). This latter result supports the finding of SKIBBA and COLLINS (1978) that gluconeogenesis is reduced in perfused rat liver if the temperature is raised to 42°C. Under normal conditions the lactate, which flows from peripheral tissues to the liver, can be used for glucose formation. This pathway of gluconeogenesis is apparently impaired by hyperthermia. From the consideration of lactate generation it can be concluded that the glycolytic rate is usually not impaired in tumors and in the liver of mammals during a hyperthermic treatment; it may even be increased.

Table 2.2. Lactate and pyruvate levels in human melanoma cells (MeWo) and their xenografts on nude mice after hyperthermia (MIRTSCH and STREFFER, unpublished data)

	MeWo cells in vitro (μmol/10^9 cells)		MeWo tumor (μmol/g tissue)	
	Control	1 h after 44°C for 1 h	Control	2 h after 43°C for 30 min
Lactate	19.5	12.5	6.6	7.8
Pyruvate	1.6	1.8	0.25	0.20
Lactate/pyruvate	12.1	6.9	26.4	39.0

If a tumor cell obtains its energy supply predominantly from glycolysis, inhibition of this pathway may considerably enhance the effect of hyperthermic cell killing. This has been demonstrated by SONG et al. (1977) and KIM et al. (1978) with 5-thio-D-glucose and with some other substances (KIM et al. 1984). On this basis it is understandable that the sensitizing effects on cell killing are especially expressed under hypoxic conditions, which induce an extreme increase in the lactate levels. KIM et al. (1984) have observed that the flavone derivative quercetin increases the thermosensitivity of HeLa cells. This drug inhibits the lactate transport across the cytoplasm membrane, produces intracellular acidification, and inhibits glycolysis (BELT et al. 1979). The decreased pH (GERWECK 1982) and the inhibition of glycolysis apparently enhance the thermosensitivity of the cells.

The pH is strongly coupled to the lactate–pyruvate ratio in cells and vice versa (STREFFER 1985). This redox ratio is also a good indicator of the status of intracellular oxygenation. As stated above, the increased rate of glycolysis with cells in vitro proves a decrease in lactate during the heat treatment and therefore also a decrease in the lactate – pyruvate ratio. However, in tumors an increase in this redox ratio is always observed after a heat treatment. This is obviously a consequence of the reduced blood supply to tumors (STREFFER 1990; VAUPEL 1990). A further consequence of these metabolic changes is the breakdown of the energy metabolism, which is mirrored by the ATP levels (STREFFER 1991). These heat effects are described further in Chap. 8.

2.2.5 Inhibition of DNA, RNA, and Protein Synthesis

It is generally assumed that radiation damage to DNA is decisive for cell killing. It is therefore of great interest whether hyperthermic treatment of cells and tissues can induce DNA damage in these cells. After heating of Ehrlich ascites tumor cells or HeLa cells at 43°C or higher temperatures in vitro, alkali-labile DNA lesions were observed (JORRITSMA and KONINGS 1984). These DNA strand breaks became apparent when the cells were incubated in an alkaline medium at 20°C for 30 min and the strand breaks were determined with the sensitive method of AHNSTRÖM and EDVARDSSON (1974). The rate of strand break production was about 1.7 times higher in Ehrlich ascites cells than in HeLa cells at an incubation temperature of 45°C. The Ehrlich ascites cells were also more thermosensitive than the HeLa cells with respect to cell killing. However, the DNA strand breaks only become measurable at a severe level of cell killing, with less than 1% cell survival (JORRITSMA and KONINGS 1984).

The authors demonstrated that the induction of strand breaks is caused by hyperthermia itself and not by other agents under these conditions. They discuss two possible mechanisms:

1. The temperature of 45°C is high enough to deposit sufficient localized energy into the DNA molecule for a direct induction of DNA strand breaks.
2. The heating may induce apurinic sites which yield strand breaks during the incubation in an alkaline medium.

However, the second possibility can probably be excluded as the number of apurinic sites formed is apparently smaller than the number of strand breaks included.

The cells used for these experiments were fast proliferating. Therefore it is also necessary to discuss the possibility that strand breaks are induced during DNA synthesis by heat-induced dissociation of nascent DNA pieces as the synthesizing complex is disintegrated or proteins of the DNA synthesizing complex (e.g., ligase) are inactivated during the heating. This proposal is supported by the finding that the activation energy for heat-induced strand breaks is 152 kcal per mole, which is typical for structural changes of proteins. In this connection it is also interesting that Ehrlich ascites cells had a shorter doubling time than HeLa cells (JORRITSMA and KONINGS 1984) and thus a higher proportion of cells were in S phase during heat treatment.

Heating of cells to 42°–45°C leads to a very sudden inhibition of DNA, RNA, and protein synthesis as measured by the incorporation of labelled precursors into these macromolecules (HAHN 1982; STREFFER 1982, 1985). In some cellular systems the synthesis of all three molecular species has been measured (MONDOVI et al. 1969; HENLE and LEEPER 1979; REEVES 1982). Generally it has been observed that the degree of inhibition correlates with the temperature at which the cells are heated. The duration of heating influences the period during which the macromolecular synthesis is affected (STREFFER 1982). Protein and RNA synthesis recover comparatively rapidly while DNA synthesis is reduced for a longer time after an identical heat treatment.

Not only the initiation of DNA synthesis in new replicons but also the elongation of the nascent DNA in these replicons is inhibited during and after a hyperthermic treatment (GERNER et al. 1979; HENLE and LEEPER 1979; WONG and DEWEY 1982). Heat gives rise to an increased amount of single-stranded DNA. DNA elongation recovers faster than replicon initiation after a heat treatment (WARTERS and STONE 1983). Therefore the prolonged depression of heat-induced DNA synthesis is apparently connected with the inhibition of the initiation processes. When cells are heated in S phase an increase in nonhistone proteins is observed in the cell nucleus, and there is an association of these proteins with the chromatin (MACKEY and ROTI ROTI 1992). Such proteins, which may interfere with the DNA polymerases, may be responsible for the effects on DNA synthesis as well as the changes in fork displacement (WONG et al. 1989). WARTERS and STONE (1983) also reported that heat treatment caused a long-term inhibition of ligation of replicative DNA fragments into chromosome-sized DNA. Nascent DNA was observed in replicated fragments with a size as small as the length of a replicon of hyperthermia.

In agreement with these data is the finding that the activity of the poly (ADP-ribose)-synthetase decreases in human melanoma cells after heating to 42° and 44°C (STREFFER et al. 1983a; TAMULEVICIUS et al. 1984). This enzyme is firmly bound to the chromatin and is involved in ligation of DNA fragments as well as in DNA repair processes (SHALL 1984). In this connection it is interesting that a correlation has been observed between inhibitors of poly (ADP-ribose)-synthetase and cell killing by heat in Chinese hamster cells (NAGLE and MOSS 1983). The observation that elevated temperatures cause chromosome aberrations in S-phase cells but not in G_1-phase cells (DEWEY et al. 1980) may be due to the inhibition of DNA ligation.

Enzymatic studies have shown that the DNA polymerase β, which is involved in unscheduled DNA synthesis for DNA repair, is more thermosensitive than the DNA polymerase α (DUBE et al. 1977). A positive correlation was observed between the hyperthermic cell killing, as well as the heat-sensitizing effect on cell killing by ionizing radiation, and the inhibition of DNA polymerase β; the correlation between cell killing and depression of DNA polymerase α was much poorer (SPIRO et al. 1982).

MIVECHI and DEWEY (1984) also studied the dependence of these processes on the pH. Chinese hamster ovary cells (CHO cells) were more thermosensitive at pH 6.65 than at pH 7.4 with respect to cell killing as well as to the loss of enzymatic activities of DNA polymerase α and β. For this pH effect a good correlation existed between cell killing and loss of DNA polymerase β but the correlation was less for DNA polymerase α.

A positive correlation of cell killing with DNA polymerase β has also been reported for thermotolerant CHO cells (DEWEY and ESCH 1982) but not for thermotolerant HeLa cells (JORRITSMA et al. 1984, 1986). Also the correlation between DNA polymerase β and cell killing does not agree with the finding that the enzyme activity is inhibited to the same degree in G_1 and S phase (SPIRO et al. 1982). The suggestion that the inactivation of DNA polymerase β is an important part of the mechanism by which heat-induced cell killing occurs is of great interest. However, the aforementioned inconsistencies should not be overlooked.

From electron microscopic observations SIMARD and BERNHARD (1967) have reported that heat treatment at 42°C destroys the structure of nucleoli, which are the sites for the synthesis of rRNA in the cell nucleus. Also the processing of the 45S RNA, a precursor of rRNA, to the functional 18S rRNA is apparently blocked by heating (WAROCQUIER and SCHERRER 1969; ASHBURNER and BONNER 1979). After recovery from a heat shock synthesis of rRNA becomes quite heat resistant (BURDON 1985). The RNA synthesis for certain proteins (heat shock proteins?) is even enhanced.

For the translational processes of protein synthesis a complex has to be formed between mRNA and ribosomes in order to build up polysomes. In mammalian cells elevated temperatures lead to a breakdown of the active polypeptide-synthesizing polysomes. McCORMICK and PENMAN (1969) reported a rapid disaggregation of polysomes when HeLa cells were heated to 42°C. PANNIERS and HENSHAW (1984) found markedly decreased levels of the initiation complex for polypeptide synthesis which is formed between the 40S ribosome subunit and methionine-tRNA in Ehrlich cells after heating at 43° for 20 min. After a short hyperthermic treatment apparently all components of the synthesizing machinery are still present, so that a reaggregation can occur and protein synthesis recovers. Phosphorylation and dephosphorylation of the initiation factor eIF-2 may play a role in this connection (BURDON 1985). BURDON (1988) observed a correlation between heat-induced depression of protein synthesis and lipid peroxidation, which might occur in membranes.

2.3 Mammalian Cell Killing by Hyperthermia

2.3.1 General Phenomena and "Dose"-Effect Curves

It is the current understanding that cancer therapy is achieved by removal or killing of neoplastic cells. This means that the reproductive ability of these cells has to be inhibited. In achieving this goal the irreversible damage in the normal tissues must be kept to a minimum so that the reduction of functional integrity is tolerable. For many normal tissues functional integrity is dependent on the number of stem cells which have survived the treatment. In tissues with low cell proliferation rates it is important that parenchymal cells survive and retain their functional capabilities, and that the tissue architecture remains undamaged.

A very important question has been asked and studied in this connection: Are malignant cells in a tumor more thermosensitive than the surrounding normal cells from which the malignant cells have probably developed? There are two phenomena which might support the assumption that malignant cells and tumors are more thermosensitive than their normal counterparts: First, it is possible that the process of malignant transformation involves a step which induces a higher thermosensitivity by itself; malignant cells are usually mutants of normal cells, and quite a number of thermosensitive mutants have been isolated. Second, the physiological conditions and the microenvironment may be altered in tumors in such a way that the thermosensitivity of the cells is enhanced (HAHN 1982); this requires further study.

Several tests have been used for the determination of cellular thermosensitivity. The proliferation of cells, the increase in cell number, and other parameters have been studied. However, the most powerful criterion is certainly the clonogenicity of stem cells. If this test is used and the survival of heated cells is plotted on a logarithmic scale against the incubation at a constant temperature, different types of dose-effect curves are observed.

The first type, which appears comparatively simple, was found after heating HeLa cells for periods up to 5 h at temperatures between 41° and 45°C (GERNER et al. 1975). The dose-effect curves are linear in a semilogarithmic plot. In this case it follows that the survival is exponential. A one-step (one-hit) reaction apparently occurs for cell killing. The curves can be described by an equation of the following type (LANDRY and MARCEAU 1978):

$$S = S_0 e^{-kt},$$

where S is the survival of clonogenic cells at any time t; S_0 is the number of clonogenic cells at the start of the experiment ($t = 0$), k is a constant representing the inactivation rate at a given temperature, and t is the duration of incubation at a given temperature. As with dose-effect curves which have been obtained for the survival after exposure to ionizing radiation, a value for the D_{37} or D_0 can be calculated from the steepness of the dose-effect curve. This value represents the time of incubation at a given temperature which results in the reduction of the cell survival to $1/e$ of the initial cell number (equal to the survival of 37% of S_0). Such exponential survival curves do not represent the regular situation, however.

Usually a different, more complex type of survival curve is observed, as was obtained for CHO cells by WESTRA and DEWEY (1971). For these experiments the cells were incubated with elevated temperatures in the range of 43.5°–46.5°C. The survival curves for the treatment at a constant treatment bend in the range of short incubation periods and apparently reach a linear shape at later incubation times if, again, the survival of the cells is plotted in a logarithmic scale against the incubation time at a constant temperature (Fig. 2.4). As in radiobiology, it is said that these dose-effect curves are characterized by a shoulder. For the exponential part of the dose-effect curve at a very low survival rate an analogous D_0 (time at the heating temperature in question which reduces the surviving cell fraction

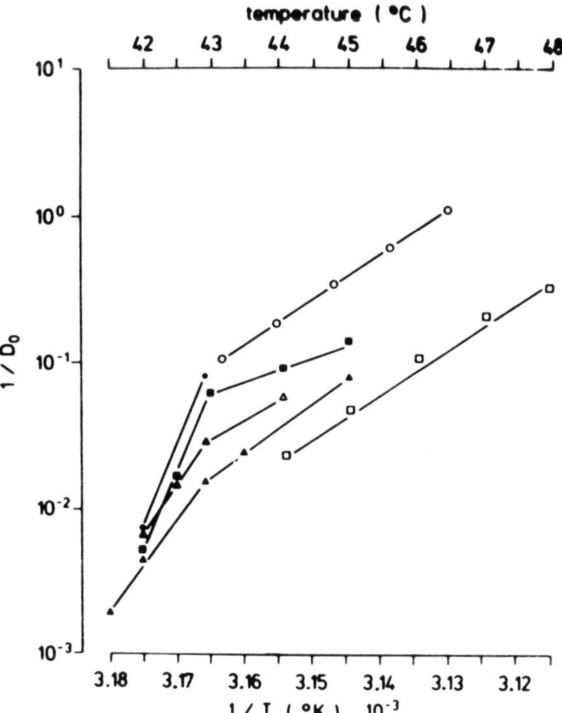

Fig. 2.5. Arrhenius plots for heat inactivation of various cell lines. On the *ordinate* the reciprocal of the D_0 value (inactivation rates) is plotted versus the reciprocal of the absolute temperature. (Redrawn from LEITH et al. 1977)

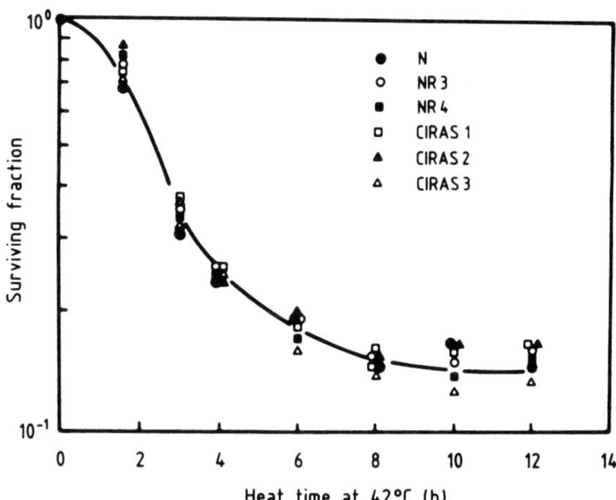

Fig. 2.6. Survival of five HRas transfected (*CIRAS 1–3, NR 3, 4*) and the normal (*N*) cell lines after heating at 45°C. (Redrawn from RAAPHORST et al. 1987)

by $1/e$) can be calculated. It is interesting that the constant of the inactivation rate which determines the steepness of the exponential part of the dose-effect curve reaches about double values when the temperature is increased by 1°C. This means by definition that the D_0 (heating time, see above) decreases to about half of the value under these conditions. The period required to reduce the cell survival to $1/e$ (37% in this range of the curve becomes shorter by a factor of 2. This correlation is observed although the constants for the inactivation rates vary over a wide range from cell line to cell line.

Again, as in radiobiology these dose-effect curves for heat-induced cell killing can be described by the multitarget, single-hit equation (DERTINGER and JUNG 1970) or by the linear-quadratic model which was proposed by KELLERER and ROSSI (1971):

$$S = 1 - (1 - \exp(D/D_0))^n$$

or

$$S = \exp(-\alpha D - \beta D^2).$$

These concepts have been used in order to fit heat-induced cell killing data (ROTI ROTI and HENLE 1979). Despite these possibilities for describing dose-effect curves for cell killing by heat in formalistic ways analogous to dose-effect curves for ionizing radiation, it must be realized that the mechanisms and targets of cell killing are completely different. Another model for the description of heat-induced cell killing has been developed by JUNG (1986). It postulates a two-step process. In the first step nonlethal lesions are produced by heat; in the second step these nonlethal lesions are converted into lethal lesions. This concept applies to heat-induced cell killing not only after single heating but also after more complex heating procedures (step-up heating, etc.).

For further analysis of the temperature dependence of cell killing the Arrhenius equation has been applied. The Arrhenius equation describes in its general form an empirical relationship between the rate of chemical reactions and the absolute temperature. Arrhenius proposed that reacting molecules must be activated to reach a transition state which is a necessary condition for the performance of the reaction. This assumption has been developed further on a thermodynamic basis for its application to enzymatic reactions (rate theory) and to the irreversible denaturation of enzyme proteins (JOHNSON et al. 1954). Using the rate theory, the activation energy and activation entropy can be calculated by plotting the logarithm of the reaction rate against the reciprocal value of the absolute temperature. PINCUS and FISHER postulated as long ago as 1931 that the heat-induced inactivation of chick embryo fibroblasts could be described by one rate-limiting step similar to a chemical reaction. Assuming a thermodynamic equilibrium the heat inactivation can be described by the following formula:

$$k = A \times \exp \frac{-H}{RT},$$

where k is the (in)activation rate which is described by the slope of the exponential part of the cell survival curve ($1/D_0$); A is a constant; H is the (in)activation enthalpy or (in)activation energy; R is the gas constant, and T is the absolute temperature.

In the same way as described above, the logarithm of $1/D_0$ can be plotted against the reciprocal value of the absolute temperature. Under these conditions linear Arrhenius plots are obtained with an inflection point between 42° and 43°C (Fig. 2.5). From the steepness of these curves the activation energy (H) for cell killing can be calculated. Usually activation energies of about 140 kcal/mole are obtained in the temperature range 43°–47°C (HENLE 1983). For temperatures below the inflection point the activation energy is considerably higher. Such analyses have been performed for numerous normal and malignant cell lines. Although the thermosensitivity of these cell lines differed greatly, in principle the same results were obtained from the Arrhenius plots.

Heat effects in vivo can generally be analyzed in the same way (HENLE 1983). The measurement of heat effects is fixed on a certain endpoint under these conditions rather than on survival curves. Quite interesting data have been obtained by comparing the heat effects on the same cells in vitro and in vivo. In the latter case ROFSTAD and BRUSTAD (1986) grew cells as a tumor on mice. In this way the Arrhenius plots were studied for cell killing of several human melanoma cell lines. Above the inflection point (41.5°–42.5°C) the activation energies were very similar (about 700 kJ/mol) for all five melanoma cell lines. However, below the inflection point a wide range of activation energies was observed (1118–2190 kJ/mol). The same melanoma cell

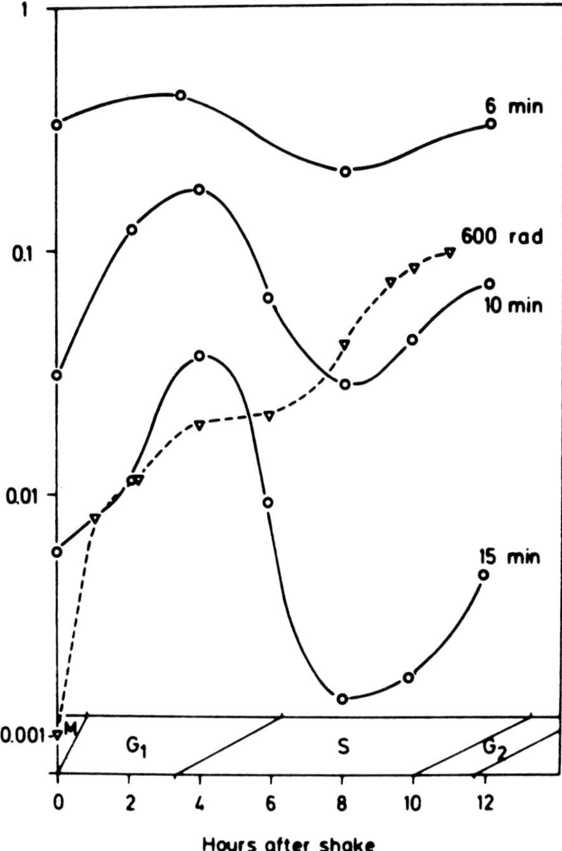

Fig. 2.7. Survival of synchronous CHO cells heated or irradiated during various phases of the cell cycle. (Redrawn from WESTRA and DEWEY 1971)

lines were also grown as tumors on nude mice and the thermosensitivity was studied in vivo in the temperature range 40.5°–44.0°C. The growth delay of the tumors was measured after heat treatment. The activation energies differed especially in the lower temperature range from those which were obtained after heating of the cells in vitro (ROFSTAD and BRUSTAD 1986). The exponential slope constant of −0.693 verifies the above-mentioned rule that after an increase in the heating temperature by 1°C the heating time must be reduced by a factor of 2 in order to achieve about the same cell-killing effect ($e^{-0.693} = 0.5$). The implications of such an analysis for the mechanism of heat-induced cell killing and tumor growth delay will be discussed later.

A third type of dose-effect curve is seen when cells are incubated at elevated temperatures which are comparatively low (usually below 43°C). The cell survival decreases after short incubation times and in their first part the dose-effect curves look very similar to those described above. However, after a longer duration of incubation the survival decreases less than expected. Therefore the survival curves bend and obtain a much shallower slope. The cell inactivation becomes smaller for a certain incubation time than is the case during the initial part of the experiment (DEWEY et al. 1977; SAPARETO et al. 1978) (Fig. 2.6). Survival curves with such a shape have been found for many cell lines after heating with mild hyperthermia.

Similar dose-effect curves have been observed in some experiments in radiobiology. In these latter cases it has been demonstrated that the shape of such survival curves after irradiation is due to mixed cell populations with cells of differing radiosensitivity (ALPER 1979; HALL 1978). After small radiation doses the dose-effect curve is determined by the more radiosensitive cells and the dose-effect curve is steep. After higher radiation doses the dose-effect curve is deter-

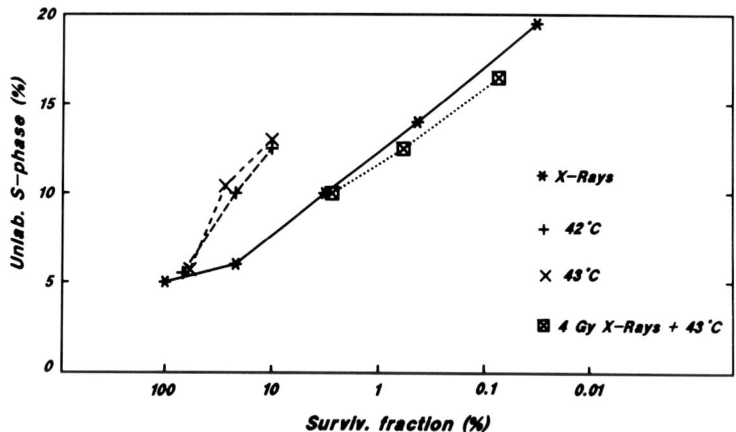

Fig. 2.8. Correlation between colony forming ability and the percentage of unlabelled S-phase cells (BrdU) after x-rays, hyperthermia, and combined treatment. Human melanoma cells (MeWo) were treated and cultured in vitro. (From ZÖLZER et al. 1993b)

mined by the less radiosensitive cell population, and the survival curve becomes shallower.

Several experiments have been undertaken with the aim of demonstrating that analogous findings can be obtained for cell survival of heterogeneous cell populations after treatment with mild hyperthermia. The results of such studies have been negative in almost all cases. From these experiments it can be concluded that protection of cell subpopulations by external environmental conditions, either physical or chemical, is very unlikely (HAHN 1982). Further, it has been discussed whether the development of such thermoresistance is of a genetic nature, being induced by mutation processes. Several authors have reported that heat-resistant cells develop after multiple and prolonged hyperthermic treatments. Under these conditions heating is usually performed over several cell generations before thermoresistant cell lines can be isolated. Thermoresistance is then passed on to subsequent cell generations (HARRIS 1967, 1969; GERNER 1983). In contrast to these phenomena the thermoresistance which has been described here and which is demonstrated by the shape of the survival curves in Fig. 2.8 is not genetically inherited; rather it is transient. Moreover, differing thermosensitivity of cells in the various phases of the cell generation cycle can be excluded, as similar dose-effect curves have been found with synchronous cells in the G_1 phase (SAPARETO et al. 1978). It has been observed that plateau phase cells also show this type of survival curve (LI and HAHN 1980). Plateau phase cells have stopped or decreased cell proliferation. Thus, most cells are found in the G_0 phase. It is generally agreed today that the cells become more thermoresistant ("thermotolerant") during such a treatment.

2.3.2 *Thermosensitivity of Normal and Malignant Cells*

Several authors have reported that malignant cells are more thermosensitive than the normal cells from which they have developed by transformation. Such observations have underlined the potential of hyperthermia as a treatment modality in tumor therapy. This subject has frequently been reviewed (CAVALIERE et al. 1967; SUIT and SHWAYDER 1974; STROM et al. 1977; HAHN 1982; GIOVANELLA 1983; STREFFER 1990). If one looks through the literature carefully and in more detail, one finds that the reported data are far from uniform. Quite often studies have tested the thermosensitivity by determining the cell number as a measure of cell survival (GIOVANELLA et al. 1973, 1976). Such data can be misleading if colony-forming ability is not investigated. GIOVANELLA et al. in fact found all malignant cells to be more thermoresistant than the normal cells.

A very early report on this problem was published by LAMBERT (1912). The author observed that mouse and rat sarcoma cells were more thermosensitive than the normal mesenchymal cells in the temperature range 42°–47°C. In these studies functional characteristics were investigated. AUERSPERG (1966) measured the uptake of vital stains and the protein content of cells, and observed that neoplastic epithelial cells were less damaged than normal fibroblasts after comparable treatments. OSSOVSKI and SACHS (1967) observed that hamster cells showed the same thermosensitivity before and after transformation by polycyclic hydrocarbons. When the hamster cells were transformed by the virus SV40 they became less thermosensitive. KACHANI and SABIN (1969) found no difference between normal hamster cells and cells after viral transformation.

CHEN and HEIDELBERGER (1969) found that transformed mouse prostate cells were more thermosensitive than the original normal cells. The transformation was performed in virto by carcinogenic hydrocarbons. In another study the thermosensitivity of Swiss mouse 3T3 cells was investigated and compared with the thermosensitivity of the transformed derivatives, 3T6 cells. The heat exposure was performed with cells in logarithmic growth; however, the proliferation kinetics were not determined. The colony-forming ability, the exclusion of the vital stain trypan blue, and the permeability of the cell membrane (efflux of phosphate) were measured. The authors observed a higher thermosensitivity of the transformed cells than of the original 3T3 cells (HAYAT and FRIEDBERG 1986).

KASE and HAHN (1975) studied the thermosensitivity of a human fibroblast cell line and compared it with the thermosensitivity of a cell line which was obtained from the fibroblasts by transformation with the virus SV40. During exponential growth the malignant cells were somewhat less thermoresistant than the normal cells. However, the difference between the two cell lines disappeared when the heating was performed at high cell densities. HAHN (1980) further studied several transformed cell lines which were all obtained by transformation from C3H 10T1/2 cells (mouse embryo fibroblasts) and compared the cell survival after heat treatment. During the exponential growth phase the original "normal" 10T1/2 cells were very slightly more resistant than the malignant cells. (The degree of malignancy was tested by the formation of tumors after injection of cells into syngeneic hosts.) However, in no case was a significantly higher thermosensitivity found with the transformed cells than with the parental cells when the cells were heated during the plateau phase.

RAAPHORST et al. (1987) also studied the thermosensitivity of C3H 10T1/2 mouse embryo cells and of transformed cells which were obtained after transfection with a plasmid containing the H-*ras* oncogene and neomycin resistance gene. The malignancy of the transformed cells was tested by injecting these cells into nude mice and by observation of tumors thereafter. The culture conditions were carefully controlled with respect to pH, oxygenation, nutrients, and cell cycle distribution. No differences were seen between the original and the transfected cells (Fig. 2.6). These very careful investigations showed no differences in thermosensitivity between the normal cells and several transformed cell lines after heating at 42°C or 45°C. No correlation existed between the malignant potential and thermosensivity. HARISIADIS et al. (1975) even found that the cell survival of hepatoma cells was higher than the survival of normal liver cells after the same heat treatment.

Several authors have studied the cell survival of cell lines from human tumors where the cells came from different individual tumors of the same tumor type. In extensive studies the thermosensitivity of 11 human melanoma cell lines was determined. The observed dose-effect curves varied tremendously. The thermosensivity of normal cells was found to be in the same range as the data from these melanoma cell lines. Exponential survival curves and survival curves with broad shoulders were found for human melanoma cells (ROFSTAD et al. 1985).

It can be concluded from these data that in some cases the transformation of cells may lead to a higher thermosensitivity but in other cases just the opposite occurs, so that the thermoresistance of the malignant cells may be higher than that of the normal cells. Especially during the plateau phase transformed cells and the parental normal cells apparently do not show differences in thermosensivitity. Also tumor cells which differ in thermosensitivity during exponential growth lose this difference in the plateau phase (VAN BEUNINGEN and STREFFER 1988).

The statement that a "selective heat sensitivity of cancer cells" exists is very optimistic and cannot be proven if the cell survival is tested after heat treatment under identical conditions in vitro. Cells which are grown and heated in vitro apparently show no characteristic difference in survival which is dependent on the malignant potential of the cells. The heterogeneity of the intrinsic thermosensitivity of individual tumor cell lines even of the same tumor entity is extremely high, so that the cell killing by heat shows a clear

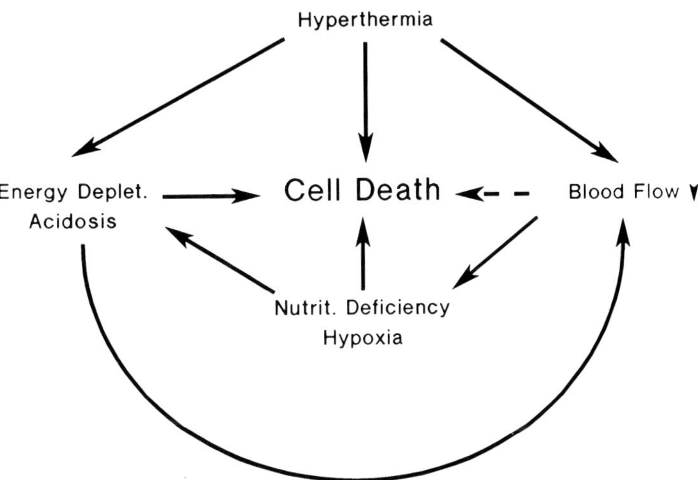

Fig. 2.9. Schematic figure for the induction of cell death by hyperthermia and interaction with other physiological as well as metabolic factors

overlap between normal cells and malignant cells. No distinction between these two groups can be made with respect to heat sensitivity, and no general therapeutic gain can be expected for tumor therapy from intrinsic thermosensitivity. However, for the heat treatment of tumors in situ the microenvironment of the tumor tissue is very important, as differences in micromilieu between normal tissues and tumors might increase the sensitivity of tumors versus normal tissues. Although these parameters will not yield a selectively higher thermosensitivity of tumors than of normal tissues, their manipulation might yield a therapeutic gain.

2.3.3 Dependence of Cell Survival on the Cell Cycle

Radiobiological studies of cellular radiosensitivity during the different phases of the cell cycle have attracted great interest as radiosensitivity changes with cell age and this might be important for the mechanisms of cell killing (ALPER 1979; HALL 1978; STREFFER and VAN BEUNINGEN 1985). Thermosensitivity of cells also changes during the cell cycle, but the highest sensitivity is usually observed during cell cycle phases other than those which have been found to be most sensitive after exposure to ionizing radiation. The general behavior with respect to heat sensitivity was first described by WESTRA and DEWEY (1971). Synchronized CHO cells were used for these experiments; the cells were synchronized by physical treatment (shaking), which allows the selective isolation of mitotic cells (TERASIMA and TOLMACH 1963a,b). The harvested cells are collected at 4°C; this treatment arrests the mitotic cells in the cell cycle. Cells from several harvests can be pooled and after raising the temperature to 37°C the cells progress through the cell cycle in an almost synchronous way.

The synchronous cell population then can be treated either with heat or with ionizing radiation during the different phases of the cell cycle. After exposure to 6.0 Gy x-rays, the lowest survival of the CHO cells was observed during mitosis. It increased during the progression of the cells through the cycle, and reached its highest value after exposures during the late S phase (WESTRA and DEWEY 1971) (Fig. 2.7). A different picture was observed for the thermosensitivity of the same synchronous CHO cells. The cells were heated at 45°C for 6, 10, or 15 min. The lowest cell survival again occurred after heating of mitotic cells. With the progression through the cell cycle the thermoresistance of the CHO cells increased and reached a maximum during the late G_1 phase. However, during the S phase the thermosensitivity increased, peaking during the second half on the S phase. Similar data have been obtained by other authors. Especially the high thermosensitivity of the S phase has been observed by quite a number of authors (SCHLAG and LÜCKE-HUHLE 1976; KIM et al. 1976; LÜCKE-HUHLE and DERTINGER 1977; BHUYAN et al. 1977). KIM et al. (1976) also found an increased thermosensitivity of cells in the G_2 phase.

After the hyperthermic treatment a division delay occurs, as has frequently been described after radiation exposure (G_2 block). This division delay is generally more pronounced after heat treatment than after irradiation when similar cell-killing effects are compared. Studies of the proliferation kinetics by cytofluorometric DNA determination and by time-lapse photography have demonstrated that the cell cycle subjected to the heat treatment is prolonged while the subsequent cell cycles of those cells which have divided once after the heat treatment have an almost normal duration (VAN BEUNINGEN et al. 1978; KURA and ANTOKU 1985). The prolongation of the first cell cycle increased in HeLa cells with heating at 44°C. A constant heat treatment induced different prolongation periods when the heating took place at different phases of the cell cycle. The longest division delay was induced by heating at the late G_1 and early S phase. These studies also showed that with increasing heating temperatures the number of cells which will never divide increases tremendously (KURA and ANTOKU 1985; DERMIETZEL and STREFFER 1992).

This behavior is quite different from the effects after radiation exposure, where most of the cells will divide after the mitotic delay and cell death usually occurs during the following cell cycles (reproductive cell death) (ALPER 1979; STREFFER and VAN BEUNINGEN 1985). Heated cells apparently die mainly during the cell cycle of treatment (interphase death). The reason for this effect is apparently inhibition of cell migration through the S phase and further arrest of cells in G_2 phase (KAL and HAHN 1976; SCHLAG and LÜCKE-HUHLE 1976; ZÖLZER et al. 1993a,b). STREFFER et al. (1983b) demonstrated that after a hyperthermic treatment a number of cells appeared which contained a DNA content equivalent to S phase but which did not incorporate ^{3}H-thymidine; these cells were defined as S_0 cells. In further experiments the proportion of S_0 cells was measured by flow cytometry after labeling melanoma cells with 5′-bromodeoxyuridine (BrdU). These studies showed that S_0 cells were produced with a much higher number after heat treatment than after X-irradiation when the number of the S_0 cells were correlated with cell survival (Fig. 2.8) (Zölzer et al. 1993a,b). The arrested S-phase cells die immediately after the heat treatment (Lücke-Huhle and Dertinger 1977; Streffer et al. 1983b). It has been suggested that the newly synthesized DNA pieces and the DNA synthesizing complex disaggregate and this effect leads to cell death (Streffer 1985). In agreement with this proposal are the findings of Dewey et al. (1971) that chromosome aberrations are induced by heat in S-phase cells, while chromosome aberrations are not observed after heating of cells in G_1 phase. The chromosomal aberrations are mainly aberrations of the chromatid type (Dewey and Li 1988). Cells heated in G_1 phase die without entering cell division or in association with abnormal divisions. This is in agreement with the finding that the number of S_0 cells is much higher after heat treatment than after X-ray exposure when the same levels of cell killing are compared (Zölzer et al. 1993). The enormous thermosensitivity of mitotic cells apparently can be explained by a disaggregation of the microtubules which form the spindle apparatus. As a consequence the heated mitotic cells cannot complete mitosis and many tetraploid cells and giant cells appear (Coss et al. 1982; van Beuningen et al. 1978; Dermietzel and Streffer 1992).

It is quite interesting that these tetraploid cells can apparently progress through a further cell cycle without mitosis. Thus quite a number of cells with a DNA content higher than tetraploid appear (van Beuningen et al. 1978). After heating a mouse mammary adenocarcinoma for 30 min at 43°C a division delay occurred for several hours; a remarkable increase of cells in G_2 phase was observed. These cells in G_2 phase apparently started to synthesize DNA without going through mitosis and later cells appeared with a DNA content which was equivalent to that of octaploid cells (G_2 phase of tetraploid cells) (George et al. 1989). Several days after the treatment the DNA histogram which mirrors the proliferation kinetics was normal again. In this connection it is interesting that no difference in thermosensitivity was found when diploid and tetraploid RIF-1 cells separated by centrifugal elutriation were compared (Rowley et al. 1987). In contrast to the above-mentioned studies of changing thermosensitivity during the cell cycle, in other studies little or no difference in thermosensitivity was found with respect to cell killing for the various cell cycle phases in HeLa cells (Palzer and Heidelberger 1973) or in kidney cells (Reeves 1972).

In general it appears that cells in late S phase and in mitosis have a high thermosensitivity. This finding is of special interest, as cells in late S phase are usually radioresistant. Thus, ionizing radiation and hyperthermia act in a complementary way in that thermosensitive cells are radioresistant and vice versa. These observations support the suggestion that the combination of ionizing radiation with hyperthermia is a very promising modality in tumor therapy.

2.3.4 Modification of Cell Survival by the Microenvironment

The micromilieu surrounding the cells is very important for their thermosensitivity (Vaupel and Kallinowski 1987; Gerweck 1985; Reinhold et al. 1985). This micromilieu is to a large extent determined by two important types of factor:

1. Physiological factors: in the case of hyperthermic treatment the blood flow plays a very important role.
2. Metabolic factors: in the case of hyperthermia energy metabolism in general plays a very important role.

It has been well established that the absence of oxygen or low oxygen pressure increases the radioresistance of cells (Alper 1979). It has also been shown frequently that, due to a lower density of blood vessels in tumors than in normal tissues, the oxygen pressure is frequently lower in tumors than in normal tissues (Vaupel et al. 1987). Therefore it has often been suggested that hypoxic cells in tumors increase the radioresistance of these tumors and that the occurrence of such cells is one important reason for the failure of radiotherapy in many cases (Hall 1978; Streffer and van Beuningen 1985). In a number of studies greater heat-induced cell killing was observed in hypoxic cells than in euoxic cells (Hahn 1974; Harisiadis et al. 1975; Kim et al. 1975; Gerweck 1977; Power and Harris 1977; Schulman and Hall 1974; Gerweck et al. 1979).

Hahn (1974) studied the cell survival of Chinese hamster cells after incubation at 43°C in the presence or absence of oxygen during heating and found that the cell killing was independent of these conditions. Bass et al. (1978) observed a slightly higher survival rate of HeLa cells when the cells were heated at 43°C under hypoxic conditions than under euoxic conditions. In these studies acute hypoxia was induced in the cells and medium by flushing the culture flasks with nitrogen instead of air. Durand (1978) investigated the survival of V79 cells grown as spheroids under hypoxic and euoxic conditions. Large spheroids in which the proliferating cells decreased became more and more thermoresistant under euoxic conditions. If hypoxia was induced, the thermosensitivity increased, however. The thermosensitivity of small spheroids was not modified by hypoxia. Durand (1978) suggests that it is not hypoxia per se that is responsible for the modified thermosensitivity but rather accompanying metabolic changes.

An interesting study was performed by Takeda et al. (1987). The authors compared the cell-killing effects of treatment with x-rays or hyperthermia at 44°C on human melanoma cells which were grown in monolayers or in spheroids of different sizes (diameter 250, 400, and 500 μm). Cell survival curves were obtained. After x-irradiation the cells in monolayers were most sensitive and radiosensitivity decreased with increasing diameter of the spheroids. After heating the lowest sensitivity was seen with monolayer cells and thermosensitivity increased with increasing diameter of the spheroids although the differences were less than after x-irradiation. These data demonstrate the low sensitivity of hypoxic cells to x-rays and just the opposite to heat. This finding favors tumor therapy by hyperthermia. The data agree with those of Durand (1978), discussed above, as the spheroids of Takeda et al. (1987) correspond to the smaller spheroids of Durand. The higher thermosensitivity of spheroids may be due not only to hypoxia but also to low pH and nutrient dificiency.

In other investigations cell respiration was used in order to reduce the oxygen in the culture medium. This was achieved by using high cell densities (Hahn 1974) or large numbers of feeder cells which were irradiated with high radiation doses (Kim et al. 1975). Under these conditions it was found that the hypoxic cells were more thermosensitive than euoxic cells. However, the experimental conditions were such that not only the oxygen but also other nutrients would have been heavily consumed. Also the pH may have changed, so interference of these parameters with hypoxia cannot be excluded. In a very careful investigation Gerweck et al. (1979) compared the modifying action of acute and chronic hypoxia on the thermosensitivity of Chinese hamster cells. It was observed that acute hypoxia did not change the cell killing which was caused by 3 h of heating at 42°C. However, increased cell killing took place when the cells were kept under chronic hypoxic conditions for 18 h and longer. Under these conditions the hypoxic cells still had a higher survival than euoxic cells after irradiation with 7.5 Gy.

As hypoxic cells in a tumor in situ will probably live longer under hypoxic conditions, the investigations of Gerweck et al. (1979) certainly represent a realistic situation for tumor therapy. In general it appears that hypoxic cells are not more resistant to hyperthermia than euoxic cells, in contrast to the situation with respect to ionizing radiation. In fact hypoxic cells in tumors may even show a higher thermosensitivity.

A broad discussion has taken place on whether the pH of the microenvironment influences cellular thermosensitivity. von Ardenne et al. (1969, 1976) have shown that glucose infusions lead to a decrease in pH in tumors and this may be responsible for increased cell killing by hyperthermia. Several studies with cell cultures have demonstrated that reduction of medium pH to approximately 7.0 and below induces increased cell death after heating of cells in vitro to 42°–45°C (Overgaard 1976; Gerweck 1977; Freeman et al. 1977; Meyer et al. 1979; Gerweck and Richards 1981).

On the other hand, Nielsen (1984) did not observe thermosensitization at 42°C with the malignant cell line L1A2 when the cells were incubated in a medium with a reduced pH of 6.5. This effect was explained by the finding that the thermosensitivity of these cells was already comparatively low at a normal pH of 7.2. With melanoma cells, too, no thermosensitization was observed at a reduced pH; however, the cells were incubated in an optimal medium (unpublished results).

Very interesting data were reported by HAHN and SHIU (1986). The authors found an increased thermosensitivity of Chinese hamster cells (HA-1) in vitro when the pH was lowered to 6.8 or 6.5, while this effect was much smaller with malignant RIF or EMT-6 cells. However, the pH effect was also much less marked with HA-1 cells when the cells were adapted to a reduced pH for several days: after adaptation of the cells to pH 6.5 for 3–4 days the thermosensitivity at pH 6.5 was about the same as that of the nonadapted cells at pH 7.2. The authors conclude, "the results strongly imply that the extracellular pH is of little importance in determining the heat response of the majority of tumor cells." The adaptation to a lowered pH was observed with exponentially growing cells as well as with plateau phase cells.

These data have to be considered in the further discussion of these problems in tumors in situ, although the situation is certainly much more complex under these conditions. In tumors hypoxia, depletion of nutrients, a possibly reduced pH, and other parameters of the microenvironment are effectively interrelated.

VEXLER and LITINSKAYA (1986) measured the intracellular pH in Chinese hamster fibroblasts and pig embryo kidney cells in vitro by a microfluorimetric technique using fluorescein diacetate. The intracellular pH (pH_i) decreased from 7.0 to 6.6 when the incubation temperature was decreased from 37°C to 22°C; however, after about 40 min at 22°C the pH_i returned to the normal value. Under hyperthermic conditions at 41°C the pH_i decreased irreversibly to the same degree. This effect was enhanced (decrease to pH_i 6.2) when the pH of the medium was reduced to 6.55. Interestingly the pH_i also decreased under hypoxic conditions and this effect was even more pronounced at 41°C. These observations underline the complex interrelation between different environmental factors. Under these conditions metabolic processes are apparently decisive for the observed alterations of pH_i which may modify the cellular thermosensitivity.

2.4 Mechanisms of Cell Killing by Heat

It has been shown and extensively discussed that hyperthermia can kill cells in the temperature range of ca. 42°–47°C. But cell killing will be remarkably enhanced if the heat exposure is combined with low LET radiation with no or only a short interval between the two modalities. Under these conditions even lower temperatures will have a strong enhancing effect on radiation-induced cell killing. These and other data suggest that the cytotoxic effect of heat alone on the one hand and the interaction of heat with ionizing radiation, the radiosensitizing effect, on the other hand are based on different mechanisms. In this chapter only the mechanisms of cell killing by heat alone will be discussed.

Several investigators have determined activation energies for cell-killing processes by means of Arrhenius plots (Fig. 2.5) (HENLE 1983). Values in the range of 140 kcal/mole were obtained for the inactivation of CHO cells in the temperature range 43°–47°C. Below 43°C a change in the slope ("break", "inflection point") of the Arrhenius plot occurred. Such Arrhenius analyses are normally used in order to determine the activation energy of a chemical reaction. Activation energies of the observed values are in the same range as those which have been found for the denaturation of proteins (PRIVALOV 1979). Therefore it has frequently been assumed that proteins are the molecules at risk for cell inactivation by heat and it can be assumed that the heat-sensitive target should be found among the cellular proteins. When the temperature is raised above 47°C the activation energy for the reaction which leads to cell inactivation changes again and is found in the range of 20–30 kcal/mole. Below and above the temperature range of 42.5°–47°C the cell-killing mechanisms of heat might be completely different from the mechanism which is active in this range.

Activation energies from such Arrhenius plots have been determined not only for cell killing in vitro but also for the heat response of transplantable tumors (OVERGAARD and SUIT 1979; NIELSEN and OVERGAARD 1982; ROFSTAD and BRUSTAD 1986). Similar results were obtained in vitro and in vivo. A very interesting study was performed by ROFSTAD and BRUSTAD (1986), who determined the activation energies for cell killing in vitro and for tumor growth delay of five human melanoma cell lines which were studied in vitro and in vivo (xenografts on nude mice). For the Arrhenius plots of both the growth delay and cell killing in the five melanomas, inflection points were observed between 42° and 43°C. The activation energies below the inflection point were generally smaller for the growth delay of the tumors than for cell killing in vitro. Above the inflection point of Arrhenius plots the activation energies were not significantly different in vivo and in vitro. Studies with cells in vitro have shown that the activation energy below the inflection point is reduced when the pH is lowered (GERWECK 1977; HENLE and DETHLEFSEN 1980). These results suggest that a reduced pH in tumors may be responsible for the smaller activation energy in tumors than in cells in vitro. In this connection it is of interest that interruption of blood flow by clamping resulted in a reduction of the activation energy for heat damage in the rat tail (MORRIS and FIELD 1985).

From these data it may be suggested that in cells at a reduced pH as well as apparently in experimental tumors the important factors for cell killing are conformational changes of proteins in the temperature range below 42°–43°C. It cannot yet be decided which proteins are decisive; they may be localized in the cytoplasmic membrane, in the cell nucleus, or in the cytoplasm, and especially in the last-mentioned case may be connected to the cytoskeleton. A transition of proteins from the native to the denatured state means a change in protein conformation (LEPOCK and KRUUV 1992). As has just been pointed out, it is not possible to name a specific individual protein which is the one whose denaturation or conformational transition is responsible for cell inactivation. Perhaps, in fact, it is not sufficient that one single protein is altered; rather it may be necessary for a group of different proteins to undergo such structural changes during heat exposure, so that various cellular processes do not function properly. Such changes could induce damage of cellular membranes with damage to compartmentation of ion gradients as well as other cellular constituents. This could lead to a collapse to the cytoskeleton or other cellular structures.

It has been demonstrated that in response to hyperthermia membranes apparently lose some of their proteins which are needed for stabilization (STREFFER 1985a,b), for transport functions (BURDON et al. 1984), or as receptors (CALDERWOOD and HAHN 1983; CALDERWOOD et al. 1985; STEVENSON et al. 1981). BORELLI et al. (1986) reported that blebing of the cytoplasmic membrane was connected with cell killing. Freeze fracture studies through electron microscopy showed that the membranes had lost their intermembrane particles, as demonstrated previously by ISSA (1985). Therefore the plasma membrane has been suggested as the critical target (HAHN 1982). Such effects would explain an increased efflux of K^+ (YI 1983; RUIFROK et al. 1984, 1985). A good correlation exists between this effect and cell killing in some investigations. Interestingly, such a correlation has not been found for the combination of x-rays and heat (RUIFROK et al. 1984; 1985; KONINGS 1987). Furthermore, membrane changes lead to an increased Ca^{2+} influx into heated cells (ANGHILARI et al. 1984; STEVENSON et al. 1981; WIEGANT et al. 1984). In this respect it is also interesting that membrane-active phenothiazine drugs can enhance heat-induced cell killing (GEORGE and SINGH 1982, 1985; SHENOY and SINGH 1985).

Other authors, however, have not found a correlation between K^+ efflux and cell killing (BOONSTRA et al. 1984; VIDAIR and DEWEY 1986). A careful study was performed by VIDAIR and DEWEY 1986). CHO cells were heated at 45°C for 30 min. This treatment caused 98% cell killing. However, the intracellular K^+ concentrations did not change within the first few hours after heating: only an intracellular Na^+ increase was observed directly after the heat treatment, which was normalized within 3 h. Up to 28 h following heating no irreversible damage occurred with respect to these ion concentrations. Similar observations were made with rat neuroblastoma cells in which the intracellular ion concentrations, including Mg^{2+} concentrations, were measured with microelectrodes (BORELLI et al. 1986; VIDAIR and DEWEY 1986). Immediately after heating the intracellular Ca^{2+} content was not significantly changed, but within the following hours an increase in Ca^{2+} occurred. This effect increased with heating dose. However, the extra- and intracellular Ca^{2+} content did not correlate with heat-induced cell killing. Therefore the authors (VIDAIR and DEWEY 1986) concluded: "These data show that an increased cellular Ca^{2+} content does not potentiate killing by heat, nor is it required for heat to cause the reproductive death." From the aforementioned data the authors also come to the same conclusion for the other ions. However, changes between free and bound Ca^{2+} within the cells may be important, and data on this topic are lacking up to now.

Although it is very tempting to conclude that the cytoplasmic membranes with their proteins are the targets for heat-induced cell killing, this is certainly not the general mechanism, as VIDAIR and DEWEY (1986) have shown. Nevertheless, a role of membranes cannot be completely ruled out. It has already been pointed out that the fluidity of membranes can modify the thermosensitivity of cells. This apparently involves a cooperative action between lipids and proteins. Besides alterations of the cytoplasmic membrane, changes of intracellular membranes occur, as has been demonstrated by electron microscopic studies (BREIPOHL et al. 1983; BORELLI et al. 1986). Especially the intracellular membranes of the endoplasmic reticulum are thermosensitive (WALLACH 1977; BREIPOHL et al. 1983). The instability of lysosomal membranes and an increase in lysosome numbers have been suggested as important phenomena in heat-induced cell killing (VON ARDENNE et al. 1969; OVERGAARD 1976). HUME et al. (1978) found an increase in lysosomal enzyme activities using histochemical methods after heating. On the other hand the lysosomal degradation of epidermal growth factor is inhibited after heating of rat embryo fibroblasts (MAGUN and FENNIE 1981). Furthermore, the biochemical determination of lysosomal enzyme activities did not reveal any heat-induced changes (TAMULEVICIUS and STREFFER 1983). Thus lysosomes seem not to be the primary target for heat-induced cell killing (HAHN 1982).

HAHN (1982) has discussed the role of ATP production through oxidative phosphorylation and mitochondrial membranes in cell killing by heat. A decrease in ATP levels has been observed in heated cells (FRANCESCONI and MAYER 1979; OHYAMA and YAMADA 1980; LUNEC and CRESSWELL 1983; MIRTSCH et al. 1984). However, at the same time the ATP turnover, and hence also the ATP synthesis, is enhanced (OHYAMA and YAMADA 1980; STREFFER 1985a,b). After severe heat damage even an increased ATP content can be observed in cells. This effect might be caused by a decrease in Na^+/K^+-ATPase (BURDON et al. 1984; MIRTSCH et al., unpublished data). Such alterations apparently differ from cell line to cell line and cannot be regarded as a general phenomenon. Damage of ATP synthesis does not seem to be a primary event in heat-induced cell killing. However, nutrient deficiency and other microenvironmental factors may potentiate heat-induced cell killing through damage to the energy metabolism.

Changes in intermediary metabolism, e.g., glycolysis, fatty acid metabolism, and the citrate cycle, can be remarkable during and after a hyperthermic treatment (STREFFER 1985b). The metabolic rates are increased during hyperthermia so that energy reservoirs are utilized and depleted. The data do not demonstrate that these alterations represent the primary events in heat-induced cell killing, but such processes can modify the microenvironment of cells, such as the pH and the amount of nutrients, in such a way that thermosensitivity increases remarkably (STREFFER 1985b). A reduction of nutrients (HAHN 1982) and inhibition of glycolysis (KIM et al. 1978, 1980, 1984; SONG et al. 1977) can sensitize the cells remarkably against heat; the latter is especially significant when glycolysis is the main pathway for energy metabolism (Fig. 2.9).

Conformational changes of proteins which form the structure of the cytoskeleton are probably responsible for the observed disturbances of the cytoskeleton, which have been described earlier. In this respect it is interesting that some of the heat shock proteins (HSPs) are apparently associated with the cytoskeleton (BURDON 1985), which might stabilize these structures. These phenomena certainly need to be substantiated by more experimental evidence. Further studies have revealed that the general organization of the tubiline cytoskeleton is not disrupted directly after hyperthermia when a comparatively mild treatment (42°C for 1 h) is used, but that the structures connecting the cytoskeleton to the nuclear envelope and other membranes may be important for the organization of the cytoskeleton. The shape of the cell changes more rapidly, the cells becoming rounded. In contrast to the mild hyperthermia (42°C) severe hyperthermic treatment (44°C for 1 h) results in complete disruption of the cytoskeleton in more than 80% of cells. Electron microscopy following immunogold labelling of the tubulin in human melanoma cells showed that the normal regular tubulin fibers were disrupted due to disaggregation of the tubulin proteins (DERMIETZEL and STREFFER 1992).

In the case of mitotic cells good evidence exists that a disaggregation of the globular proteins of the spindle apparatus occurs which inhibits regular mitosis and induces cell death (COSS et al. 1982). The mechanism is probably analogous to that discussed for the cytoskeleton above.

Changes in RNA and DNA as well as the heat-induced inhibition of their biosynthesis have also been discussed in connection with cell death (HAHN 1982; STREFFER 1982). Heat-induced changes in the conformation of DNA and RNA or other damage to these molecules generally seem to occur only at higher temperatures than those which have been considered here. RNA synthesis, like general protein synthesis, recovers relatively rapidly. It is not known whether the synthesis of certain specific proteins or RNA species, for instance mRNA, is inhibited longer than has been observed in general. The same situation is more or less found for DNA synthesis. However, the recovery of this process is much slower and apparently ligation of newly synthesized DNA pieces is delayed (WARTERS and STONE 1983). In this respect it is of interest that poly (ADP-ribose) synthetase is inhibited after heating cells in vitro (STREFFER et al. 1983a; TAMULEVICIUS et al. 1984) and inhibitors of this enzyme enhance heat-induced cell killing (NAGLE and MOSS 1983). This long delay and the conformational changes of the DNA synthesizing complex as well as of the DNA structure in these newly synthesized regions may induce disaggregation of the DNA structure and chromosomal aberrations, which have been observed after heating cells in S phase but not G_1 phase (DEWEY et al. 1971; DEWEY 1988). These conditions leat to the induction of S_0 cells (ZÖLZER et al. 1993a,b). Thus, cell death of S-phase cells is probably caused through these mechanisms. However, S-phase cells are a special case and even in a tumor most cells are generally not found in S phase. In this regard it is interesting that alkali-labile DNA lesions were induced by heat with an activation energy of 152 kcal/mol (JORRITSMA and KONINGS 1984).

With respect to the cell nucleus it is interesting that an increase in nuclear protein content occurs after hyperthermic treatment of cells due to migration of proteins from the cytoplasm (ROTI ROTI 1982; WARTERS et al. 1986). This increase correlates with cell killing. The new proteins from a complex with the chromatin and may interfere with the formation of the DNA replication complex (WARTERS and ROTI ROTI 1982). It was further demonstrated that the increased binding of nuclear nonhistone protein correlated with cell killing but also that the release of the bound protein during the post-heat period may be important (KAMPINGA et al. 1987). Thus the release of protein bound to the cell nucleus after heating was faster in thermotolerant cells and was retarded when cells were sensitized by procaine. The mechanism of these processes was further studied with subnuclear units on the DNA superstructure known as nucleoids, which possess tertiary (superhelical coiling) and quaternary (superhelical domains) levels of DNA organization. It is asssumed that nucleoids consist of supercoiled DNA loops which are free of protein and which are attached to a protein backbone for stabilization of the superhelical structure of DNA. Isolation of such nucleoids from heat-treated cells demonstrated that the protein to DNA ratio is increased in comparison to nucleoids from untreated cells (ROTI ROTI and PAINTER 1982; SIMPSON et al. 1987). The increased nuclear protein after heat treatment is apparently covalently bound to the nucleoids. However, it is not clear whether this binding is due to a protein–protein or a protein–DNA interaction (SIMPSON et al. 1987). Hyperthermia inhibited the recovery from this damage and it is suggested that a proteolytic enzyme is inhibited which is involved in maintaining a normal protein to DNA ratio in these nucleoids (SIMPSON et al. 1987). The nature of these proteins as well as the mechanism by which these processes induce cell killing remain unclear at present. Recently is has been shown these proteins are mainly associated with the nuclear matrix (ROTI ROTI et al. 1993); this finding may shed more light on the mechanism involved.

In conclusion, it remains a very intriguing possibility that the proposed conformational changes of proteins in the various cellular structures constitute a more general mechanism of heat-induced cell killing. This would also explain the most important modifications of cellular thermosensitivity. The micromilieu with its pH and ion concentration is very important for protein conformation, as has been described above. In order to maintain the micromilieu and with it the conformation of proteins as well as the cellular structures in general, energy is steadily needed; this fact would explain the modifications of cellular sensitivity by metabolism. Also the development of thermotolerance with the synthesis of HSPs is in agreement with this proposal. Furthermore, the trigger mechanism of thermotolerance shows an activation energy of about 120 kcal/mole (LI et al. 1982) which would be in line with the suggestion regarding heat-induced protein denaturation. Such a mechanism would furthermore explain why heat effects, including cell death, develop rapidly (for instance in comparison to the effects of ionizing radiation), as the conformational changes will occur during heating and can lead to irreversible loss of these structure. Regeneration, if it is possible at all, needs time. As a consequence changes in membrane function and the cytoskeleton, possible nuclear damage, and other effects will occur which lead to disturbances of vital cellular functions. If these alterations are severe and continue for a longer period, they become irreversible and cells die. Besides these effects the rate of a number of metabolic reactions increases during heating. The heat-induced depletion of energy reservoirs or disturbances of energy metabolism will modify and strongly enhance the thermosensitivity of cells (Fig. 2.9).

2.5 Summary

- Heating of cells in the temperature range of 42 to 45°C induces conformational changes of certain proteins and not of nucleic acids. These changes are dependent on the pH values.
- These conformational changes lead to alterations of multimolecular structures like cytoskeleton, membranes and also of structures in the cell nucleus.
- In the temperature range of 40 to 45°C a hyperthermic treatment increases metabolic rates. This has been clearly shown for the glycolytic pathway.
- Under hypoxic conditions the stimulation of glycolysis increases the lactate levels in the tissues especially in tumors. The increase of the lactate levels decreases pH and has an impact on blood flow.
- Under conditions of sufficient oxygen supply the lactate can be metabolised via pyruvate and acetyl CoA in the citrate cycle. However heat induced changes of the multimolecular structures make the citrate cycle and especially oxidative phosphorylation very vulnerable to a hyperthermia treatment. Therefore energy metabolism and ATP supply is reduced.
- There exist apparently no differences between normal and malignant cells with respect to intrinsic heat sensitivity.
- These metabolic changes lead to alterations of the microenvironment in tumors and has an impact on heat induced cell death. These changes contribute to a sensitization against heat.
- Conformational changes of the enzyme complexes for DNA synthesis as well as for DNA repair are also very important in this connection.
- Cell killing by heat is apparently induced and modified by these molecular changes.

References

Ahnström G, Edvardsson KA (1974) Radiation-induced single-strand breaks in DNA determined by rate of alkaline strand separation and hydroxylapatite chromatography: an alternative to velocity sedimentation. Taylor & Francis, London. Int J Radiat Biol 26: 493–497

Alper T (1979) Cellular radiobiology. Cambridge University Press, Cambridge

Anghilari LJ, Crone-Escanye MC, Marchal C, Robert J (1984) Plasma membrane changes during hyperthermia: probable role of ionic modification in tumor cell death. In: Overgaard J (ed) Hyperthermic oncology, vol I, pp 49–52

von Ardenne M (1982) Hyperthermia and cancer therapy. Adv Pharmacol Chemother 10: 339

von Ardenne M, Reitnauer P (1976) Verstärkung der mit Glukoseinfusion erzielbaren Tumorübersäuerung in vivo durch NAD. Arch Geschwulstforsch 30: 319–330

von Ardenne M, Chaplain R, Reitnauer P (1969) Selektive Krebszellenschädigung durch eine Attackenkombination mit Übersäuerung, Hyperthermie, Vitamin A, Dimethylsulfoxid und weiteren die Freisetzung lysosomaler Enzyme fördernden Agenzien. Arch Geschwulstforsch 33: 331–344

Ashburner M, Bonner JJ (1979) The induction of gene activity in *Drosophila* by heat shock. Cell 17: 241–254

Auersperg N (1966) Differential heat sensitivity of cells in tissue culture. Nature 209: 415–416

Bass H, Moore JL, Coakely WT (1978) Lethality in mammalian cells due to hyperthermia under oxic and hypoxic conditions. Int J Radiat Biol 33: 57–67

Belt JA, Thomas JA, Buchsbaum RN, Racker E (1979) Inhibition of lactate transport and glycolysis in Ehrlich ascites tumor cells by bioflavonoids. Biochemistry 18: 3506–3511

van Beuningen D, Streffer C (1988) Importance of thermotolerance for radiothermotherapy as assessed using two human melanoma cell lines. Recent Results Cancer Res 109: 203–213

van Beuningen D, Molls M, Schulz S, Streffer C (1978) Effects of irradiation and hyperthermia on the development of preimplanted mouse embryos in vitro. In: Streffer C (eds) Cancer therapy by hyperthermia and radiation. Urban & Schwarzenberg, Baltimore, pp 151–153

Bhuyan BK, Day KJ, Edgerton CE, Ogunbase O (1977) Sensitivity of different cell lines and of different phases in the cell cycle to hyperthermia. Cancer Res 37: 3780–3784

Boonstra J, Schamhart DHJ, de Laat SW, van Wijk R (1984) Analysis of K^+ and Na^+ transport and intracellular contents during and after heat shock and their role in protein synthesis in rat hepatoma cells. Cancer Res 44: 955–960

Borelli MJ, Wong RSL, Dewey WC (1986) A direct correlation between hyperthermia-induced membrane blebbing and survival in synchronous G_1 CHO cells. J Cell Physiol 126: 181–190

Bowler K, Duncan CJ, Gladwell RT, Davison TF (1973) Cellular heat injury. Comp Biochem Physiol (A) 45: 441–450

Breipohl W, van Beuningen D, Ummels M, Streffer C, Schönfelder B (1983) Effect of hyperthermia on the intestinal mucosa of mice. Verh Anat Ges 77: 567–569

Burdon RH (1985) Heat shock proteins. In: Overgaard J (ed) Hyperthermic oncology, 1984, vol 2. Taylor & Francis, London, pp 223–230

Burdon RH (1988) Hyperthermic toxicity and the modulation of heat damage to cell protein synthesis in HeLa cells. Recent Results Cancer Res 109: 1–8

Burdon RH, Cutmore CMM (1982) Human heat shock gene expression and the modulation of plasma membrane Na^+/K^+ ATPase activity. FEBS Lett 140: 45–48

Burdon RH, Kerr SM, Cutmore CMM, Munro J, Gill V (1984) Hyperthermia, Na^+/K^+ ATPase and lactic acid production in some human tumour cells. Br J Cancer 49: 437–445

Calderwood St. K, Hahn GM (1983) Thermal sensitivity and resistance of insulin-receptor binding. Biochim Biophys Acta 756: 1–8

Calderwood St. K, Bump EA, Stevenson MA, van Kersen I, Hahn GM (1985) Investigation of adenylate energy charge, phosphorylation potential, and ATP concentration in cells stressed with starvation and heat. J Cell Physiol 124: 261–268

Cavaliere R, Ciocatto EC, Giovanella BC, Heidelberger C, Johnson RO, Moricca G, Rossi-Fanelli A (1967) Selective heat sensitivity of cancer cells (biochemical and clinical studies). Cancer 20: 1351–1381

Chen TT, Heidelberger C (1969) Quantitative studies on the malignant transformation of mouse prostate cells by carcinogenic hydrocarbons in vitro. Int J Cancer 4: 166–178

Coss RA, Dewey WC, Bamburg JR (1982) Effects of hyperthermia on dividing Chinese hamster ovary cells and on microtubules in vitro. Cancer Res 42: 1059–1071

Cress AE, Culver PS, Moon TE, Gerner EW (1982) Correlation between amounts of cellular membrane components and sensitivity to hyperthermia in a variety of mammalian cell lines in cultures. Cancer Res 42: 1716–1721

Dennis WH, Yatvin MB (1981) Correlation of hyperthermic sensitivity and membrane microviscosity in *E. coli* K1060. Int J Radiat Biol 39: 265–271

Dermietzel R, Streffer C (1992) The cytoskeleton and proliferation of melanoma cells under hyperthermal conditions. A correlative double immuno-labelling study. Strahlenther Onkol 168: 593–602

Dertinger H, Jung H (1970) Molekulare Strahlenbiologie. Springer, Berlin Heidelberg New York

Dewey WC (1988) Hyperthermic effects studied in vitro. In: Fielden EM, Fowler JF, Hendry JH, Scott D (eds) Radiation research. Taylor and Francis, London, pp 954–959

Dewey WC (1989) The search for critical cellular targets damaged by heat. Radiat Res 120: 191–204

Dewey WC, Esch JL (1982) Transient thermal tolerance: cell killing and polymerase activities. Radiat Res 92: 611–614

Dewey WC, Li XL (1988) Cell cycle effects: killing, division delay, and chromosomal aberrations. In: Sugahara T, Saito M (eds) 5th International symposium on Hyperthermic Oncology, Kyoto (Abstracts), Taylor & Francis, London, p 20

Dewey WC, Westra A, Miller HH (1971) Heat-induced lethality and chromosomal damage in synchronized Chinese hamster cells treated with 5-bromodeoxyuridine. Int J Radiat Biol 20: 505–520

Dewey WC, Hopwood LE, Sapareto SA, Gerweck LE (1977) Cellular responses to combinations of hyperthermia and radiation. Radiology 123: 463–474

Dewey WC, Freeman ML, Raaphorst GP et al. (1980) Cell biology of hyperthermia and radiation. In: Meyn RE, Withers HR (eds) Radiation biology in cancer research. Raven Press, New York, pp 589–623

Dube DK, Seal G, Loeb LA (1977) Differential heat sensitivity of mammalian DNA polymerase. Biochem Biophys Res Commun 76: 483–487

Durand RE (1978) Potentiation of radiation lethality by hyperthermia in a tumor model: effects of sequence, degree and duration of heating. Int J Radiat Oncol Biol Phys 4: 401–406

Francesconi R, Mayer M (1979) Heat- and exercise-induced hyperthermia: effects on high-energy phosphate. Aviat Space Environ Med 50: 799–802

Freeman ML, Dewey WC, Hopwood LE (1977) Effect of pH on hyperthermic cell survival. J Natl Cancer Inst 58: 1837–1839

George KC, Singh BB (1982) Synergism of chlorpromazine and hyperthermia in two mouse solid tumours. Br J Cancer 45: 309–313

George KC, Singh BB (1985) Hyperthermic response of a mouse fibrosarcoma as modified by phenothiazine drug. Br J Cancer 51: 737–738

George KC, Streffer C, Pelzer T (1989) Combined effects of x-rays, Ro-03-8799 and hyperthermia on growth, necrosis and cell proliferation in a mouse tumour. Int J Radiat Oncol Biol Phys 16: 1119–1122

Gerner EW (1983) Thermotolerance: In: Storm FK (ed) Hyperthermia and cancer therapy. G.K. Hall, Boston, Mass, pp 141–162

Gerner EW (1984) Definition of thermal dose. In Overgaard J (ed) Hyperthermic oncology, vol 2. Taylor & Francis, London, pp 245–251

Gerner EW, Connor WG, Boone MLM, Doss JD, Mayer EG, Miller RG (1975) The potential of localized heating as an adjunct to radiation therapy. Radiology 116: 433–489

Gerner EW, Holmes PW, McCullough JA (1979) Influence of growth state on several thermal responses of EMT-6/Az tumor cells in vitro. Cancer Res 39: 981–986

Gerweck LE (1977) Modification of cell lethality at elevated temperatures: the pH effect. Radiat Res 70: 224–235

Gerweck LE (1982) Effect of microenvironmental factors on the response of cells to single and fractionated heat treatments. NCJ Monogr 61: 19–25

Gerweck LE (1985) Environmental and vascular effect. In: Overgaard J (ed) Hyperthermic oncology, vol 2. Taylor & Francis, London, pp 253–262

Gerweck LE, Richards B (1981) Influence of pH on the thermal sensitivity of cultured human glioblastoma cells. Cancer Res 41: 845–849

Gerweck LE, Nygaard TG, Burlett M (1979) Response of cells to hyperthermia under acute and chronic hypoxic conditions. Cancer Res 39: 966–972

Gerweck LE, Richards B, Michaels HB (1982) Influence of low pH on the development and decay of 42°C thermotolerance in CHO cells. Int J Radiat Oncol Biol Phys 8: 1935–1941

Giovanella BC (1983) Thermosensitivity of neoplastic cells in vitro. In: Storm FK (ed) Hyperthermia and cancer therapy. GK Hall, Boston, Mass, pp 55–62

Givoanella BC, Morgan AC, Stehlin JA, Williams LJ (1973) Selective lethal effect of supranormal temperatures on mouse sarcoma cells. Cancer Res 33: 2568–2578

Giovanella BC, Stehlin JS, Morgan AC (1976) Selective lethal effects of supranormal temperatures on human neoplastic cells. Cancer Res 36: 3944–3950

Guffy MM, Rosenberger JA, Simon J, Burns CP (1982) Effect of cellular fatty acid alteration on hyperthermic sensitivity in cultured L1210 murine leukemia cells. Cancer Res 42: 3625–3630

Hahn GM (1974) Metabolic aspects of the role of hyperthermia in mammalian cell inactivation and their possible relevance to cancer treatment. Cancer Res 34: 3117–3123

Hahn GM (1980) Comparison of the malignant potential of 10T1/2 cells and transformants with their survival responses to hyperthermia and to amphotericin B. Cancer Res 40: 3763–3767

Hahn GM (1982) Hyperthermia and cancer. Plenum Press, New York

Hahn GM, Shiu EC (1983) Effect of pH and elevated temperature on the cytotoxicity of some chemotherapeutic agents on Chinese hamster cells in vitro. Cancer Res 43: 5789–5791

Hahn GM, Shiu EC (1986) Adaptation to low pH modifies thermal and thermo-chemical response of mammalian cells. Int J Hyperthermia 2: 379–387

Hall E (1978) Radiobiology for the radiologist. Harper & Row, Hagestown, Md

Harisiadis L, Hall EJ, Kraljevic U, Borek C (1975) Hyperthermia: biological studies at the cellular level. Radiology 117: 447–452

Harris M (1967) Temperature-resistant variants in clonal populations of pig kidney cells. Exp Cell Res 46: 301–314

Harris M (1969) Growth and survival of mammalian cells under continuous thermal stress. Exp Cell Res 56: 382–386

Hayat H, Friedberg I (1986) Heat-induced alterations in cell membrane permeability and cell inactivation of transformed mouse fibroblasts. Int J Hyperthermia 2: 369–378

Henle KJ (1983) Arrhenius analysis of thermal responses. In: Storm FK (ed) Hyperthermia and cancer therapy. GK Hall, Boston, Mass, pp 47–53

Henle KJ, Dethlefsen LA (1980) Time-temperature relationships for heat-induced cell killing of mammalian cells. Ann NY Acad Sci 335: 234–253

Henle KJ, Leeper DB (1979) Effects of hyperthermia (45°C) on macromolecular synthesis in Chinese hamster ovary cells. Cancer Res 39: 2665–2674

Hume SP, Rogers MA, Field SB (1978) Two qualitatively different effects of hyperthermia on acid phosphatase staining in mouse spleen, dependent on the severity of the treatment. Int J Radiat Biol 34: 401–409

Isbruch, C (1986) Untersuchungen zum Glukosestoffwechsel menschlicher Melanomzellen in vitro nach Hyperthermie, Bestrahlung und Glukosegabe. Inaugural-Dissertation, Universität-Gesamthochschule Essen

Issa M (1985) Hyperthermie am Dünndarm der Maus. Eine elektronenmikroskopische Untersuchung. Dissertation, Essen

Jähde E, Rajewsky MF (1982) Sensitization of clonogenic malignant cells to hyperthermia by glucose-mediated, tumour-selective pH reduction. J Cancer Res Clin Oncol 104: 23–30

Johnson FH, Eyring H, Polisar MJ (1954) The kinetic basis of molecular biology. John Wiley, New York

Jorritsma JBM, Konings AWT (1984) The occurrence of DNA strand breaks after hyperthermic treatments of mammalian cells with and without radiation. Radiat Res 98: 198–208

Jorritsma JBM, Konings AWT (1986) DNA lesions in hyperthermic cell killing: effects of thermotolerance, procaine and erythritol. Radiat Res 106: 89–97

Jung H (1986) A generalized concept for cell killing by heat. Radiat Res 106: 56–72

Kachani ZFC, Sabin AB (1969) Reproductive capacity and viability at higher temperatures of various transformed hamster cell lines. J Natl Cancer Inst 43: 469–480

Kal HB, Hahn GM (1976) Kinetic responses of murine sarcoma cells to radiation and hyperthermia in vivo and in vitro. Cancer Res 36: 1923–1929

Kampinga HH, Luppes JG, Konings AWT (1987) Heat-induced nuclear protein binding and its relation to thermal cytotoxicity. Int J Hyperthermia 3: 459–465

Kase K, Hahn GM (1975) Differential heat response of normal and transformed human cells in tissue culture. Nature 255: 228–230

Kellerer AM, Rossi HH (1971) RBE and the primary mechanism of radiation action. Radiat Res 47: 15–34

Kim SH, Kim JH, Hahn EW (1975) Enhanced killing of hypoxic tumor cells by hyperthermia. Br J Radiol 48: 872–874

Kim SH, Kim JH, Hahn EW (1976) The enhanced killing of irradiated HeLa cells in synchronous culture by hyperthermia. Radiat Res 66: 337–345

Kim SH, Kim JH, Hahn EW (1978) Selective potentiation of hyperthermia killing of hypoxic cells by 5-thio-D-glucose. Cancer Res 38: 2935–2938

Kim SH, Kim JH, Hahn EW, Ensign NA (1980) Selective killing of glucose and oxygen-deprived HeLa cells by hyperthermia. Cancer Res 40: 3459–3462

Kim JH, Kim SH, Alfieri A, Young CW (1984) Quercetin, an inhibitor of lactate transport and a hyperthermic sensitizer of HeLa cells. Cancer Res 44: 102–106

Konings AWT (1987) Effects of heat and radiation on mammalian cells. Radiat Phys Chem 30: 339–349

Konings AWT, Penninga P (1985) On the importance of the level of glutathione and the activity of the pentose phosphate pathway in heat sensitivity and thermotolerance. Int J Radiat Biol 48: 409–422

Konings AWT, Ruifrok ACC (1985) Role of membrane lipids and membrane fluidity and thermotolerance of mammalian cells. Radiat Res 102: 86–98

Kura S, Antoku S (1985) Time-lapse photographic studies of heated HeLa cells. In: Abe M, Takahashi M, Sugahara T (eds) Hyperthermic in cancer therapy. Nippon Hoshasen Kiki Kogyokai, Tokyo, pp 192–193

Lambert RA (1912) Demonstration of the greater susceptibility to heat of sarcoma cells. JAMA 59: 2147–2148

Landry J, Marceau N (1978) Rate-limiting events in hyperthermic cell killing. Radiat Res 75: 573–578

Lee SY, Ryn KH, Kang MS, Song CW (1986) Effect of hyperthermia on the lactic acid and beta-hydroxybutyric acid content in tumours. Int J Hyperthermia 2: 213–222

Leeper DB (1985) Molecular and cellular mechanisms of hyperthermia alone or combined with other modalities. In: Overgaard J (ed) Hyperthermic oncology 1984. Taylor & Francis, London, vol. 2, pp 9–40

Lepock JR (1982) Involvement of membranes in cellular responses to hyperthermia. Radiat Res 92: 433–438

Lepock JR (1991) Protein denaturation: its role in thermal killing. In: Dewey WC, Edington M, Fry RJM, Hall EJ,

Whitmore GF (eds) Radiation research: a twentieth-century perspective. Academic Press, New York, pp 992–998

Lepock JR, Kruuv J (1992) Mechanisms of thermal cytotoxicity. In: Gerner EW, Cetas TC (eds) Hyperthermic oncology Proceedings of the 6th International Congress on Hyperthermic Oncology, Tucson, Arizona, April 27 – May 1, 1992. Arizona Board of Regents, pp 9–16

Lepock JR, Cheng KH, Al-Qysi H, Kruuv J (1983) Thermotropic lipid and protein transitions in Chinese hamster lung cell membranes: relationship to hyperthermic cell killing. Can J Biochem Cell Biol 61: 421–427

Li GC, Hahn GM (1980) Adaptation to different growth temperatures modifies some mammalian cell survival responses. Exp Cell Res 128: 475–485

Li GC, Shiu EC, Hahn GM (1980) Similarities in cellular inactivation by hyperthermia or by ethanol. Radiat Res 82: 257–268

Li GC, Petersen NS, Mitchell HK (1982) Induced thermal tolerance and heat shock protein synthesis in Chinese hamster ovary cells. Int J Radiat Oncol Biol Phys 8: 63–67

Lin PS, Turi A, Kwock L, Lu RC (1982) Hyperthermia effect on microtubule organization. Natl Cancer Inst Monogr 61: 57–60

Lücke-Huhle C, Dertinger H (1977) Kinetic response of an in vitro "turmor model" (V99 spheroids) to 42°C hyperthermia. Eur J Cancer 13: 23–28

Lunec J, Cresswell SR (1983) Heat-induced thermotolerance expressed in the energy metabolism of mammalian cells. Radiat Res 93: 588–597

Mackey MA, Roti Roti JL (1992) A model of heat-induced clonogenic cell death. J Theor Biol 156: 133–146

Magun BE, Fennie CW (1981) Effects of hyperthermia on binding, internalization and degradation of epidermal growth factor. Radiat Res 86: 133–146

Massicotte-Nolan P, Glofcheski DJ, Kruuv J, Lepock JR (1981) Relationship between hyperthermic cell killing and protein denaturation by alcohols. Radiat Res 87: 284–299

McCormick W, Penman SH (1969) Regulation of protein synthesis in HeLa cells: translation at elevated temperatures. J Mol Biol 39: 315–333

Mehdi SQ, Recktenwald DJ, Smith LM, Li GC, Armour EP, Hahn GM (1984) Effect of hyperthermia on murine cell surface histocompatibility antigens. Cancer Res 44: 3394–3397

Meyer KR, Hopwood LE, Gillette EL (1979) The thermal response of mouse adenocarcinoma cells at low pH. Eur J Cancer 15: 1219–1222

Mirtsch Sch, Streffer C, van Beuningen D, Rebmann A (1984) ATP metabolism in human melanoma cells after treatment with hyperthermia (42°C). In: Overgaard J (ed) Hyperthermic oncology 1984. Taylor & Francis, London, vol. 2, pp 19–22

Mivechi NF, Dewey WC (1984) Effect of glycerol and low pH on heat-induced cell killing and loss of cellular DNA polymerase activities in Chinese hamster overy cells. Radiat Res 99: 352–362

Mondovi B, Strom R, Rotilio G et al. (1969) The biochemical mechanism of selective heat sensitivity of cancer cells. I. Studies on cellular respiration. Eur J Cancer 5: 129–136

Morris CC, Field SB (1985) The relationship between heating time and temperature for rat tail necrosis with and without occlusion of the blood supply. Int J Radiat Biol 47: 41–48

Nagle WA, Moss AJ Jr (1983) Inhibitors of poly (ADP-ribose) synthetase enhance the cytotoxicity of 42°C and 45°C hyperthermia in cultured Chinese hamster cells. Int J Radiat Biol 44: 475–481

Nagle WA, Moss AJ, Baker ML (1982) Increased lethality at 42°C for hypoxic Chinese hamster cells heated under conditions of energy deprivation. Natl Cancer Inst Monogr 61: 107–110

Nielsen OS (1984) Franctionated hyperthermia and thermotolerance. Dan Med Bull 31: 376–390

Nielsen OS, Overgaard J (1982) Influence of time and temperature on the kinetics of thermotolerance in L1A2 cells in vitro. Cancer Res 42: 4190–4196

Ohyama H, Yamada T (1980) Reduction of rat thymocyte interphase death by hyperthermia. Radiat Res 82: 342–351

Ossovski L, Sachs L (1967) Temperature sensitivity of polyoma virus: induction of cellular DNA synthesis and multiplication of transformed cells at high temperatures. Proc Natl Acad Sci USA 58: 1938–1945

Overgaard J (1976) Ultrastructure of a murine mammary carcinoma exposed to hyperthermia in vivo. Cancer Res 36: 983–995

Overgaard J, Suit H (1979) Time-temperature relationship in hyperthermic treatment of malignant and normal tissue in vivo. Cancer Res 39: 3248–3253

Palzer R, Heidelberger C (1973) Influence of drugs and synchrony on the hyperthermic killing of HeLa cells. Cancer Res 33: 422–427

Panniers R, Henshaw EC (1984) Mechanism of inhibition of polypeptide chain initiation in heat-shocked Ehrlich ascites tumour cells. Eur J Biochem 140: 209–214

Pincus G, Fischer A (1931) The growth and death of tissue cultures exposed to supranormal temperatures. J Exp Med 54: 323–332

Power J, Harris J (1977) Response of extremely hypoxic cells to hyperthermia: survival and oxygen enhancement ratios for exponential and plateau-phase cultures. Radiology 123: 767–770

Privalov PL (1979) Stability of proteins. Adv Protein Chem 33: 167–241

Raaphorst GP, Spiro IJ, Azzam EJ, Sargent M (1987) Normal cells and malignant cells transfected with the H-*ras* oncogene have the same heat sensitivity in culture. Int J Hyperthermia 3: 209–216

Reeves O (1982) Mechanism of acquired resistance to acute heat shock in cultured mammalian cells. J Cell Physiol 79: 157–159

Reinhold HS, Wike-Hooley JL, van den Berg AP, van den Berg-Blok A (1985) Environmental factors, blood flow and microcirculation. In: Overgaard J (ed) Hyperthermic oncology 1984, vol 2. Taylor & Francis, London, pp 41–52

Rofstad EK, Brustad T (1986) Arrhenius analysis of the heat response in vivo and in vitro of human melanoma xenografts. Int J Hyperthermia 2: 359–368

Rofstad EK, Wahl A, Tveit KM, Monge OR, Brustad T (1985) Survival curves after X-ray and heat treatments for melanoma cells derived directly from surgical specimens of tumours in man. Radiother Oncol 4: 33–44

Roti Roti JL (1982) Heat-induced cell death and radiosensitization: molecular mechanisms. Natl Cancer Inst Monogr 61: 3–9

Roti Roti JL, Henle KJ (1979) Comparison of two mathematical models for describing heat-induced cell killing. Radiat Res 78: 522–531

Roti Roti JL, Turkel N, Laszlo A (1993) Heat-induced alterations which may play a role in radieseusitization of Hela cells. In: Hyperthermic Oncology, Gerner EW and Cetas Th.C (eds) Arizona Board of Regents, pp 99–101

Roti Roti JL, Painter RB (1982) Effects of hyperthermia on the sedimentation of nucleoids from HeLa cells in sucrose gradients. Radiat Res 89: 166–175

Rowley R, Joyner DE, Stewart JR (1987) In vitro response to hyperthermia or X-irradiation of diploid and tetraploid RIF-1 cells separated by centrifugal elutriation. Int J Hyperthermia 3: 235–244

Ruifrok ACC, Kanon B, Hulstaart CE, Konings AWT (1984) Permeability change of cells treated with hyperthermia alone and in combination with x-irradiation. In: Overgaard J (ed) Hyperthermic oncology, vol I. Taylor and Francis, London, pp 65–68

Ruifrok ACC, Kanon B, Konings AWT (1985a) Correlation between cellular survival and potassium loss in mouse fibroblasts after hyperthermia alone and after a combined treatment with X-rays. Radiat Res 101: 326–331

Ruifrok ACC, Kanon B, Konings AWT (1985b) Correlation of colony forming ability of mammalian cells with potassium content after hyperthermia under different experimental conditions. Radiat Res 103: 452–454

Ruifrok ACC, Kanon B, Konings AWT (1986) Na^+/K^+ ATPase activity in mouse lung fibroblasts and HeLa S-3 cells during and after hyperthermia. Int J Hyperthermia 2: 51–59

Ruifrok ACC, Kanon B, Konings AWT (1987) Heat-induced K^+ loss, trypan blue uptake, and cell lysis in different cell lines: effect of serum. Radiat Res 109: 303–309

Sapareto SA, Hopwood L, Dewey W, Raju M, Gray J (1978) Effects of hyperthermia on survival and progression of Chinese hamster ovary cells. Cancer Res 38: 393–400

Schlag H, Lücke-Huhle C (1976) Cytokinetic studies on the effect of hyperthermia on Chinese hamster lung cells. Eur J Cancer 12: 827–831

Schubert B, Streffer C, Tamulevicius P (1982) Glucose metabolism in mice during and after whole-body hyperthermia. Natl Cancer Inst Monogr 61: 203–205

Schulman N, Hall E (1974) Hyperthermia: its effect on proliferative and plateau phase cell cultures. Radiology 113: 207–209

Shall S (1984) ADR-ribose in DNA repair: a new component of DNA excision repair. Adv Radiat Biol 11: 1–69

Shenoy MA, Singh BB (1985) Temperature dependent modification of radiosensitivity following hypoxic cytocidal action of dechlorpromazine. Radiat Environ Biophys 24: 113–117

Simard R, Bernhard W (1967) A heat-sensitive cellular function located in the nucleolus. J Cell Biol 34: 61–76

Simpson ThA, La Russa PG, Mullins DW, Daugherty JP (1987) Restoration of hyperthermia-associated increased protein to DNA ratio of nucleoids. Int J Hyperthermia 3: 49–62

Singer SJ, Nicolson GI (1972) The fluid mosaic model of the structure of cell membranes. Science 175: 720–731

Skibba JL, Collins FG (1978) Effect of temperature on biochemical functions in the isolated perfused rat liver. J Surg Res 24: 435–441

Song CW, Clement SS, Levitt SH (1977) Cytotoxic and radiosensitizing effects of 5-thio-d-glucose hypoxic cells. Radiology 123: 201–205

Spiro IJ, Denman DL, Dewey WC (1982) Effect of hyperthermia on CHO DNA polymerase-α and β. Radiat Res 89: 134–139

Stevenson MA, Minton KW, Hahn GM (1981) Survival and concanavalin-A-induced capping in CHO fibroblasts after exposure to hyperthermia, ethanol, and X-irradiation. Radiat Res 86: 467–478

Streffer C (1963) Reaktivität und Struktur von Aminosäuren und Proteinen (Cystein and β-Galaktosidase). Dissertation, Universität Freiburg i.Br

Streffer C (1982) Aspects of biochemical effects by hyperthermia. Natl Cancer Inst Monogr 61: 11–16

Streffer C (1985a) Mechanism of heat injury. In: Overgaard J (ed) Hyperthermic oncology 1984. Taylor & Francis, London, vol 2, pp 213–222

Streffer C (1985b) Metabolic changes during and after hyperthermia. Int J Hyperthermia 1: 305–319

Streffer C (1987) Biological basis for the use of hyperthermia in tumour therapy. Strahlentherapie 163: 416–419

Streffer C (1988) Aspects of metabolic changes of hyperthermia. Recent Results Cancer Res 107: 7–16

Streffer C (1990) Biological basis of thermotherapy (with special reference to oncology). In: Gautherie M (ed) Biological basis on oncologic thermotherapy. Springer, Berlin Heidelberg New York, pp 1–71

Streffer C, van Beuningen D (1985) Zelluläre Strahlenbiologie und Strahlenpathologie (Ganz- und Teilkörperbestrahlung). In: Diethelm L, Heuck F, Olsson O, Strnad F, Vieten H, Zuppinger A (eds) Handbuch der medizinischen Radiologie, vol xx. Springer Berlin Heidelberg New York, pp 1–39

Streffer C, Tamulevicius P, Schmidt K (1983a) Poly (ADPR) synthetase activity in melanoma cells after hyperthermia and radiation. Radiat Res 94: 589 (abstract)

Streffer C, van Beuningen D, Bertholdt G, Zamboglou N (1983b) Some aspects of radiosensitization by hyperthermia: neutrons and x-rays. In: Kano E (ed) Fundamentals of cancer therapy by hyperthermia, radiation and chemicals. MAG Bros, Tokyo, pp 121–134

Strom R, Crifo C, Rossi-Fanelli A, Mondovi B (1977) Biochemical aspects of heat sensitivity of tumor cells. In: Rossi-Fanelli A, Cavaliere R, Mondovi B, Morrica G (eds) Selective heat sensitivity of cancer cells. Springer, Berlin Heidelberg New York, pp 7–35

Suit HD, Shwayder M (1974) Hyperthermia: potential as an anti-tumor agent. Cancer 34: 122–129

Takeda M, Majima H, Okada S, Suzuki N, Kubodera A (1987) Surviving fractions and cure-rate in spheroids by x-rays or heat. In: Onoyama, Y (ed) Hyperthermic oncology '86 in Japan. MAG Bros, Tokyo, pp 157–158

Tamulevicius P, Streffer C (1983) Does hyperthermia produce increased lysosomal enzyme activity? Int J Radiat Biol 43: 321–327

Tamulevicius P, Schmidt K, Streffer C (1984) The effects of X-irradiation, hyperthermia and combined modality treatment on poly (ADPR) synthetase activity in human melanoma cells. Radiat Res 100: 65–77

Terasima T, Tolmach LJ (1963a) Variations in several responses of HeLa cells to X-irradiation during the division cycle. Biophys J 3: 11–33

Terasima T, Tolmach LJ (1963b) X-ray sensitivity and DNA synthesis in synchronously dividing populations of HeLa cells. Science 140: 490–492

von Ardenne M (1982) Hyperthermia and cancer therapy Adv Pharmacol Chemother 10: 339

von Ardenne M, Reitnauer P (1976) Verstärkung der mit Glukoseinfusion erzielbaren Tumorübersäuerung in vivo durch NAD. Arch Geschwulstforsch 30: 319–330

von Ardenne M, Chaplain R, Reitnauer P (1969) Selektive Krebszellenschädigung durch eine Attackenkombination mit Übersäuerung, Hyperthermie, Vitamin A, Dimethylsulfoxid und weiteren die Freisetzung lysosomaler Enzyme fördernden Agenzien. Arch Geschwulstforsch 33: 331–344

Vaupel P, Kallinowski F (1987) Physiological effects of hyperthermia. In: Streffer C (ed) Hyperthermia and the therapy of malignant tumors. Recent Results in Cancer Research, vol 104. Springer, Berlin Heidelberg New York, pp 71–109

Vaupel P (1990) Pathophysiological mechanisms of hyperthermia in cancer therapy. In: Gautherie M (ed) Biological basis of oncologic thermotherapy. Springer, Berlin, Heidelberg New York, pp 73–134

Verma SP, Wallach DFH (1976) Erythrocyte membranes undergo cooperative, pH-sensitive state transitions in the physiological temperature range: evidence from Raman spectroscopy. Proc Natl Acad Sci USA 73: pp 3558–3561

Vexler AM, Litinskaya LL (1986) Changes in intracellular pH induced by hyperthermia and hypoxia. Int J Hyperthermia 2: 75–81

Vidair CA, Dewey WC (1986) Evaluation of a role of Na^+, K^+, Ca^{2+}, and Mg^{2+} in hyperthermic cell killing. Radiat Res 105: 187–200

Volk T, Jähde E, Fortmeyer HP, Glüsenkamp K-H, Rajewsky MF (1993) pH in human tumour xenografts: effect of intravenous administration of glucose. Br J Cancer 68: 492–500

van Beuningen D, Streffer C (1988) Importance of thermotolerance for radiothermotherapy as assessed using two human melanoma cell lines. Recent Results Cancer Res 109: 203–213

van Beuningen D, Molls M, Schulz S, Streffer C (1978) Effects of irradiation and hyperthermia on the development of preimplanted mouse embryos in vitro. In: Streffer C Cancer therapy by hyperthermia and radiation. Urban & Schwarzenberg, Baltimore, pp 151–153

Wallach DHF (1977) Basic mechanisms in tumor thermotherapy. J Mol Med 2: 381–403

Wallach DHF (1978) Action of hyperthermia and ionizing radiation on plasma membranes: In: Streffer C, van Beuningen D, Dietzel F et al. (eds) Cancer therapy by hyperthermia and radiation. Urban & Schwarzenberg, Munich, pp 19–28

Wallenfels K, Streffer C (1964) Chemische Reaktivität von Proteinen. In: "14. Colloquium der Gesellschaft für Physiologische Chemie in Mosbach/Baden". Springer, Berlin Göttingen Heidelberg, pp 6–40

Wallenfels K, Streffer C (1966) Das Dissoziationsverhalten von Cystein und verwandten SH-Verbindungen. Biochem Z 346: 119–132

Warburg O, Wind F, Negelein E (1926) Über den Stoffwechsel von Tumoren im Körper Klin Wochenschr 5: 829–834

Warocquier R, Scherrer K (1969) RNA metabolism in mammalian cells at elevated temperature. Eur J Biochem 10: 362–370

Warters RL, Roti Roti JL (1982) Hyperthermia and the cell nucleus. Radiat Res 92: 458–462

Warters RL, Stone OL (1983) Effects of hyperthermia on DNA replication in HeLa cells. Radiat Res 93: 71–84

Warters RL, Brizgys LM, Sharma R, Roti Roti JL (1986) Heat shock (45°C) results in an increase of nuclear matrix protein mass is HeLa cells. Int J Radiat Biol 50: 253–268

Weber G (1983) Biochemical strategy of cancer cells and the design of chemotherapy: G.H.A. Glowes memorial lecture. Cancer Res 43: 3466–3492

Westra A, Dewey WC (1971) Heat shock during the cell cycle of Chinese hamster cells in vitro. Int J Radiat Biol 19: 467–477

Wiegant F, Karelaars A, Blok F, Linnemanns W (1984) Effects of extracellular Ca^{2+} concentrations upon hyperthermia induced cell death. In: Overgaard J (ed) Hyperthermic oncology, vol 1. Taylor & Fancis, London, pp 3–6

Wong RSL, Dewey WC (1982) Molecular studies on the hyperthermic inhibition of DNA synthesis in Chinese hamster ovary cells. Radiat Res 92: 370–395

Wong RSL, Kapp LN, Dewey WC (1989) DNA fork displacement rate measurements in heated Chinese hamster ovary cells. Biochim Biophys Acta 1007: 224–227

Yatvin MB (1977) The influence of membrane lipid composition and procaine on hyperthermic death of cells. Int J Radiat Biol 32: 513–521

Yatvin MB, Cree TC, Elson CE, Gipp JJ, Tegmo I-M, Vorpahl JW (1982) Probing the relationship of membrane "fluidity" to heat killing of cells. Radiat Res 89: 644–646

Yatvin MB, Abuirmeileh NM, Vorphal JW, Elson CE (1983) Biological optimization of hyperthermia: modification of tumor membrane lipids. Eur J Cancer 19: 657–663

Yi PN (1983) Hyperthermia-induced intracellular ionic level changes in tumor cells. Radiat Res 93: 534–544

Zölzer F, Streffer C, Pelzer T (1993a) Induction of quiescent S-phase cells by irradiation and/or hyperthermia. I. Time and dose dependence. Int J Radiat Biol 63: 69–76

Zölzer F, Streffer C, Pelzer T (1993b) Induction of quiescent S-phase cells by irradiation and/or hyperthermia. II. Correlation with colony forming ability. Int J Radiat Biol 63: 77–82

3 Thermotolerance

P. BURGMAN, A. NUSSENZWEIG, and G.C. LI

CONTENTS

3.1 Introduction

One of the most interesting aspects of thermal biology in the mammalian system is the response of heated cells to subsequent heat challenges. Mammalian cells, when exposed to a nonlethal heat shock, have the ability to acquire a transient resistance to one or more subsequent exposures at elevated temperatures. This phenomenon has been termed thermotolerance (GERNER and SCHNEIDER 1975; HENLE and LEEPER 1976). It has been studied most extensively in mammalian cells, largely because of the interest in the use of heat as an adjuvant technique for the treatment of some human cancers (HAHN 1982). The clinical application of hyperthermia, in general, involves multiple exposures of tumors to elevated temperatures. Clearly, it is important to know whether a past treatment affects the response of cells to a subsequent heat exposure. Therefore, the kinetics of induction and decay of thermotolerance are of great interest. Furthermore, it is equally important to determine whether the radiation (or drug) sensitivity of cells surviving hyperthermic exposures has been modified. Many studies have examined the response of thermotolerant cells to drugs or x-irradiation (see Chaps. 4 and 5 in this volume).

The mechanism(s) for the development of thermotolerance is not well understood, but earlier experimental evidence suggests that protein synthesis may play a role in its manifestation. On the molecular level, heat shock activates a specific set of genes, so-called heat shock genes, and results in the preferential synthesis of heat shock proteins (hsps). Heat shock response, specifically the regulation, expression, and functions of hsps, has been extensively studied in the past decades, and has attracted the attention of a wide spectrum of investigators ranging from molecular and cell biologists to radiation and hyperthermia oncologists. There is a large body of data supporting the hypothesis that hsps play important roles in modulating cellular response to heat shock or other environmental stress, and are involved in the development of thermotolerance.

This review summarizes our current knowledge on the induction of thermotolerance by heat shock and other environmental stresses, the biochemical and molecular mechanisms for the induction of thermotolerance, the role of hsps in the development of thermotolerance, and the characterization of transiently thermotolerant cells.

3.2 Induction of Thermotolerance

Exposure of mammalian cells to temperatures above 40°C leads to a gradual loss of the cells' reproductive capacity (reproductive cell death). The amount of cell killing is dependent on the temperature and the duration of the exposure (Fig. 3.1). However, it has been shown that

P. BURGMAN, PhD, Departments of Medical Physics and Radiation Oncology, Memorial Sloan-Kettering Cancer Center, 1275 York Avenue, New York, NY 10021, USA
A. NUSSENZWEIG, PhD, Departments of Medical Physics and Radiation Oncology, Memorial Sloan-Kettering Cancer Center, 1275 York Avenue, New York, NY 10021, USA
G.C. LI, PhD, Departments of Medical Physics and Radiation Oncology, Memorial Sloan-Kettering Cancer Center, 1275 York Avenue, New York, NY 10021, USA

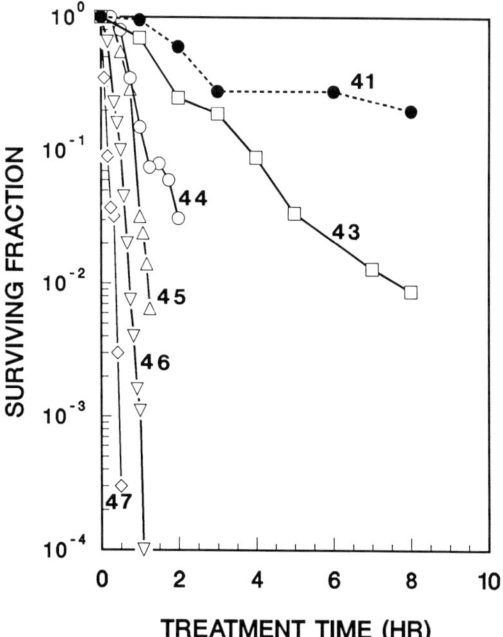

Fig. 3.1. Survival curves for human 293 cells heated at different temperatures for varying periods: ●, 41°C; □, 43°C; ○, 44°C; △, 45°C; ▽, 46°C; ◇, 47°C. The surviving fraction was determined by the colony formation assay (Li, unpublished)

cells exposed to a nonlethal heat treatment can develop a transient resistance against a subsequent heat challenge, a phenomenon termed thermotolerance (Gerner and Schneider 1975; Henle and Leeper 1976). In vitro, thermotolerance can be induced by either a long (1–20 h) exposure to a low hyperthermic temperature (<43°C), or a short (<1 h) exposure to a higher hyperthermic temperature followed by incubation at 37°C. The amount of thermotolerance expressed depends on the temperature and duration of the first heat treatment, as well as on the length of the interval between the two heat treatments (Li et al. 1982a; Li and Hahn 1980). An example is shown in Fig. 3.2. These data indicate that at temperatures of 43°C and higher, thermotolerance does not develop during the first heat exposure. A subsequent incubation at 37°C is required for its expression. On the other hand, if the initial treatment is at 41°C, thermotolerance is almost completely developed at the end of the first heat treatment.

Based on these data an operational model for the development of thermotolerance was formulated (Fig. 3.3) (Li and Hahn 1980). In this model, thermotolerance is divided into three complementary processes: an initial event ("trigger"), the expression of resistance ("development"), and the gradual disappearance of resistance ("decay"). Each of these components may have its own temperature dependence as well as dependence on other factors such as pH and nutrients. Conceptually, the three components of thermotolerance may be considered to be

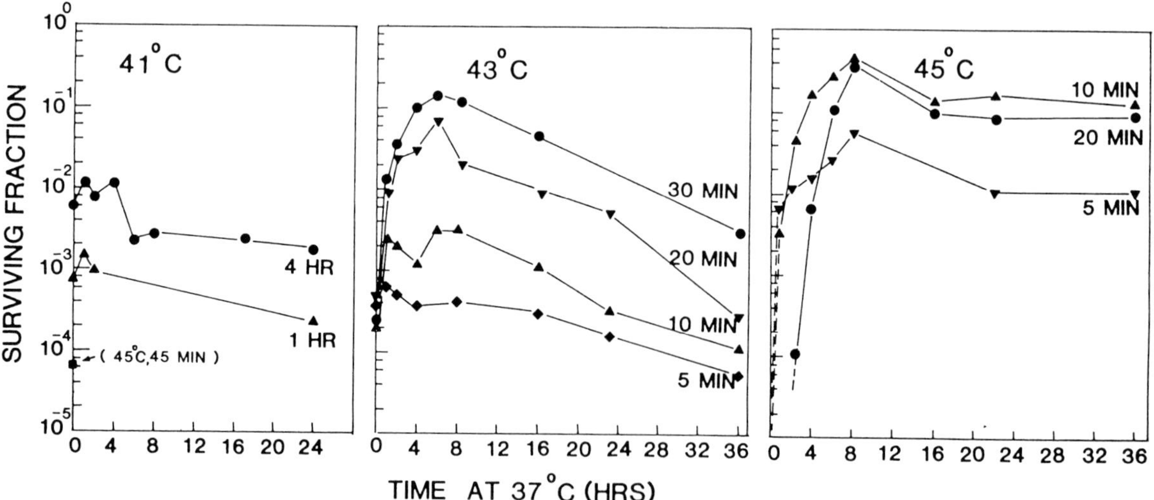

Fig. 3.2. Kinetics of induction of thermotolerance in plateau-phase HA-1 cells. Cells were initially exposed to the designated temperature for the duration noted. In each case the second heat treatment was 45°C for 45 min. The surviving fractions are plotted as a function of the duration of the 37°C incubations between the first and second heat treatments. Note that survival at 0 h is at (or near) maximum if the initial treatment was 41°C. This is in contrast to the survival kinetics following the initial treatments at higher temperatures, where survival at 0 time is minimal; an incubation interval at 37°C is required before thermotolerance manifests itself (Li et al. 1982a)

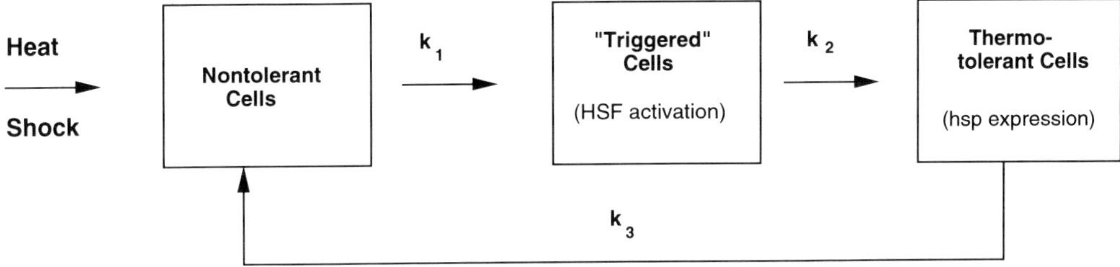

Fig. 3.3. Phenomenological model of thermotolerance development and decay. Thermotolerance develops in two steps: First, a triggering event (e.g., heat shock) converts nontolerant cells to the triggered state. Thermotolerance then develops at a rate determined by the highly temperature sensitive constant, k_2. Finally, thermotolerant cells reconvert to their sensitive state at a slow rate governed by k_3

independent processes. However, independent measurements of each component are not always possible.

Thermotolerance develops in at least two steps. First, the triggering event converts normal cells to the triggered state with a rate constant k_1. This process very likely involves the activation of the heat shock transcription factor, HSF1 (Lis and Wu 1993; Morimoto 1993). Second, these triggered cells are converted to thermotolerant cells with a rate constant k_2. Above 43°C, $k_2 = 0$; the triggered cells remain sensitive, and only after being transferred to 37°C do they convert to thermotolerant cells. This thermotolerant state, in general, is associated with the elevated expression of hsps and enhanced protection against and faster recovery from thermal damage. Finally, thermotolerant cells all reconvert to their sensitive state at a slower rate governed by rate constant k_3.

Thermotolerance can also be induced by treatment of cells with a variety of chemicals followed by a drug-free period before the heat challenge. A list showing some examples of the thermotolerance-inducing chemicals is given in Table 3.1.

As shown in Fig. 3.4, pretreatment with heat or chemicals induces not only thermotolerance but also resistance against the toxic action of the tested chemicals. This development of cross-resistance suggests similarities in the mechanism of induction of tolerance by heat and chemicals,

Table 3.1. Relation between induction of thermotolerance and induction of hsp synthesis

Thermotolerance inducing treatment	Hsp synthesis	Reference
Heat	+	Laszlo (1988b), Li (1983)
Heavy metals	+	Li and Mivechi (1986)
Ethanol	+	Boon-Niermeijer et al. (1988), Burgman et al. (1993), Henle et al. (1986), Li (1983), Li and Hahn (1978)
Sodium/arsenite	+	Crete and Landry (1990), Kampinga et al. (1992), Li (1983)
Procaine, lidocaine	+	Hahn et al. (1985)
Aliphatic alcohols (C_5–C_8)	+	Hahn et al. (1985)
Dinitrophenol[a]	0	Boon-Niermeijer et al. (1986), Haveman et al. (1986)
	+[c]	Ritossa (1962, 1963)
CCP[a]	+	Haveman et al. (1986)
Puromycin[b]	+	Lee and Dewey (1987)
Prostaglandin A	+	Amici et al. (1993)

+, increased; 0, unaffected

[a] No induction of thermotolerance or hsp synthesis was observed by Rastogi et al. (1988); this might, however, have been due to the long interval between DNP or CCP treatment and test heating, and the low concentrations of CCP and DNP used.

[b] Only at intermediate concentrations of puromycin (3–30 μg/ml) that inhibit protein synthesis by 15%–80%; not at higher concentrations.

[c] Induction of new puffs in *Drosophila* salivary gland giant chromosomes was observed, a phenomenon shown to be involved in the induction of synthesis of new proteins (Tissieres et al. 1974).

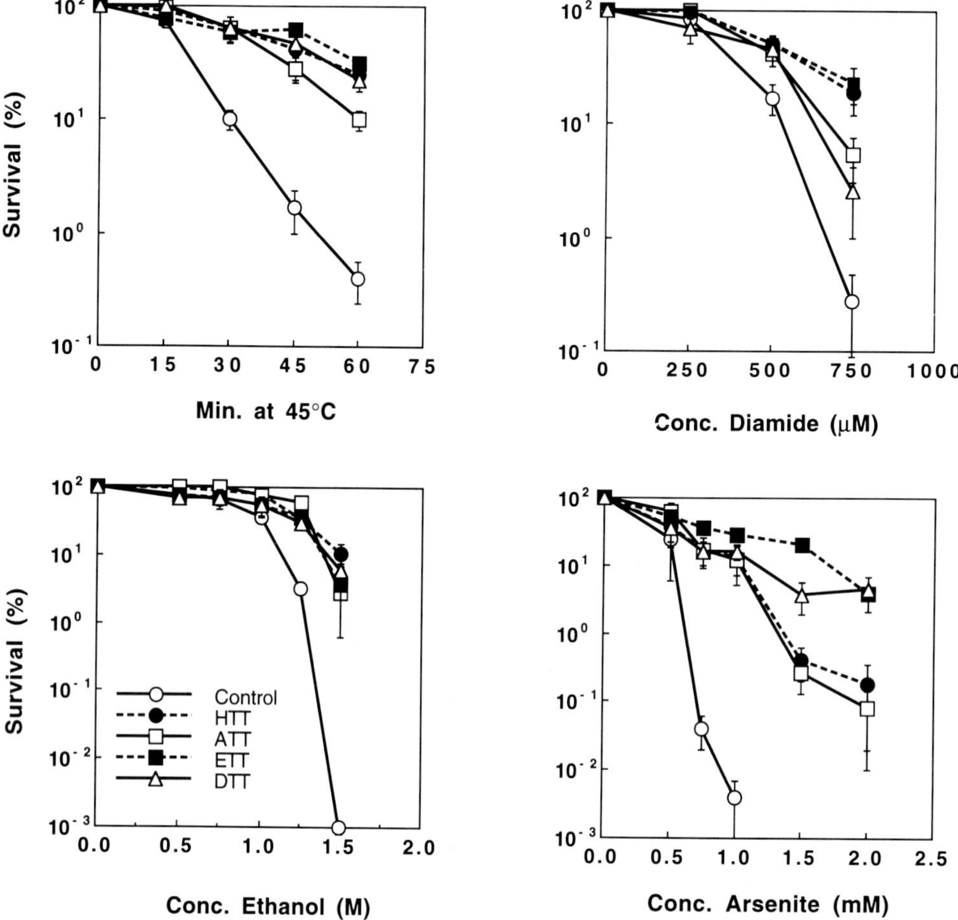

Fig. 3.4. Stress-induced resistance against the cytotoxicity of heat, sodium arsenite, diamide, and ethanol. HeLa S3 cells were pretreated with heat (15 min 44°C + 5 h 37°C: *HTT*), sodium arsenite (1 h 100 μM + 5 h 37°C: *ATT*), diamide (1 h 500 μM + 5 h 37°C: *DTT*), or ethanol (1 h 6% + 4 h 37°C: *ETT*), or left untreated (*Control*) before exposure to heat (45°C) or 1-h incubations at 37°C with different concentrations of sodium arsenite, diamide, or ethanol. Survival data are corrected for the toxicity of the tolerance-inducing treatments. (KAMPINGA, et al., 1995-personal communication)

and is indicative of the existence of one mechanism capable of protecting the cells against a wide variety of stresses.

3.3 Role of Heat Shock Proteins in the Development of Thermotolerance

When cells are exposed to a heat shock a specific set of proteins, hsps, is preferentially synthesized. Since this set of proteins can be induced after exposure of cells to a variety of other stresses, these proteins are also referred to as stress proteins (sps). These (h)sps are usually identified by their molecular mass, e.g., (h)sp27 is a heat shock protein with a molecular mass of 27 000 daltons.

In mammals, hsps with molecular masses of 27 (28), 40, 47, 56, 60 (58), 70, 90, and 110 kD are synthesized. A list of these hsps, with their cellular localization before and after heat shock, and (if known) their function, is shown in Table 3.2. The most extensively studied hsps with respect to their role in thermotolerance and cullular heat senstivity are hsp27 (CRETE and LANDRY 1990; LANDRY et al. 1989), hsp70 (ANGELIDIS et al. 1991; LI 1985; LI et al. 1991), and hsp90 (BANSAL et al. 1991; YAHARA et al. 1986). The role of the other hsps in thermotolerance and cellular heat resistance is unclear as yet. It has, however, been reported that in yeast hsp104 (the yeast homologue of hsp110) is required for the development of thermotolerance (SANCHEZ and LINDQUIST 1990).

Table 3.2. Intracellular localization of the main mammalian hsps under physiological conditions and after heat stress

hsp	Localization		Remarks	References
	Normal	After HT		
28	Cytoplasm near Golgi apparatus	Cytoplasm Nucleus	Increased phosphorylation after stress, forms aggregates	CRETE and LANDRY (1990), WELCH (1990), Arrigo et al. (1988)
40	Cytoplasm	Cytoplasm Nucleus	Co-localizes with hsp70, homology with *E. coli* DnaJ	OHTSUKA et al. (1990), HATTORI et al. (1992)
47	Endoplasmic reticulum	Endoplasmic reticulum	Basic pI, binds collagen	NAGATA et al. (1986), NAGATA and YAMADA (1986)
56	Cytoplasm	Cytoplasm	Found in complexes with hsp70/hsc70, hsp90, and steroid receptors	SANCHEZ (1990), SANCHEZ et al. (1990)
60	Mitochondria	Mitochondria	Catalyzes protein assembly, homology with GroEL	FRYDMAN and HARTL (1994), MIZZEN et al. (1989), OSTERMANN et al. (1989)
72 (hsp70)	Cytoplasm	Cytoplasm Nucleus Nucleoli	In primates constitutively expressed, in other mammals only after stress; dissociates some protein aggregates	LINDQUIST and CRAIG (1988), MORIMOTO et al. (1990), WELCH (1990)
73 (hsc70)	Cytoplasm	Cytoplasm Nucleus Nucleoli	Related to hsp72; associated with steroid receptors; involved in translocation of proteins across cellular membranes	LINDQUIST and CRAIG (1988), MORIMOTO et al. (1990), WELCH (1990)
90	Cytoplasm	Cytoplasm Nucleus	Associated with several receptors and protein kinases, dissociates from complex after heat shock	PRATT (1990), COLLIER and Schlesinger (1986), BOHEN and YAMAMOTO (1994)
110	Nucleus Nucleoli	Nucleus Nucleoli	May protect ribosome production during prolonged heating	KOCHEVAR et al. (1991), LINDQUIST and CRAIG (1988)

Stress-induced activation of genes coding for hsps has been shown for almost all cells and organisms studied so far. Only undifferentiated cells such as mammalian embryos before the 16- to 32-cell stage (BANERJI et al. 1984, 1987; DURA 1981; MULLER et al. 1985; WITTIG et al. 1983) show no heat shock response. Comparison of heat shock genes and proteins from different species has shown that hsps are among the most highly conserved proteins in nature (BARDWELL and CRAIG 1984, 1987; HUNT and MORIMOTO 1985; MORIMOTO and MILARSKI 1990; MORIMOTO et al. 1990; WELCH 1990). For example, the human hsp70 and its *E. coli* homologue DnaK are approximately 50% identical at the amino acid level (BARDWELL and CRAIG 1984; LINDQUIST and CRAIG 1988).

Although hsps were first noticed because of their increased synthesis upon heat treatment, most heat shock proteins are abundantly expressed under physiological conditions, and many are essential for cell viability (GEORGOPOULOS et al. 1990; LINDQUIST and CRAIG 1988). It has been shown that hsps are involved in processes like protein folding, assembly of proteins into oligomeric structures, and translocation of proteins across cellular membranes (see, e.g., CRAIG 1990; HENDRICK and HARTL 1993; MORIMOTO and MILARSKI 1990; PELHAM 1990; WELCH 1990; and Table 3.2). Hsps bind noncovalently and reversibly to a wide variety of hydrophobic protein surfaces that are transiently exposed during these processes, and this interaction shields the partially unfolded and denatured polypeptides from their tendency to form aggregates.

Heat shock proteins are also thought to be involved in the development of thermotolerance (LANDRY et al. 1989; LASZLO 1988a,b; LI and MAK

1985, 1989). In mammalian cells good correlations were reported for thermotolerance development and (a) hsp70 synthesis (HATAYAMA et al. 1991; LASZLO 1988b; LI 1985), (b) hsp27 synthesis (LEE et al. 1991), and (c) hsp27 phosphorylation (CRETE and LANDRY 1990; LANDRY et al. 1991). Conversely, reduction of the level of hsp70, either by competitive inhibition of hsp70 gene expression (JOHNSTON and KACEY 1988) or by microinjection of cells with antibodies against hsp70 (KHAN and SOTELO 1989; RIABOWOL et al. 1988), resulted in an enhanced thermosensitivity. Reduction of the cellular hsp90 levels have also been shown to increase thermosensitivity in mouse L cells (BANSAL et al. 1991), while an increased hsp90 expression resulted in stable heat resistance in CHO cells (YAHARA et al. 1986).

Recently, it has been reported that transfection of cells with genes coding for hsp27 (LANDRY et al. 1989) or hsp70 (ANGELIDIS et al. 1991; LI et al. 1991), which results in constitutive expression of the genes, confers heat resistance. Preliminary data in our laboratory show that transfection of rat cells with a gene coding for mycobacterial hsp65 (a homologue of the mammalian hsp60) also confers heat resistance to the transfected cells (BURGMAN et al., unpublished results). These data provide direct evidence for a causal relation between the expression of hsps and an increased heat resistance.

The mechanism by which hsps confer heat resistance is not clear. It is likely, however, that hsps perform similar functions during stress conditions as during physiological conditions, such as to bind to the improperly folded proteins and to prevent their aggregation. This protective mechanism has been shown for hsp27 (JAKOB et al. 1993), hsp90 (WIECH et al. 1992), and DnaK, the *E. coli* homologue of the mammalian hsp70 (LIBEREK et al. 1991). Thus the presence of extra hsps during heat shock probably reduces the amount of damage that is induced in thermotolerant cells.

A second possibility is that hsps are involved in the repair of heat-denatured proteins. It has been shown in vitro that DnaK can reactivate heat-inactivated RNA polymerase (SKOWYRA et al. 1990), and in collaboration with the *E. coli* hsps DnaJ and GrpE can renature heat-denatured lambda repressor (GAITANARIS et al. 1990). Thus the presence of extra hsps might accelerate the repair of heat-induced damage in thermotolerant cells.

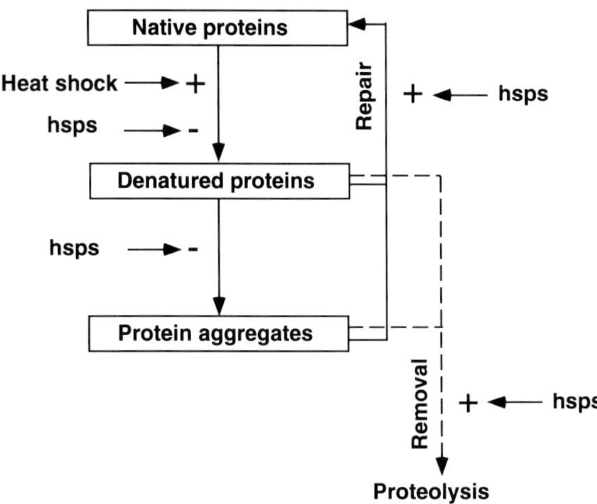

Fig. 3.5. Possible role(s) of hsps in the protection against and restoration from heat-induced protein denaturation and aggregation (− indicates retardation; + indicates enhancement). (Adapted from KAMPINGA 1993)

To summarize, it has been shown in vitro that hsps are capable of preventing aggregation of heat-denatured proteins and are capable of "repair" of heat-denatured proteins. Assuming that hsps perform the same functions in vivo, this would (at least partially) explain the increased heat resistance in cells with an increased amount of hsps. A schematic diagram showing these possible roles of hsps is shown in Fig. 3.5.

Additionally, hsps (especially the hsp70 family) may facilitate the degradation of denatured proteins, and in this way assist in the removal of the heat-induced damage. For a recent review on the involvement of hsps in lysosomal degradation of proteins, see DICE et al. (1994).

3.4 Biochemical and Molecular Mechanisms for Induction of Thermotolerance

Heat and most of the chemical inducers of thermotolerance have been shown to cause protein damage (HIGHTOWER 1980; VOELLMY 1985). Furthermore, the thermodynamics of the induction of the heat shock response have been shown to be consistent with protein denaturation (LI et al. 1982a). It has been suggested that intracellular accumulation of abnormal proteins acts as the trigger for the induction of thermotolerance (HIGHTOWER 1980; MUNRO and PELHAM 1985). Over the years this hypothesis has been supported by experimental data such as:

1. The synthesis of large amounts of abnormal proteins induced a heat shock response in *E. coli* (GOFF and GOLDBERG 1985).
2. Drosophila cells that produce truncated, non-functional actin molecules constitutively synthesize hsps (OKAMOTO et al. 1986).
3. Incubation of mammalian cells with amino acid analogs, which causes synthesis of abnormal proteins, induces a heat shock response (LASZLO and LI 1993; LI and LASZLO 1985).
4. Incubation of cells with puromycin in concentrations that inhibit protein synthesis by 15%–80% and cause the accumulation of truncated proteins, induces a heat shock response (LEE and DEWEY 1987).
5. Microinjection of denatured proteins into frog oocytes results in the activation of heat shock genes, whereas the injection of the same proteins in their native form does not activate these genes (ANANTHAN et al. 1986).
6. In situ cross-linking of intracellular proteins with alkylating agents or sulfhydryl compounds induces a heat shock response and the development of thermotolerance in CHO cells (LEE and HAHN 1988).

These results reinforce the hypothesis that the presence of abnormal proteins in the cell acts as a signal that triggers the heat shock response.

The first step in the heat shock response is the activation of heat shock genes. In eukaryotic cells, this activation process is mediated by a transcription factor known as heat shock factor (HSF) (MORIMOTO 1993; MORIMOTO et al. 1992). In unstressed cells, HSF is present in both the cytoplasm and the nucleus in a monomeric form that has no DNA binding activity. Upon heat shock, HSF assembles into a trimer and binds to the heat shock element (HSE), a specific DNA recognition sequence located in the 5′-flanking sequences of heat shock genes. In addition to trimerization and acquisition of DNA-binding competence, HSF exhibits, a stress-dependent phosphorylation that is thought to regulate its transcriptional activity (LARSON et al. 1988; SARGE et al. 1993). The heat-induced transcriptional response attenuates upon return to 37°C; this attenuation is accompanied by conversion of the active trimeric form of HSF to the non-DNA binding monomer and by a return to the normal subcellular distribution. In eukaryotic cells, the conversion of HSF from its monomeric inactive form to the trimeric active form is though to be controlled by a regulatory protein. It has been hypothesized that hsps themselves may negatively regulate the expression of heat shock genes via an autoregulatory loop (MORIMOTO 1993; MORIMOTO et al. 1992; SORGER 1991). A model of this autoregulatory loop is shown in Fig. 3.6. According to this hypothesis, the increased number of misfolded proteins induced by heat shock sequesters hsp70/hsc70, resulting in the activation of HSF (MORIMOTO 1993; MORIMOTO et al. 1992). In this model the transcriptional activity of heat responsive genes is entirely regulated by HSF. However, recent results from our group indicate a role for a second, negative regulator of heat shock gene expression (LIU et al. 1993).

3.5 Characterization of Thermotolerant Cells

So far, thermotolerance has only been discussed in terms of an increased survival after a heat

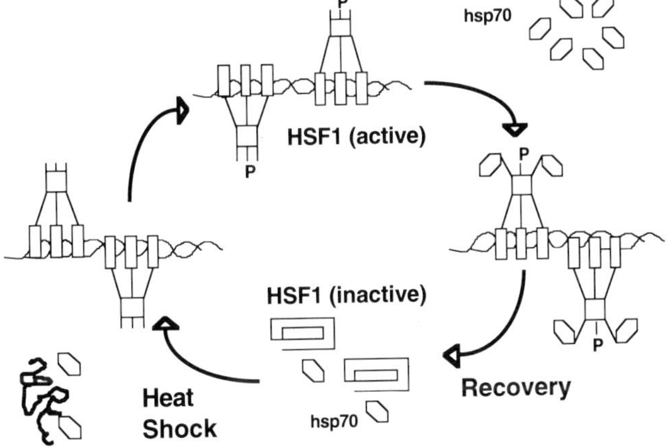

Fig. 3.6. Hypothetical autoregulatory loop for the expression of heat shock genes. In the unstressed cell, HSF1 is maintained in the monomeric, non-DNA-binding form through interactions with hsp70. Upon heat shock, hsp70 is sequestered by denatured protein, and HSF1 assembles into trimers which bind to heat shock elements and become phosphorylated. Transcriptional activation of the heat shock genes leads to increased levels of hsp70 and the formation of an HSF1–hsp70 complex. Finally, HSF1 dissociates from the HSE and is converted into its monomeric non-DNA binding form. (Redrawn from MORIMOTO 1993)

treatment. However, cell killing is the consequence of heat-induced damage to structures/functions within cells and the cell's capacity to repair this damage. When cells are heated, the absorption of energy is evenly distributed over the cell, resulting in damage to virtually all cellular structures/functions [see, e.g., LASZLO (1992) and Chap. 2 in this volume]. In thermotolerant cells, however, many of these structures/functions show an increased resistance against heat-induced alterations (Table 3.3).

The data listed in Table 3.3 show that thermotolerance develops for nuclear, cytoplasmic, and membrane properties. Thus within the cell there seems to be no spatial preference for the expression of tolerance. This led some authors to the conclusion that thermotolerance might represent a nonspecific protection of all parts of the cell (MINTON et al. 1982). There is, however, an increasing amount of data to suggest that the development of thermotolerance is much more specific than previously assumed. For example, when thermotolerance is induced by a sodium arsenite, diamide, or ethanol treatment, it has been shown that thermotolerance only develops in cellular fractions that are damaged during the thermotolerance-inducing treatment (Table 3.4). Thus the subcellular localization of the induced resistance appears to correspond with the localization of the damage induced during the tolerance-inducing treatment.

Several other reports in the literature also support the idea of a (spatial) correlation between damage and the expression of tolerance:

1. LUNEC and CRESSWELL (1983) observed an enhanced resistance of the ATP synthesis in thermotolerant cells, but only in a cell line (L5178Y-S) in which the ATP synthesis was affected by the tolerance-inducing heat treatment. In another cell line (Ehrlich ascites) this treatment had no effect on the ATP synthesis, and in the thermotolerant cells no enhanced resistance of this proces was observed.

Table 3.3. Characterization of the thermotolerant mammalian cell: molecules, cellular structures, or functions that are protected after a mild heat shock

Macromolecules, cellular structure and function	References
DNA	
Polymerase activity[a]	CHU and DEWEY (1987), DIKOMEY et al. (1987)
Synthesis	VAN DONGEN et al. (1984)
RNA	
rRNA synthesis	BURDON (1986), NOVER et al. (1986)
Splicing	YOST and LINDQUIST (1986)
Protein	
Synthesis	HAHN and SHIU (1985), MIZZEN and WELCH (1988), SCIANDRA and SUBJECK (1984)
Denaturation	LEPOCK et al. (1990), NGUYEN et al. (1989), PINTO et al. (1991)
Removal of aggregates	KAMPINGA et al. (1989), WALLEN and LANDIS (1990)
Membrane	
Con A capping	STEVENSON et al. (1981)
Na^+/K^+-ATPase[b]	ANDERSON and HAHN (1985), BURDON and CUTMORE (1982)
Permeability	MAYTIN et al. (1990)
Insulin receptors	CALDERWOOD and HAHN (1983)
Cytoplasm	
Cytoskeletal reorganization	WIEGANT et al. (1987)
cAMP levels	CALDERWOOD et al. (1985)
ATP levels[c]	LUNEC and CRESSWELL (1983)
Cell cycle progression	VAN DONGEN et al. (1984)

[a] Not observed by KAMPINGA et al. (1985) or JORRITSMA et al. (1986)
[b] ANDERSON and HAHN observed thermotolerance development for the ouabain binding capacity only; the heat sensitivity of the ATP hydrolyzing activity was unchanged in thermotolerant cells
[c] Only in L5178Y-S cells; no resistance was observed in Ehrlich ascites cells

Table 3.4. Comparison of the damage and resistance induced in the membrane fraction (PF) and the nuclear fraction of HeLa S3 cells by different resistance-inducing agents

	TTR_{10}	Damage to membranes (by agent)	Enhanced resistance of membranes	Damage to nuclei (by agent)	Enhanced resistance of nuclei
C	(1.0)				
HTT	2.3	Yes	Yes	Yes	Yes
ATT	1.8	Yes[a]	Yes	No	No
DTT	2.5	ND	No	Yes	Yes
ETT	2.3	No	No	Yes	Yes

As a measure for the induced thermotolerance, the thermotolerance ratio is given (TTR_{10}: ratio of heating times required to reduce survival to 10%). Thermotolerance is induced as described in the legend to Fig. 3.4. Data from BURGMAN et al. (1993) and KAMPINGA et al. (1995, personal communication)

ND, not determined

[a] Taken from YIH et al. (1991)

2. NGUYEN et al. (1989), using firefly luciferase-transfected cells, found that heat treatments that decreased the luciferase activity but not protein synthesis in these cells, induced an increased heat resistance of the luciferase activity but not of the protein synthesis. After a priming treatment at a higher temperature (45°C instead of 42°C), both activities were impaired and in the thermotolerant cells resistance against a subsequent heat treatment was observed for both the luciferase activity and the protein synthesis.

3. Data reported by ANDERSON and HAHN (1985) indicate that the correlation between damage and induced resistance might even hold true for multidomain proteins in which the domains differ in heat sensitivity. These authors, working on Na^+/K^+-ATPase, reported that thermotolerance could be induced in a heat-sensitive domain of the protein (the ouabain-binding domain) without changing the heat sensitivity of a more heat-resistant domain (the ATP-hydrolyzing domain).

For all cellular proteins/structures/functions that have been studied it has been shown that thermotolerance can be induced. However, there are indications that thermotolerance is not a nonspecific protection of the entire cell, but is restricted to those targets in the cell that have been damaged during the thermotolerance-inducing treatment.

This direct correlation between damage and tolerance may open the possibility to study more directly the role of inactivation of different proteins/structures in hyperthermic cell killing.

The role of hsps in this protective mechanism is unclear. KAMPINGA et al. (1995-personal communication), using HeLa S3 cells, report a correlation between an enhanced resistance against heat-induced protein denaturation and an enhanced level of hsp70 in a crude membrane fraction. However, no correlation between heat resistance and the (enhanced) presence of hsps was found for the nuclear fraction isolated from the same cells.

3.6 Conclusion

Cells exposed to a nonlethal heat treatment, develop a transient increased resistance against a subsequent treatment. The correlation between the accumulation of hsps and the induction of thermotolerance suggests a vital role for hsps in thermotolerance. The fact that cells become permanently heat resistant when transfected with hsp70, and conversely, that cells become thermal sensitive when the levels of hsp70 are reduced, directly demonstrates the importance of hsp70 for the cellular heat sensitivity. Similarly, it has been shown that hsp27 and hsp90 have thermal protective functions. Heat shock has been shown to induce an increase in the number of denatured proteins which (according to Morimoto's hypothesis), through the depletion of the cellular hsp70 pool, might trigger the activation of HSF, which could result in the transcriptional activation of heat shock genes and the synthesis of additional hsps. This enhanced level of hsps facilitates the repair and the removal of the heat induced damage and can protect the cell against a subsequent heat treatment. Furthermore, thermotolerance can be detected on all levels in the cell (enzyme activity to cell survival) and a (spatial) relation might exist between the induction of damage and the expression of thermotolerance.

3.7 Summary

- Cells exposed to a nonlethal heat treatment develop a transient resistance against a subsequent heat treatment (thermotolerance)
- In thermotolerant cells, an enhanced thermal resistance can be observed for various cellular structures and functions, assuming that the particular structures/functions are damaged by the thermotolerance inducing treatment.
- Heat shock proteins (either constitutively present or newly synthesized) play a vital role in the development of thermotolerance
- Heat shock proteins can protect against protein denaturation, facilitate the recovery of heat-induced damage, and assist in the removal of denatured proteins.
- Thermal protective roles have been shown for hsp27, hsp70, and hsp90.
- The development of thermotolerance is triggered by heat induced protein denaturation.

References

Amici C, Palamara T, Santoro MG (1993) Induction of thermotolerance by prostaglandin A in human cells. Exp Cell Res 207: 230–234

Ananthan J, Goldberg AL, Voellmy R (1986) Abnormal proteins serve as eukaryotic stress signals and trigger the activation of heat shock genes. Science 232: 522–524

Anderson RL, Hahn GM (1985) Differential effects of hyperthermia on the Na^+,K^+-ATPase of Chinese hamster ovary cells. Radiat Res 102: 314–323

Angelidis CE, Lazaridis I, Pagoulatos GN (1991) Constitutive expression of heat-shock protein 70 in mammalian cells confers thermoresistance. Eur J Biochem 199: 35–39

Arrigo AP, Suhan JP, Welch WJ (1988) Dynamic changes in the structure and intracellular locale of the mammalian low-molecular-weight heat shock protein. Mol Cell Biol 8: 5059–5071

Banerji SS, Theodorakis NG, Morimoto RI (1984) Heat shock-induced translational control of HSP70 and globin synthesis in chicken reticulocytes. Mol Cell Biol 4: 2437–2448

Banerji SS, Laing K, Morimoto RI (1987) Erythroid lineage-specific expression and inducibility of the major heat shock protein HSP70 during avian embryogenesis. Genes Dev 1: 946–953

Bansal GS, Norton PM, Latchman DS (1991) The 90-kDa heat shock protein protects mammalian cells from thermal stress but not from viral infection. Exp Cell Res 195: 303–306

Bardwell JCA, Craig EA (1984) Major heat shock gene of *Drosophila* and the *Escherichia coli* heat-inducible dnaK gene are homologous. Proc Natl Acad Sci USA 81: 848–852

Bardwell JCA, Craig EA (1987) Eukaryotic M_r 83 000 heat shock protein has a homologue in *Escherichia coli*. Proc Natl Acad Sci USA 84: 5177–5181

Bohen SP, Yamamoto KR (1994) Modulation of steroid receptor signal transduction by heat shock proteins. In: Morimoto RI, Tissières A, Georgopoulos C (eds) The biology of heat shock proteins and molecular chaperones. Cold Spring Harbor Laboratory Press, New York, pp 313–334

Boon-Niermeijer EK, Tuyl M, Van der Scheur H (1986) Evidence for two states of thermotolerance. Int J Hyperthermia 2: 93–105

Boon-Niermeijer EK, Souren JEM, De Waal AM, Van Wijk R (1988) Thermotolerance induced by heat and ethanol. Int J Hyperthermia 4: 211–222

Burdon RH (1986) Heat shock and the heat shock proteins. Biochem J 240: 313–324

Burdon RH, Cutmore CMM (1982) Human heat shock gene expression and the modulation of Na^+,K^+-ATPase activity. FEBS Lett 140: 45–48

Burgman PWJJ, Kampinga HH, Konings AWT (1993) Possible role of localized protein denaturation in the induction of thermotolerance by heat, sodium-arsenite, and ethanol. Int J Hyperthermia 9: 151–162

Calderwood SK, Hahn GM (1983) Thermal sensitivity and resistance of insulin-receptor binding. Biochim Biophys Acta 756: 1–8

Calderwood SK, Stevenson MA, Hahn GM (1985) Cyclic AMP and the heat shock response in Chinese hamster ovary cells. Biochem Biophys Res Commun 126: 911–916

Chu GL, Dewey WC (1987) Effect of cycloheximide on heat-induced cell killing, radiosensitization, and loss of cellular DNA polymerase activities in Chinese hamster ovary cells. Radiat Res 112: 575–580

Collier NC, Schlesinger MJ (1986) The dynamic state of heat shock proteins in chicken embryo fibroblasts. J Cell Biol 103: 1495–1507

Craig EA (1990) Role of hsp70 in translocation of proteins across membranes. In: Morimoto RI, Tissieres A, Georgopoulos C (eds) Stress proteins in biology and medicine. Cold Spring Harbor Laboratory Press, New York, pp 279–286

Crete P, Landry J (1990) Induction of hsp27 phosphorylation and thermoresistance in chinese hamster cells by arsenite, cycloheximde, A23187, and EGTA. Radiat Res 121: 320–327

Dice JF, Agarraberes F, Kirven-Brooks M, Terlecky LJ, Terlecky SR (1994) Heat-shock 70-kD proteins and lysosomal proteolysis. In: Morimoto RI, Tissières A, Georgopoulos C (eds) The biology of heat shock proteins and molecular chaperones. Cold Spring Harbor Laboratory Press, New York, pp 137–151

Dikomey E, Becker W, Wielckens K (1987) Reduction of DNA-polymerase β activity of CHO cells by single and combined heat treatments. Int J Radiat Biol 52: 775–785

Dura JM (1981) Hsp synthesis is induced only after treatment at blastoderm and later stages in development. Mol Gen Genet 184: 73–79

Frydman J, Hartl F-U (1994) Molecular chaperone functions of hsp70 and hsp60 in protein folding. In: Morimoto RI, Tissières A, Georgopoulos C (eds) The biology of heat shock proteins and molecular chaperones. Cold Spring Harbor Laboratory Press, New York, pp 251–283

Gaitanaris GA, Papavassiliou AG, Rubock P, Silverstein SJ, Gottesman ME (1990) Renaturation of denatured λ repressor requires heat shock proteins. Cell 61: 1013–1020

Georgopoulos C, Ang D, Liberek K, Zylicz M (1990) Properties of the *E. coli* heat shock proteins and their role in bacteriophage lambda growth. In: Morimoto RI, Tissieres A, Georgopoulus C (eds) Stress proteins in biology and medicine. Cold Spring Harbor Laboratory Press, New York, pp 191–222

Gerner EW, Schneider MJ (1975) Induced thermal resistance in HeLa cells. Nature 256: 500–502

Goff SA, Goldberg LA (1985) Production of abnormal proteins in *E. coli* stimulates transcription of *lon* and other heat-shock genes. Cell 41: 587–595

Hahn GM (1982) Hyperthermia and cancer. Plenum Press, New York

Hahn GM, Shiu EC (1985) Protein synthesis, thermotolerance and step down heating. Int J Radiat Oncol Biol Phys 11: 159–164

Hahn GM, Shiu EC, West B, Goldstein L, Li GC (1985) Mechanistic implications of the induction of thermotolerance in Chinese hamster cells by organic solvents. Cancer Res 45: 4138–4143

Hatayama T, Kano E, Taniguchi Y, Nitta K, Wakatsuki T, Kitamura T, Imahara H (1991) Role of heat-shock proteins in the induction of thermotolerance in Chinese hamster V79 cells by heat and chemical agents. Int J Hyperthermia 7: 61–74

Hattori H, Liu Y-C, Tohnai I, et al. (1992) Intracellular localization and partial amino acid sequence of a stress-inducible 40 kDa protein in HeLa cells. Cell Struct Funct 17: 77–86

Haveman J, Li GC, Mak JY, Kipp JB (1986) Chemically induced resistance to heat treatment and stress protein synthesis in cultured mammalian cells. Int J Radiat Biol 50: 51–64

Hendrick JP, Hartl F-U (1993) Molecular chaperone functions of heat-shock proteins. Annu Rev Biochem 62: 349–384

Henle KJ, Leeper DB (1976) Interaction of hyperthermia and radiation in CHO cells: recovery kinetics. Radiat Res 66: 505–518

Henle KJ, Moss AJ, Nagle WA (1986) Temperature-dependent induction of thermotolerance by ethanol. Radiat Res 108: 327–335

Hightower LE (1980) Cultured animal cells exposed to amino acid analogues or puromycin rapidly synthesize several polypeptides. J Cell Physiol 102: 407–427

Hunt C, Morimoto RI (1985) Conserved features of eukaryotic hsp70 genes revealed by comparison with the nucleotide sequence of human hsp70. Proc Natl Acad Sci USA 82: 6455–6459

Jakob U, Gaestel M, Engel K, Buchner J (1993) Small heat shock proteins are molecular chaperones. J Biol Chem 268: 1517–1520

Johnston RN, Kacey BL (1988) Competitive inhibition of hsp70 gene expression causes thermosensitivity. Science 242: 1551–1554

Jorritsma JBM, Burgman P, Kampinga HH, Konings AWT (1986) DNA-polymerase activity in heat killing and hyperthermic radiosensitization of mammalian cells, as observed after fractionated heat treatments. Radiat Res 105: 307–319

Kampinga HH (1993) Thermotolerance in mammalian cells: protein denaturation, aggregation and stress proteins. J Cell Sci 104: 11–17

Kampinga HH, Jorritsma JBM, Konings AWT (1985) Heat-induced alterations in DNA polymerase activity of HeLa cells and of isolated nuclei. Relation to cell survival. Int J Radiat Biol 47: 29–40

Kampinga HH, Turkel-Uygur N, Roti Roti JL, Konings AWT (1989) The relationship of increased nuclear protein content induced by hyperthermia to killing of HeLa S3 cells. Radiat Res 117: 511–522

Kampinga HH, Brunsting JF, Konings AWT (1992) Acquisition of thermotolerance induced by heat and arsenite in HeLa cells: multiple pathways to induce tolerance? J Cell Physiol 150: 406–415

Khan NA, Sotelo J (1989) Heat shock stress is deleterious to CNS cultured neurons microinjected with anti-HSP70 antibodies. Biol Cell 65: 199–202

Kochevar DT, Aucoin MM, Cooper J (1991) Mammalian heat shock proteins: an overview with a systems perspective. Toxicol Lett 56: 243–267

Landry J, Chretien P, Lambert H, Hickey E, Weber LA (1989) Heat shock resistance conferred by expression of the human HSP27 gene in rodent cells. J Cell Biol 109: 7–15

Landry J, Chretien P, Laszlo A, Lambert H (1991) Phosphorylation of HSP27 during development and decay of thermotolerance in Chinese hamster cells. J Cell Physiol 147: 93–101

Larson JS, Schuetz TJ, Kingston RE (1988) Activation in vitro of sequence-specific DNA binding by a human regulatory factor. Nature 335: 372–375

Laszlo A (1988a) Evidence for two states of thermotolerance in mammalian cells. Int J Hyperthermia 4: 513–526

Laszlo A (1988b) The relationship of heat-shock proteins, thermotolerance, and protein synthesis. Exp Cell Res 178: 401–414

Laszlo A (1992) The effects of hyperthermia on mammalian cell structure and function. Cell Prolif 25: 59–87

Laszlo A, Li GC (1993) Effect of amino acid analogs on the development of thermotolerance and on thermotolerant cells. J Cell Physiol 154: 419–432

Lee K-J, Hahn GM (1988) Abnormal proteins as the trigger for the induction of stress responses: heat, diamide, and sodium arsenite. J Cell Physiol 136: 411–420

Lee YJ, Dewey WC (1987) Induction of heat shock proteins in Chinese hamster ovary cells and development of thermotolerance by intermediate concentrations of puromycin. J Cell Physiol 132: 1–11

Lee YJ, Curetty L, Corry PM (1991) Differences in preferential synthesis and redistribution of hsp70 and hsp28 families by heat and sodium arsenite in Chinese hamster ovary cells. J Cell Physiol 149: 77–87

Lepock JR, Frey HE, Heynen MP, Nishio J, Waters B, Ritchie KP, Kruuv J (1990) Increased thermostability of thermotolerant CHL V79 cells as determined by differential scanning calorimetry. J Cell Physiol 142: 628–634

Li GC (1983) Induction of thermotolerance and enhanced heat shock protein synthesis in Chinese hamster fibroblasts by sodium arsenite and by ethanol. J Cell Physiol 115: 116–122

Li GC (1985) Elevated levels of 70000 dalton heat shock protein in transiently thermotolerant Chinese hamster fibroblasts and in their stable heat resistant variants. Int J Radiat Oncol Biol Phys 11: 165–177

Li GC, Hahn GM (1978) Ethanol-induced tolerance to heat and to adriamycin. Nature 274: 699–701

Li GC, Hahn GM (1980) A proposed operational model of thermotolerance based on effects of nutrients and the initial treatment temperature. Cancer Res 40: 4501–4508

Li GC, Laszlo A (1985) Amino acid analogs while inducing heat shock proteins sensitize CHO cells to thermal damage. J Cell Physiol 122: 91–97

Li GC, Mak JY (1985) Induction of heat shock protein synthesis in murine tumors during the development of thermotolerance. Cancer Res 45: 3816–3824

Li GC, Mak JY (1989) Re-induction of hsp70 synthesis: an assay for thermotolerance. Int J Hyperthermia 5: 389–403

Li GC, Mivechi NF (1986) Thermotolerance in mammalian systems: a review. In: Anghileri LJ, Robert J (eds) Hyperthermia in cancer treatment. CRC Press, Boca Raton, Fl, pp 59–77

Li GC, Fisher GA, Hahn GM (1982a) Induction of thermotolerance and evidence for a well-defined, thermotropic cooperative process. Radiat Res 89: 361–368

Li GC, Fisher GA, Hahn GM (1982b) Modification of the thermal response by D2O. II. Thermotolerance and the specific inhibition of development. Radiat Res 92: 541–551

Li GC, Li L, Liu Y-K, Mak JY, Chen L, Lee WMF (1991) Thermal response of rat fibroblasts stably-transfected with the human 70 kDa heat shock protein-encoding gene. Proc Natl Acad Sci USA 88: 1681–1685

Liberek K, Skowyra D, Zylicz M, Johnson C, Georgopoulos C (1991) The *Escherichia coli* DnaK chaperone, the 70-kDa heat shock protein eukaryotic equivalent, changes conformation upon ATP hydrolysis, thus triggering its dissociation from a bound target protein. J Biol Chem 266: 14491–14496

Lindquist S, Craig EA (1988) The heat shock proteins. Annu Rev Genet 22: 631–677

Lis J, Wu C (1993) Protein traffic on the heat shock promoter: parking, stalling, and trucking along. Cell 74: 1–4

Liu RY, Kim D, Yang S-H, Li GC (1993) Dual control of heat shock response: involvement of a constitutive heat shock element-binding factor. Proc Natl Acad Sci USA 90: 3078–3082

Lunec J, Cresswell SR (1983) Heat-induced thermotolerance expressed in the energy metabolism of mammalian cells. Radiat Res 93: 588–597

Maytin EV, Wimberly JM, Anderson RR (1990) Thermotolerance and the heat shock response in normal human keratinocytes in culture. J Invest Dermatol 95: 635–642

Minton KW, Karmin P, Hahn GM, Minton AP (1982) Non-specific stabilization of stress-susceptible proteins by stress-resistant proteins: a model for the biological role of heat shock proteins. Proc Natl Acad Sci USA 79: 7107–7111

Mizzen LA, Welch WJ (1988) Characterization of the thermotolerant cell. I. Effects on protein synthesis activity and the regulation of heat-shock protein 70 expression. J Cell Biol 106: 1105–1116

Mizzen LA, Chang C, Garrels JG, Welch WJ (1989) Identification, characterization and purification of two mammalian stress proteins present in the mitochondria: one related to hsp70, the other to GroEL. J Biol Chem 264: 20664–20675

Morimoto RI (1993) Cells in stress: transcriptional activation of heat shock genes. Science 259: 1409–1410

Morimoto RI, Milarski KL (1990) Expression and function of vertebrate hsp70 genes. In: Morimoto RI, Tissieres A, Georgopoulos C (eds) Stress proteins in biology and medicine. Cold Spring Harbor Laboratory Press, New York, pp 323–360

Morimoto RI, Tissieres A, Georgopoulos C (1990) The stress response, function of the proteins, and perspectives. In: Morimoto RI, Tissieres A, Georgopoulos C (eds) Stress proteins in biology and medicine. Cold Spring Harbor Laboratory Press, New York, pp 1–36

Morimoto RI, Sarge KD, Abravaya K (1992) Transcriptional regulation of heat shock genes: a paradigm for inducible genomic responses. J Biol Chem 267: 21987–21990

Muller WU, Li GC, Goldstein LS (1985) Heat does not induce synthesis of heat shock proteins or thermotolerance in the earliest stage of mouse embryo development. Int J Hyperthermia 1: 97–102

Munro S, Pelham HRB (1985) What turns on heat shock genes. Nature 317: 477–478

Nagata K, Yamada KM (1986) Phosphorylation and transformation sensitivity of a major collagen-binding protein of fibroblasts. J Biol Chem 261: 7531–7536

Nagata K, Saga S, Yamada KM (1986) A major collagen-binding protein of chick embryo fibroblasts is a novel heat shock protein. J Cell Biol 103: 223–229

Nguyen VT, Morange M, Bensaude O (1989) Protein denaturation during heat shock and related stress. J Biol Chem 264: 10487–10492

Nover L, Munsche D, Neumann D, Ohme K, Scharf KD (1986) Control of ribosome biosynthesis in plant cell cultures under heat-shock conditions. Ribosomal RNA. Eur J Biochem 160: 297–304

Ohtsuka K, Masuda A, Nakai A, Nagata K (1990) A novel 40-kDa protein induced by heat shock and other stresses in mammalian and avian cells. Biochem Biophys Res Commun 166: 642–647

Okamoto H, Hiromi Y, Ishikaw E, Yamada T, Isoch K, Mackawa H, Hotta Y (1986) Molecular characterization of mutant actin genes which induce heat-shock proteins in *Drosphila* flight muscles. EMBO J 5: 589–596

Ostermann J, Horwich AL, Neupert W, Hartl F-U (1989) Protein folding in mitochondria requires complex formation with hsp60 and ATP hydrolysis. Nature 341: 125–130

Pelham HRB (1990) Functions of the hsp70 protein family: an overview. In: Morimoto RI, Tissieres A, Georgopoulos C (eds) Stress proteins in biology and medicine. Cold Spring Harbor Laboratory Press, New York, pp 287–299

Pinto M, Morange M, Bensaude O (1991) Denaturation of proteins during heat shock. J Biol Chem 266: 13941–13946

Pratt WB (1990) At the cutting edge: interaction of Hsp90 with steroid receptors: organizing some diverse observations and presenting the newest concepts. Mol Cell Endocrinol 74: C69–C76

Rastogi D, Nagle WA, Henle KJ, Moss AJ, Rastogi SP (1988) Uncoupling of oxidative phosphorylation does not induce thermotolerance in cultured Chinese hamster cells. Int J Hyperthermia 4: 333–344

Riabowol KT, Mizzen LA, Welch WJ (1988) Heat shock is lethal to fibroblasts microinjected with antibodies against hsp70. Science 242: 433–436

Ritossa FM (1962) A new puffing pattern induced by heat shock and DNP in *Drosophila*. Experientia 18: 571–573

Ritossa FM (1963) New puffs induced by temperature shock, DNP and salicylate in salivary chromosomes of *Drosophila melanogaster*. Drosophila Inf Service 37: 122–123

Sanchez ER (1990) Hsp56: a novel heat shock protein associated with untransformed steroid receptor complexes. J Biol Chem 265: 22067–22070

Sanchez ER, Hirst M, Scherrer LC, et al. (1990) Hormone-free mouse glucocorticoid receptors overexpressed in Chinese hamster ovary cells are localized to the nucleus and are associated with both hsp70 and hsp90. J Biol Chem 265: 20123–20130

Sanchez Y, Lindquist SL (1990) Hsp104 required for induced thermotolerance. Science 248: 1112–1115

Sarge KD, Murphy SP, Morimoto RI (1993) Activation of heat shock gene transcription by heat shock factor 1 involves oligomerization, acquisition of DNA-binding activity, and nuclear localization and can occur in the absence of stress. Mol Cell Biol 13: 1392–1407

Sciandra JJ, Subjeck JR (1984) Heat shock proteins and protection of proliferation and translation in mammalian cells. Cancer Res 44: 5188–5194

Skowyra D, Georgopoulos C, Zylicz M (1990) The *E. coli* DnaK gene product, the Hsp70 homolog, can reactivate heat-inactivated RNA polymerase in an ATP-dependent manner. Cell 62: 939–944

Sorger PK (1991) Heat shock factor and the heat shock response. Cell 65: 363–366

Stevenson MA, Minton KW, Hahn GM (1981) Survival and concavalin-A induced capping in CHO-fibroblasts after exposure to hyperthermia, ethanol and x-irradiation. Radiat Res 86: 467–478

Tissieres A, Mitchell HK, Tracy U (1974) Protein synthesis in the salivary glands of *Drosophila melanogaster*. Relation to chromosome puffs. J Mol Biol 84: 389–398

Van Dongen G, Van de Zande L, Schamhart D, Van Wijk R (1984) Comparative studies on the heat-induced thermotolerance of protein synthesis and cell cycle division in synchronized mouse neuroblastoma cells. Int J Radiat Biol 46: 759–769

Voellmy R (1985) The heat shock protein genes: a family of highly conserved genes with a superbly complex expression pattern. Bioessays 1: 213–217

Wallen CA, Landis M (1990) Removal of excess nuclear protein from cells heated in different physiological states. Int J Hyperthermia 6: 87–95

Welch WJ (1990) The mammalian stress response: cell physiology and biochemistry of stress proteins. In: Morimoto RI, Tissieres A, Georgopoulos C (eds) Stress proteins in biology and medicine. Cold Spring Harbor Laboratory Press, New York, pp 223–278

Wiech H, Buchner J, Zimmermann R, Jakob U (1992) Hsp90 chaperones protein folding in vitro. Nature 358: 169–170

Wiegant FAC, Van Bergen en Henegouwen PMP, Van Dongen G, Linnemans WAM (1987) Stress induced thermotolerance of the cytoskeleton of mouse neuroblastoma N2A cells and rat Reuber H35 hepatoma cells. Cancer Res 47: 1674–1680

Wittig S, Hensse S, Keitel C, Elsner C, Wittig B (1983) Heat shock gene expression is regulated during teratocarcinoma cell differentiation and early embryonic development. Dev Biol 96: 507–514

Yahara I, Iida H, Koyasu S (1986) A heat shock-resistant variant of Chinese hamster cell line constitutively expressing heat shock protein of M_r 90 000 at high level. Cell Struct Funct 11: 65–73

Yih L-H, Huang H, Jan KY, Lee T-C (1991) Sodium arsenite induces ATP depletion and mitochondrial damage in HeLa cells. Cell Biol Int Rep 46: 253–264

Yost HJ, Lindquist S (1986) RNA splicing is interrupted by heat shock and is rescued by heat shock protein synthesis. Cell 45: 185–193

4 Interaction of Heat and Radiation In Vitro and In Vivo

A.W.T. KONINGS

CONTENTS

4.1 Introduction

From in vitro as well as from animal studies there is convincing evidence that the tumor response to ionizing radiation is improved by temporary exposure to hyperthermic temperatures. In this review no attempt will be made to give a historical overview of hyperthermic radiosensitization; excellent texts on this topic already exist. Rather, the sections on in vitro radiosensitization will focus on recent ideas concerning the concept of critical targets, the identity of targets, and possible mechanisms of action. The part of the text devoted to the in vivo situation has been kept short. For more extensive reading, other reviews, e.g., the article by HORSMAN and OVERGAARD (1989), are available. Some remarks are included on recent developments using interstitial techniques and on the use of positron emission tomography in tumor-bearing animals to monitor results of therapy.

A.W.T. KONINGS, PhD, Department of Radiobiology, University of Groningen, Bloemsingel 1, NL-9713 BZ Groningen, The Netherlands

4.2 Molecular and Cellular Mechanisms of the Interaction of Heat and Radiation In Vitro

4.2.1 Cell Damage by Radiation Alone Versus Damage by Heat Alone

4.2.1.1 Energy Deposition

The direct damage to cellular molecules or to structural entities in the cell that is caused by ionizing radiation is different from that produced by hyperthermia. This is due to the fact that the nature of energy deposition during these treatments is fundamentally different. In the case of ionizing radiation a number of *localized high-energy depositions* occur, while with hyperthermia all molecules in the cell absorb the applied energy more or less *evenly*. In order to kill a cell 10^3- to 10^5-fold more energy has to be expended by hyperthermia than by ionizing radiation (HAHN 1982; ROTI ROTI and LASZLO 1988). A target theory has been developed for radiation damage to cells as a tool for calculating and quantifying radiosensitivity (HUTCHINSON and POLLARD 1961). Because cellular and subcellular studies on hyperthermic damage are often performed at radiobiological laboratories, the idea that heat inactivates specific targets, which subsequently leads to cell killing, has entered into the literature without critical evaluation. However, the target concept as developed for damage by ionizing radiation cannot simply be applied to damage by hyperthermia.

In the case of ionizing radiation, the microlocalization of the energy absorption in the cell has led to the notion of a "target volume," which often corresponds to the true volume of a molecule. Due to the ionizing nature of the radiation, the target molecule undergoes a chemical reaction. The molecule may lose an electron or a hydrogen atom, and reactive radical intermediates (single electron compounds) are formed. In the case of hyperthermia no localized high-energy depositions occur in the cell and no ionizing events take place in the molecules. As regards cellular damage during hyperthermia, it is probably more realistic to consider heat damage to groups of molecules that undergo structural changes. Some authors use the terms "lesion" and "target" as a more abstract concept. JUNG (1986, 1991) assumes that heat initiates nonlethal lesions that can be converted into lethal lesions. LEPOCK et al. (1988, 1990) introduced the term "hypothetical critical target" for hyperthermic cell killing. In this model they assume that the rate of hyperthermic cell killing corresponds to the rate of hyperthermic inactivation of this target. In both models it is necessary not only to consider the lesion or target as a single molecule, but also as structural entities in the cell.

4.2.1.2 Critical Damage to Molecules and Structural Entities in the Cell

4.2.1.2.1 Ionizing Radiation. Given at clinically relevant doses, ionizing radiation will damage many molecules in the cell (Table 4.1), including proteins, saccharides, lipids, and DNA. In recent years most attention has been focused on DNA and lipids. DNA has attracted such interest because the integrity of this molecule is essential for the successful functioning of the cell in terms of transmitting genetic information and because alterations in this molecule may interfere with replication. The latter is of special importance for proliferating cells. The bilayer of lipids in the cellular membranes is the most important structural entity separating compartments in the cell and constituting the boundary between the cellular contents and the environment.

Table 4.1. Molecular targets for cell killing after radiation, hyperthermia or the combined treatment

Molecules	Treatments		
	Radiation	Hyperthermia	Combination
DNA	yes[1]	no[2]	yes
Proteins	no	yes[3]	yes[4]
Lipids	no/yes(?)[5]	no[6]	no

[1] Reproductive death; [2] Only at high doses (≥43°C); [3] Set of critical proteins, accumulated damage above a certain threshold; [4] Protein aggregates on the nuclear matrix prevent DNA repair; [5] Not in reproductive death; possibly in interphase death; [6] Not as a primary target; lipids may modify the heat sensitivity of proteins

Although membranes may be critical subcellular targets under certain conditions, a number of independent experiments have pointed to DNA as the main target for radiation-induced cell death. With a microdosimetry approach, using ionizing radiation of different penetration depths, it can be shown that little lethal damage occurs when the energy is only absorbed by the outer cellular membrane and by the cytoplasm (see COLE et al. 1980). WARTERS and HOFER (1977) reported experiments in which cellular DNA was labelled with ^{3}H-thymidine or ^{125}I-iododeoxyuridine, and in other cells the outer membrane was labelled with ^{125}I-labelled concanavalin A. It could be demonstrated that when the radiation source was on the membrane, there was very little radiation damage to the cell in terms of LD_{50}. Incorporation of bromodeoxyuridine into DNA of living cells increases radiosensitivity. Under many circumstances cell killing by ionizing radiation appears to correlate with induction of chromosomal aberrations (DEWEY and SAPARETO 1978). It is not yet known what types of damage to the DNA molecule have to be considered the critical lesions, although irreparable double-strand breaks have to be one of the most important (see FRANKENBERG-SCHWAGER 1989).

With regard to membrane lipids it can be stated that polyunsaturated fatty acids are the most radiosensitive ones and that α-tocopherol can efficiently protect these membrane lipids against radiation damage (KONINGS et al. 1979). When cellular membranes are enriched by these radiosensitive lipids there is, however, no further decrease in reproductive capacity after radiation, even when these cells are depleted of α-tocopherol (WOLTERS and KONINGS 1982, 1984, 1985; GEORGE et al. 1983). When doses above 20 Sv are delivered to proliferating cells, interphase death may become an important mode of cell death. If loss of intracellular potassium and uptake of trypan blue are accepted as evidence for interphase death at high doses, it can be shown (WOLTERS and KONINGS 1985) that the lipids of membranes are a determining factor in this process (for review see also KONINGS 1987a). This is illustrated in Fig. 4.1. One has to conclude that membrane lipids are not the critical entities in cells leading to radiation-induced reproductive death; however, these components might play an important role in interphase death at high doses.

The ultimate radiosensitivity of a cell is dependent on the extent of repair of radiation

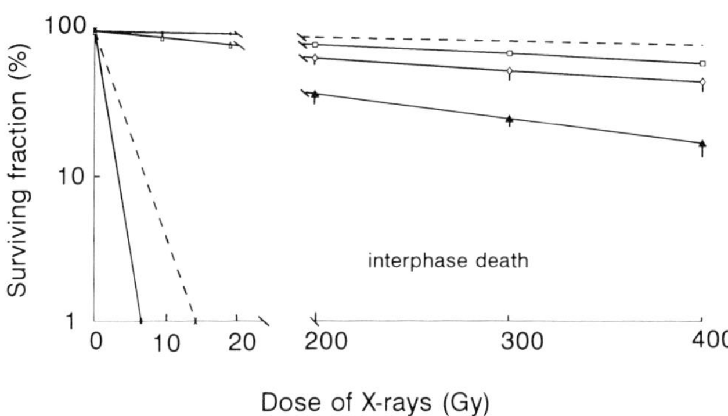

Fig. 4.1. Effect of membrane modification on radiation-induced reproductive death and radiation-induced interphase death of proliferating mouse fibroblast LM cells. Clonogenic ability and loss of intracellular potassium were determined as endpoints. Extensive loss of clonogenic ability (reproductive death) was seen at relatively low x-ray doses (<15 Gy), while loss of potassium (>50%) was observed at higher (>200 Gy) doses. The cellular membranes of the fibroblasts were modified by substitution of polyunsaturated fatty acyl (PUFA) chains. The antioxidant status of the cells was changed via depletion of GSH. The *broken lines* indicate x-irradiation under anoxic conditions. The *solid lines* indicate oxic conditions. The clonogenic ability of the cells did not change as a result of the modifications. PUFA substitution and GSH depletion in PUFA cells markedly increased the radiosensitivity in terms of potassium loss. □, normal cells, GSH depleted or not; ◇, PUFA cells not GSH depleted; ▲, GSH-depleted PUFA cells

damage. Both the DNA and the lipids of the cell can be repaired after radiation treatment. While there is an abundant supply of data on repair of DNA damage (see, e.g., PEAK et al. 1988), data on repair of membrane lipids are very scarce. FONCK et al. (1982a,b) could show in lymphosarcoma cells in vitro and in vivo that, after a dose of 5 Gy of x-rays, an immediate increase in lipid turnover took place that lasted about 50 min.

4.2.1.2.2 Hyperthermia. When cells are heated all macromolecules may be affected. Even at modest hyperthermic doses (43°C for less than 30 min) lipids may be fluidized and proteins may be denatured. However, in most cases direct DNA breaks cannot be detected at such dose levels (DIKOMEY 1982; JORRITSMA and KONINGS 1984; WARTERS and BRIZGYS 1987). Because the structure of the lipid bilayer and that of proteins are easily altered by hyperthermia, membranes have been, and still are, of interest as critical structures in cellular heat damage. It is possible to enhance the hyperthermic sensitivity of cells by introducing more of the fluidizing polyunsaturated fatty acids into the membrane phospholipids. Especially for bacteria this approach has led to spectacular results (YATVIN 1977). In the case of eukaryotic cells, the effects of lipid substitutions are less dramatic. The fluidity of phospholipids in membranes can also be modified by cholesterol. There are indications in the literature that cholesterol content in membranes might influence the cellular heat sensitivity. This is, however, not always found.

One has to realize that lipids and proteins in membranes are in dynamic equilibrium with each other. The physical state of the lipid component of the membrane may have significant effects on the properties of the proteins and as such modulate their conformation and activity. It is expected that the heat dose necessary for denaturation of membrane proteins is dependent on the nature of the surrounding lipids (for further discussion see KONINGS 1988). So, specific lipids present in domains around heat-sensitive proteins may be of importance for cellular heat sensitivity, when the function of these proteins is critical for cell survival. Modification of the heat sensitivity of a membrane Ca-ATPase by replacement of lipids could be shown by CHENG et al. (1987). Sometimes very extensive lipid substitutions are necessary to influence the heat sensitivity of critical proteins (KONINGS 1988). This seems to be the case for the mouse fibroblasts illustrated in Fig. 4.2. The polyunsaturated fatty acyl (PUFA) chains of the phospholipids of these cells changed from 8% in normal cells to about 40% in the modified cells. This membrane modification was accompanied by a clear change in fluidity in all membrane fractions. The difference in heat sensitivity was, however, very small. When the normal fibroblasts were given a mild heat

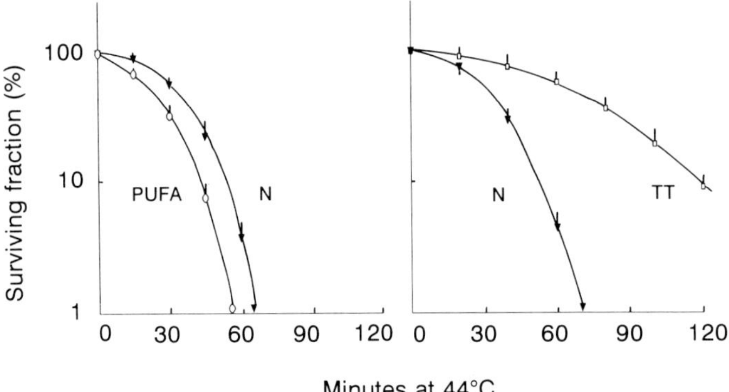

Fig. 4.2. Effect of membrane modification on cellular heat sensitivity. The clonogenic ability of normal (*N*) and PUFA-substituted mouse fibroblast LM cells was determined after exposure to 44°C. *Left panel*: extensive enrichment of PUFA (from 8% in N cells to 40% in PUFA cells) in the cellular membranes leads to a modest increase in heat sensitivity. *Right panel*: normal fibroblasts (*N*) were made thermotolerant (*TT*), which resulted in a clear difference in heat sensitivity; no change in overall lipid composition could be found. (Redrawn from KONINGS and RUIFROK 1985)

treatment to induce thermotolerance, the overall lipid composition in all membranes of the thermotolerant cells was not changed. If gross lipid modification was the primary endogenous mechanism for the cells to regulate their cellular heat sensitivity, one might expect the overall lipid composition in thermotolerant cells to be different from that in control cells. There is, of course, always a minor possibility that during the development of thermotolerance, lipid changes (rigidifying) around specific proteins take place which are not noticed during the determination of the overall lipid composition (KONINGS and RUIFROK 1985).

From the existing literature the most reasonable conclusion at present seems to be that proteins are the critical macromolecules for cell killing by heat. In those cases where membranes are suspected to be the heat-critical cellular structures, it is concluded that membrane proteins and not membrane lipids are the primary critical molecules leading to cell death. The lipids must be considered as modifiers of protein heat sensitivity. This notion is consistent with the finding (e.g., DEWEY et al. 1971) that the rates of inactivation (cell killing) for heat treatments at different temperatures, calculated from the slope of the exponential part of survival curves and used to construct Arrhenius plots, yield activation energies around 140 kcal/mole, a value observed (JOHNSON et al. 1954) for protein denaturation. The activation energy for membrane lipids is much lower (MASSICOTTE-NOLAN et al. 1981).

4.2.1.3 Heat-Induced Protein Denaturation

As discussed above, DNA double-strand breaks are among the most important critical radiation lesions in the cell. Proteins in membranes and in other cellular compartments are the critical molecules for heat damage.

The search for the identity of these cellular proteins determining hyperthermic cell killing has only started recently. During hyperthermia many proteins will be denatured in all cellular compartments. Only a part of them will be critical in the process of heat induced cell killing. When a set of critical proteins is damaged such, that a certain threshold is exceeded the cell will be killed. The degree of cell killing depends on the extent of protein damage beyond the threshold. In thermotolerant cells the heat sensitive proteins have become (partly) resistant. The accumulated damage is less then and more cells will survive. Spectroscopic studies using fluorescent and spin labels demonstrate that protein conformational changes occur in Chinese hamster lung V79 cells in the plasma and mitochondrial membrane proteins at temperatures above 40°C (LEPOCK et al. 1983). Transitions observed (LEPOCK et al. 1988) with differential scanning calorimetry (DSC) starting at 40°–45°C resemble those of proteins. With electron spin resonance (ESR) techniques it could be shown (BURGMAN and KONINGS 1992) that a number of membrane proteins had acquired heat resistance during the development of thermotolerance. With thermal gel analysis three of these proteins could be identified. Their apparent molecular masses were 55, 70, and 94 kDa. Strong evidence is available (KONINGS 1993) that heat shock proteins (HSPs), especially HSP72, play a role in induced heat resistance of membrane proteins. When heat-induced denaturation of proteins takes place in the different cellular compartments, the denatured proteins tend to aggregate. As long ago as 1978 reports were published (ROTI ROTI and WINWARD 1978; TOMASOVIC et al. 1978) indicating an increase in protein in nuclear structures isolated from heated cells. We now know that soluble nuclear proteins that are lost during standard procedures for the isolation of nuclei or nuclear structures, are co-isolated as protein aggregates in the isolates of heated cells. Depending on the initial heat dose, partial or total disaggregation of the proteins may take place after the heating, a process that has been shown (KAMPINGA et al. 1987) to be faster in thermotolerant cells. There is strong evidence that HSPs participate in the recovery of this protein damage, as well as in the prevention of protein aggregation (for a recent review see KAMPINGA 1993).

4.2.2 Cell Damage by the Combined Treatment

4.2.2.1 Hyperthermic Radiosensitization

When heat and radiation treatments are performed simultaneously, more than additive effects on cell killing are observed. The cells are killed by heat alone and by enhanced radiation damage. The synergistic component of the latter effect can be quantified by the thermal enhancement ratio (TER). This ratio may be expressed on the basis of isodose or isoeffect. To understand the radiobiological effects of heat radiosensitization, the isoeffect concept is more appropriate, the TER being defined as the ratio of the radiation dose required to produce a certain biological effect (e.g., 90% cell killing) and the radiation dose which in combination with hyperthermia leads to the same effect. The TER increases with heat dose, but may become saturated. When cell cycle dependency is determined, sensitization essentially follows the heat sensitivity of the cells and not the radiosensitivity.

Separation of the modalities in time leads to a decrease in the TER. In most cases recovery to normal cell radiosensitivity occurs more rapidly when radiation is followed by heat than vice versa. This is illustrated in Fig. 4.3. Apparently the critical lesions induced by radiation show more rapid repair than those induced by heat.

4.2.2.2 Effect of Thermotolerance and Step-Down Heating on the TER

When a combined treatment is preceded by a hyperthermic dose the extent of heat radiosensitization is often influenced. This is the case when the heat sensitivity of the cells is modified by the prior heat treatment. When the cells are pretreated with a heat dose at a temperature lower than or identical to the second dose, a temporary state of thermotolerance (TT) may develop. A short exposure to a high temperature may, however, increase the effect of a subsequent heating at a lower temperature, thus resulting in a temporary state of increased thermosensitivity. The latter approach is referred to as step-down heating (SDH).

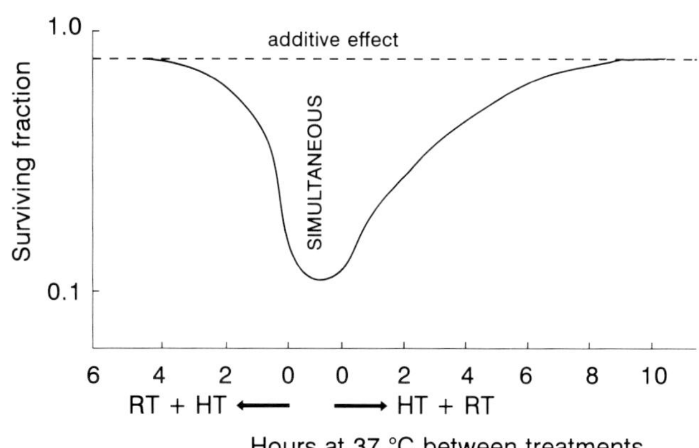

Fig. 4.3. Effect of separation of hyperthermia and radiation on cell survival. Asynchronous cells received radiation before, during, or after hyperthermia. The curve is drawn from data obtained from a number of different publications (see KONINGS 1987b)

A review of the literature (KONINGS 1987b) on the effect of TT on TER has revealed that about half of the published papers report a reduction of TER, while the other half do not show such an effect. At least three possibilities can be put forward to explain this non-uniformity. Firstly, there are indications that the phenomenon is cell line dependent and related to the presence and induction of certain HSPs (see Sect. 4.2.2.4). Secondly, in a number of cases the treatment may not have been truly simultaneous. The decline in TER after the heat treatment in thermotolerant cells is often faster than in non-thermotolerant cells. Thirdly, in some cases the initial heat treatment may have selectively killed S-phase cells, leaving a clonogenic population of cells that are more radiosensitive.

Only limited data are available on the effect of SDH on TER. Most publications (see LINDEGAARD 1992) have shown a higher TER when SDH preceded the combined treatment.

4.2.2.3 Low-Dose-Rate Irradiation at Mild Hyperthermic Temperatures

Although only a few publications are available concerning dose rate effects on the TER, most studies (BEN HUR et al. 1974; HARISIADIS et al. 1978; GERNER et al. 1983; LING and ROBINSON 1989) show a higher TER at low dose rates (LDR). It seems that appropriate heat treatments can totally eliminate the sparing effect of LDR in the range of 0.08–130 Gy/h. Because it is not always possible during clinical practice to achieve sufficiently high temperatures, it is important to know whether mild hyperthermia can still reduce the LDR sparing effect. The in vitro data obtained until now (ARMOUR et al. 1991; CORRY et al. 1993) are promising, TERs for temperatures as low as 41°C are between 1.5 and 2.5, depending on heat/radiation exposure. Optimal TERs are obtained when hyperthermia is present at all times during irradiation. The situation with human tissue may be advantageous as compared with the situation in rodents, because human cells seem to be different in terms of the development of TT in the temperature range 40°–42°C. As a consequence, they are more heat responsive at 41°C than the rodent cells. The human cells are, however, considered to be intrinsically more heat stable than the rodent cells.

4.2.2.4 Mechanisms of Action

As mentioned above, hyperthermia not only reduces survival directly (heat cytotoxicity), but also enhances radiosensitivity by increasing the slope and decreasing the shoulder of the radiation survival curve (DEWEY et al. 1977). From an analysis using the linear quadratic model, DIKOMEY and JUNG (1991) concluded (for CHO cells) that thermosensitization is predominantly due to an enhancement of cell killing of the α-term type at the lower temperature range (<43°C), while at higher temperatures both (α and β) modes of cell killing are altered by heat to a similar extent.

The number of radiation-induced DNA lesions is not enhanced by hyperthermia, provided that the heat-induced lesions (only at ≥43°C, see JORRITSMA and KONINGS 1984) are subtracted. Hyperthermic radiosensitization is generally considered to result from thermal effects on the repair of radiation-induced damage. Exposure to hyperthermic temperatures can influence both the initial rate and the extent of DNA strand break rejoining.

As can be seen in Fig. 4.4, exposure to a temperature of 42°C or higher progressively diminishes the rate of repair (JORRITSMA and KONINGS 1983). From the slopes in this figure an activation energy of about 140 kcal/mole can be calculated, which approximates the activation energy for hyperthermic cell killing. So it seems that protein denaturation is a critical process in heat killing and in heat radiosensitization.

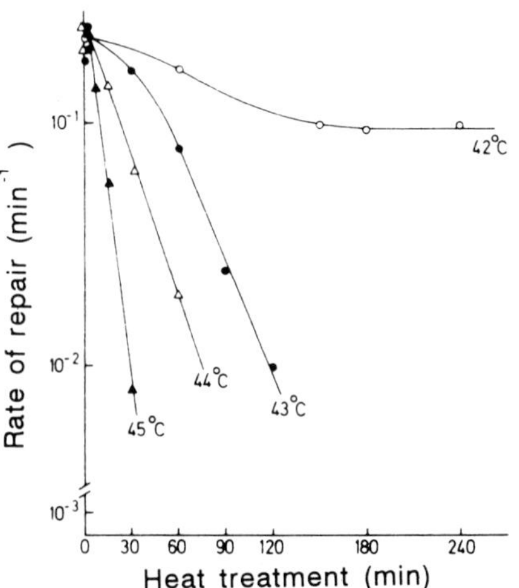

Fig. 4.4. Effect of hyperthermia on the kinetics of the repair of DNA strand breaks $(t_{1/2})^{-1}$. (From JORRITSMA and KONINGS 1983)

DIKOMEY and FRANZKE (1992) have studied DNA repair kinetics of CHO cells in considerable detail. This is illustrated in Fig. 4.5. Irradiation with 9 Gy of x-rays produced about 3000 strand breaks per cell. After radiation, three-phase repair kinetics have been proposed by these authors, with a fast, an intermediate, and a slow component. The slow component, which is exponential for $t \geqslant 120$ min, with a repair half-time of about 170 min, is considered to concern repair of double strand breaks – about 6% of all strand breaks induced (extrapolation of the final slope in Fig. 4.5). For the heated cells the half-time of repair of double strand breaks is doubled, yielding now about 20% double strand breaks (extrapolation). The additional double strand breaks are assumed to be formed during repair incubation at 37°C arising from lesions which disappear at 37°C with a half-time of about 17 min. It is suggested (JUNG and DIKOMEY 1993) that cell killing is related to the formation of these additional double strand breaks. Hyperthermia may decrease the extent of DNA break rejoining, but this is difficult to prove when low doses of radiation are given. For a dose of 50 Gy, however, it could clearly be shown (MILLS and MEYN 1983) in CHO cells that 43°C heat treatment for 1 h resulted in a doubling of the residual number of strand breaks when the two modalities were applied simultaneously. Separation of the heat and radiation treatment (Fig. 4.6) diminishes the extra residual damage and yields a picture that indicates an inverse proportionality to cell survival (compare with Fig. 4.3).

The above-mentioned observations combined with others tempt one to conclude that hyperthermic radiosensitization is caused by heat effects on the DNA repair machinery, resulting in inhibition of effective repair and formation of new lesions during the repair period.

A clear correlation between hyperthermic inhibition of strand break repair and radiosensitization (survival) is, however, not always found. This is, for example, the case for fractionated

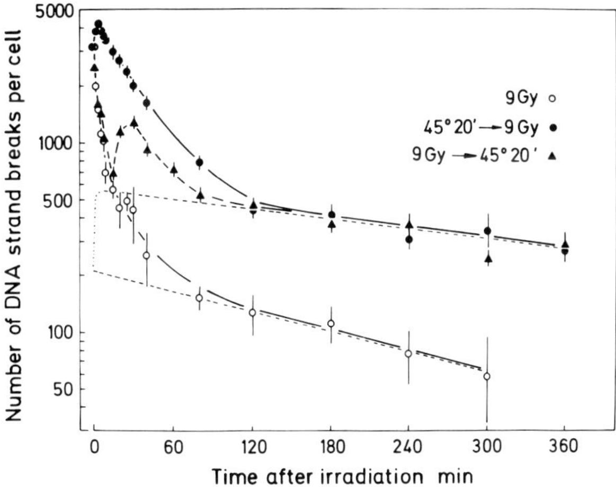

Fig. 4.5. Effect of hyperthermia on repair of DNA strand breaks. CHO cells were heated prior to or immediately after irradiation. The number of DNA strand breaks plotted represents the sum of single and double strand breaks. (From DIKOMEY and FRANZKE 1992)

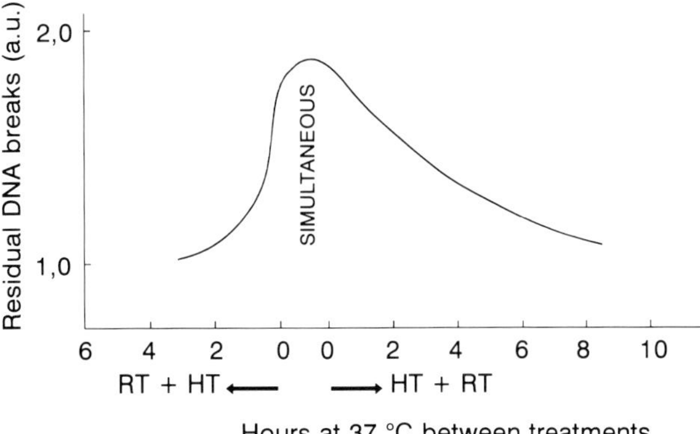

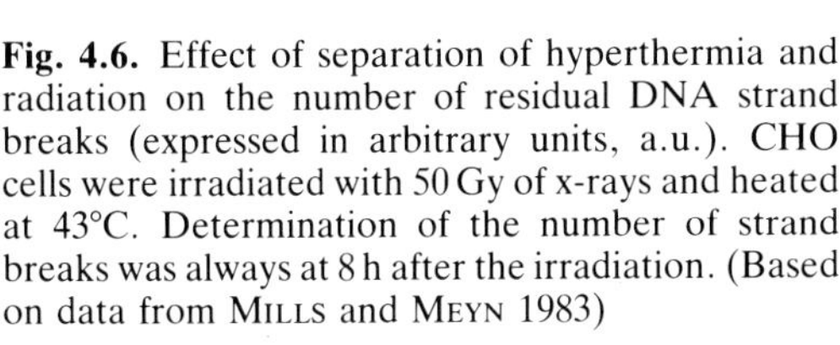
Fig. 4.6. Effect of separation of hyperthermia and radiation on the number of residual DNA strand breaks (expressed in arbitrary units, a.u.). CHO cells were irradiated with 50 Gy of x-rays and heated at 43°C. Determination of the number of strand breaks was always at 8 h after the irradiation. (Based on data from MILLS and MEYN 1983)

heat treatments (JORRITSMA et al. 1985) and for modifiers of the heat effect, such as polyols (JORRITSMA and KONINGS 1986). It must, however, be realized that the different assays which have been used to determine DNA damage are not always comparable. In most cases it is not exactly known what type of DNA lesions are measured and whether these are the critical lesions for cell survival. In this respect it may be mentioned that low-temperature hyperthermia (<42°C) accelerates the rejoining of single and double strand breaks (BEN HUR and ELKIND 1974; DIKOMEY 1982; WARTERS et al. 1987; WARTERS and AXTELL 1992) while a clear radiosensitization (survival) is caused by these heat treatments.

If the inhibition of DNA repair by heat treatments above 42°C is causing the observed enhanced radiosensitivity, then the question arises as to the mechanism of this inhibition. At the moment there are two popular theories based on the phenomenon of heat induced protein denaturation in the cell nucleus. Both, either, or neither of these may hold true or be applicable only in special situations. One of the possibilities is thermal inactivation of repair enzymes; the second is reduced accessibility to the damaged sites for the repair enzymes.

With respect to the first-mentioned option, DNA polymerase β is of particular interst, since this repair enzyme has been found to be very heat sensitive (DUBE et al. 1977). Thermal inactivation of DNA polymerase has been postulated repeatedly as a mechanism to explain heat radiosensitization, but there is still not consensus. In a recent report concerning this issue (DIKOMEY and JUNG 1993), the increase in radiosensitivity caused by various kinds of single and combined heat treatments was studied in CHO cells and related to the heat-induced loss of this repair enzyme. The TER for 90% cell killing correlated well with the polymerase β activity for single heating at temperatures exceeding 41.5°C and for thermotolerant cells. This is in agreement with results of previous reports (JORRITSMA et al. 1985; MIVECHI and DEWEY 1985; DIKOMEY and JUNG 1988). However, the relationship did not hold for single heating at temperatures below 41.5°C and for step-down heating leading to thermosensitization, which is similar to the findings previously reported by JORRITSMA et al. (1986) and KAMPINGA et al. (1989a).

The possible restriction of accessibility of the repair system to damaged (heated) sites was mentioned by WARTERS and ROTI ROTI as long ago as 1979. Recent studies using a DNA supercoiling assay (KAMPINGA et al. 1988b) reported the "masking" of DNA damage by hyperthermia. Inhibition of repair and masking of DNA damage were gradually reduced during the recovery period after the hyperthermic treatment. The time course of this recovery was similar to that observed for the reduction of protein aggregates formed during heating in the cell nucleus. It had been shown previously (KAMPINGA et al. 1987) that thermotolerant cells recovered faster from heat-induced protein aggregation than non-thermotolerant cells. A good correlation was observed (KAMPINGA et al. 1989c) between the kinetics of protein aggregation/disaggregation (area under the curve, AUC) and heat-induced cell killing. When kinetic data on nuclear protein aggregation/disaggregation, TER, and residual DNA damage are compared (KONINGS 1993) for normal and thermotolerant HeLa S_2 cells, when hyperthermia and radiation are separated in time (0–6 h), a suggestive similarity is apparent. No correlation could be established, however, (KAMPINGA et al. 1989a) between inactivation and recovery of DNA polymerase β with TER under the same experimental conditions. Lipid modification did not influence thermal radiosensitization (WOLTERS et al. 1987).

Recently SAKKERS et al. (1993) showed that hyperthermia selectively affects repair of cyclobutane pyrimidine dimers (CPDs) in transcriptionally active genes in UV-irradiated fibroblasts. Hyperthermia had no effect, however, on an inactive non-matrix-associated locus. Because heat-induced nuclear protein aggregation mainly occurs at the nuclear matrix, these results suggest that limited damage accessibility and not inactivation of repair enzymes is the cause of DNA repair inhibition. This agrees with earlier data (KAMPINGA et al. 1989d) on the importance of protein aggregation to DNA anchor points on the nuclear matrix (topo-isomerase II sites). Because only preliminary data (KAMPINGA et al. 1989a; KONINGS 1993) are available with respect to the relation between the extent of heat-induced nuclear protein aggregates and TER, it is too early to draw a general conclusion on this issue. If such a relation can be quantitated, the presence and induction of certain HSPs are probably of major importance for the phenomenon of cellular heat radiosensitization.

4.3 Interaction of Heat and Radiation in Tumor-Bearing Animals

4.3.1 Heat Cytotoxicity and Heat Radiosensitization

Numerous studies have clearly demonstrated that heat can enhance the radiation sensitivity of animal tumors [for reviews see, e.g., OVERGAARD (1978) and STREFFER and VAN BEUNINGEN (1987)] and normal tissues (FIELD and BLEEHEN 1979; HUME 1985). The modalities have, of course, to be given in such a way that a clear therapeutic gain is obtained. There is currently no general consensus concerning the best protocols for avoiding unacceptable normal tissue damage under conditions leading to complete tumor cure.

The action of heat and radiation in vivo is more complicated than in the in vitro situation. In vitro the two components in cell killing are radiosensitization and heat toxicity. In vivo, especially the latter component is dependent on several physiological factors. Radioresistant hypoxic cells are found in many solid tumors (MOULDER and ROCKWELL 1984) and are more heat sensitive than the well-oxygenated cells. During hyperthermia oxygenated tumor cells may become more heat sensitive because of damage to the tumor vascular system. It is assumed (REINHOLD et al. 1978) that the cytotoxic action of hyperthermia is less marked in normal tissue because its vasculature is less heat sensitive. TANAKA (1993) could modify the heat sensitivity of murine tumors by applying the vasoactive drug, hydralazine. The tumor blood flow decreased dramatically after injection, while the flow in the surrounding blood vessels was only slightly affected.

While the TER in vitro is mostly defined in terms of enhanced radiosensitivity (heat cytotoxicity subtracted), for the in vivo situation heat cytotoxicity is mostly included too. The lack of in vivo data makes it difficult to reach a general conclusion concerning the contribution of both components to the overall effect. One may expect that at low heat doses the radiosensitizing effect will be dominant, especially with truly simultaneous treatment.

4.3.2 Sequence and Spacing of the Modalities

It is generally agreed that maximal TERs (heat cytotoxicity included!) in vivo are obtained when radiation and hyperthermia are applied simultaneously. The decrease in TER when an interval is introduced varies between individual tumors and also between different normal tissues. This is probably mainly caused by tissue physiology (e.g., vasculature) especially affecting heat cytotoxicity. In Fig. 4.7 TERs in a C3H mouse mammary carcinoma and its surrounding skin are shown as a function of time interval and sequence between hyperthermia and radiation. Local tumor control and moist desquamation in skin were used as biological endpoints of the assays (OVERGAARD et al. 1987). The TER remaining in the tumor after a 4-h separation is most likely a consequence of heat that kills radioresistant hypoxic cells. It is obvious that little therapeutic advantage is to be expected from a simultaneous treatment, if the tumor and normal tissue are heated to the same degree.

4.3.3 Effect of Thermotolerance and Step-Down Heating

In general thermotolerance has no effect on the response to radiation alone, but does reduce the

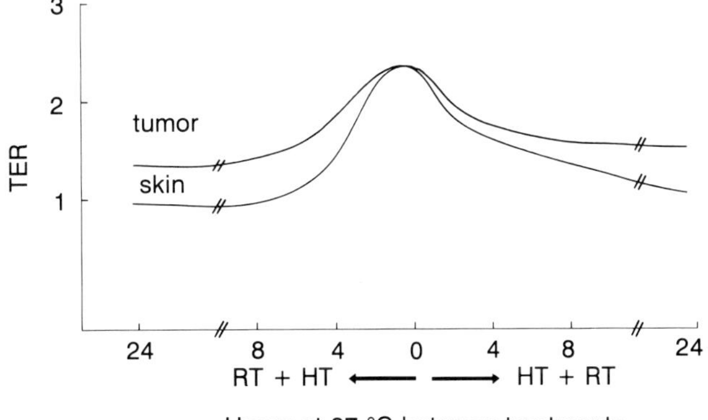

Fig. 4.7. Effect of separation of hyperthermia and radiation on tumor control and skin damage. Local control of mouse mammary carcinoma in C3H mice and degree of moist dequamation in surrounding skin in 50% of the treated animals were taken as endpoints for the determination. (Redrawn from OVERGAARD et al. 1987)

TER in most tumors and normal tissues (for review see HORSMANN and OVERGAARD 1989). The influence of thermotolerance on the interaction between heat and radiation is more pronounced when heat and radiation are given sequentially (NIELSEN et al. 1983). The TER was found by these authors to be maximal 5 days after thermotolerance induction (complete disappearance of TT). To avoid interference by thermotolerance, flavonoids, and in particular quercetin, may be used (NAGATA and HOSOKAWA 1993). This compound is nontoxic to mice and therefore promising for clinical use. Also amino acid analogs can inhibit thermotolerance (LI and LASZLO 1985).

NISHIMURA and URANO (1993) have investigated the effect of hyperthermia on fractionated radiotherapy in mice bearing a fibrosarcoma in the foot. Tumor response was studied by tumor growth (TG) and TCD_{50} (50% tumor control dose) assays. One heat treatment at 43.5°C for 45 min in a water bath was combined independently or simultaneously with fractionated doses. Five and ten fractions were used for TG and TCD_{50} assays, respectively. Normal tissue damage was scored as acute foot reactions. TER was greatest when heat was administered with the last radiation dose in the TG assay and with the first dose in the TCD_{50} assay. The size of the hypoxic cell fraction during the overall radiation treatment may be the cause of this result. Significant thermal sensitization of the skin reaction was observed at all times. These experiments suggest that heat is best given with the first radiation fraction to effectively kill hypoxic cells.

As compared with single temperature heating, SDH generally increases the TER of both tumor tissue and normal tissue. Furthermore, SDH may cause significantly higher TER values in the tumor, suggesting a therapeutic gain (LINDEGAARD and OVERGAARD 1988). These authors found that the TER value decreased when an interval was allowed between radiation and SDH and was lost completely in normal tissues within a 3-h interval. In tumors the decrease was slower, suggesting an enhanced effect of SDH with respect to radiation-resistant hypoxic cells. SDH has never been used clinically because it is difficult to achieve the high temperature needed. The development of scanned-focussed ultrasound, however, does offer the possibility of a short (10-min) increase in temperature (HAHN 1993). After this initial treatment, continuous low-temperature heating could be achieved even via whole-body heating.

4.3.4 Interstitial Radiation Combined with (Interstitial) Hyperthermia

As discussed in Sect. 4.2.2, heat radiosensitization of cells in vitro is very effective when heat is combined with low-dose-rate (LDR) irradiation. Only a few published studies have analyzed this in tumor-bearing animals. A review of these experiments has recently been given by HAHN (1991). SAPOZINK et al. (1983) combined continuous ultra-LDR irradiation with radiofrequency hyperthermia in RIF-1 tumors of C3H mice. Low-dose-rate irradiation up to 180 Gy did not cure any of the tumors; however, combining 80 Gy with hyperthermia (44°C for 30 min) did. Two heat exposures appeared to be better than one; three were not better than two. In conjunction with hyperthermia, internal irradiation, i.e., brachytherapy with iridium-192, is essentially equivalent to fractionated irradiation given from a source with much higher dose rates (MOORTHY et al. 1984; BAKER et al. 1987).

A particularly relevant study has been performed recently by JONES et al. (1989). Irradiation of a breast carcinoma was accomplished by placing a noninvasive cap containing three iodine-125 seeds over the tumor. Dose rates ranged from 14 to 40 cGy/h with a variation in the total dose between 830 and 2378 cGy over the treatment period (48–72 h). Heating with a waterbath was given before, after, or in the middle of the irradiation. The best results were obtained after heating in the middle. Heating after the radiation was the least effective.

Interstitial hyperthermia combined with interstitial radiation has the logistic advantage that catheters implanted to serve as source holders for the radiation can also be used for the heating. Only a few animal studies have been published on this topic (MILLER et al. 1978; PAPADOPOULOS et al. 1989; RUIFROK et al. 1991; VAN HOOIJE et al. 1993). In all these cases TERs of about 1.5 were found when the two modalities were given at (almost) the same time.

Recently the use of multiple short pulses of radiation has been proposed (BRENNER and HALL 1991; VISSER and LEVENDAG 1992) in order to simulate continuous LDR irradiation. Such a brachytherapy modality would allow the application of multiple interstitial hyperthermia treatments between the brachytherapy "pulses." At present there are no animal experiments in which LDR irradiation or fractionated doses have been combined with long-duration mild-temperature

(39°–41°C) hyperthermia. In vitro investigations (Sect. 4.2.2) have provided a strong basis for such an approach (ARMOUR et al. 1993).

4.3.5 *Positron Emission Tomography*

There is great interest in methods that may predict the outcome of a cancer treatment during the initial period of the protocol. The conventional techniques of diagnostic radiology, x-ray computed tomography, nuclear magnetic resonance imaging and ultrasonography, detect a tumor only by its physical attributes (e.g., shape, size). PET is a noninvasive tool able to monitor quantitatively metabolic activities in tissues. Only a few investigators have applied positron-emitting tracers in experiments with tumor-bearing animals. One study (DAEMEN et al. 1991) has been published on PET measurements after hyperthermia. Heat-induced inhibition of protein synthesis in the tumor was monitored by PET using L-(1-^{11}C)tyrosine and correlated with growth delay of a rhabdomyosarcoma tumor in Wag/Rij rats. It was concluded that the acute (30–90 min after treatment) effects of hyperthermia can be monitored by PET with a predictive outcome in terms of tumor regression. When the same type of experiment was performed (DAEMEN et al. 1992) after radiation and radiation plus hyperthermia, a different picture emerged. No acute effects could be observed, either with L-(1-^{11}C) tyrosine or with ^{18}FDG (fluorodeoxyglucose). Later effects (after days) on tracer uptake appeared to correlate with changes in tumor volume. It may be expected that when ^{11}C-thymidine is used as the positron-emitting compound it will be possible to measure early radiation responses because, in contrast to protein synthesis, DNA synthesis is inhibited at clinically relevant radiation doses.

4.4 Summary

- Molecular targets for cell killing by radiation are essentially different from those in hyperthermia, because of the different nature of energy absorption.
- DNA is the molecular target for cell killing by radiation. Proteins for cell killing by hyperthermia. Lipids can modulate the heat sensitivity of proteins.
- Cellular radiosensitization is caused by protein denaturation and aggregation on the nuclear matrix.
- Hsp's regulate cellular radiosensitization by influencing the protein denaturation/aggregation/disaggregation process in the cell nucleus.
- Most in vitro studies show a higher TER at low dose rates (LDR).
- A considerable TER can be reached when long duration low temperature (41°C) is combined with LDR.
- Thermotolerance generally reduces the TER in vitro as well as in vivo (tumors and normal tissues).
- Heat may be best given with the first radiation fraction during fractionated radiotherapy because of the killing of hypoxic cells.

References

Armour EP, Wang Z, Corry PM, Martinez A (1991) Sensitization of rat 9L gliosarcoma cells to low dose rate irradiation by long duration 41°C hyperthermia. Cancer Res 51: 3088–3095

Armour EP, Corry P, Wang Z, McEachern D, Martinez A (1993) An in vitro basis for combining "long duration-mild temperature hyperthermia" with low-dose-rate and fractionated radiation. In: Proceedings of the 41st annual meeting of the RRS and the 13th annual meeting of the NAHS, March 1993, Dallas, Texas, pp 16: S-01-2

Baker DG, Sager HT, Constable WC (1987) The response of a solid tumor to X-radiation as modified by dose rate, fractionation, and hyperthermia. Cancer Invest 5: 409–416

Ben Hur E, Elkind MM (1974) Thermally enhanced radioresponse of cultured Chinese hamster cells: damage and repair of single-stranded DNA and a DNA complex. Radiat Res 59: 484–495

Ben Hur E, Bronk VB, Elkind MM (1974) Thermally enhanced radioresponse of cultured Chinese hamster cells: Inhibition of repair of sublethal damage and enhancement of lethal damage. Radiat Res 58: 38–51

Brenner DJ, Hall EJ (1991) Conditions for the equivalence of continuous to pulsed low dose rate brachytherapy. Int J Radiat Oncol Biol Phys 20: 181–190

Burgman PWJJ, Konings AWT (1992) Heat induced protein denaturation in the particulate fraction of HeLa S3 cells; effect of thermotolerance. J Cell Physiol 153: 88–94

Cheng KH, Lepock JR, Hui SW, Lepock JR (1987) Protection of the membrane Ca-ATPase by cholesterol from thermal activation Cancer Res 47: 1255–1262

Cole A, Meyn RE, Chen R, Corry PM, Hittelman W (1980) Mechanisms for cell injury. In: Meyn RE, Withers HR (eds) Radiation biology in cancer research. Raven Press, New York, pp 33–58

Corry PM, Armour EP, Wang Z (1993) Thermo-brachytherapy biology. In: Proceedings of the 41st annual meeting of the RRS and the 13th annual meeting of the NAHS, March 1993, Dallas, Texas. p 121: S-12-1

Daemen BJG, Elsinga PhH, Mooibroek J, Paans AMJ, Wieringa A, Konings AWT, Vaalburg W (1991) PET measurements of hyperthermia-induced suppression of protein synthesis in tumors in relation to effects on tumor growth. J Nucl Med 32: 1587–1592

Daemen BJG, Elsinga PH, Paans AMJ, Wieringa RA, Konings AWT, Vaalburg W (1992) Radiation-induced inhibition of tumor growth as monitored by PET using L-[1-^{11}C]tyrosine and fluorine-18-fluorodeoxyglucose. J Nuclear Med 33(3): 373–379

Dewey WC, Sapareto SA (1978) Radiosensitization by hyperthermia occurs through an increase in chromosomal aberrations. In: Streffer C (ed) Cancer therapy by hyperthermia and radiation. Urban and Schwarzenberg, Baltimore, pp 149–150

Dewey WC, Westra A, Miller H, Nagasawa H (1971) Heat-induced lethality and chromosomal damage in synchronized Chinese hamster cells treated with 5-bromodesoxyuridine. Int J Radiat Biol 20: 505–520

Dewey WC, Hopwood LE, Sapareto SA, Gerweck LE (1977) Cellular responses to combinations of hyperthermia and radiation. Radiology 123: 463–474

Dikomey E (1982) Effect of hyperthermia at 42 and 45°C on repair of radiation-induced DNA strand breaks in CHO cells. Int J Radiat Biol 41: 603–614

Dikomey E, Franzke J (1992) Effect of heat on induction and repair of DNA strand breaks in X-irradiated CHO cells. Int J Radiat Biol 61: 221–233

Dikomey E, Jung H (1988) Correlation between polymerase B activity and thermal radiosensitization in CHO cells. Recent Results Cancer Res 9: 35–41

Dikomey E, Jung H (1991) Thermal radiosensitization in CHO cells by prior heating at 41°–46°C. Int J Radiat Biol 59: 815–825

Dikomey E, Jung H (1993) Correlation between thermal radiosensitization and heat-induced loss of DNA polymerase β activity in CHO cells. Int J Radiat Biol 63: 215–221

Dube EK, Seal G, Loeb LA (1977) Differential heat sensitivity of mammalian DNA polymerases. Biochem Biophys Res Commun 76: 483–487

Field SB, Bleehen NM (1979) Hyperthermia in the treatment of cancer. Cancer Treat Rev 6: 63–94

Fonck K, Scherphof GL, Konings AWT (1982a) Control of fatty acid incorporation in membrane phospholipids; X-ray-induced changes in fatty acid uptake by tumor cells. Biochim Biophys Acta 692: 406–414

Fonck K, Scherphof GL, Konings AWT (1982b) The effect of X-irradiation on membrane lipids of lymphosarcoma cells in vivo and in vitro. J Radiat Res 23: 371–384

Frankenberg-Swager M (1989) Review article: review of repair kinetics for DNA damage induced in eukaryotic cells in vitro by ionizing radiation. Radiother Oncol 14: 307–320

George AM, Lunec J, Cramp WA (1983) Effect of membrane fatty acid changes on the radiation sensitivity of human lymphoid cells. Int J Radiat Biol 43: 363–378

Gerner EW, Oval JH, Manning MR, Sim DA, Bowden GT, Hevezi JM (1983) Dose rate dependence of heat radiosensitization. Int J Radiat Oncol Biol Phys 9: 1401–1404

Hahn GM (1982) Hyperthermia and Cancer. Plenum Press, New York

Hahn GM (1991) Brachytherapy and hyperthermia:biological rationale. In: Handl-Zeller L (ed) Interstitial hyperthermia. Springer, Wien New York, pp 1–9

Hahn GM (1993) Biological rationale for new clinical trials. In: Gerner EW, Cetas TC (eds) Hyperthermic oncology 1993, vol 2. Plenaty and symposia lectures. Proceedings of the 6th International Congress on hyperthermic oncology. Tucson, Arizon 1992, Arizon a Board of Regents, pp 79–81

Harisiadis L, Sung C, Kessaris L, Hall E (1978) Hyperthermia and low dose rate irradiation. Radiology 12: 195–198

Horsman MR, Overgaard J (1989) Thermal radiosensitization in animal tumors: the potential for therapeutic gain. In: Urano M, Douple EB (eds) Hyperthermia Oncol 2: 113–145

Hume SP (1985) Experimental studies of normal tissue response to hyperthermia given alone or combined with radiation. In: Overgaard J (ed) Hyperthermic oncology. Taylor and Francis, London, pp 53–70

Hutchinson F, Pollard E (1961) Target theory and radiation effects on biological molecules. In: Errera M, Forssberg A (eds) Mechanisms in radiobiology, Vol 1. Academic Press, New York, pp 71–91

Johnson FH, Eyring H, Palissar MI (1954) The kinetic basis of molecular biology. Wiley New York, pp 215–285

Jones EL, Lyons BE, Douple EB, Dain BJ (1989) Thermal enhancement of low dose rate irradiation in a murine tumour system. Int J Hyperthermia 5: 509–523

Jorritsma JBM, Konings AWT (1983) Inhibition of repair of radiation-induced strand breaks by hyperthermia, and its relationship to cell survival after hyperthermia. Int J Radiat Biol 43: 505–516

Jorritsma JBM, Konings AWT (1984) Radiosensitization by hyperthermia in thermotolerant cells and its relationship with the repair of DNA strand breaks. Radiat Res 98: 198–208

Jorritsma JBM, Konings AWT (1986) DNA lesions in hyperthermic cell killing: effects of thermotolerance, procaine and erythritol. Radiat Res 106: 89–97

Jorritsma JBM, Kampinga HH, Scaf AHJ, Konings AWT (1985) Strand break repair, DNA polymerase activity and heat radiosensitization in thermotolerant cells. Int J Hyperthermia 1: 131–145

Jorritsma JBM, Burgman P, Kampinga HH, Konings AWT (1986) DNA polymerase activity in heat killing and hyperthermic radiosensitization of mammalian cells as observed after fractionated heat treatments. Radiat Res 105: 307–319

Jung H (1986) A generalized concept for cell killing by heat. Radiat Res 106: 56–72

Jung H (1991) A generalized concept for cell killing by heat. Effect of chronically induced thermotolerance. Radiat Res 127: 235–242

Jung H, Dikomey E (1993) Mechanisms of thermal radiosensitization. Effect of heat on induction and repair of DNA strand breaks in X-irradiated CHO cells. In: Gerner EW, Cetas TC (eds) Hyperthermic oncology 1993. pp 103–108

Kampinga HH (1993) Thermotolerance in mammalian cells: protein denaturation and aggregation and stress proteins (a commentary) J Cell Sci 104: 11–17

Kampinga HH, Luppes JG, Konings AWT (1987) Heat-induced nuclear protein binding and its relation to thermal cytotoxicity. Int J Hyperthermia 3: 459–465

Kampinga HH, Wright WD, Konings AWT, Roti Roti JL (1988) The interaction of heat and radiation effecting the ability of nuclear DNA to undergo supercoiling changes. Radiat Res 116: 114–123

Kampinga HH, Keij JF, Van der Kruk G, Konings AWT (1989a) Interaction of hyperthermia and radiation in tolerant and nontolerant HeLa S3 cells: role of DNA polymerase inactivation. Int J Radiat Biol 55: 423–433

Kampinga HH, Wright WD, Konings AWT, Roti Roti JL (1989b) Changes in the structure of nucleoids isolated from heat-shocked HeLa cells. Int J Radiat Biol 56: 369–382

Kampinga HH, Turkel-Uygur N, Roti Roti JL, Konings AWT (1989c) The relationship of increased nuclear protein content induced by hyperthermia to killing of HeLa cells. Radiat Res 117: 511–522

Kampinga HH, Vander Kruk G, Konings AWT (1989d) Reduced DNA break formation and cytotoxicity of the toporsomerase II duy 4′-(9′-Acridinylamino) multanesulfon-m-ansidide when combined with hyperthermia in human and rodent cell lines. Cancer Res 49: 1712–1717

Konings AWT (1987a) Role of membrane lipid composition in radiation-induced death of mammalian cells. In: Walden TL, Hughes HN (eds) Prostaglandin and lipid metabolism in radiation injury. Plenum Press, New York, pp 29–44

Konings AWT (1987b) Effects of heat and radiation on mammalian cells. Radiat Phys Chem 30: 339–349

Konings AWT (1988) Membranes as targets for hyperthermic cell killing. Recent Results Cancer Res 109: 9–21

Konings AWT (1993) Thermal radiosensitization: role of heat shock proteins in heat-induced alterations of protein conformation. In: Gerner EW, Cetas TC (eds) Hyperthermic oncology 1993, pp 109–114

Konings AWT, Ruifrok ACC (1985) Role of membrane lipids and membrane fluidity in thermosensitivity and thermotolerance of mammalian cells. Radiat Res 102: 86–98

Konings AWT, Damen J, Trieling WB (1979) Protection of liposomal lipids against radiation-induced oxidative damage. Int J Radiat Biol 34: 343–350

Lepock JR, Cheng K-H, Al-Qysi H et al. (1983) Thermotropic lipid and protein transitions in Chinese hamster lund cell membranes: relationship to hyperthermic cell killing. Can J Biochem Cell Biol 61: 421–427

Lepock JR, Frey HE, Rodahl M, Kruuv J (1988) Thermal analysis of CHL V79 cells using differential scanning calorimetry: implications for hyperthermic cell killing and the heat-shock response. J Cell Physiol 137: 14–24

Lepock JR, Frey HE, Heynen MP, Nishio J, Waters B (1990) Increased thermostability of thermotolerant CHL V79 cells as determined by differential scanning calorimetry. J Cell Physiol 142: 628–634

Law MP (1981) The induction of thermal resistance in the ear of the mouse by heating at temperatures ranging from 41.5 to 45.5°C. Radiat Res 85: 126–134

Li GC, Laszlo AJ (1985) Amino acid analogs, while inducing heat shock proteins, sensitize CHO cells to thermal damage. J Cell Physiol 122: 91–97

Lindegaard JC (1992) Thermosensitization induced by step-down heating. A review on heat-induced sensitization to hyperthermia alone or hyperthermia combined with radiation. Int J Hyperthermia 8: 561–586

Lindegaard JC, Overgaard J (1988) Effect of step-down heating on hyperthermic radiosensitization in an experimental tumor and a normal tissue in vivo. Radiother Oncol 11: 143–151

Ling CC, Robinson E (1989) Moderate hyperthermia and low dose rate irradiation. Radiat Res 114: 379–384

Massicotte-Nolan P, Glofcheski DJ, Kruuv J, Lepock JR (1981) Relationship between hyperthermic cell killing and protein denaturation by alcohols. Radiat Res 87: 284–299

Miller RC, Leith JC, Veomett RC, Gerner EW (1978) Effects of interstitial radiation alone, or in combination with localized hyperthermia on the response of a mouse mammary carcinoma. Radiat Res 19: 175–180

Mills MD, Meyn RE (1983) Hyperthermic potentation unrejoined DNA breaks following irradiation. Radiat Res 95: 327–338

Mivechi NF, Dewey WC (1985) DNA polymerase α and β activities during the cell cycle and their role in heat radiosensitization in Chinese hamster ovary cells. Radiat Res 103: 337–350

Moorthy CR, Hahn EW, Kim JH, Feingold SM, Alfieri AA, Hilaris BS (1984) Improved response of a murine fibrosarcoma (Meth-A) to interstitial radiation when combined with hyperthermia. Int J Radiat Oncol Biol Phys 10: 2145–2148

Moulder JE, Rockwell S (1984) Hypoxic fractions of solid tumors. Int J Radiat Oncol Biol Phys 10: 695–712

Nagata K, Hosokawa N (1993) Flavonoids inhibit the expression of heat shock proteins and the acquisition of thermotolerance: inhibition of the activation of heat shock factor is a key mechanism. In: Gerner EW, Cetas TC (eds) Hyperthermic oncology 1993, pp 57–64

Nielsen OS, Overgaard J, Kamura T (1983) Influence of thermotolerance on the interaction between hyperthermia and radiation in a solid tumor in vivo. Br J Radiol 56: 267–273

Nishimura Y, Urano M (1993) Thermal radiosensitization in fractionated radiotherapy of a spontaneous murine fibrosarcoma. In: Gerner EW, Cetas TC (eds) Hyperthermic oncology 1993, pp 119–124

Overgaard J (1978) The effect of local hyperthermia alone and in combination with radiation on solid tumors. In: Streffer C (ed) Cancer therapy by hyperthermia and radiation. Urban and Schwarzenberg, Baltimore, pp 49–62

Overgaard J, Nielsen OS, Lindegaard JC (1987) Biological basis for rational design of clinical treatment with combined hyperthermia and radiation. In: Field SB, Franconi C (eds) Physics and technology of hyperthermia. Martinus Nijhoff, Amsterdam, pp 54–79

Papadopoulos D, Kimler BF, Estes NC, Durham FJ (1989) Growth delay effect of combined interstitial hyperthermia and brachytherapy in a rat solid tumor model. Anticancer Res 9: 45–47

Peak MJ, Peak JG, Blazek ER (1988) Symposium report. Radiation-induced DNA damage and repair: Argonne National Laboratory Symposium, Argonne, Illinois. Int J Radiat Biol 54: 513–520

Reinhold HS, Blackiewics B, Berg-Blok A (1978) Decrease in tumor microcirculation during hyperthermia. In: Streffer C, van Beuningen D, Dietzel F (eds) Cancer therapy by hyperthermia and radiation. Schwarzenberg, Baltimore, pp 231–232

Roti Roti JL, Lazslo A (1988) The effects of hyperthermia on nuclear macromolecules. In: Urano M, Douple E (eds) Hyperthermia and oncology. VSP, Zeist, pp 13–56

Roti Roti JL, Winward RT (1978) The effects of hyperthermia on the protein-to-DNA ratio of isolated HeLa cell chromatin. Radiat Res 74: 155–169

Ruifrok ACC, Levendag PC, Lakeman RF, Deurloo IKK, Visser AG (1991) Combined treatment with interstitial hyperthermia and interstitial radiotherapy in an animal tumor model. Int J Radiat Oncol Biol Phys 20: 1281–1286

Sakkers RJ, Filon AR, Brunsting JF, Kampinga HH, Mullenders LHF, Konings AWT (1993) Heat-shock treatment selectively affects induction and repair of cyclobutane pyrimidine dimers in transcriptionally active genes in ultraviolet-irradiated human fibroblasts. Radiat Res 135: 343–350

Sapozink MD, Palos B, Goffinet DR, Hahn GM (1983) Combined continuous ultra low dose rate irradiation and radiofrequency hyperthermia in the C3H mouse. Int J Radiat Oncol Biol Phys 9: 1357–1367

Streffer C, Van Beuningen D (1987) The biological basis for tumour therapy by hyperthermia and radiation. Recent Results Cancer Res 104: 24–70

Tanaka Y (1993) Modification of thermal Radiosensitization using hydralazine in vivo. In: Gerner EW, Cetas TC (eds) Hyperthermic oncology 1993, pp 115–118

Tomasovic SP, Turner GN, Dewey WC (1978) Effect of hyperthermia on non-histone proteins isolated with DNA. Radiat Res 73: 535–552

Van Hooije CMC, Van Geel CAJF, Visser AG, Kaatee RSJP, Van den Aardweg PC, Levendag PC (1993) Interstitial hyperthermia and interstitial radiotherapy in an animal tumor model: effects of sequential treatment and of thermal dose. Proceedings of the 13th conference of ESHO, Brussels, Belgium, p 59

Visser AG, Levendag PC (1992) Pulsed dose rate brachytherapy: treatment set-up and choice of fractionation. In: Mould RF (ed) International brachytherapy. Proceedings 7th International Brachytherapy Working Conference, Baltimore/Washington, USA. Nucletron International BV, Veenendaal, pp 501–504

Warters RL, Axtell J (1992) Repair of DNA strand breaks at hyperthermic temperatures in Chinese hamster ovary cells. Int J Radiat Biol 61: 43–48

Warters RL, Brizgys LM (1987) Apurinic site induction in the DNA of cells heated at hyperthermic temperatures. J Cell Physiol 133: 144–150

Warters RL, Roti Roti JL (1979) Excision of X-ray-induced thymine damage in chromatin from heated cells. Radiat Res 79: 113–121

Warters RL, Hofer KG (1977) Radionuclide Toxicity in Cullmed Mammalian. Cells Radiat Res 69: 348–358

Warters RL, Lyons BW, Axtell-Bartlett J (1987) Inhibition of repair of radiation-induced DNA damage by thermal shock in Chinese hamster ovary cells. Int J Radiat Biol 51: 505–517

Wolters H, Konings AWT (1982) Radiation effects on membranes. III. The effect of X-irradiation on survival of mammalian cells substituted by polyunsaturated fatty acids. Radiat Res 92: 474–482

Wolters H, Konings AWT (1984) Radiosensitivity of normal and polyunsaturated fatty acid supplemented fibroblasts after depletion of glutathione. Int J Radiat Biol 46: 161–168

Wolters H, Konings AWT (1985) Membrane radiosensitivity of fatty acid supplemented fibroblasts as assayed by the loss of intracellular potassium. Int J Radiat Biol 48: 963–973

Wolters H, Kelholt D, Konings AWT (1987) Effect of hyperthermia on the repair of subbethal radiation damage in normal and membrane fatty acid substituted fibroblasts. Radiat Res 109: 294–302

Yatvin MB (1977) The influence of membrane lipid composition and procaine on hyperthermic death of cells. Int J Radiat Biol 32: 513

5 Interaction of Heat and Drugs In Vitro and In Vivo

O. DAHL

CONTENTS

5.1 Introduction

The intention of this chapter is to review existing experimental data on combinations of cytotoxic drugs and hyperthermia. The focus will be on those drugs which are the most likely candidates for potentiation by hyperthermia, and attention will be drawn to findings which may form a basis for the design of clinical studies.

5.2 Drugs Potentiated by Heat

5.2.1 *Alkylating Agents*

It is now 25 years since the first report of an increased effect of *nitrogen mustard* (5 mg/kg) on a rat sarcoma when given in conjunction with heating to above 42°C (SUZUKI 1967). The monofunctional alkylating agent *methyl methanesulfonate* also killed more Chinese hamster cells in culture above 41°C, at which temperature a decrease in the shoulder of the survival curve and a steeper final slope were observed (BEN-HUR and ELKIND 1974). A similar potentiation of the effect of methyl dimethanesulfonate was also observed at 41°–42°C in rat Yoshida sarcoma cells in vitro and grown as tumours in vivo (DICKSON and SUZANGAR 1974). The mechanisms of action of this drug were enhanced production of DNA single strand breaks and also reduced repair of DNA strand breaks after heat exposure (BRONK et al. 1973; BEN-HUR and ELKIND 1974).

For Chinese hamster cells exposed to *thio-TEPA* in culture, proportionally less cells survived as the temperature increased between 35°C and 42°C (JOHNSON and PAVELEC 1973). The activation energies calculated from Arrhenius plots for thio-TEPA concentrations of 5 and 10 mg/ml were 36.8 and 32.9 kcal/mol, respectively. The result is compatible with an alkylating reaction and much lower than the activation energy for hyperthermia alone, i.e., 185 kcal/mol.

In vitro *melphalan* was more active at 42°C against several human fibroblast strains, with more varying results among melanoma lines (GOSS and PARSONS 1977). In Chinese hamster cells the cytotoxicity was increased fourfold at 42°C compared with 37°C, despite a net increase in the intracellular drug level of only 20% at 42°C (BATES and MACKILLOP 1989). Increased efficacy was observed when melphalan was combined with hyperthermia (43°C for 1 h) in Lewis lung carcinoma cells in vitro and in mice (JOINER et al. 1982). Also in a human breast tumor xenograft in nude mice, hyperthermia (42.5°C for 20 min) combined with melphalan reduced growth of tumors compared with melphalan alone (SENAPATI et al. 1982). Melphalan given with whole-body hyperthermia (41°C for 45 min) on KHT or RIF-1 tumors grown intramuscularly in the legs of mice preferentially killed tumor cells compared with

O. DAHL, MD, University of Bergen, Department of Oncology, Haukeland Hospital, N-5021 Bergen, Norway

the effect on normal bone marrow cells (HONESS and BLEEHEN 1985a). This therapeutic gain contrasts with the results obtained with cisplatin, BCNU, CCNU, and cyclophosphamide in the same tumor (HONESS and BLEEHEN 1982a, 1985b).

The dose of *cyclophosphamide* needed to cure 50% of Lewis lung carcinomas in mice was reduced from 170 mg/kg to 100 mg/kg when cyclophosphamide was combined with hyperthermia (42.5°C for 30 min) (HAZAN et al. 1981). Simultaneous whole-body hyperthermia (41°C for 45 min) and cyclophosphamide (100 mg/kg) in RIF-1 tumors yielded a growth delay similar to that achieved after 150 mg/kg cyclophosphamide alone (HONESS and BLEEHEN 1982a). However, a parallel increased effect on bone marrow in the same leg was observed, giving no therapeutic gain. When we grew our transplanted rat glioma BT_4A in the leg of rats, we observed seven complete responses, four of which were permanent cures, in eight rats after local water bath hyperthermia (44°C for 60 min) in combination with cyclophosphamide (200 mg/kg), in contrast to only nine partial responses in ten rats receiving cyclophosphamide alone, and no objective responses after hyperthermia alone (DAHL and MELLA 1983). In the C3H mouse mammary carcinoma, too, the supra-additive effect increased with heating time at 43.5°C and cyclophosphamide dose (MONGE et al. 1988). Human melanomas and breast tumors grown as xenografts in nude mice responded better when cyclophosphamide was combined with hyperthermia than when the drug was given alone (SENAPATI et al. 1982).

Ifosphamide, an analogue of cyclophosphamide, was also more cytotoxic at 43°C than at 37°C when tested on uterine cervical cancer cells in culture (FUJIWARA et al. 1984). Human breast carcinoma (MX1/3) and human sarcoma (S117) xenografts in nude mice both showed only a transient growth delay when given either cyclophosphamide or ifosphamide, while the same drug doses in combination with hyperthermia (43°C for 1 h) resulted in complete tumor regressions (WIEDEMANN et al. 1992a).

The alkylating antibiotic *mitomycin C* combined with hyperthermia in vitro produced a steeper exponential part of the survival curve with a dose modifying factor of 1.5 at 10% survival at 41°C, and 2.6 at 42°C (BARLOGIE et al. 1980). When EMT6 tumor cells grown in vitro were exposed to mitomycin C (1.0 and 10 μM for 1–6 h) in combination with hyperthermia (41°–43°C for 1–6 h), an additive effect was observed for oxygenated tumor cells while a synergistic effect was observed in hypoxic tumor cells, especially after exposure for 6 h (TEICHER et al. 1981). In these cells a 30%–50% increase in the rate of formation of reactive alkylating species was observed at 41°–43°C compared to controls at 37°C, but there was no difference between 42° and 43°C. For the murine fibrosarcoma (FSa-IIC) only a limited dose modification (factor, 1.2) of mitomycin C was seen when hyperthermia (43°C for 30 min) was applied following administration of the drug, demonstrating an additive effect (HERMAN et al. 1990). In C3H mouse mammary carcinoma the thermal enhancement ratios for mitomycin C and cyclophosphamide were 2.8 and 1.6, respectively (MONGE et al. 1988).

5.2.2 Nitrosoureas

Despite increased hydrolytic decay of the nitrosoureas *BCNU*, *CCNU*, and *methyl-CCNU* at elevated temperatures, a temperature-dependent reduction of survival was seen when Chinese hamster cells were heated at temperatures of 41°–43°C in vitro (HAHN 1978). The activation energies (18–24 kcal/mol) calculated from Arrhenius plots indicated an alkylating reaction. In the mouse fibrosarcoma FSa-II the activation energies at pH 6.7 and 7.4 were 53 and 51 kcal/mol for BCNU, again supporting an alkylating reaction (URANO et al. 1991). In vivo thermochemotherapy also enhanced the effect on FSa-II tumors. The positive effect of a combination of BCNU and heat (42.4°–43.3°C) was confirmed in Chinese hamster ovary cells in vitro (HERMAN 1983b). In EMT6 mouse tumors treated with BCNU (20 mg/kg) and local water bath heating (43°C for 1 h) a potentiation of different endpoints such as cell survival, growth delay, and cure was observed (TWENTYMAN et al. 1978). In our rat glioma BT_4A, combination of BCNU 20 mg/kg and local hyperthermia (44°C for 1 h) produced objective tumor regression in all rats, with cures in eight of ten animals, whereas no cures were observed when single modalities were used (DAHL and MELLA 1982). Similarly, in mice with RIF tumors grown on the foot, BCNU (40 mg/kg) with concomitant heat (45°C for 30 min) resulted in cures in nine of ten animals (NEILAN and HENLE 1989). As originally described by HAHN and SHIU (1983), we found that an intraperitoneal glucose dose before heat and BCNU or ACNU increased the effect of these combinations (SCHEM et al. 1989; SCHEM and DAHL 1991).

Experiments failed to demonstrate that an improved therapeutic response occurred in mice with Lewis lung carcinomas when treatment with CCNU or methyl-CCNU was supplemented by whole-body hyperthermia (41°C for 30 min) (ROSE et al. 1979). However, local heat (42.5°C for 1 h) enhanced the effect of methyl-CCNU in Lewis lung carcinoma (ZIMBER et al. 1986). Heat (41°–42°C) did not increase the effect of methyl-CCNU on human colon cancer xenografts in nude mice (OSIEKA et al. 1978). In contrast, a synergistic effect on survival occurred when mice with an intracerebrally transplanted ependymoblastoma were treated with whole-body hyperthermia (40°C for 2 h) and CCNU (8–16 mg/kg) (THUNING et al. 1980). For B16 melanoma and Lewis lung carcinoma treated in vivo and scored in an agar colony assay after graded doses of CCNU at 43°C for 1 h, the thermal enhancement rate was 1.6, whereas it was 2.4 after melphalan (JOINER et al. 1982). When the relatively nitrosourea-insensitive RIF-1 fibrosarcoma and the more sensitive KHT sarcoma were treated with BCNU (5–15 mg/kg) or BCNU (10–15 mg/kg) combined with whole-body hyperthermia (41°C for 45 min), there was no therapeutic gain when the effect on tumors was compared with that on the bone marrow stem cells (HONESS and BLEEHEN 1982a, 1985a). This confirms that mouse bone marrow cells are especially sensitive to temperature elevations combined with BCNU in vitro (O'DONNEL et al. 1979). In B16 melanoma cells in mice, the combination of hyperthermia and CCNU or melphalan produced not only an enhanced growth delay, but interestingly a noticeable reduction in the number of metastases (VICENTE et al. 1990).

Both B16 melanoma and C24 human malignant melanoma tumors showed a synergistic effect when the water-soluble ACNU (10 mg/kg) was given in combination with hyperthermia (43°C for 30 min) in three repeated doses every other day, whereas no such effect was observed with CCNU and methyl-CCNU in vivo (YAMADA et al. 1984). However, the combination of hyperthermia with ACNU yielded only a slight synergistic effect on human malignant melanoma cells in vitro (SOMEYA et al. 1990). In our glioblastoma line (BT_4An) in rats we found that the effect of ACNU (10 mg/kg) on foot tumors was clearly potentiated by heat (44°C for 45 min), this potentiation being further increased by a glucose load (SCHEM and DAHL 1991). For rats heated (42.4°C for 45 min) with BT_4An tumors in the brain, combination with ACNU (15 mg/kg) resulted in 50% increased life span (SCHEM et al. 1991). However, when ACNU (18 mg/kg) was administered intra-arterially and combined with the same heat treatment, survival increased by 100% and was significantly better than with the same drug dose given intravenously (SCHEM et al. 1991).

5.2.3 *Cisplatin, Carboplatin, and Analogues*

When normal bone marrow cells and P388 lymphocytic leukemia cells were analyzed for survival after heating of mouse legs in a water bath (42.3°C for 30–60 min), hyperthermia was found to increase the cytotoxicity of *cisplatin* (5 mg/kg) on leukemia cells by a factor of 100 while no synergistic effect was observed in bone marrow cells (ALBERTS et al. 1980). Heat alone and cisplatin alone reduced survival by 20% and 25%, respectively. In culture, significant enhancement of cisplatin cytotoxicity at elevated temperatures has been clearly demonstrated by several investigators (BARLOGIE et al. 1980, FISHER and HAHN 1982, HERMAN 1983a). Hyperthermia (40.4°–41.8°C) markedly enhanced the efficacy of cisplatin and carboplatin in human lymphoblastic leukemia cells in vitro (COHEN and ROBINS 1987, COHEN et al. 1989). However, whole-body hyperthermia in mice with L1210 leukemia yielded no differential effect between malignant cells and normal bone marrow stem cells (DE NEVE et al. 1991), as also reported earlier (HONESS and BLEEHEN 1985a).

In the BT4A tumor, where cisplatin and hyperthermia alone only transiently retarded growth, cures were observed after combination therapy (MELLA 1985). The effect increased with increasing temperature (41°–44°C) and cisplatin dose (2–4 mg/kg). Interestingly, hyperthermia alone induced central tumor necrosis, while the thermochemotherapy especially caused cell death in the well-vascularized tumor periphery, which implies a spatial cooperation. There were no increased local side-effects, but there was a substantial increase in systemic toxicity for the combined treatment at the higher drug dose (4 mg/kg). Further analyses showed that even an increased core temperature to 41°C produced a significant increase in cisplatin-induced renal damage in rats

(Mella et al. 1987). This finding has been confirmed in another rat model (Wondergem et al. 1988). A significant enhancement ratio was obtained when cisplatin was given 15 min before heat (40.5°C); an optimum ratio of 3 seemed to be reached at 42.5°C, with no further increase at 43.5°C (Lindegaard et al. 1992).

Cisplatin produces intrastrand cross-links. Alkaline elution demonstrated a significant increase in DNA cross-linking caused by cisplatin at 42°–43°C (Meyn et al. 1980; Herman and Teicher 1988), and Arrhenius plot analysis showed the activation energy for the chemical reaction of cisplatin to be 44 kcal/mol in the range 37°–41°C in the murine fibrosarcoma FSa-II (Urano et al. 1990). When intraperitoneal cisplatin (5 mg/kg) was added to regional abdominal hyperthermia, the cytotoxicity was increased by a factor of 4 at 40°C and a factor of 6 at 43°C compared to 37°C (Los et al. 1991). The increased toxicity correlated with an increased intracellular platinum concentration.

In spontaneous canine and feline tumors intralesional cisplatin (1.8 mg per cm^3 tumor) combined with 42°C for 30 min once a week for 4 weeks resulted in complete response in four of ten tumors (Theon et al. 1991). Injection of cisplatin into melanomas in mice was also synergistic when combined with local heat (42.5°C) (Kitamura et al. 1992).

When *carboplatin* and the new analogue *iproplatin* (CHIP) were administered at different concentrations in vitro in a human ovarian adenocarcinoma cell line, a tenfold decrease in drug concentration yielded similar survival when the temperature was raised by 3°C in the temperature range 37°–43°C (Xu and Alberts 1988). In vitro both carboplatin and the analogue *tetraplatin* showed thermal enhancement above 40°C, with maximal thermal enhancement at 42°C and no further increase at 43°C (Cohen and Robins 1990), which is a similar finding to that reported by Lindegaard et al. (1992) for cisplatin. The antitumor activity and normal tissue toxicity of carboplatin given with whole-body hyperthermia (41.5°C for 2 h) were similar to cisplatin in the rat F344 fibrosarcoma, but carboplatin was less nephrotoxic than cisplatin (Ohno et al. 1991). A therapeutic gain with a therapeutic ratio of 3.0 for carboplatin was reported, in contrast to a ratio of 0.8 for cisplatin. In our glioma BT_4A or glioblastoma line BT_4An we found a striking parallel effect both in vitro and in vivo: both local toxicity and weight loss following thermochemotherapy were comparable for carboplatin and cisplatin (Schem et al. 1992). Other experimental platinum complexes have also been tested in combination with hyperthermia, and found to have a comparable or even larger effect than cisplatin (Herman et al. 1989, 1990a, 1990b; Teicher et al. 1989).

5.2.4 Anthracyclines

For *doxorubicin* the cytotoxicity was increased in Chinese hamster cells (Hahn et al. 1975; Hahn and Strande 1976), FM3A mammary carcinoma cells (Mizuno et al. 1980), Chinese hamster V79 cells (Roizin-Towle et al. 1982), and in our BT_4C glioma cell line (Dahl 1982). This positive effect could not be confirmed in uterine cancer cells (Fujiwara et al. 1984). In EMT6 spheroids doxorubicin cytotoxicity was not increased after 1 h at 43°C, but a significant enhanced effect was observed after heating at 42°C for 6 h (Morgan and Bleehen 1980).

The same discrepancy has also been reported in animal studies. An enhanced effect was only achieved at doxorubicin doses so high as to be incompatible with survival of mice bearing two different mammary carcinomas (Overgaard 1976; Marmor et al. 1979). When local hyperthermia (43°C for 1 h) and doxorubicin (10 mg/kg) were combined to treat the 16/C mouse mammary carcinoma, increased tumor growth delay was observed despite similar drug uptake with and without heating (Magin et al. 1980). In BT_4A tumors grown on the leg of rats, an enhanced growth delay was observed when hyperthermia (44°C for 1 h) and doxorubicin (7 mg/kg) or the less cardiotoxic analogue *4-epirubicin* (7 mg/kg) were given, but no cures occurred (Dahl 1983).

In P388 leukemia cells, hyperthermia (43°C for 1 h) showed only an additive effect on survival in vitro and there was no increased growth delay compared to doxorubicin alone in animals; furthermore there was no difference in drug uptake with and without heating in this tumor (van der Linden et al. 1984). In mice bearing C3H carcinoma on the foot only an additive effect was observed when doxorubicin (8 mg/kg) was combined with hyperthermia at 43.5°C (Monge et al. 1988). Whole-body hyperthermia (41.5°C for 2 h), when given in combination with doxorubicin (5 mg/kg i.v.), increased the effect on tumors by a factor of 1.6, but at the same time increased leukopenia and thrombocytopenia by a factor of 1.3, late cardiac toxicity by a factor of 2.4, and renal toxicity by a factor of 4.3 (WONDERGEM et al. 1991; NEWMAN et al. 1992). Thus no therapeutic gain was found in this system.

In vitro a short exposure to *mitoxantrone* inhibited proliferation of WIDR colon carcinoma cells when the temperature was raised from 37°C to 42°C, this effect being at least in part related to increased drug uptake (WANG et al. 1984). When the human breast carcinoma MX1 or human sarcoma S117 was transplanted to nude mice, local hyperthermia (42°–43°C for 1 h) significantly enhanced the effect of mitoxantrone (3 mg/kg) given twice a week (WIEDEMANN et al. 1992b). In both cell lines complete tumor regression was achieved only in the combined modality groups, without increasing side-effects of the drug alone. Mitoxantrone has also been tested in various spontaneous neoplasms in dogs (OGILVIE et al. 1991). Mouse mammary FM3A carcinoma cells were sensitized to *aclacinomycin A* when combined with hyperthermia at 42°–43°C, but the effect of *daunomycin* was not enhanced (MIZUNO et al. 1980).

Thus the sensitivity for anthracyclines seems to vary with cell type and growth conditions, and also seems to be dependent on drug scheduling.

5.2.5 Bleomycin

Survival curves for graded doses of *bleomycin* or increased exposure times to bleomycin at normal temperature are usually biphasic, an initial sensitive part being followed by a resistant tail. When bleomycin is combined with heat a threshold usually appears; thus there is only slight enhancement of cell killing at temperatures up to 40°–41°C in culture, but above 42°–43°C a marked potentiation occurs, with reduction of the resistant tail for Chinese hamster cells (HAHN et al. 1975; HERMAN 1983b; ROIZIN-TOWLE et al. 1982; DOGRAMATZIS et al. 1991), EMT6 cells (HAR-KEDAR 1975, MARMOR et al. 1979, MORGAN and BLEEHEN 1982, MIRCHEVA et al. 1986), HeLa cells (RABBANI et al. 1978), and a murine fibrosarcoma FSa-IIC (TEICHER et al. 1988). In the latter cell line bleomycin was substantially more toxic towards normally oxygenated cells at 37°C, but this difference in killing was not observed at 42° and 43°C. Comparison of the effectiveness of bleomycin and *peplomycin* in 13 different human tumors grown in monolayer culture at normal temperature and after hyperthermic treatment (40.5°C for 2 h) revealed a thermal enhancement effect for both bleomycin and *peplomycin* in three of the 13 samples (NEUMANN et al. 1989). When human bone marrow stem cells (CFU-C) were subjected to the same procedure, peplomycin was less toxic towards the normal cells. There was no difference between normal and hyperthermic incubation, indicating a possible therapeutic benefit of using bleomycin even at a temperature around the threshold temperature. An increased sensitivity of most leukemia cells and Chinese hamster V79 cells was demonstrated when they were exposed to bleomycin (0.1 mg/ml) at a temperature of 40°C (KANO et al. 1988). This could imply that leukemia cells have a lower threshold for thermochemotherapy than most other solid tumors.

In vivo a super-additive interaction occurred when local hyperthermia (>43°C for 30–60 min) was combined with bleomycin (7–100 mg/kg) for the treatment of Lewis lung carcinoma in mice (MAGIN et al. 1979). Marked enhancement was also observed in KHT tumors when bleomycin (7 and 15 mg/kg) was combined with heat (42° and 43°C for 30 min) (MARMOR et al. 1979). In this tumor even cures were observed. When EMT6 tumors were heated in vivo and assayed in vitro, a synergistic interaction was confirmed. A positive interaction has also been reported in a mouse adenocarcinoma (VON SZCZEPANSKI and TROTT 1981), a mouse squamous cell carcinoma (HASSANZADEH and CHAPMAN 1982), RIF tumors (NEILAN and HENLE 1989), and the fibrosarcoma FSa-II when the tumor was heated in vivo (URANO et al. 1988a). In the latter study there was a biphasic response, and the authors noted that above 42.5°C the benefit of combined treatment appeared to disappear, the effect above this temperature being caused by hyperthermia alone. Tumor growth time was similarly prolonged by combination of bleomycin (10–30 mg/kg) with 41.5°C for 1 h and 43.5°C for 30 min, but 1 h at 43.5°C further increased the effect, probably by an additive effect (URANO and KHAN 1989). Glucose injection before the administration of hyperthermia and bleomycin enhanced tumor responses, probably via a reduction of pH. In our glioma BT_4A, the doubling time increased from 5.7 days for control to 6.2 days for bleomycin (20 mg/kg), 11 days for hyperthermia alone (44°C for 60 min), and 28.1 days for combined treatment, but we did not observe any cures as a result of the combination of these two modalities (DAHL and MELLA 1982). No increase in local side-effects was seen, but rats in the combined modality group had a significantly reduced weight.

Bleomycin is of particular interest for combination with hyperthermia as this drug by itself has no bone marrow suppressing effect in humans and hence can be included in any hyperthermia schedule. As this drug has a threshold effect, it does not seem to be a candidate for combination with whole-body hyperthermia, and even with local hyperthermia there are areas where the temperature is in the range of 40°C (PILEPICH et al. 1989).

5.2.6 *Actinomycin D*

Actinomycin D chiefly interacts with RNA. In Chinese hamster cells exposure for less than 30 min at 43°C reduced cell survival, with further heating deminishing the cell killing (DONALDSON et al. 1978). This resistance was probably caused by an initial increased drug uptake followed by reduced actinomycin D in the cells. In EMT6 cells in vitro no enhancement was observed when actinomycin D was given in combination with heat (HAR-KEDAR 1975), in contrast to the results in leukemic cells (GIOVANELLA et al. 1970; MIZUNO et al. 1980) and a murine fibrosarcoma (YERUSHALMI 1978).

5.2.7 *Antimetabolites and Vinca Alkaloids*

Antimetabolite drugs are dependent on intact cellular functions to be metabolized and transported to the enzymes whose function they block. Hyperthermia at least transiently reduce cellular metabolism. It is therefore not surprising that frequently used antimetabolites like *5-fluorouracil* and *methotrexate* have only a limited increased effect at elevated temperatures. Thus Chinese hamster cells were not sensitized by methotrexate after heating (43°C for 1 h) in vitro (HAHN and SHIU 1983) and a negative report was also given for rats with VX2 carcinoma (MUCKLE and DICKSON 1973). In a Chinese hamster methotrexate-resistant cell line, exposure to 43°C but not 41°C or 42°C for 1 h increased the killing by 50%, probably as a consequence of reduced synthesis of dihydrofolate reductase caused by heat (HERMAN et al. 1981).

Early studies with 5-fluorouracil indicated a significantly increased effect when the drug was given in combination with heat in a murine ependymoblastoma in vivo (SUTTON 1971); similarly, human pancreatic carcinoma xenografted in nude mice and treated with 5-fluorouracil and hyperthermia at 43.5°C responded more favorably than after 5-fluorouracil alone (SHIU et al. 1983). However, other largely negative studies have been published (see DAHL and MELLA 1990). In the case of *cytosine arabinoside* (ROSE et al. 1979; MIZUNO et al. 1980) and *phosphoracetyl aspartate*, too, no benefit has been reported to accrue from combination with heat (ROIZIN-TOWLE et al. 1982).

Also, studies of *vinblastine* and *vincristine* failed to demonstrate enhanced efficacy due to heat (DAHL and MELLA 1990).

5.2.8 *Etoposide*

Hyperthermia (40°–42.5°C for 30–90 min) did not increase the cytotoxicity of etoposide on cultured human lymphoblasts (VOTH et al. 1988). In another study etoposide had no supra-additive effect in combination with hyperthermia (41.8°C for 10–30 min) on a human T-cell lymphoblastic cell line in culture (COHEN et al. 1989). However, in FSaIIC sarcoma cells in culture a dose-modifying factor of 2 was demonstrated by heating at 43°C for 30 min (PFEFFER et al. 1990). In animals etoposide was less effective than cisplatin in combination with radiation and heat (tumor growth delay 14 days vs 25 days) in FSaII tumours, but when added to the trimodality cisplatin/radiation/hyperthermia the drug yielded a significantly longer growth delay (34 days). Caution has been expressed regarding the combination of etoposide and hyperthermia as hyperthermia actually decreased etoposide cytotoxicity in Chinese hamster cells (DYNLACHT et al. 1994) and heating (40°C for 30 min for 4 days) did not add to the effect of etoposide alone in a murine bladder carcinoma (ILZUMI et al. 1989).

The finding that etoposide was unstable when heated at 43°C for 90 min, in contrast to 41°C for 90 min, may be of relevance for the failure of higher temperatures to enhance the effect of this drug (VOTH et al. 1988). Upon the addition of hyperthermia there is no change in DNA single strand breaks caused by the topoisomerase II effects of etoposide (DYNLACHT et al. 1994, BERTRAND et al. 1991). With our present knowledge etoposide should probably be given as an additive, independent modality in combination with hyperthermia. The topoisomerase I inhibitors camptothecin and topotecan also failed to exhibit enhanced cytotoxicity towards EMT-6 cells in culture upon heating at 42° and 43°C (TEICHER et al. 1993). However, the same authors reported that in vivo local hyperthermia (43°C for 30 min) enhanced the killing of FSaIIC tumor cells.

5.2.9 Hypoxic Cell Sensitizers

Hypoxic cell sensitizers include electron-affinic drugs which are potent radiosensitizers of hypoxic cells (ADAMS 1978). These drugs mimic the electrophilic effect of oxygen and act as stabilizers for unstable oxygen radicals caused by ionizing radiation. The prototype drugs metronidazole and misonidazole (ADAMS 1978) have the advantage over oxygen that they are not readily metabolized, and therefore can penetrate deeper into tumors where cells are hypoxic because oxygen cannot reach them. In addition to the oxygen mimicking actions with ionizing radiation, some nitroimidazoles may also be metabolized under hypoxic conditions (nitroreduction) to release a range of toxic and nontoxic metabolites and thus become selectively cytotoxic for hypoxic cells (ADAMS et al. 1980). Recently bifunctional analogues have been introduced which also have an alkylating effect.

As regards combinations of hyperthermia and radiation, these two modalities might both have an independent effect or heat may function as a radiosensitizer (OVERGAARD 1989). Heat may selectively kill hypoxic cells by a direct effect or indirectly by destruction of vasculature. The combination with nitroimidazole derivatives may be especially effective in radioresistant hypoxic cells. Most in vivo studies have demonstrated that local hyperthermia simultaneously administered with misonidazole and irradiation significantly increases the tumor response (OVERGAARD 1980; HOFER et al. 1981; BLEEHEN et al. 1988; WONG 1994). The pharmacokinetics of radiosensitizers have been studied under whole-body hyperthermia (HONESS et al. 1980, WALTON et al. 1986). A decrease in plasma clearance and an increase in area under the concentration curve have been demonstrated, but also a decrease in tumor and tumor/plasma concentration for misonidazole. The reduced tumor concentration may be explained by an increased hypoxic metabolism at higher temperatures (WALTON et al. 1989). It has been underlined that the optimal temperature for hypoxic metabolism of misonidazoeles is about 41°C in FSAII tumors (WONG 1994). OVERGAARD (1980) provided evidence that misonidazole is most effective when given simultaneously with heat and radiation, which suggests that thermal enhancement of misonidazole radiosensitization is more important than thermal potentiation of the misonidazole hypoxic effect.

A major clinical problem with nitroimidazoles is their neurotoxicity. For the newer analogues which are less prone to penetrate the blood brain barrier, gastrointestinal toxicity has been observed. The future role of radiosensitizers is still an open question, although a recent randomized study has shown promising results of nimorazole treatment in patients with head and neck cancer (OVERGAARD et al. 1991).

Lonidamine has a limited antitumor effect by itself, but can potentiate the action of both radiation and chemotherapeutic drugs as well as hyperthermia (KIM et al. 1984; RAAPHORST et al. 1991a,b). Its mechanism of action is chiefly on mitochondria by inhibition of oxidative phosphorylation and aerobic glycolysis, in combination with radiation it may inhibit repair of potentially lethal damage. Lonidamine may be added to other effective combinations to improve the efficacy.

5.2.10 Biological Agents

Cytokines are naturally occurring polypeptides with regulating or signalling effects. By use of recombinant techniques it is now possible to produce pure cytokines in sufficient quantities for clinical application. Despite the fact that these substances are natural in origin, cytokines are potent drugs, sometimes causing severe side-effects. The cytokines are of particular interest in relation to hyperthermia, as fever is mediated by several cytokines, including interleukin-1α, interleukin 1β, interleukin-6, tumor necrosis factor α

(TNF-α), and the interferons (KAPPEL et al. 1991).

5.2.10.1 Interferons

The term "interferon" is used for a family of related proteins induced by viral infections or different pyrogens. Three interferons are isolated from different cells: leukocytes produce interferon α (IFN-α), fibroblasts produce interferon β (IFN-β) and T-helper cells excrete interferon γ (IFN-γ). In culture mild heat (39.4°C) enhanced the antiproliferative effect of murine IFN-γ (tenfold) on B16 melanoma cells, but the effect was less pronounced (2.9- and 3.4-fold, respectively) for IFN-α and IFN-β (FLEICHMANN et al. 1986). Thus fever may maximize the effect of at least IFN-γ. In the same tumor system a considerably more enhanced effect was observed (153-fold increase) when IFN-γ was combined with IFN-α and IFN-β at the same temperature (FLEICHMANN et al. 1986a). When mice bearing B16 melanoma tumors were heated by whole-body hyperthermia at about 39°C, the antitumor activity of IFN-γ again was more effective than that of IFN-α (2.9- vs 1-fold) (ANJUM and FLEICHMANN 1992). Following local injection of murine recombinant IFN-β in combination with local hyperthermia (43°C for 15 min) a growth delay was observed (NAKAYAMA et al. 1993). These authors reported that the effect was related to a modulation of the local immune response by a reduction of NK cells seen after IFN-β alone, and an augmentation of T-cell infiltration. Also in vitro IFN-β and heat exerted a greater antitumor effect against a Rous sarcoma virus-induced mouse malignant glioma (RSV glioma) (KUROKI et al. 1987). In a human renal carcinoma transplanted to nude mice, IFN-α combined with 44°C for 30 min caused complete disappearance of the tumor in five of ten mice, in contrast to no effect of each modality alone (ONISHI et al. 1989). It is also of interest that the combination of IFN-α and hyperthermia at 42° and 43°C has been launched as a method for bone marrow purging based on the finding that the combination enhances killing among myeloid leukemic cell lines, while normal CFU-GMs appear to be significantly protected (MORIYAMA et al. 1991). The conclusion based on the literature is that the different types of IFN may have selective effects on different tumors. An enhanced effect may be shown at temperatures considered unsatisfactory for hyperthermic cell killing. If a selective efficacy in tumors can be confirmed, IFNs may become very interesting options in some tumors.

5.2.10.2 Tumor Necrosis Factor

Recombinant tumor necrosis factor α, r-TNFα, is currently used in clinical studies as an antitumor agent (LEJEUNE et al. 1993). The principal mechanism of action of TNFα seems to be damage to endothelial cells resulting in vascular leakage with hemoconcentration and increased interstitial pressure and production of thrombosis and hemorrhages in tumors (KALLINOWSKI et al. 1989, SRINIVASAN et al. 1990). Blood stasis and vascular permeability induced by TNF were significantly enhanced when TNF was combined with hyperthermia (40°C for 30 min) in a murine Meth-A fibrosarcoma (UMENO et al. 1994) and (40.5°, 42.0°, or 43.5°C for 23 min) in human gastric adenocarcinoma transplanted to nude mice (FUJIMOTO et al. 1992). The local accumulation of neutrophils has suggested that the neutrophils may mediate the endothelial damage (SRINIVASAN et al. 1990). Recent studies may indicate a role of nitric oxide in leukocyte adhesion and vasodilation (ÄNGGÅRD 1994). Direct DNA fragmentation resembling apoptosis has also been observed in cells exposed to TNF (TOMASOVIC et al. 1994).

Use of TNF in combination with hyperthermia (long term at low temperature or short term at higher temperatures) resulted in a synergistic effect in L-M cells in vitro (WATANABE et al. 1988), in different tumors given TNFα i.v. (Meth-A fibrosarcoma, WATANABE et al. 1988; L929 fibroblasts and EMT6 tumor cells, TOMASOVIC et al. 1994), and in several human carcinoma cell lines (KLOSTERGAARD et al. 1992; LEE et al. 1993). When TNF-α was injected directly into RIF-1 tumors (SRINIVASAN et al. 1990) and a murine bladder tumor MTB-2 (ILZUMI et al. 1989), an enhanced effect of hyperthermia (42.5°C and 40°C for 30 min, respectively) was observed. However, no enhanced effect on a murine B-cell lymphoma in culture was seen when hyperthermia (43.5°C for 30 min) was combined with TNF (10–100 U/ml) (DE DAVIES et al. 1990). Also in vivo i.v. TNF (1000 units/mouse) in combination with heating (43.5°C for 20 min) showed no enhanced effect on a murine bladder carcinoma KK-47 in athymic mice (AMANO et al. 1990), and a similar finding has also been reported in a fibrosarcoma (OHNO et al. 1992). Thus the effect of TNF may be selective. It seems to be important that TNFα is administered before hyperthermia, like most cytotoxic drugs (TOMASOVIC et al. 1992). TNF has also been introduced for trimodality therapy in combination with hyperthermia and drugs or radiation (see Sect. 5.7).

5.3 Timing and Sequence

HAHN (1979) reported a much better effect when hyperthermia (43°C for 1 h) and BCNU exposure for 1 h in vitro were given simultaneously than when there was an interval up to ±6 h. Similar findings were also reported for cisplatin (FISHER and HAHN 1982), melphalan (ZUPI et al. 1984; WALLNER et al. 1986), BCNU (HAHN 1979; O'DONNEL et al. 1979), carboplatin (COHEN and ROBINS 1987), and bleomycin (HOU and MARUYAMA 1990) in culture.

In the case of our experimental rat brain tumor grown on the foot of rats exposed to water bath hyperthermia (44°C for 1 h), we observed a significant enhancement of i.p. cyclophosphamide (200 mg/kg), BCNU (20 mg/kg), and cisplatin (3 mg/kg) for time intervals of ±24 h (DAHL and MELLA 1983, MELLA and DAHL 1985). We saw no increase in local side-effects, as had been previously reported (HONESS and BLEEHEN 1982b). Also in mice bearing mammary carcinomas, bleomycin (15 mg/kg) (MA et al. 1985), cyclophosphamide (100 mg/kg) and mitomycin C (3 mg/kg) (MONGE et al. 1988) and cisplatin (6 mg/kg) (LINDEGAARD et al. 1992) were most effective when given just before hyperthermia, ensuring maximal drug concentration during heating.

No consistent difference has been shown favouring drug administration before or after heat; thus the optimal timing seems to be simultaneous or administration of the drug immediately before hyperthermia. Interestingly, a study of the pharmacokinetics of cisplatin given 1 h before the beginning of, at the end of, and 1 h after hyperthermia treatment at 43°C for 1 h did not show any significant difference in the time profiles of cisplatin in the plasma, but the mean tumor cisplatin concentration in rats which received drug at the beginning of hyperthermia was statistically greater than in those animals given cisplatin at the end of the heat treatment (AUSMUS et al. 1992).

In many of the above studies only an additive effect was observed when the two modalities were separated in time. It therefore seems important to give simultaneous therapy to obtain the maximal effect from the combination.

5.4 Side-effects

Generally, no increase in local side-effects has been reported when systemic drugs have been given in conjunction with local hyperthermia; an exception is adverse skin reactions after local hyperthermia at 44°C combined with cyclophosphamide and BCNU (HONESS and BLEEHEN 1982b; DAHL and MELLA 1982). The LD_{10} was reduced when mice were treated with cyclophosphamide, methyl-CCNU, and vincristine in combination with hyperthermia (ROSE et al. 1979). Increased liberation of catecholamines after injection of doxorubicin during whole-body hyperthermia was associated with ventricular irritability and cardiac dysfunction in patients (KIM et al. 1979). As stated above, we saw a substantial increase in renal toxicity with core temperatures above 41°C in combination with cisplatin in rats (MELLA et al. 1987). BCNU combined with local heat (44°C for 1 h), giving a systemic temperature of about 41°C, increased death associated with urinary tract toxicity at high doses (30 mg/kg) (DAHL and MELLA 1982). It has also been reported that heat recalled skin damage caused by prior bleomycin therapy (KUKLA and MCGUIRE 1982). When several alkylating agents and nitrosoureas were tested in a tumor against normal bone marrow, a therapeutic gain was only observed for melphalan after whole-body hyperthermia (41°C for 45 min) (HONESS and BLEEHEN 1982a, 1985a). These results underline the possibility that systemic hyperthermia may enhance specific side-effects of drugs.

5.5 Thermal Tolerance

Hyperthermia induces a transient resistance to subsequent heating, termed thermal tolerance. The degree of thermal tolerance is dependent on the primary heat dose (temperature and duration). When doxorubicin was combined with heat, an initial increase in cell killing was seen for longer exposure times in vitro followed by substantially reduced cell killing, in Chinese hamster cells

(43°C) (HAHN and STRANDE 1976) and BT_4C cells (41°C) (DAHL 1982). In BT_4C cells the same effect was seen in cells exposed to simultaneous therapy and in cells exposed to heating before drug exposure. In EMT6 cells preheating (40°C for 3h) reduced cell killing by bleomycin and BCNU, but not by doxorubicin (MORGAN et al. 1979); however, preheating at 37°C had no effect on any of these drugs. In contrast, preheating at 43°C sensitized EMT6 cells to bleomycin and BCNU, but protected them against doxorubicin toxicity. Earlier studies indicated an increased uptake response, with an initial increase in doxorubicin uptake for exposure times below 30 min, followed by a reduced cellular concentration of doxorubicin relative to that at 30 min (HAHN and STRANDE 1976; YAMANE et al. 1984). This could explain the observed development of heat-induced drug resistance, similar to thermal tolerance, during continuing heating (HAHN and STRANDE 1976, MIZUNO et al. 1980; DAHL 1982). Recent studies have also revealed elevated HSP70 and HSP27 levels to be associated with doxorubicin resistance through a mechanism not associated with multidrug resistance as heat did not induce P170 glycoprotein (CIOCCA et al. 1992).

Preheating at 43°C for various times enhanced the cytotoxicity of cisplatin in culture when it was given immediately after heating, but this enhancement decreased within 24h to less than additive level (MAJIMA et al. 1992). Bleomycin followed the same kinetics except that the immediate preheating enhancement was much less. In Chinese hamster cells exposure to cisplatin and carboplatin prevented the development of thermal tolerance after priming heating (42°C) during step-up experiments and continuous heating at 42°C (OHTSUBO et al. 1990).

In vivo hyperthermia (41.5°C for 1 h) alone and combined with cyclophosphamide (100 mg/kg alone) induced resistance to cyclophosphamide both alone and combined with heat in FSa-II tumors (URANO et al. 1988b). Thus five fractions were not more effective than a single fraction. Although in C3H mouse mammary carcinomas the relative effect (drug enhancement ratio) for cyclophosphamide and mitomycin C was higher in thermotolerant cells, the absolute effect was lower in these cells (MONGE and ROFSTAD 1989). These authors also reported a potentially improved therapeutic ratio for fractionated heating (MONGE and ROFSTAD 1991). Chemosenitivity for BCNU was also dependent on the interval following hyperthermia in BT_4An tumors, but there was no clear relation between thermal tolerance and chemosensitivity during normothermia (MELLA 1990). Thermal tolerance influenced the effect of thermochemotherapy 168h after primary heat exposure.

We can conclude that cells rendered thermotolerant by prior heating have largely unchanged or slightly reduced sensitivity for drugs alone but have generally reduced sensitivity for thermochemotherapy. In thermotolerant cells the reduced hyperthermia effect is therefore the dominant factor. These facts should be taken into consideration when designing experimental and clinical studies.

5.6 Drug Resistance

Cytotoxic drugs can induce drug resistance through several mechanisms: induction of p-glycoprotein, induction of detoxifying enzymes, transport changes, or amplification of target structures. After multiple drug exposures or exposure to prolonged low concentrations, many researchers have produced stable drug-resistant cell sublines. In Chinese hamster ovary cells hyperthermia was suggested as a method of overcoming drug resistance, as mitomycin C cytotoxicity was enhanced by hyperthermia (42°–43.5°C) in both a sensitive and a resistant subline (WALLNER et al. 1987). An increased uptake of mitomycin C was found in both lines at 43.5°C, but the difference from normal temperatures was less in the resistant cell line. Hyperthermia (>42°C) potentiated cell killing in BCNU-sensitive and BCNU-resistant gliomas (DA SILVA et al. 1991), as did heat (41°C) in Mer(+) nitrosourea-resistant human tumor cells exposed to CCNU alone or combined with heat (MULCAHY et al. 1988). In melphalan-resistant and -sensitive human rhabdomyosarcomas grown in athymic nude mice, melphalan plus hyperthermia (42°C for 70 min) increased equally the effect of melphalan in both cell lines (therapeutic enhancement rates of 1.7 in the resistant and 1.5 in the sensitive cells) (LASKOWITZ et al. 1992), confirming the earlier report of BATES and MACKILLOP (1990) in Chinese hamster ovary cells. Heat-induced alterations in glutathione or melphalan were not responsible for the thermochemotherapy effect. Reversal of drug-induced resistance has also been reported in several cell lines for cisplatin (DE GRAEFF et al.

Table 5.1. Reported mechanisms for potentiation of cytotoxic drugs by hyperthermia (for references, see also DAHL 1994)

Drug	Cellular target	Mechanisms
Doxorubicin	Membranes	Increased drug uptake
	DNA	Increased oxygen radical production
		Interaction with topoisomerase II
	Proteins	Enzyme damage
	Pharmacology	Increased half-life (reduced excretion)
Mitoxantrone	Membranes	Increased uptake
	DNA	Interaction with topoisomerase II
Alkylating agents	DNA (strand breaks)	No repair of double stranded breaks
		Reduced repair of single stranded breaks
Thiotepa	DNA	Rate of alkylation
Melphalan	Membranes	Increased uptake
Cyclophosphamide	Pharmacology	Increased half-life
Ifosfamide		
Mitomycin C	DNA	Increased oxygen radical production
BCNU	DNA	Increased oxygen radical production
		Increased strand breaks
Cisplatin	Membranes	Increased uptake
	Pharmacology	Increased peripheral protein binding
	DNA	Increased oxygen radical production
		Increased strand breaks
		Apoptosis
Bleomycin	DNA	Reduced repair
		Increased oxygen radical production
Lonidamide	Mitochondria	Decreased respiration
		Damage of membrane enzymes

1988; MANSOURI et al. 1989) and doxorubicin and mitoxantrone (JUVEKAR and CHITNIS 1991). It has been shown that multidrug resistance is not associated with a greater likelihood of development of thermotolerance during hyperthermia, and multidrug-resistant cells do not display reduced sensitivity to hyperthermia (UCKUN et al. 1992).

5.7 Trimodality Therapy

Most curative chemotherapy is currently given as combinations of several drugs. DOUPLE et al. (1982) reported that together cisplatin, heat, and radiation were better than two modalities. In two human bladder cancer lines, heat (43°C) significantly enhanced the effect of cisplatin, mitomycin C, and particularly bleomycin (NAKAJIMA and HISAZUMI 1987). HERMAN and co-workers have, in many papers, supported the use of trimodality therapy (HERMAN and TEICHER 1988; HERMAN et al. 1990a, 1991). They propose the use of maximally tolerated radiation as the basic therapy as this is the single most effective local therapy. Heat and drugs should then be given as adjuvant therapy in the combination most effective for the particular tumor. Recently studies addressing combination of two drugs with hyperthermia have been published: When cisplatin (5 mg/kg i.p.) was followed by hyperthermia and 3 Gy radiation on day 1, with five subsequent daily doses of 3 Gy, a growth delay of 25 days resulted. When this triple therapy was combined with mitomycin C, a growth delay of 44 days resulted, and the authors could show that toxicity was most pronounced in the additional cell killing of hypoxic cells (HERMAN et al. 1991).

In vitro etoposide and mild heating (40°C for 30 min) enhanced the cytotoxicity of a constructed tumor necrosis factor (rTNF-S) (ILZUMI et al. 1989). In three human colon tumor cell lines in culture TNF enhanced the effect of carboplatin, while hyperthermia (42°C for 2 h), which had a minimal effect alone, further enhanced the effect of the combination, resulting in 3–4 log decreased survival in two of the cell lines (KLOSTERGAARD et al. 1992). TNFα also increased the therapeutic efficacy of whole-body hyperthermia (2h at 41.5°C) and cisplatin or carboplatin in rats (OHNO et al. 1992, SAKAGUCHI et al. 1994). The human colon carcinoma HT-29 exhibited synergistic cell killing when rhTNF-α and rhINF-γ were combined with heat at 42°C for 15 min, but given together as trimodality therapy only additive effects of the two combinations were reported (LEE et al. 1993). Despite the preclinical promise, more information concerning the effect of two modalities, drugs or radiation with heat, should be provided in phase II studies before trimodality therapy is generally used. It is difficult to exclude the possibility that additive effects on tumors will be achieved only at the expense of increased side-effects in the clinic.

5.8 Mechanisms of Interaction

Hyperthermia induces many different cellular effects, including alterations in plasma membranes, proteins and DNA. The mechanisms of interaction between chemotherapeutic drugs and hyperthermia have recently been reviewed (for detailed references, see DAHL 1994). Increased uptake of alkylating agents like thio-TEPA and nitrogen mustard, as well as melphalan, has been shown in vivo, but for the last-mentioned drug there was no differential uptake in tumors and normal tissues. There is also increased uptake of cisplatin in several tumors, including both sensitive and resistant sublines, parallel with an increased efficacy. Doxorubicin has been extensively studied and in many cell lines shows increased uptake and increased cell killing; however, increased cell killing without increased cellular uptake and increased uptake with no increased efficacy have also been reported. For cells with similar drug uptake with and without hyperthermia, those cells exposed to hyperthermia were more readily killed than the unheated cells, providing evidence that drug uptake is not the only factor involved in increased cell killing by the combination (RICE and HAHN 1987). Despite an increased effect at temperatures above 43°C, no increased uptake of bleomycin was shown in three animal studies.

Involvement of DNA damage in the interactive effect is indicated both directly, by single strand breakage and neutral nuclear sedimentation assays as well as indirectly by calculation of activation energies compatible with degradation or depurination of DNA. DNA undergoes conformal and topological changes during many cellular processes such as replication and transcription. DNA topoisomerase II causes protein-linked DNA breaks essential for cellular replication. Several cytotoxic drugs such as doxorubicin, mitoxantrone, and the podophyllin derivatives etoposide and tenoposide are classified as topoisomerase II poisons as they interfere with the breakage/rejoining reaction of topoisomerase II by trapping a key reaction intermediate termed "the cleavage complex." The drugs binding to this enzyme may act indirectly on DNA in a manner which possibly is related to a primary effect of hyperthermia on nuclear proteins. Primary damage to membranes is one of the oldest theories explaining hyperthermic cell damage (YATVIN and CRAMP 1993). Membrane damage could explain increased drug uptake. However, newer evidence shows that membrane effects are secondary to primary characteristic fragmentation of DNA caused by endonucleases by a process termed programmed cell death or apoptosis (BARRY et al. 1990). In their study with 90% cell killing apoptosis was seen after exposure for 18h to methotrexate and 48–72h to other cytotoxic agents, but DNA digestion started 30 min after heating (43°C for 60 min). Even the induction of endonucleases may be only a first, though important step, as a variety of nuclear proteins including topoisomerase I and II and poly(ADP-ribose) polymerase are degraded concomitantly with the fragmentation of DNA (KAUFMANN 1989). Many drugs like cisplatin, etoposide, methotrexate and vinca alkaloids may induce apoptosis. Not all of them are necessarily potentiated by heat. Recent findings imply that different heat shock proteins have regulatory effects on the tertiary structure of cellular proteins playing key roles in the nucleus.

Alkylating agents bind directly to DNA, forming DNA adducts. Hyperthermia has been shown to inhibit repair of the strand breaks induced by several chemotherapeutic agents: methyl methanesulfonate, and bleomycin. This impaired repair has been associated with inhibition of polymerase β, which is involved in DNA repair. Whether there is a direct effect on the enzyme or whether the effect on the enzyme is impaired due to an excess of nuclear proteins caused by hyperthermia remains unclear.

Oxidation-reduction reactions and electron transfer are central to many cellular functions.

Production of reactive oxygen radicals is probably the basic mechanism underlying radiation effects in cells. Both radiation and hyperthermia can alter the amount of glutathione (GSH), which is the major cellular oxygen radical detoxifier, together with cysteine in proteins. Production of oxygen radicals has now been shown for several anticancer drugs such as doxorubicin, bleomycin, mitomycin C, BCNU, chlorambucil, and cisplatin.

Reduced protein synthesis is reversible and therefore not likely to be the cause of cellular death. Arrhenius plot analysis and calculation of activation energy suggest that denaturation of protein structures, possibly related to membrane structures, or protein interaction with DNA may be involved. Of all the drugs tested, only etoposide and possibly amsacrine seem to be inactivated by heat. There is also hydrolytic degradation of the nitrosoureas BCNU, CCNU, melphalan, and chlorambucil, but this does not result in less effect when the drugs are administered immediately before hyperthermia.

There have been several experimental studies aimed at measuring pharmacokinetic parameters such as difference in activation or inactivation of drug and calculation of area under the concentration curve, but as yet no general conclusions can be drawn.

In summary, as yet no exact mechanism of action is known for hyperthermia alone. When it is given together with drugs the most likely mechanisms are an increased effect of drugs and heat on DNA, probably partially mediated by nuclear proteins (apoptosis) or oxygen radicals and increased drug uptake into cells.

5.9 Conclusions

This review of experimental data clearly demonstrates that the combination of heat and chemotherapeutic drugs potentially has a clinically useful role, possibly also in combination with local radiation. Present knowledge justifies further clinical trials in this field. Unfortunately, the clinical use of hyperthermia and drugs has hitherto been limited. Often the combination is offered to patients with advanced tumors in a multidrug setting, where any possible benefit is difficult to assess.

Based on the experimental studies in vitro and in vivo, it seems appropriate to select drugs like the alkylating agents, the nitrosoureas, and cisplatin or carboplatin or possibly bleomycin at higher temperatures for further clinical studies.

5.10 Summary

- Many cytotoxic drugs are potentiated in vitro and in vivo by combination with hyperthermia.
- The most promising drugs are the alkylating agents, nitrosoureas, cisplatin, and carboplatin.
- Close timing, i.e., administration of the drug immediately before or during hyperthermia, seems to be the optimal schedule.
- The exact mechanisms of action are not known, but increased drug uptake, DNA effects, and primary protein damage are involved.
- Trimodality therapy, i.e. combination of local radiation and heat with one or more drugs, is promising in animal studies, but assessment of the contribution of each modality is not easy.
- Thermal tolerance, i.e., transient heat-induced thermal resistance, also causes transient resistance to combinations of hyperthermia and drugs, but less to drugs alone.
- Reducing the extracellular pH will increase the effect of at least some cytotoxic drugs (cisplatin, nitrosoureas, bleomycin) in combination with hyperthermia.
- The following drugs should be used with caution: antimetabolites (5-fluorouracil and methotrexate), vinca-alkaloids, daunomycin, and actinomycin D.
- Etoposide (and perhaps other podophyllin derivatives) and amsacrin should not be combined with hyperthermia as the drug effects may be reduced when combined with heat.
- Drug-specific side-effects can be enhanced by hyperthermia.

References

Adams GE (1978) Hypoxic cell sensitizers for radiotherapy. Int J Radiat Oncol Biol Phys 4: 135–141

Adams GE, Stratford IJ, Wallace RG, Wardman P, Watts ME (1980) Toxicity of nitro compounds toward hypoxic mammalian cells. J Natl Cancer Inst 64: 555–560

Alberts DS, Peng YM, Chen GHS, Moon TE, Cetas TC, Hoescheie JD (1980) Therapeutic synergism of hyperthermia-cis-platinum in a mouse tumor model. J Natl Cancer Inst 65: 445–461

Amano T, Kumini K, Nakashima K, Uchibayashi T, Hisazumi H (1990) A combined therapy of hyperthermia and tumor necrosis factor for nude mice bearing KK-47 bladder cancer. J Urol 144: 370–374

Ånggård E (1994) Nitric oxide: mediator, murderer, and medicine. Lancet 343: 1199–1206

Anjum A, Fleischmann WR Jr (1992) Effect of hyperthermia on the antitumor actions of interferons. J Biol Regul Homeost Agents 6: 75–86

Ausmus PL, Wilke AV, Frazier DL (1992) Effects of hyperthermia on blood flow and cis-diamminedichloroplatinum(II) pharmacokinetics in murine mammary adenocarcinomas. Cancer Res 52: 4965–4968

Barlogie B, Corry PM, Drewinco B (1980) In vitro thermochemotherapy of human colon cancer cells with cis-dichlorodiammineplatinum(II) and mitomycin C. Cancer Res 40: 1165–1168

Barry MA, Behnke CA, Eastman A (1990) Activation of programmed cell death (apoptosis) by cisplatin, other anticancer drugs, toxins and hyperthermia. Biochem Pharmacol 40: 2353–2362

Bates DA, MacKillop WJ (1989) The effect of hyperthermia on the uptake and cytotoxicity of melphalan in Chinese hamster ovary cells. Int J Radiat Oncol Biol Phys 16: 187–191

Bates DA, MacKillop WJ (1990) The effect of hyperthermia in combination with melphalan on drug-sensitive and drug-resistant CHO cells in vitro. Br J Cancer 62: 183–188

Ben-Hur E, Elkind MM (1974) Thermal sensitization of Chinese hamster cells to methyl methanesulfonate: relation of DNA damage and repair to survival response. Cancer Biochem Biophys 1: 23–32

Bertrand R, Kerrigan D, Sarang M, Pommier Y (1991) Cell death induced by topoisomerase inhibitors. Role of calcium in mammalian cells. Biochem Pharmacol 42: 7–85

Bleehen NM, Walton MI, Workman P (1988) Interactions of hyperthermia with hypoxic cell sensitizers. Recent Results Cancer Res 109: 136–148

Bronk BV, Wilkins RJ, Regan JD (1973) Thermal enhancement of DNA damage by an alkylating agent in human cells. Biochem Biophys Res Commun 52: 1064–1071

Ciocca DR, Fuqua SA, Lock Lim S, Toft DO, Welch WJ, McGuire WL (1992) Response of human breast cancer cells to heat shock and chemotherapeutic drugs. Cancer Res 52: 3648–3654

Cohen JD, Robins HI, Schmitt CL (1989) Tumoricidal interactions of hyperthermia with carboplatin and etopocide. Cancer Letters 44: 205–210

Cohen JD, Robins HI (1987) Hyperthermic enhancement of cis-diammine-1, 1-cyclubutane dicarboxylate platinum(II) cytotoxicity in human leukemia cells in vitro. Cancer Res 47: 4335–4337

Cohen JD, Robins HI (1990) Thermal enhancement of tetraplatin and carboplatin in human leukaemic cells. Int J Hyperthermia 6: 1013–1017

Cohen JD, Robins HI, Schmitt CL (1989) Tumoricidal interactions of hyperthermia with carboplatin, cisplatin and etoposide. Cancer Lett 44: 205–210

Dahl O (1982) Interaction of hyperthermia and doxorubicin on a malignant, neurogenic rat cell line (BT_4C) in culture. Natl Cancer Inst Monogr 61: 251–253

Dahl O (1983) Hyperthermic potentiation of doxorubicin and 4'-epi-doxorubicin in a transplantable neurogenic rat tumor (BT_4A) in BD IX rats. Int J Radiat Oncol Biol Phys 9: 203–207

Dahl O (1994) Mechanisms of thermal enhancement of chemotherapeutic cytotoxicity. In: Urano M, Douple E (eds) Hyperthermia and Oncology, vol 4, VSP, Utrecht, pp 9–28

Dahl O, Mella O (1982) Enhancement effect of combined hyperthermia and chemotherapy (bleomycin, BCNU) in a neurogenic rat tumour (BT_4A) in vivo. Anticancer Res 2: 359–364

Dahl O, Mella O (1983) Effect of timing and sequence of hyperthermia and cyclophosphamide on a neurogenic rat tumour (BT_4A) in vivo. Cancer 52: 983–987

Dahl O, Mella O (1990) Hyperthermia and chemotherapeutic agents. In: Field SB, Hand JW (eds) An introduction to the practical aspects of clinical hyperthermia. Taylor & Francis, London, pp 108–142

Da Silva VF, Feely M, Raaphorst GP (1991) Hyperthermic potentiation of BCNU toxicity in BCNU-resistant human glioma cells. J Neurooncol 11: 37–41

de L Davies C, Basham TY, Anderson RL, Hahn GM (1990) Changes in the expression of idiotype antigen on murine B-cell lymphoma after hyperthermia alone and in combination with interferon and tumour necrosis factor. Int J Cancer 45: 500–507

DeGraeff A, Slebos RJ, Rodenhius S (1988) Resistance to cisplatin and analogues: mechanisms and potential clinical implications. Cancer Chemother Pharmacol 22: 325–332

De Neve W, Fortan L, Van Den Berghe D, Storme G (1991) Modulation of cis- and carboplatin cytotoxicity by whole-body hyperthermia: absence of a differential and increased DNA-protein cross-link formation (meeting abstract). Strahlenther Onkol 167: 352

Dickson JA, Suzangar M (1974) In vitro – in vivo studies on the susceptibility of the solid Yoshida sarcoma to drugs and hyperthermia (42 degrees). Cancer Res 34: 1263–1274

Dogramatzis D, Nishikawa K, Newman RA (1991) Interaction of hyperthermia with bleomycin and liblomycin: effects on CHO cells in vitro. Anticancer Res 11: 359–364

Donaldson SS, Gordon LF, Hahn GM (1978) Protective effect of hyperthermia against the cytotoxicity of actinomycin D on Chinese hamster cells. Cancer Treat Rep 62: 1489–1495

Douple EB, Strohben JW, de Sieyes DC, Alborough DP, Trembley BS (1982) Therapeutic potentiation of cis-dichlorodiammineplatinum(II) and radiation by interstitial microwave hyperthermia in a mouse tumour. Natl Cancer Inst Monogr 61: 259–262

Dynlacht JR, Wong RS, Albright N, Dewey WC (1994) Hyperthermia can reduce cytotoxicity from etoposide without a corresponding reduction in the number of topoisomerase II-DNA cleavage complexes. Cancer Res 54: 4129–4137

Fisher GA, Hahn GM (1982) Enhancement of cis-platinum(II) diamminedichloride cytotoxicity by hyperthermia. Natl Cancer Inst Monogr 61: 255–257

Fleischmann WR Jr, Fleischmann CM, Gindhart TD (1986) Effect of hyperthermia on the antiproliferative activities of murine α-, β-, and γ-interferon: Differential enhancement of murine γ-interferon. Cancer Res 46: 8–13

Fleischmann WR Jr, Fleischmann CM, Gindhart TD (1986a) Effect of hyperthermia on combination interferon treatment: Enhancement of the antiproliferative activity against murine B-16 melanoma. Cancer Res 46: 1722–1726

Fujimoto S, Kobayashi K, Takahashi M, Konno C, Kokubun M, Ohta M, Shrestha RD, Kiuchi S (1992) Effects on tumour microsirculation in mice of misonidazole and tumour necrosis factor plus hyperthermia. Br J Cancer 65: 33–36

Fujiwara K, Kohno I, Miyao J, Sekiba K (1984) The effect of heat on cell proliferation and the uptake of anticancer drugs into tumour. In: Overgaard J (ed) Hyperthermic oncology 1984, vol 1. Taylor & Francis, London, pp 405–408

Giovanella BC, Lohman WA, Heidelberger C (1970) Effects of elevated temperatures and drugs on the viability of L1210 leukemia cells. Cancer Res 30: 1623–1631

Goss P, Parsons PG (1977) The effect of hyperthermia and melphalan on survival of human fibroblast strains and melanoma cell lines. Cancer Res 37: 152–156

Hahn GM (1978) Interactions of drugs and hyperthermia in vitro and in vivo. In: Streffer C (ed) Cancer therapy by hyperthermia and radiation. Urban & Schwarzenberg, Munich, pp 72–79

Hahn GM (1979) Potential for therapy of drugs and hyperthermia. Cancer Res 39: 2264–2268

Hahn GM, Shiu EC (1983) Effect of pH and elevated temperatures on the cytotoxicity of some chemotherapeutic agents on Chinese hamster cells in vitro. Cancer Res 43: 5789–5791

Hahn GM, Strande DP (1976) Cytotoxic effects of hyperthermia and adriamycin on Chinese hamster cells. J Natl Cancer Inst 57: 1063–1067

Hahn GM, Braun J, Har-Kedar I (1975) Thermochemotherapy: synergism between hyperthermia (42–43 degrees) and adriamycin (or bleomycin) in mammalian cell inactivation. Proc Natl Acad Sci USA 72: 937–940

Har-Kedar I (1975) Effect of hyperthermia and chemotherapy in EMT6 cells. In: Wizenberg MJ, Robinson JE (eds) Proceedings International Symposium on Cancer Therapy by Hyperthermia and Radiation, ACR Washington DC, pp 91–93

Hassanzadeh M, Chapman IV (1982) Thermal enhancement of bleomycin-induced growth delay in a squamous carcinoma of CBA/Ht mouse. Eur J Clin Oncol 18: 795–797

Hazan G, Ben-Hur E, Yerushalmi A (1981) Synergism between hyperthermia and cyclophosphamide in vivo: the effect of dose fractionation. Eur J Cancer 6: 681–684

Herman TS (1983a) Effect of temperature on the cytotoxicity of vindesine, amsacrine, and mitoxantrone. Cancer Treat Rep 67: 1019–1022

Herman TS (1983b) Temperature dependence of adriamycin, cis-diamminedichloroplatinum, bleomycin, and 1,3-bis(2-chloroethyl)-1-nitrosourea cytotoxicity in vitro. Cancer Res 43: 365–369

Herman TS, Teicher BA (1988) Sequencing of trimodality therapy (cis-diamminedichloroplatinum(II)/hyperthermia/radiation) as determined by tumor growth delay and tumor cell survival in the FSaIIc fibrosarcoma. Cancer Res 48: 2693–2697

Herman TS, Teicher BA, Chan V, Collins LS, Abrams MJ (1989) Effect of heat on the cytotoxicity and interaction with DNA of a series of platinum complexes. Int J Radiat Oncol Biol Phys 16: 443–449

Herman TS, Teicher BA, Pfeffer MR, Khandekar VS (1990a) Interaction with hyperthermia of platinum complexes of triaminotriphenylmethane dyes. Int J Hyperthermia 6: 629–639

Herman TS, Teicher BA, Pfeffer MR, Khandekar VS, Alvarez-Sotomayor E (1990b) Interaction of platinum complexes of thiazin and xanthine dyes with hyperthermia. Cancer Chemother Pharmacol 26: 127–134

Herman TS, Teicher BA, Holden SA (1990c) Trimodality therapy (drug/hyperthermia/radiation) with BCNU or mitomycin C. Int J Radiat Oncol Biol Phys 18: 375–382

Herman TS, Teicher BA, Holden SA (1991) Addition of mitomycin C to cis-diamminedichloroplatinum(II)/hyperthermia/radiation therapy in the FSaIIC fibrosarcoma. Int J Hyperthermia 7: 893–903

Hofer KG, MacKinnon AR, Schubert AL, Lehr JE, Grimmett EV (1981) Radiosensitization of tumors and normal tissues by combined treatment with misonidazole and heat. Radiology 141: 801–809

Honess DJ, Workman P, Morgan JE, Bleehen NM (1980) Effects of local hyperthermia on the pharmacokinetics of misonidazole in the anesthetized mouse. Br J Cancer 41: 529–540

Honess DJ, Bleehan NM (1982a) Sensitivity of normal mouse marrow and RIF-1 tumour to hyperthermia combined with cyclophosphamide or BCNU: a lack of therapeutic gain. Br J Cancer 46: 236–248

Honess DJ, Bleehen NM (1982b) Effects of the combination of hyperthermia and cytotoxic agents on the skin of the mouse foot. In: Arcangeli G, Mauro F (eds) Proceedings of the first meeting of the European Group of Hyperthermia in Radiation Oncology. Masson, Milan, pp 151–155

Honess DJ, Bleehen NM (1985a) Potentiation of melphalan by systemic hyperthermia in mice: therapeutic gain for mouse lung microtumours. Int J Hyperthermia 1: 57–68

Honess DJ, Bleehen NM (1985b) Thermochemotherapy with cisplatinum CCNU, BCNU, chlorambucil and melphalan on murine marrow and two tumours: therapeutic gain for melphalan only. Br J Radiol 58: 63–72

Hou D-Y, Maruyama Y (1990) Enhanced killing of human small cell lung cancer by hyperthermia and indium-111-bleomycin complex. J Surg Oncol 44: 5–9

Ilzumi T, Yazaki T, Waku M, Soma G-I (1989) Immunochemotherapy for murine bladder tumour with a human recombinant tumour necrosis factor (rTNF-S), VP-16 and hyperthermia. J Urol 142: 386–389

Johnson HA, Pavelec M (1973) Thermal enhancement of thio-TEPA cytotoxicity. J Natl Cancer Inst 50: 903–908

Joiner MC, Steel GC, Stephens IC (1982) Response of two mouse tumours to hyperthermia with CCNU or melphalan. Br J Cancer 45: 17–26

Juvekar AS, Chitnis MP (1991) Circumvention of drug resistance of P388/R cells by the combination of adriamycin and mitoxanthrone with hyperthermia (42°C). Neoplasma 38: 207–211

Kano E, Furukawa-Furuya M, Kajimoto-Kinoshita KNT, Picha P, Sugimoto K, Ohtsubo T, Tsuji K, Tsubouchi S, Kondo T (1988) Sensitivities of bleomycin-resistant variant cells enhanced by 40°C hyperthermia in vitro. Int J Hyperthermia 4: 547–553

Kappel M, Diamant M, Hansen MB, Klokker M, Pedersen BK (1991) Effects of in vitro hyperthermia on the proliferative response of blood mononuclear cell subsets, and detection of interleukins 1 and 6, tumour necrosis factor-alpha and interferon-gamma. Immunology 73: 304–308

Kallinowski F, Schaefer G, Tyler G, Vaupel P (1989) In vivo targets of recombinant human tumour necrosis factor-α: blood flow, oxygen consumption and growth of isotransplanted rat tumours. Br J Cancer 60: 555–560

Kaufmann SH (1989) Induction of endonucleolytic DNA cleavage in human acute myelogenous leukemia cells by etoposide, camptothecin, and other cytotoxic anticancer drugs: a cautionary note. Cancer Res 49: 5870–5878

Kim JH, Kim SH, Alifieri A, Young CW, Silvestrini B (1984) Lonidamine: A hyperthermic sensitizer of HeLa cels in culture and of the Math-A tumor in vivo. Oncology 41: Suppl 1, pp 30–35

Kim YD, Lees DE, Lake CR, Wang-Peng J, Schuette W, Smith R, Bull J (1979) Hyperthermia potentiates doxorubicin-related cardiotoxic effects. JAMA 241: 1816–1817

Kitamura K, Kuwano H, Matsuda H, Toh Y, Masuda H, Sugimachi K (1992) Synergistic effects of intratumor administration of cis-diamminedichloroplatinum(II) combined with local hyperthermia in melanoma bearing mice. J Surg Oncol 51: 188–194

Klostergaard J, Leroux E, Siddik ZH, Khodadadian M, Tomasovic SP (1992) Enhanced sensitivity of human colon tumor cell lines in vitro in response to thermochemoimmunotherapy. Cancer Res 52: 5271–5277

Kuroki M, Tanaka R, Hondo H (1987) Antitumour effect of interferon combined with hyperthermia against experimental brain tumour. Int J Hyperther 3: 527–534

Kukla L, Mc Guire WP (1982) Heat-induced recall of bleomycin skin changes. Cancer 50: 2283–2284

Laskowitz DT, Elion GB, Dewhirst MW, Griffith OW, Savina PM, Blum MR, Prescott DM, Bigner DD, Friedman HS (1992) Hyperthermia-induced enhancement of melphalan activity against a melphalan-resistant human rhabdomyosarcoma xenograft. Radiat Res 129: 218–223

Lee YJ, Hou Z, Curetty L, Cho JH, Corry PM (1993) Synergistic effect of cytokine and hyperthermia on cytotoxicity in HT-29 cells are not mediated by alterations of induced protein levels. J Cell Physiol 155: 27–35

Lejeune FJ, Li'enard D, Leyvraz S, Mirimanoff RO (1993) Regional therapy of melanoma. Eur J Cancer 29A: 606–612

Lindegaard JC, Radacic M, Khalil AA, Horsman MR, Overgaard J (1992) Cisplatin and hyperthermia treatment of a C3H mammary carcinoma in vivo. Acta Oncol 31: 347–351

Los G, Sminia P, Wondergem J, Mutsaers PHA, Haveman J, ten Bokkel Huinink D, Smals O, Gonzalez-Gonzalez D, McVie JG (1991) Optimisation of intraperitoneal cisplatin therapy with regional hyperthermia in rats. Eur J Cancer 27: 472–477

Ma F, Hiraoka M, Jo S, Akuta K, Nishimura Y, Takahashi M, Abe M (1985) Response of mammary tumours of C3H/He mice to hyperthermia and bleomycin in vivo. Radiat Med 3: 230–233

Magin RL, Sisik BI, Cysyk RL (1979) Enhancement of bleomycin activity against Lewis lung tumors in mice by local hyperthermia. Cancer Res 39: 3792–3795

Magin RL, Cysyk RL, Litterst CL (1980) Distribution of adriamycin in mice under conditions of local hyperthermia which improve systemic drug therapy. Cancer Treat Rep 64: 203–210

Majima H, Kashiwado K, Egawa S, Suzuki N, Urano M (1992) Interaction between the kinetics of thermotolerance and effect of cis-diamminedichloroplatinum(II) or bleomycin given at 37 or 43°C. Int J Hyperthermia 8: 431–442

Mansouri A, Henle KJ, Benson AM, Moss AJ, Nagle WA (1989) Characterization of a cisplatin-resistant subline of murine RIF-1 cells and reversal of drug resistance by hyperthermia. Cancer Res 49: 2674–2678

Marmor JB, Kozak D, Hahn GM (1979) Effects of systemically administered bleomycin or adriamycin with local hyperthermia. Cancer Treat Rep 63: 1279–1290

Mella O (1985) Combined hyperthermia and cis-diamminedichloroplatinum in BD IX rats with transplanted BT_4A tumours. Int J Hyperthermia 1: 171–183

Mella O (1990) Fractionated hyperthermia in vivo: thermotolerance, sensitivity to BCNU and thermochemotherapy in the BT4An rat glioma. Int J Hyperthermia 6: 253–260

Mella O, Dahl O (1985) Timing of combined hyperthermia and 1,3-bis(2-chloroethyl)-1-nitrosourea or cis-diamminedichloroplatinum in BD IX rats with BT4A tumours. Anticancer Res 5: 259–264

Mella O, Eriksen R, Dahl O, Laerum OD (1987) Acute systemic toxicity of combined cis-diamminedichloroplatinum and hyperthermia in the rat. Eur J Cancer Clin Oncol 23: 365–373

Meyn RE, Corry PM, Fletcher SE, Demetriades M (1980) Thermal enhancement of DNA damage in mammalian cells treated with cis-diamminedichloroplatinum(II). Cancer Res 40: 1136–1139

Mircheva J, Smith PJ, Bleehen NM (1986) Interaction of bleomycin, hyperthermia and a calmodulin inhibitor (trifluoperazine) in mouse tumour cells. I. In vitro cytotoxicity. Br J Cancer 53: 99–103

Mizuno S, Amagai M, Ishida A (1980) Synergistic cell killing by antitumor agents and hyperthermia in cultured cells. Gann 71: 471–478

Monge OR, Rofstad EK (1989) Thermochemotherapy in vivo of a C3H mouse mammary carcinoma: thermotolerant tumours. Int J Hyperthermia 5: 579–587

Monge OR, Rofstad EK (1991) Fractionated thermochemotherapy in vivo of a C3H mouse mammary carcinoma. Radiother Oncol 21: 171–178

Monge OR, Rofstad EK, Kaalhus O (1988) Thermochemotherapy in vivo of a C3H mouse mammary carcinoma: single fraction heat and drug treatment. Eur J Cancer Clin Oncol 24: 1661–1669

Morgan JE, Bleehen NM (1982) A comparison of the interaction between hyperthermia and bleomycin on the EMT6 tumour as a monolayer or spheroids in vitro and in vivo. In: Arcangeli G, Mauro F (eds) Proceedings of the first meeting of the European Group of Hyperthermia in radiation oncology. Masson, Milan, pp 165–170

Morgan JE, Honess DJ, Bleehen NM (1979) The interaction of thermal tolerance with drug cytotoxicity in vitro. Brit J Cancer 39: 422–428

Moriyama Y, Goto T, Nikkuni K, Aoki A, Furukawa T, Narita M, Koyama S, Kishi K, Takahashi M, Shibata A (1991). Alpha-interferon broadens the difference between surviving fractions of normal and leukemic progenitor cells in vitro by heat: its application to marrow purging. Bone Marrow Transplant 8: 301–305

Muckle DS, Dickson JA (1973) Hyperthermia (42°C) as an adjuvant to radiotherapy and chemotherapy in the treatment of the allogeneic VX2 carcinoma in the rabbit. Br J Cancer 27: 307–315

Mulcahy RT, Gipp JJ, Tanner MA (1988) Sensitization of nitrosourea-resistant Mer(+) human tumor cells to *N*-

(2-chloroethyl)-N'-cyclohexyl-N-nitrosourea by mild (41°C) hyperthermia. Cancer Res 48: 1086–1090

Nakajima K, Hisazumi H (1987) Enhanced radioinduced cytotoxicity of cultured human bladder cells using 43°C hyperthermia and anticancer drugs. Urol Res 15: 255–260

Nakayama J, Toyofuku K, Urabe A, Taniguchi S, Hori Y (1993) A combined therapeutic modality with hyperthermia and locally administered rIFN-β inhibited the growth of B16 melanoma in association with the modulation of cellular infiltrates. J Deratol Sci 6: 240–246

Neilan BA, Henle KJ (1989) In vivo response of murine RIF tumors to thermochemotherapy. J Med 20: 107–112

Neumann HA, Herrmann DB, Fiebig HH, Engelhardt R (1989) Treatment of human clonogenic tumor cells and bone marrow progenitor cells with bleomycin and peplomycin under 40.5°C hyperthermia in vitro. Eur J Cancer Clin Oncol 25: 99–104

Newman RA, Dogramatzis D, Benvenuto JA, Trevino M, Stephens LC, Wondergem J, Strebel R, Baba H, Bull JM (1992) Effect of whole-body hyperthermia on pharmacokinetics and tissue distribution of doxorubicin. Int J Hyperthermia 8: 79–85

O'Donnel JF, McKoy WS, Makuch RW, Bull JM (1979) Increased in vitro toxicity to mouse bone marrow with 1,3-bis(2-chloroethyl)-1-nitrosourea and hyperthermia. Cancer Res 39: 2547–2549

Ogilvie GK, Obradovich JE, Elmslie RE, Vail DM, Moore AS, Straw RC, Dickinson K, Cooper MF, Withrow SJ (1991) Efficacy of mitoxantrone against various neoplasms in dogs. J Am Vet Med Assoc 198: 1618–1621

Ohno S, Strebel FR, Stephens C, Siddik ZH, Makino M, Klostergaard J, Tomasovic SP, Kokhar AR, Bull JM (1992) Increased therapeutic efficacy induced by tumor necrosis factor α combined with platinum complexes and whole-body hyperthermia in rats. Cancer Res 52: 4096–4101

Onishi T, Machida T, Mori Y, Ilzuka N, Masuda F, Mochizuki S, Tsukamoto H, Harada N (1989) Hyperthermia with simultaneous administration of interferon using established human renal carcinoma heterotransplanted in nude mice. Br J Urol 63: 227–232

Ohno S, Siddik ZH, Baba H, Stephens LC, Strebel FR, Wondergem J, Khokhar AR, Bull JM (1991) Effect of carboplatin combined with whole body hyperthermia on normal tissue and tumor in rats. Cancer Res 51: 2994–3000

Ohtsubo T, Chang SW, Tsuji K, Picha P, Saito H, Kano E (1990) Effects of cis-diamminedichloroplatinum (CDDP) and cis-diammine(1, 1-cyclobutanedicarboxylate)platinum (CBDCA) on thermotolerance development and thermosensitivity of the thermotolerant cells. Int J Hyperthermia 6: 1031–1039

Osieka R, Magin RL, Atkinson ER (1978) The effect of hyperthermia on human colon cancer xenografts in nude mice. In: Streffer C (ed) Cancer therapy by hyperthermia and radiation. Urban & Schwarzenberg, Munich, pp 287–290

Overgaard J (1976) Combined adriamycin and hyperthermia treatment of a murine mammary carcinoma in vivo. Cancer Res 36: 3077–3081

Overgaard J (1980) Effect of misonidazole and hyperthermia on the radiosensitivity of a C3H mouse mammary carcinoma and its surrounding normal tissue. Br J Cancer 41: 10–21

Overgaard J (1989) The current and potential role of hyperthermia in radiotherapy. Int J Radiat Oncol Biol Phys 16: 535–549

Overgaard J, Sand Hansen H, Lindeløv B, Overgaard M, Jørgensen K, Rasmussen B, Berthelsen A (1991) Nimorazole as a hypoxic radiosensitizer in the treatment of supraglottic larynx and pharynx carcinoma. First report from the Danish Head and Neck Cancer Study (DAHANCA) protocol 5–85. Radiother Oncol 20: 143–149

Pfeffer MR, Teicher BA, Holden SA, Al-Achi A, Herman TS (1990) The interaction of cisplatin plus etoposide with radiation $\pm$ hyperthermia. Int J Radiat Oncol Biol Phys 19: 1439–1447

Pilepich MV, Jones KG, Emami BN, Perez CA, Fields JN, Myerson RJ (1989) Interaction of bleomycin and hyperthermia – results of a clinical pilot study. Int J Radiat Oncol Biol Phys 16: 211–213

Raaphorst GP, Feeley MM, Danjoux CE, Martin L, Maroun J, DeSantis AJ (1991) The effect of lonidamine (LND) on radiation and thermal responses of human and rodent cell lines. Int J Radiat Oncol Biol Phys 20: 509–515

Raaphorst GP, Feeley MM, Martin L, Danjoux CE, Maroun J, DeSantis AJ (1991a) Enhancement of sensitivity to hyperthermia by lonidamine in human cancer cells. Int J Hyperther 7: 763–722

Rabbani B, Sondhaus CA, Swingle KF (1978) Cellular response to hyperthermia and bleomycin: effect of time sequencing and possible mechanisms. Proceedings of the international symposium on cancer therapy by hyperthermia and radiation. American College of Radiology, Washington DC, 1975

Rice GC, Hahn GM (1987) Modulation of adriamycin transport by hyperthermia as measured by fluorescence-activated cell sorting. Cancer Chemother Pharmacol 20: 183–187

Roizin-Towle L, Hall EJ, Capuano L (1982) Interaction of hyperthermia and cytotoxic agents. Natl Cancer Inst Monogr 61: 149–151

Rose WC, Veras GH, Laster WR Jr, Schabel FM Jr (1979) Evaluation of whole-body hyperthermia as an adjunct to chemotherapy in murine tumors. Cancer Treat Rep 63: 1311–1325

Sakaguchi Y, Makino M, Kaneko T, Stephens LC, Strebel FR, Danhauser LL, Jenkins GN, Bull JMC (1994) Therapeutic efficacy of long duration-low temperature whole body hyperthermia when combined with tumor necrosis factor and carboplatin in rats. Cancer Res 54: 2223–2227

Schem BC, Dahl O (1991) Thermal enhancement of ACNU and potentiation of thermochemotherapy with ACNU by hypertonic glucose in the BT_4AN rat glioma. J Neurooncol 10: 247–252

Schem BC, Mella O, Dahl O (1989) Potentiation of combined BCNU and hyperthermia by pH reduction in vitro and hypertonic glucose in vivo in the BT-4 rat glioma. Int J Hyperthermia 5: 707–715

Schem BC, Kronen-Krossnes B, Mella O, Dahl O (1991) Intra-arterial ACNU and local brain hyperthermia in rat BT_4AN gliomas (meeting abstract). Strahlenther Onkol 167: 356

Schem BC, Mella O, Dahl O (1992) Thermochemotherapy with cisplatin or carboplatin in the BT-4 rat glioma in

vitro and in vivo. Int J Radiat Oncol Biol Phys 23: 109–114
Senapati N, Houchens D, Ovejera A, Beard R, Nines R (1982) Ultrasonic hyperthermia and drugs as therapy for human tumor xenografts. Cancer Treat Rep 66: 1635–1639
Shiu MH, Cahan A, Fogh J, Fortner JG (1983) Sensitivity of xenografts of human pancreatic adenocarcinomas in nude mice to heat and heat combined with chemotherapy. Cancer Res 43: 4014–4018
Someya T, Nogita T, Yamada K, Tsuchida T, Watanabe R, Otsuka F (1990) Antiproliferative effect of hyperthermia and ACNU on cultured human malignant melanoma cells. J Dermatol 17: 303–306
Srinivasan JM, Fajarda L, Hahn GM (1990) Mechanism of antitumor activity of tumor necrosis factor α with hyperthermia in a tumor necrosis factor α-resistant tumor. J Natl Cancer Inst 82: 1904–1910
Sutton CH (1971) Tumour hyperthermia in the treatment of malignant gliomas of the brain Trans Am Neurol Assoc 96: 195–199
Suzuki K (1967) Application of heat to cancer chemotherapy – experimental studies. Nagoya J Med Sci 30: 1–21
Teicher BA, Holden SA, Khandakar V, Herman TS (1993) Addition of a topoisomerase I inhibitor to trimodality therapy [cis-diamminedichloroplatinum(II)/heat/radiation] in a murine tumor. J Cancer Res Clin Oncol 119: 645–651
Teicher BA, Kowal CD, Kennedy KA, Sartorelli AC (1981) Enhancement by hyperthermia of the in vitro cytotoxicity of mitomycin C toward hypoxic tumor cells. Cancer Res 41: 1096–1099
Teicher BA, Herman TS, Holden SA (1988) Combined modality therapy with bleomycin, hyperthermia, and radiation. Cancer Res 48: 6291–6297
Teicher BA, Herman TS, Pfeffer MR, Alvarez-Sotomayor E, Khandekar VS (1989) Interaction of PtCl-4(Fast Black)-2 with hyperthermia. Cancer Res 49: 6208–6213
Theon AP, Madewell BR, Moore AS, Stephens C, Krag DN (1991) Localized thermocisplatin therapy: a pilot study in spontaneous canine and feline tumours. Int J Hyperthermia 7: 881–892
Thuning CA, Bakir NA, Warren J (1980) Synergistic effect of combined hyperthermia and a nitrosourea in treatment of a murine ependymoblastoma. Cancer Res 40: 2726–2729
Tomasovic SP, Barta M, Klostergaard (1992) Temporal dependence of hyperthermic augmentation of macrophage-TNF production and tumor cell-TNF sensitization. Int J Hyperther 5: 625–639
Tomasovic SP, Vasey TA, Story MD, Stephens LC, Klostergaard J (1994) Cytotoxic manifestations of the interaction between hyperthermia and TNF: DNA fragmentation. Int J Hyperther 10: 247–262
Twentyman PR, Morgan JE, Donaldson J (1978) Enhancement by hyperthermia of the effect of BCNU against the EMT6 mouse tumor. Cancer Treat Rep 62: 439–443
Uckun FM, Mitchell JB, Obuz V, Chandan Langlie M, Min WS, Haissig S, Song CW (1992) Radiation and heat sensitivity of human T-lineage acute lymphoblastic leukemia (ALL) and acute myeloblastic leukemia (AML) clones displaying multidrug resistance (MDR). Int J Radiat Oncol Biol Phys 23: 115–125
Umeno H, Watanabe N, Yamauchi N, Tsuji N, Okamoto T, Niitsu Y (1994) Enhancement of blood stasis and vascular permeability in Meth-A tumors by administration of hyperthermia in combination with tumor necrosis factor. Jpn J Cancer Res 85: 325–330
Urano M, Kahn J (1989) The effect of bleomycin administered in combination with hyperthermia on a C3H mouse fibrosarcoma. Int J Hyperthermia 5: 377–382
Urano M, Kahn J, Kenton LA (1988a) Effect of bleomycin on murine tumor cells at elevated temperatures and two different pH values. Cancer Res 48: 615–619
Urano M, Kahn J, Kenton LA (1988b) Thermochemotherapy-induced resistance to cyclophosphamide Br J Cancer 57: 295–297
Urano M, Kahn J, Kenton LA (1990) The effect of cis-diamminedichloroplatinum(II) treatment at elevated temperatures on murine fibrosarcoma, FSa-II. Int J Hyperthermia 6: 563–570
Urano M, Majima H, Miller R, Kahn J (1991) Cytotoxic effect of 1,3 bis (2-chloroethyl)-*N*-nitrosourea at elevated temperatures: Arrhenius plot analysis and tumour response. Int J Hyperthermia 7: 499–510
Van der Linden PWG, Sapareto SA, Corbett TH, Valeriote FA (1984) Adriamycin and heat treatments in vitro and in vivo. In: Overgaard J (ed) Hyperthermic oncology, 1984, vol 1. Taylor & Francis, London, pp 449–452
Vicente V, Gomez M, Ochotorena MM, Cremades A, Canteras M (1990) Thermochemotherapy for B16 melanoma: combination therapy of hyperthermia, melphalan, and CCNU in mice. Pigment Cell Res 3: 1–7
Von Szczepanski L, Trott KR (1981) The combined effect of bleomycin and hyperthermia on the adenocarcinoma 284 of the C3H mouse. Eur J Cancer Clin Oncol 17: 997–1000
Voth B, Sauer H, Willmans W (1988) Thermostability of cytostatic drugs in vitro and thermosensitivity of cultured human lymphoblasts against cytostatic drugs. Recent Results Cancer Res 107: 170–176
Wallner KE, DeGregorio MW, Li GC (1986) Hyperthermic potentiation of cis-diamminedichloroplatinum-(II) cytotoxicity in Chinese hamster ovary cells resistant to the drug. Cancer Res 46: 6242–6245
Wallner KE, Banda M, Li GC (1987) Hyperthermic enhancement of cell killing by mitomycin C in mitomycin C resistant Chinese hamster ovary cells. Cancer Res 47: 1308–1312
Walton MI, Bleehen NM, Workman P (1986) Effects of localized tumour hyperthermia on pimonidazole (Ro 03-8799) pharmacokinetics in mice. Br J Cancer 59: 667–673
Walton MI, Bleehen NM, Workman P (1989) Stimulation by localized hyperthermia of reductive bioactivation of 2-nitroimidazole benznidazole in mice. Cancer Res 49: 2351–2355
Wang BS, Lumanglas AL, Ruszala-Mallon V, Wallace RE, Durr FE (1984) Effect of hyperthermia on the sensitivity of human colon carcinoma cells to mitoxantrone (MX). Proc Am Assoc Cancer Res 25: 341
Watanabe N, Niitsu Y, Umeno H, Sone H, Neda H, Yamauchi N, Maeda M, Urushizaki I (1988). Synergistic cytotoxic and antitumor effects of recombinant human tumor necrosis factor and hyperthermia. Cancer Res 48: 650–653
Wiedemann G, Roszinski S, Biersack A, Weiss C, Wagner T (1992a) Local hyperthermia enhances cyclophosphamide, ifosfamide and cis-diamminedichloroplatinum

cytotoxicity on human-derived breast carcinoma and sarcoma xenografts in nude mice. J Cancer Res Clin Oncol 118: 129–135

Wiedemann G, Mella O, Roszinski S, Weiss C, Wagner T (1992b) Hyperthermia enhances mitoxantrone cytotoxicity on human breast carcinoma and sarcoma xenografts in nude mice. Int J Radiat Oncol Biol Phys 24: 669–673

Wondergem J, Bulger RE, Strebel FR, Newman RA, Travis EL, Stephens LC, Bull JMC (1988) Effect of cis-diamminedichloroplatinum(II) combined with whole body hyperthermia on renal injury. Cancer Res 48: 440–446

Wondergem J, Stephens LC, Strebel FR, Baba H, Ohno S, Siddik ZH, Newman RA, Bull JM (1991) Effect of adriamycin combined with whole body hyperthermia on tumor and normal tissues. Cancer Res 51: 3559–3567

Wong K-H (1994) Enhancement of radiosensitization and chemosensitization of nitroimidazoles by local hyperthermia. In: Urano M, Douple E (eds) Hyperthermia and Oncology, Vol 4. Chemopotentiation by hyperthermia. VSP, Utrecht, pp 285–319

Xu MJ, Alberts DS (1988) Potentiation of platinum analogue cytotoxicity by hyperthermia. Cancer Chemother Pharmacol 21: 191–196

Yamada K, Someya T, Shimada S, Ohara K, Kukita A (1984) Thermochemotherapy for malignant melanoma: combination therapy of ACNU and hyperthermia in mice. J Invest Dermatol 82: 180–184

Yamane T, Koga S, Maeta M, Hamazone R, Karino T, Oda M (1984) Effects of in vitro hyperthermia on concentration of adriamycin in Ehrlich ascites cells. In: Overgaard J (ed) Hyperthermic Oncology 1984, Vol 1. Taylor & Francis, London, pp 409–476

Yatvin MB, Cramp WA (1993) Role of cellular membranes in hyperthermia: some observations and theories reviewed. Int J Hyperthermia 9: 165–185

Yerushalmi A (1978) Combined treatment of a solid tumour by local hyperthermia and actinomycin D. Br J Cancer 37: 827–832

Yerushalmi A, Hazan G (1979) Control of Lewis lung carcinoma by combined treatment with local hyperthermia and cyclophosphamide: preliminary results. Isr J Med Sci 15: 462–463

Zimber A, Lurie H, Hazan G, Perk K (1986) Enhancement of methyl-CCNU and cyclophosphamide inhibition of Lewis lung carcinoma in mice by local hyperthermia. Ann NY Acad Sci 463: 366–368

Zupi G, Badaracco G, Cavaliere R, Natali PG, Greco C (1984) Influence of sequence on hyperthermia and drug combination. In: Overgaard J (ed) Hyperthermic Oncology 1984, Vol 1. London, Taylor & Francis, pp 429–432

6 Thermal Dosimetry

M.W. Dewhirst

CONTENTS

6.1 Introduction

Implementation of thermal dosimetry requires three steps. First, it is necessary to use accurate thermometers. This subject is covered in Chap. 15 of this volume. Second, it is necessary to use a measure of treatment effect that has biological significance (i.e., there is a quantitative relationship between the measure of treatment delivered and the cytotoxic effect of the treatment). A large database from in vitro and in vivo models has provided useful concepts for this aspect of dosimetry, although recent data from human cells suggest that some key revisions to the concepts may be necessary. In this chapter the relations between temperature, time at temperature, and cytotoxicity will be reviewed. In addition, factors that are known to influence the accuracy of these measures of effect will be presented, along with an emphasis on their clinical relevance.

The third step of dosimetry is to be able to describe the treatment delivered. This is perhaps the most difficult step. Methods to accomplish this task are not straightforward, particularly as long as invasive thermometry is required such that only a small part of the heated volume is sampled. Sources of sampling error will be reviewed and methods to minimize errors will be emphasized. In spite of problems with sampling error, significant progress has been made recently in the interpretation of invasive thermometric data. A review of the evolution of thinking about interpretation of thermal dosimetric data will be presented, along with recommendations for current implementation.

Finally, new methods of dosimetry are under development that involve the combined use of limited invasive thermometry with heat transfer modeling. This potentially powerful approach to dosimetry may allow for much greater knowledge of the complete temperature distribution along with more realistic prediction of the cytotoxic effect of treatment on a given tumor, taking into account various patient-related and treatment-related factors that influence overall cytotoxicity.

6.2 Cellular Basis for Thermal Isoeffect Dose

6.2.1 Cell Survival Curves and the Arrhenius Relationship

It is well established in in vitro cell systems that thermal cytotoxicity is a function of both temperature and time. It is also known that there is an exponential relationship between the rate of cell kill (as described by the slope of a heat cell survival curve) and temperature. The biophysical relationship between temperature and rate of cell kill has commonly been depicted using an Arrhenius plot (Fig. 6.1) (Field and Morris 1983; Sapareto and Dewey 1984).

For most murine cell lines and for in vivo-derived murine data a biphasic plot is obtained that has a "breakpoint" around 43°C. Above the breakpoint the amount of time needed to reach an isoeffect is halved for every degree of temperature rise. For example, 60 min at 43°C will yield

M.W. Dewhirst, DVM, PhD, Tumor Microcirculation Laboratory, Department of Radiation Oncology, Duke University Medical Center, P.O. Box 3455, Durham, NC 27710, USA

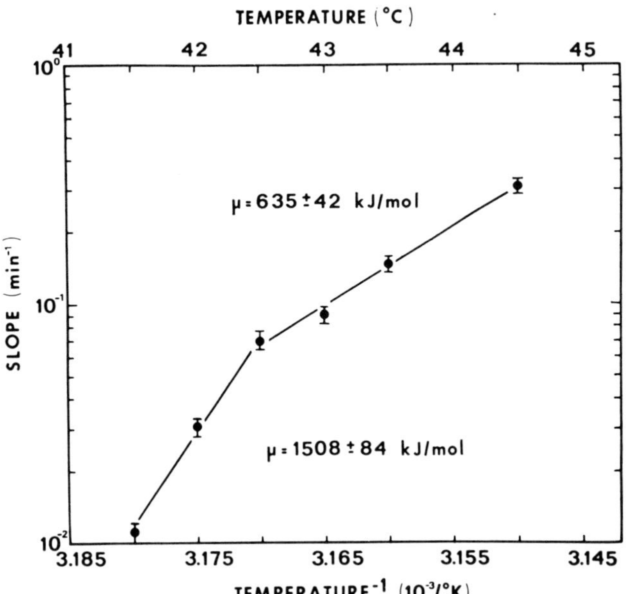

Fig. 6.1. Arrhenius plot depicting the time-temperature relationships for heat killing in vivo. In this application, the authors determined the dependence of tumor regrowth time on time of heating at a range of temperatures. Linear relationships were observed between the regrowth times and time of heating. The Arrhenius plot, therefore, depicts the slope of these relationships as a function of temperature. Note that there is a "break" in the plot that occurs at about 42.5°C. The change in slope below the breakpoint is due to thermotolerance induction during heating. (From Nielson and Overgaard 1982)

the same amount of damage as 30 min at 44°C. This relationship above the breakpoint is remarkably consistent over many cell lines and in vivo systems.

The break in the Arrhenius plot is thought to be due to the development of thermotolerance during heating. Because different cell lines and tissues have variable rates of thermotolerance induction, the slope of the Arrhenius plot below the breakpoint is not as consistent as it is above the breakpoint. For Chinese hamster ovary (CHO) cells, the slope changes to a factor of 4 in the rate of cell kill for every degree temperature drop below the breakpoint. For example, the same amount of cell kill can be obtained by heating for 60 min at 43°C as can be obtained by heating at 42°C for 4 h. Field and Morris (1983) reviewed data from a number of murine in vivo systems and found that overall, the slope relationship below the break was more consistent with a factor of 6 than a factor of 4. Recent studies evaluating the thermal sensitivity of human cell lines indicate that the characteristics of the Arrhenius plot may be somewhat different for human cells. It is evident that the breakpoint for human cells is probably nearer to 44°C (Roizin-Towle and Pirro 1991; Hahn et al. 1989). Interestingly, however, the slope below the breakpoint may be less than the factor of 4 that has been observed for CHO cells. The implication of these two observations is that human cells are more resistant to heat killing above 43°C while being more sensitive to killing at temperatures below 42°C (Armour et al. 1993). Since temperature distributions tend to average <42°C in the clinic, this is encouraging news, particularly for strategies that involve long-duration heating.

The relationships between rates of cell kill and temperature led to the introduction of a dosimetric concept that has been given the name "thermal isoeffect dose" (Sapareto 1987). This method of dosimetry does not use a physical dose unit (such as the Gray for radiation dose), because the amount of cell kill that is induced is not a consequence of how much energy is delivered to a system. It is instead the consequence of the actual temperatures achieved from the energy deposition. The thermal isoeffect dose method uses the Arrhenius relationship to convert any time temperature history to an equivalent number of minutes at a standard temperature, such as 43°C (Sapareto and Dewey 1984). This potentially powerful tool allows for standardization of time-temperature data retrieved from the clinic, where temperatures within a tumor may vary by several degrees during a single treatment session. Theoretically the method allows for standardization of data reporting across patients even if the duration of heating and temperatures achieved vary from patient to patient:

$$\text{CEM 43 } T_{90} = \Sigma(\Delta t)R^{(43-\bar{T})},$$

where CEM 43 T_{90} = cumulative equivalent minutes at a T_{90} converted to 43°C, Δt = time increments at which thermal data are acquired during treatment, $\bar{T}$ = average temperature over the time interval Δt, and $R = 0.25$ when $T < 43$°C and 0.5 when it is ⩾43°C.

Although the concept of thermal isoeffect dose, as shown above, is simple, its use in the clinic cannot be cavalierly recommended. There are a number of treatment- and tumor-related factors that could influence accurate interpretation of such data. In 1987, a symposium on thermal isoeffect dose was held in conjunction with the North American Hyperthermia Society Meeting. The consensus of that meeting was that the concept should not be used, except in the context of experimental protocols, and that additional research was necessary to investigate methods to determine the accuracy of the method in the clinic (SAPARETO 1987). More recent analyses of human clinical trial data suggest that this method may have great potential, even with the inherent sources of potential error (OLESON et al. 1993).

A fundamental limitation to the concept of using an Arrhenius plot as the basis for calculating thermal isoeffect dose is that the analysis does not account for the shoulder on the heat survival curve. For cell lines with large shoulders, or shoulder widths that vary with temperature, the Arrhenius calculation would overestimate the amount of cytotoxicity for a given thermal history. This problem has been addressed by MACKEY and ROTI ROTI (1992), who consider thermal sensitivity in a different manner. In this application, they characterize any population of cells by a parameter ε, which is normally distributed within a population of cells. They assume that cells below an arbitrary cut-off value of ε will be unable to divide and form a colony. As temperature is elevated, the frequency distribution of ε value trends downward at a rate that is controlled by the temperature and prior thermal history. This approach has been successfully used to predict thermal sensitivity of S-phase cells, based on models developed from synchronized G_1 cells.

6.2.2 *Thermotolerance*

Thermotolerance is a factor that may have a profound and complicated influence on the Arrhenius relationship. Development of thermotolerance during heating can have an important influence on the slope of the relationship below the breakpoint (i.e., <43°C, or 44°C for human cells). Variations in the slope of the Arrhenius plot in this region that deviate from the model used could lead to large over- or underestimates of cell kill (Fig. 6.2).

For example, if the slope below the break is a factor of 4, as has been observed by SAPARETO and DEWEY (1984) for CHO cells, then 60 min of heating at 42°C would be equivalent to 15 min at the standard of 43°C. If the slope is a factor of 6, as has been suggested by FIELD and MORRIS (1983) for murine in vivo systems, then 60 min of heating at 42°C would only be equivalent to 10 min of heating at 43°C. The most important question that needs to be addressed, however, is: What is the slope of the Arrhenius plot below the breakpoint for human cells? Interestingly, recent studies that have examined cell survival of human cell lines at temperatures below the breakpoint have demonstrated quite clearly that thermotolerance induction during heating does not occur to the same extent as that observed with murine and hamster cell lines (Fig. 6.3) (ARMOUR et al. 1993).

These recent observations need to be confirmed in additional human cell lines, but the implications are encouraging. If thermotolerance is not induced to the same extent, then a slope of 2–3

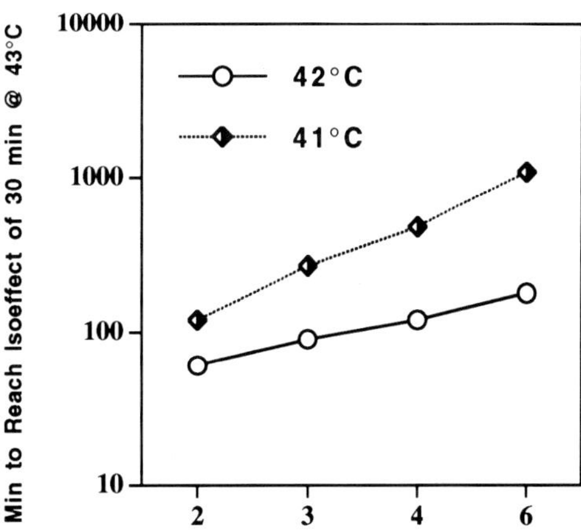

Fig. 6.2. Effect of differences in slope of the Arrhenius plot on time to reach an isoeffect, as compared with 30 min of heating at 43°C. Accurate determination of the slope of this relationship is important for application of thermal dosimetric concepts. If the slope below the breakpoint is near 2 for human cells, as has been suggested by some authors (ARMOUR et al. 1993), then 120 min at 41°C would be equivalent to 30 min at 43°C. On the other hand, if the slope is a factor of 6, as has been suggested by other authors (FIELD and MORRIS 1983), then more than 1000 min of heating would be needed to achieve the isoeffect

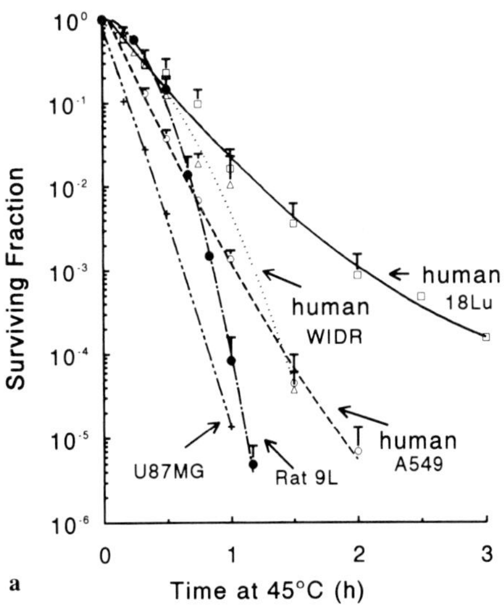

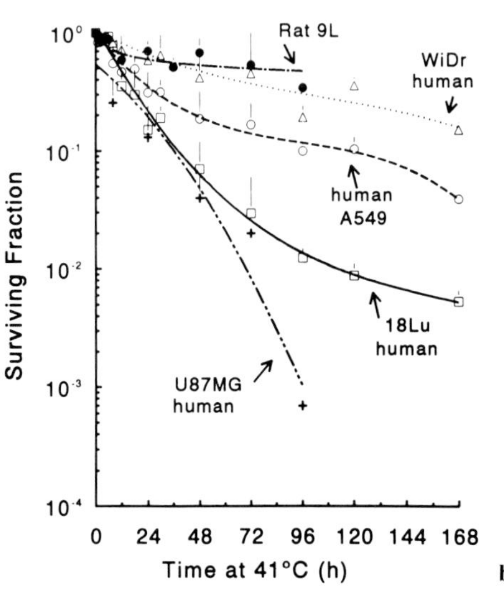

Fig. 6.3. **a** Hyperthermic cell survival after 45°C heating of human and rat cell lines. The sensitivity of three of the human cell lines is less than the rat cell line at this temperature. **b** Hyperthermic cell survival after 41°C heating of human and rat cell lines. The sensitivity of all of the human cell lines is greater than the rodent cell line at this temperature. These results taken together indicate that human cells are more sensitive than rat cells to hyperthermic cell killing at low temperature, and more resistant at high temperature. Furthermore, this would indicate that the slope of the Arrhenius plot below the breakpoint will be shallower than would be predicted by studies done with rodent cell lines. (From Armour et al. 1993)

below the breakpoint may be more accurate. The clinical implication of this result could mean that temperatures below 43°C are more cytotoxic than was previously appreciated. Interestingly, the heat sensitivity of human cells may be less than that of rodent cell lines at temperatures ≥43°–44°C (e.g., they may have a breakpoint that is nearer to 44°C than 43°C (Roizin-Towle and Pirro 1991). The clinical relevance of this feature of human tumor cell heat sensitivity and estimates of thermal isoeffect dose is probably small because it is extremely difficult to achieve temperatures exceeding 43°C in anything but small volumes of most tumors.

Thermotolerance development between two heat treatments could also confound interpretation of isoeffect dose calculations involving the second heat. The persistence of thermotolerance would have the effect of reducing the rate of cell kill for any given temperature, including those above the breakpoint. The effect of this form of thermotolerance on the Arrhenius plot is to shift the entire curve down and to the right, indicating that a higher temperature is needed to achieve the same rate of cell kill (Fig. 6.4).

Since thermotolerance that develops after heating is dependent upon the severity of the initial heat treatment and the amount of time that has elapsed between the two heat treatments, correction of the estimate of thermal isoeffect dose delivered could be very complicated. The complexity of this effect was elegantly shown by Nielson and Overgaard (1982), who examined the amount of time at 43°C to cure a murine tumor, as influenced by the prior thermal history (Fig. 6.5). In this analysis it is readily seen that the amount of thermotolerance induced is directly related to the initial heat exposure. Secondly, the time needed for thermotolerance to decay is longer for higher initial thermal exposures. Since temperatures achieved in human tumors are typically quite nonuniform, it is likely that differing levels of thermotolerance will be encountered and correction of the calculation of thermal isoeffect dose would vary in each part of the tumor, as related to its thermal history on the previous treatment. Although this aspect of thermal dosimetry seems formidable, its importance in the clinic is probably minimal. First, it is very difficult to achieve high temperatures in all but small volumes of most tumors. Secondly, for those volumes in which high temperatures do occur, there is also significant thermal cytotoxicity, such that only a few cells might survive to become thermotolerant (Dewey 1993). In many clinical series it has been shown that descriptors of the treatment related to the majority of the tumor volume (such as the 10th percentile or T_{90}) are at

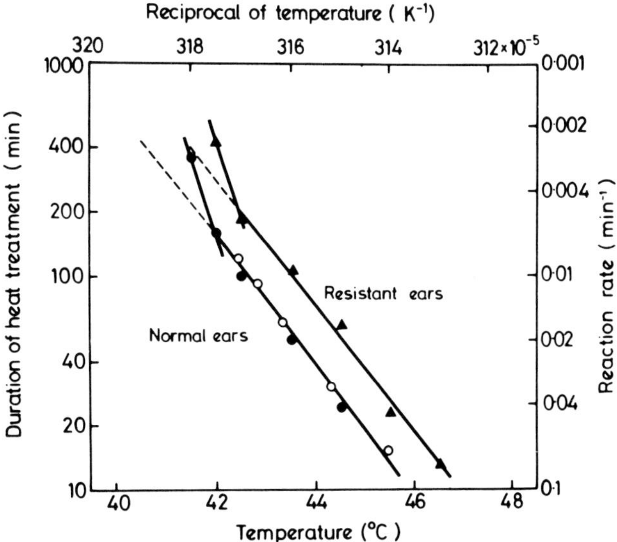

Fig. 6.4. Relationship between heating time and temperature in normal and previously heated (43.5°C, 20 min) mouse ears. This plot relates the duration of heating to achieve 50% incidence of ear necrosis at various temperatures, and is an alternate method of plotting an Arrhenius relationship. The studies on the previously heated ears were performed at 24 h after the first heat, which was the time of maximum thermotolerance. It is important to note that the shift in the Arrhenius plot is equivalent to 1°C, and that the two curves are parallel. The parallel nature of the curves means that a relatively simple conversion could be made to correct isoeffect dose calculations for thermotolerance if it could be detected or predicted to occur clinically as a result of fractionated hyperthermia treatments. (From LAW 1979)

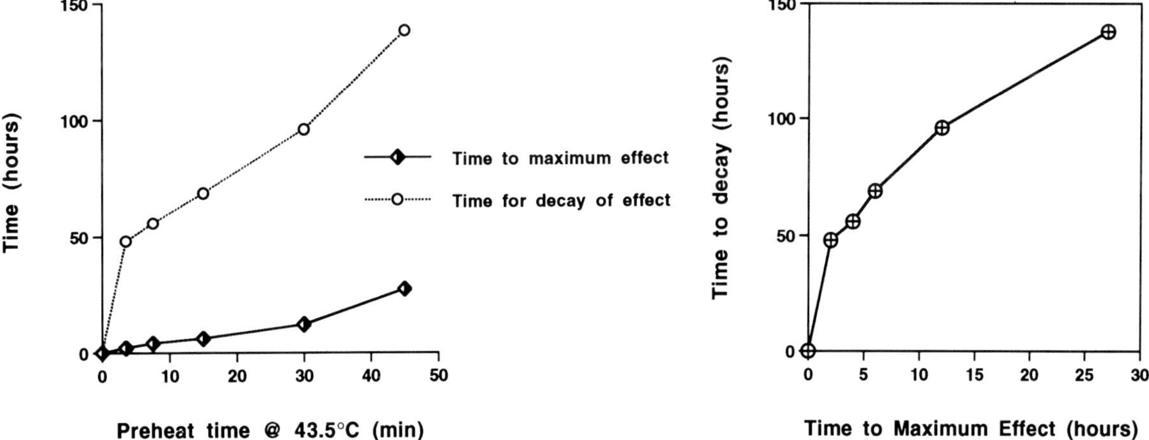

Fig. 6.5. a Time course of thermotolerance induction and decay in a murine tumor model, based on varying times of heating at 43.5°C. The time to maximum induction and time to decay of tolerance are both dependent upon the severity of an initial heat treatment. The total amount of tolerance that was induced in these experiments, which used tumor growth delay as an endpoint, was independent of the thermal exposure. This indicates that even the smallest heat shock was sufficient to induce a maximal level of thermotolerance. **b** Relationship between the time to maximum thermotolerance expression and time to decay of thermotolerance. Both sets of data are abstracted from NIELSEN and OVERGAARD (1982)

41°C or less. Given that thermotolerance induction in this temperature range is not large in human cell lines in the first place, it is not likely that thermotolerance induction will have much impact on the calculation of thermal isoeffect dose. Additionally, most clinical protocols utilize interfraction intervals of 72 h or greater. This is adequate time to allow for decay of most thermotolerance, such that a correction for a second heat is probably unnecessary.

6.2.2.1 pH and Bioenergetics

The effect of pH on thermal sensitivity is complex. Acute lowering of extracellular pH has been clearly demonstrated to enhance the thermal sensitivity of cells, particularly below 43°C (GERWECK 1977). This enhancement of sensitivity is linked to a delay in the onset of thermotolerance (GERWECK et al. 1982). The effect on the Arrhenius relationship is to make the slope of the curve more shallow below the breakpoint (i.e., closer to a factor of 2 change in heating time for every degree temperature change). Since tumors are frequently acidotic, early observations of this effect raised hopes that hyperthermia would be selectively cytotoxic to tumor cells. However, classic studies by HAHN and SHIU (1985) and COOK and FOX (1988) subsequently indicated that chronic exposure to low pH conditions causes cells to lose the pH sensitization effect. Chronic exposure to low pH conditions is likely to be more typical of cells residing in tumors. The implication of this more recent observation is that the resting pH of the tumor is unlikely to affect the accuracy of the calculation of thermal isoeffect dose.

Depletion of glucose has also been shown to sensitize cells to hyperthermia. (LANKS et al. 1988). Chronic exposure studies of glucose depletion have not been done, however. Thus, it is not known whether such environmental conditions would allow cells to resume thermal sensitivity more typical of normoglycemic cells.

6.2.2.2 Step-down Heating

Step-down heating refers to the scenario where temperatures rise above the breakpoint and then subsequently drop below the breakpoint during the same treatment session. Step-down heating has been observed during clinical treatments, either as a result of turning power down in response to patient pain, or subsequent to vasodilation induced by the heating. Even though it occurs, it is not likely to be of great importance clinically. The main effect of step-down heating is to delay the onset of thermotolerance, such that the cytotoxicity of the lower temperature is greater than would be expected, based on an uncorrected Arrhenius calculation. As with the pH effect, step-down heating makes the slope of the Arrhenius plot below the breakpoint less steep. If a correction is not made for this effect when it occurs, the amount of cytotoxicity from a thermal exposure will be underestimated. However, it must be recognized that even though step-down heating has been observed, it does not occur uniformly throughout a tumor volume. As discussed above, temperatures high enough to create step-down heating probably only occur in very small volumes of tumor and any mistake in isoeffect dose which might occur as a result of such error would be insignificant, relative to the whole tumor volume.

6.2.2.3 Position of the Breakpoint

Recent studies with human cell lines indicate that the break in the Arrhenius plot may be nearer to 44°C and the slope below the break appears to be less than 4 (ARMOUR et al. 1993; ROIZIN-TOWLE and PIRRO 1991; HAHN et al. 1989). These observations mean that human cells are probably more thermally resistant than rodent cells at temperatures above 44°C, but they are more sensitive to hyperthermia at temperatures below the breakpoint. The difference in thermosensitivity below the breakpoint is probably due to reduced thermotolerance induction. Given the uncertainties in temperature measurement that occur clinically, it is not likely that these subtle variations in time-temperature relationships will be important in using thermal isoeffect dose in the clinic.

6.2.2.4 Variations in Thermal Sensitivity by Histology

There is no question that the thermal sensitivity of tumor cells varies (FIELD and MORRIS 1983). These variations in absolute thermal sensitivity mean that the degree of thermal cytotoxicity that results from a defined thermal isoeffect dose calculation will not be the same across various histological types and perhaps not even within the same histological type. If this were a major factor in controlling thermal response in the clinic, then one might expect that the dose calculation method would not work in the clinical setting. However, this has not been the case. In a recent review of the Duke University clinical series, strong relationships between thermal isoeffect dose calculations were seen for soft tissue sarcomas and miscellaneous superficial tumors. The goodness of fit of the models was better for soft tissue sarcomas than for the superficial tumors, which may in part have been due to greater histological heterogeneity in the latter group. Larger variations in tumor size may also have contributed.

6.2.2.5 Thermal Isoeffect Dose Summary

A compilation of the effects of various factors on the Arrhenius plot and subsequent thermal isoeffect dose calculations is shown in Table 6.1 and Fig. 6.6. Theoretically, these effects might be enough to make the isoeffect dose calculation method invalid for interpreting thermal data derived from the clinic. As will be seen in the following sections, however, this method seems to work in spite of these limitations.

6.3 Integration of Dosimetric Principles into Clinical Practice

Hyperthermic dosimetry in the clinic has undergone a revolution in understanding and application

Table 6.1. Factors that influence accuracy of thermal isoeffect dose calculations

Factor	Comment	Effect on calculation (if not accounted for)
Cell type or histology	Absolute thermal sensitivity varies	Isoeffect calculations may not be accurate across histologic types
Thermotolerance	Rate of cell kill is reduced.	Predicted dose will be too high.
Acid pH	Rate of thermotolerance induction is reduced and sensitivity increased	Predicted dose will be too low
Low glucose	Same as above	Same as above
Step-down heating	Rate of thermotolerance induction is reduced	Predicted dose below breakpoint will be too low
Shoulder on heat-survival curve	Not accounted for*	Predicted dose will be too high

* Isoeffect dose formula described in this chapter and suggested by Sapareto and Dewey, 1984.

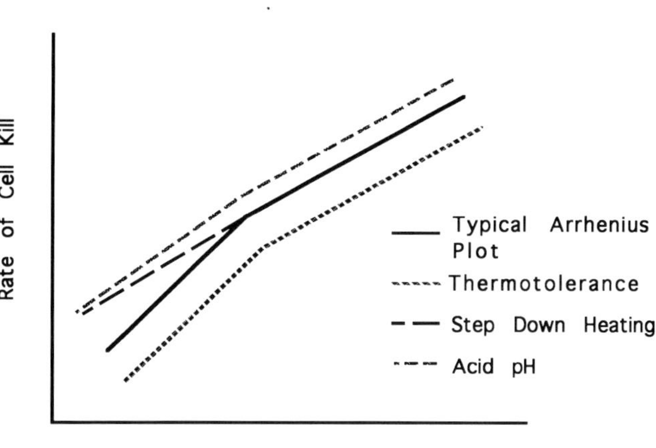

Fig. 6.6. Summary figure pictorially demonstrating the effects of various modifiers on the shape and position of the Arrhenius plot. Thermotolerance will reduce the rate of cell killing for a set temperature, as compared with non-thermotolerant cells. The effect on the Arrhenius plot is to shift it down and to the right, but parallel with the original curve, both above and below the breakpoint. Step down heating prevents the development of thermotolerance during heating, so the slope of the plot does not change below the breakpoint that is observed for control cells that are not subjected to step down heating. Acid pH creates sensitization to thermal cell killing both above and below the breakpoint, although the effect is somewhat larger below the breakpoint because acid pH also delays the onset of thermotolerance

over the past 15 years. We have progressed from not measuring temperatures at all, to limited unstandardized procedures to quality controlled rigorous standards for thermometry. This change in understanding of how to measure temperatures in human patients came from carefully planned prospective thermal dose evaluation trials, as discussed in DEWHIRST et al. (1993). These latter trials have set the stage for how to write treatment prescriptions for hyperthermia that are verifiable from invasive temperature measurements.

6.3.1 Temperature Sampling Theory

It has been recognized since modern hyperthermia trials began that invasive temperature measurements will only give a selected and potentially biased view of the full temperature distribution within a tumor. In early hyperthermia trials many investigators were so skeptical about the validity of invasive measurements that they preferred to perform no thermometry at all, or at the most would only use one or two points/tumor. For example, approximately 30% of the patients in the RTOG randomized study (81-04; hyperthermia + radiation vs radiation alone for superficial tumors) had no thermometry performed (PEREZ et al. 1989). In spite of the obvious problems with sparse temperature sampling, several investigators began to systematically compare various measures of the temperature distribution with treatment outcome. Results prior to 1988 were nicely reviewed by VALDAGNI et al. (1988). In general, it was found that simple descriptors, such as the the minimum average temperature, often correlated with treatment outcome as assessed by response rates and duration of local control. In more recent series, these descriptors still carry significant prognostic importance even for duration of local control (COX and KAPP 1992). Even though there were many technical differences between institutions in exactly how the thermometry was performed, the consistency in the relation between treatment outcome and some measure of temperature clearly pointed to the need to measure temperature in all patients and to establish guidelines for standardization in thermometry. These observations, along with the failure of RTOG 81-04 to show a therapeutic advantage for hyperthermia, dictated that careful thermometry should be performed in all patients. Standards for thermometry in hyperthermia clinical trials have been established (DEWHIRST et al. 1990). Until recently, however, there has not been an established method for writing a hyperthermia treatment prescription, even when temperatures are measured in a standard fashion. Thus, the measurements were of no value in controlling the treatment of any individual patient. A method for writing a treatment prescription has recently been proposed, but has not been adopted universally (OLESON et al. 1993).

Until the mid-1980s no one attempted to analytically assess how to measure temperatures in tumors or to evaluate the effect that any measurement strategy would have on assessing the true temperature distribution in a heated volume. Ideas relating to sampling theory were first introduced by DEWHIRST et al. in 1987 and were later expanded by EDELSTEIN-KESHET et al. (1989). These concepts are related to the use of integrated frequency distributions that were first utilized by the Hyperthermia Equipment Evaluation Study (SAPOZINK et al. 1988). The relationship between a standard frequency distribution and an integrated distribution is shown in Fig. 6.7.

The fundamental problem has been that thermometry has typically been obtained via linear maps or multipoint from preplaced catheters that are introduced into the tumor. Most commonly, such catheters are placed through the center of a tumor and the resulting data are a linear profile, with equal spacing between measured points. If one computes a frequency distribution from such data, it will not reflect the true volume temperature distribution, since the majority of the measurements are obtained from the center of the tumor, which represents the minority of the volume. In an ideal spherical tumor, with concentric isotherms, it is possible to cube the integrated frequency distribution to obtain a more realistic assessment of the volume temperature distribution (EDELSTEIN-KESHET et al. 1989). In fact, small perturbations in the shape of a tumor away from a true spherical shape, or slight variations in the isotherms away from concentricity, do not affect the estimate of the volume frequency distribution very much, as long as the thermometry catheter passes through the center of the tumor volume. It was this observation that led, in part, to the generation of the thermometry standards that have been established by the RTOG for bulky tumors (DEWHIRST et al. 1990).

Even though standards have been established for hyperthermia thermometry, a systematic

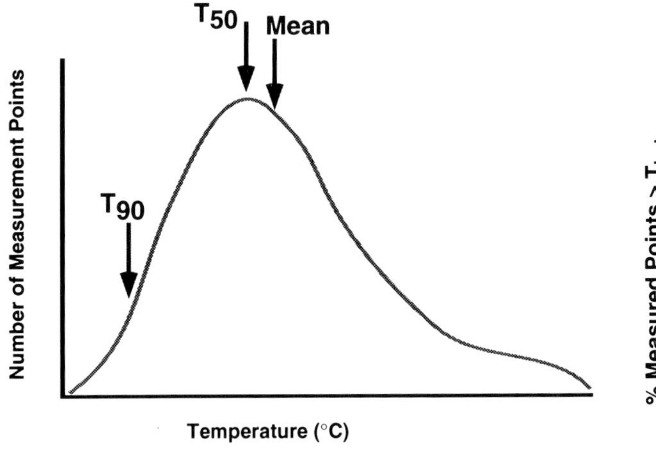

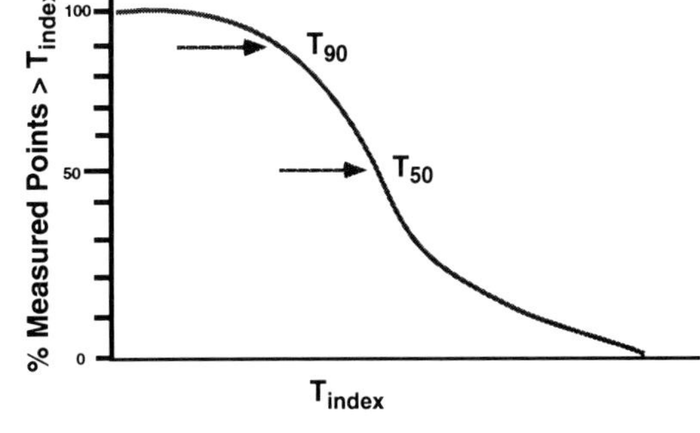

Fig. 6.7. **a** Idealized view of a frequency distribution of measured temperatures. During a hyperthermia session, linearly mapped temperature data can be visualized as a frequency distribution that has a mean and median (T_{50}). Typically the median is lower than the mean because the frequency distribution is not normally distributed. A descriptor of the lower end of the frequency distribution that has often been used in the reporting of this type of data is the tenth percentile, or the T_{90}. **b** Integrated frequency distribution of temperatures. In most clinical reports, the frequency distribution is reported in this form, which plots the fraction of measured points that exceed a given threshold temperature (index temperature) as a function of temperature. The locations of the T_{50} and T_{90} are shown

evaluation of sources of error in assessment of the temperature distribution has not been made until recently. We have evaluated the effect of various treatment- and patient-related variables on the estimates of the temperature distribution as described by the T_{90} (10th percentile) or T_{50} (median) (Samulski, Clegg, Rosner, Dewhirst, unpublished observations, 1994). This study was performed by creating a series of "computer tumors," which had random shapes and perfusion distribution patterns. Both low- and high-perfusion cases were considered. These simulated tumors were subjected to a simulated microwave field (based on modeled and verified measurements from a dielectrically loaded waveguide) and the resulting temperature distributions were calculated, using heat transfer modeling. Once the "true" temperature distributions were determined, simulated thermometry catheters were introduced into the tumors in various orientations. The measured temperatures were converted to frequency distributions and compared with the "real" temperature distribution. Inherent factors that were considered in these studies included the shape of the tumor and the magnitude of perfusion. Temperature sampling variables included the orientation of the catheter as it enters the tumor, its proximity to the true geometric center, spacing between measured points along a catheter, number of catheters, measurement error in the thermometer, and mis-assignment of a position as being tumor when it is really normal tissue.

The two patient-related variables had the greatest influence on the estimate of the true temperature distribution, whereas the variations in sampling methodology had relatively little influence. Distance between measured points and noise in the measurement and proximity to the geometric center of the tumor had almost no influence on the estimate, as long as these parameters were within RTOG guidelines (maximum errors of the estimate of T_{90} were less than 0.2°C). It was clear from the analysis that significant gain could be made by using two, as opposed to one, catheter; however, the addition of a third catheter did not afford any better estimate of the temperature distribution than using two. Cubing the frequency distribution, as was suggested by Edelstein-Keshet et al. (1989), had the effect of reducing the error in the estimate. Mis-assignment of a position as being in tumor, when it was really in normal tissue, had a larger influence on the T_{90} than the T_{50}.

The angle of the catheter, relative to the surface of the tumor, had a large influence on the measurement, which was attributed to effects of the tumor shape on the temperatures sampled. The maximum error in T_{90} could be as large as 1°C, for example. This effect could be minimized to some extent by making certain that the thermometry catheter passed through a long rather than a short axis of the tumor. Similarly, there was much greater error in the estimate of the distribution in the high-perfusion cases. The important conclusion to be drawn from these studies was that use of RTOG guidelines would keep sources of measurement error to much less than the sources of error that are inherent to the tumor (geometry and perfusion). In the best case it is likely that these two uncontrollable sources of noise in the estimate of the temperature distribution will add 0.5°–1.0°C potential error in the estimate of T_{90} for a given patient (Table 6.2).

The only way to make further improvement in the assessment of the true temperature distribution would be to develop noninvasive thermometry or to use heat transfer modeling to gain better three-dimensional temperature distribution data (CLEGG et al. 1994).

6.3.2 *Thermometric Indices of Treatment Efficacy*

6.3.2.1 Historic Overview

The correlation of thermometric information with estimates of treatment efficacy were first reported by DEWHIRST et al. (1982) using pet animals with cancer that were treated with hyperthermia and radiation. The concepts were further refined by that group in subsequent reports (DEWHIRST et al. 1983, 1984a,b; DEWHIRST and SIM 1986). In these early studies, thermometry was limited to three to ten intratumoral points and standardization of thermometer location was used although thermal mapping was not routinely practiced. In these early reports minimum and average temperature were found to be significantly correlated with both response rate and duration of local control; minimum temperature was most strongly correlated with treatment outcome. Maximum intratumoral temperature was correlated with the incidence of thermal injury (DEWHIRST and SIM 1986). Although these simple estimates of the temperature distribution were related to treatment outcome, the goodness of fit of logistic regression analyses was not high. This suggested that more complete thermometric data might be needed to be more precise about the adequacy of treatment for a given patient. These early studies used a conversion of the thermometric data to isoeffect dose, but this approach was later criticized because of the potential pitfalls in the estimate of thermal isoeffect dose, as discussed above.

Following the initial reports in the pet animal studies, a number of subsequent reports verified the relationship between minimum measured temperature or average temperature and treatment outcome in human patients. In some studies thermal isoeffect dose was used and in others temperature only was used (VALDAGNI et al.

Table 6.2. Influence of thermometry procedures and tumor-related variables on accuracy of estimates of temperature frequency distribution[1]

Parameter	Range of Errors in Descriptor	
	T_{90}	T_{50}
Tumor geometry	O to 0.5°C	−1.0 to 0°C
Tumor perfusion	−0.5 to −1.5°C	−1.0 to −2.5°C
Number of thermometry catheters	±0.1°C	±0.2°C
Spacing of thermometry points in catheter	0.1 to 0.6°C	0.1 to 0.4°C
Offset (distance from geometric center, as set by RTOG[2])	−0.2 to 0.3°C	0 to 0.7°C
SAR pattern	<0.1°C	<0.1°C
Noise in temperature measurement	<0.1°C	<0.1°C

[1] Based on unpublished computer simulations by the author and collaborators (Clegg; Samulski; Rosner) of ten tumor geometries and two different types of perfusion patterns
[2] From: DEWHIRST et al. 1990

1988). More recently, minimum temperature continues to be strongly correlated with duration of local control in patients with chest wall recurrences treated with thermoradiotherapy (KAPP et al. 1992).

In an attempt to more accurately characterize the true temperature distribution, OLESON et al. (1989) performed an interesting analysis in patients with soft tissue sarcomas. In this study, they reasoned that the majority of volume of a tumor resides in the outer 20% of the radius. Thus, for this particular set of patients, in which the geometry is reasonably spherical, they used a two-parameter model, based on the temperature at the edge of the tumor and the average slope of the temperature profile in the outer 2 cm of the tumor radius. The reasoning was that in the case of a high edge temperature, it is not necessary to have a steep temperature profile from the edge toward the center. In contrast, in the case of a low edge temperature, a steep profile would be needed to heat this outer volume of tumor. This two-parameter model was able to accurately distinguish patients that responded favorably to the preoperative course of themoradiotherapy. Two factors contributed to the inability to translate this model to a more general case. First, it was recognized that it is difficult to accurately determine where the edge of a tumor resides, even with CT guidance. Second, most tumors are not spherical, so extrapolation to the general case is not possible.

Given the problems inherent in the edge–slope analysis above, the hyperthermia group at Duke embarked on a series of studies to utilize the frequency distribution of temperatures, as described above. Both the T_{90} and the T_{50} were found to be strongly correlated with treatment outcome (LEOPOLD et al. 1992). Other investigators have verified the utility of these indices for prediction of treatment outcome (ISSELS et al. 1991; SNEED et al. 1991; COX and KAPP 1992). However, a basic problem with the use of only temperature as a treatment efficacy index is that it ignores the time factor, which should also be taken into consideration. In addition, it ignores the logarithmic relationship between rate of cell kill and temperature.

In partial response to this problem, the cumulative minutes that the T_{90} or T_{50} exceeds various threshold temperatures were used for prediction of treatment outcome (Fig. 6.7) (LEOPOLD et al. 1992).

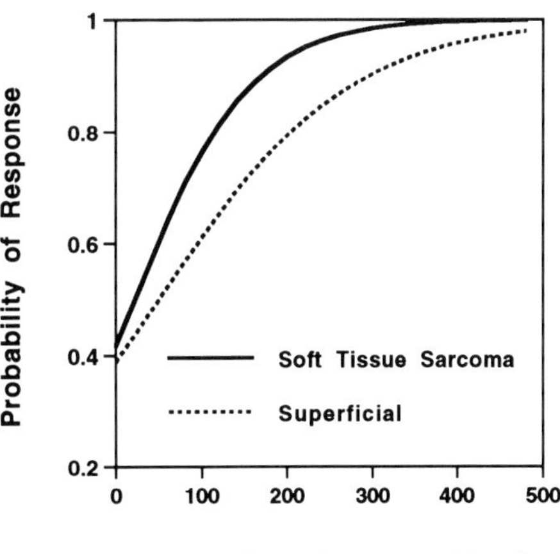

Fig. 6.8. Probability of tumor response for soft tissue sarcomas and superficial tumors as a function of the cumulative minutes that the T_{90} exceeds 40.5°C. These data are replotted using logistic regression evaluations of data from previously published reports (LEOPOLD et al. 1992, 1993) and sums the total time over all treatments received. In both studies this parameter was a statistically significant predictor of treatment outcome. However, the analysis assumes a threshold temperature as being clinically efficacious (e.g., 40.5°C). Thus, a tumor that has a T_{90} of 40.4°C would be deemed to have no therapeutic benefit, while one with a T_{90} of 40.5°C would be considered to be successfully treated

Although this approach was quite successful, the basic limitation was that one was forced to choose an arbitrary threshold temperature to judge treatment success from failure. In examining univariate analyses for superficial tumors, for example, it was found that any temperature between 39.5° and 43°C was a statistically significant threshold temperature. If one picked 41°C as the critical threshold temperature, then any temperature below that threshold would have no therapeutic value. Clearly, this method of analysis provided no clear way to distinguish between good and bad therapy, and as a result it could not be used to write a treatment prescription that could be complied with. For example, if 300 cumulative minutes with a T_{90} greater than 41°C were required to place a patient into a high-risk category for a good response, then a patient with 300 cumulative minutes with a T_{90} of 40.8° or 40.9°C would be considered a failure. It is unlikely that a few tenths of a degree will be that important in governing treatment outcome, based on what is known about hyperthermia cytotoxicity in vitro.

It was for these reasons that Oleson and coworkers went back to the use of the thermal isoeffect dose to reconsider the issue of treatment prescription writing (OLESON et al. 1993). In the most recent analysis, this group has used the cumulative minutes of the T_{90} or T_{50}, converted to equivalent minutes at 43°C, as estimators of treatment efficacy. This method alleviates the need for assignment of an arbitrary threshold temperature and has been useful in predicting treatment outcome in patient groups with soft tissue sarcomas and miscellaneous superficial tumors. It has been possible to utilize this approach to estimate the isoeffective dose needed to increase the probability of response over what is estimated from radiation alone. For example, in superficial tumors, a T_{90} of 10 equivalent minutes at 43°C was predicted to increase the probability of CR by 25%, over what is estimated for radiation alone (Fig. 6.8).

In the Duke superficial tumor series, the average T_{90} was about 2 equivalent minutes at 43°C. Thus, one would want to increase the isoeffective dose by a factor of 5 to justify the initiation of a phase III study. This could be achieved by increasing the time by 5 or by increasing the average T_{90} temperature from 39.4°C to 40.6°C (1.2°C). T_{50} was used for soft tissue sarcomas while T_{90} was used for superficial tumors in order to use the descriptor that gave the highest $\chi 2$ value in univariate logistic regression analyses. However, in a subsequent analysis, T_{90} was used for both patient groups and the consistency in prediction of treatment outcome between the two groups is remarkable (DEWEY 1994).

The importance of these most recent analyses cannot be overstated. In 1987, the recommendation of the hyperthermia community was that thermal isoeffect dose should not be used in routine clinical applications because of the potential sources of error in the calculation, as described above. However, continued work at the basic science level and in the clinic has pointed to the fact that many of these sources of error are not important clinically, thus leading the way for reestablishment of the use of thermal isoeffect dose in combination with a descriptor of the temperature frequency distribution as a means of writing and verifying a treatment prescription for hyperthermia. Additional clinical studies utilizing this approach to data analysis would strengthen this argument further, particularly in studies where the duration of heating during single sessions is variable. A summary of the limitations of thermometric indices of hyperthermic treatment efficacy is shown in Table 6.3.

6.4 Summary

- Accuracy in thermal dosimetry focuses on two concepts. The first is that the unit used to

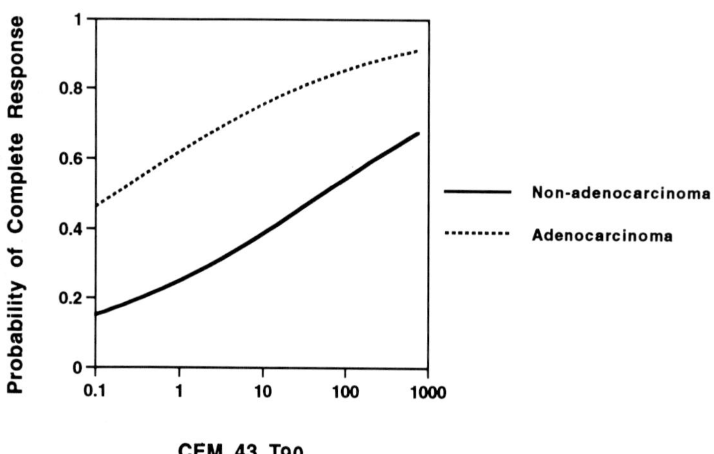

Fig. 6.9 Probability of tumor response for superficial tumors as a function of the cumulative equivalent minutes at 43°C that the T_{90} reaches over a course of therapy. In this type of analysis the T_{90} at each minute of therapy is converted to equivalent minutes at 43°C. These data are then summed over the entire course of therapy. The advantage of this type of analysis is that there is no need to assume a threshold of treatment success, as was shown in Fig. 6.7. In addition, the analysis takes into account the time of heating as well as the temperature achieved, including factoring in the exponential relationship between temperature and rate of cell killing. These data are replotted from published logistic regression analyses of clinical data (OLESON et al. 1993)

Table 6.3. Limitations of some thermometric indices of hyperthermic treatment[1] that have been correlated with treatment outcome

Index	Features			
	Statistically imprecise	Geometrically biased	Does not include time as factor	Does not consider change in rate of cell kill with temperature
Minimum Temperature	√		√	√
Average Temperature	√	√	√	√
T_{90} (10th percentile)		√	√	√
T_{50} (median)		√	√	√
Edge temperature vs. slope	√		√	√
Min $T_{90} > T_{index}$		√		√
CEM 43°T_{90}		√		

[1] Obtained from linear maps

describe the treatment should have some thermal biologic meaning. This requirement is different than units used to describe radiation dose, which are based solely on a physical measurement of energy deposited in matter. The reason for this is that thermal effects are not based directly on the amount of energy deposited, but instead are based on the temperatures that are achieved, the duration of the hyperthermic exposure and a number of modifiers, such as environmental pH, thermotolerance, etc. The thermal isoeffect dose method (Sapareto and Dewey 1984) has been used successfully to describe treatment outcome, although additional work is needed to define the exact nature of this isoeffect dose calculation method for human tumor cells. Additional models may also warrant investigation (Mackey and Roti Roti 1992).

- The second requirement for accurate thermal dosimetry is to be able to accurately determine the full three-dimensional temperature distribution. None of the methods that rely solely on mapped temperature measurements is capable of achieving this requirement, as all of them have some geometric biases. Even if the full three-dimensional temperature distribution is known, there is not a well-defined method for describing it in a way that gives optimal predictive power as to the therapeutic effect. Simple frequency distribution measurements, such as the minimum monitored temperature and the T_{90} have been used with some success, but these are likely not the optimal descriptors.
- Future goals in clinical thermal dosimetry need to focus in two directions. First, it is necessary to develop means to obtain more accurate three-dimensional temperature distribution data. Two methods that show great promise in this arena are heat-transfer modeling and noninvasive thermometry.

A second step that is needed is to prove that escalation of thermal dose leads to improvement in treatment outcome. This requires a prospective test of thermal dosimetric concepts on a more sophisticated level than merely increasing the number of hyperthermia fractions (Oleson et al 1993). Prospective thermal dose escalation trials, based on CEM 43 T_{90} concepts are currently underway, for example.

- It is anticipated that significant improvement in our understanding of how to successfully implement thermal dosimetry will emerge in the next 5–10 years as a result of progress in all of the above-mentioned arenas of inquiry.
- Areas of future inquiry that are needed to improve current methods of thermal dosimetry:
  Accurate measures of the biologic effects of hyperthermia, and its modifiers on human tumor cell cytotoxicity
  Accurate measures of true three-dimensional temperature distributions in human tumors
  Prospective trials that test new thermal dosimetric concepts.

References

Armour EP, McEachern D, Wang Z, Corry PM, Martinez A (1993) Sensitivity of human cells to mild hyperthermia. Cancer Res 53: 2740–2744

Clegg ST, Samulski TV, Murphy K, Rosner G, Dewhirst MW (1994) Inverse techniques in hyperthermia: a sensitivity study. IEEE Trans Biomed Eng 41: 373–382

Cook JA, Fox MH (1988) Effects of acute pH 6.6 and 42.0°C heating on the intracellular pH of Chinese hamster ovary cells. Cancer Res 48: 496–502

Cox RS, Kapp DS (1992) Correlation of thermal parameters with outcome in combined radiation therapy-hyperthermia trials. Int J Hyperthermia 8: 719–732

Dewey WC (1994) Arrhenius relationships from the molecule and cell to the clinic. Int J Hyperthermia 10: 457–483

Dewhirst MW, Sim DA (1986) Estimation of therapeutic gain in clinical trials involving hyperthermia and radiotherapy. Int J Hyperthermia 2: 165–178

Dewhirst MW, Connor WG, Moon TE, Roth HB (1982) Response of spontaneous animal tumors to heat and/or radiation: Preliminary results of a phase III trial. J Natl Cancer Inst Monogr 61: 395–397

Dewhirst MW, Connor WG, Sim DA, Wilson S, DeYoung D, Parsells JL (1983) Correlation between initial and long term responses of spontaneous pet animal tumors to heat and radiation or radiation alone. Cancer Res 43: 5735–5741

Dewhirst MW, Gross JF, Sim D, Arnold P, Boyer D (1984a) The effect of rate of heating and cooling prior to heating on tumor and normal tissue microcirculatory blood flow. Biorheology 21: 539–558

Dewhirst MW, Sim D, Sapareto S, Connor WG (1984b) Importance of minimum tumor temperature in determining early and long-term responses of spontaneous canine and feline tumors to heat and radiation. Cancer Res 44: 43–50

Dewhirst MW, Winget JM, Edelstein-Keshet L et al. (1987) Clinical application of thermal isoeffect dose. Int J Hyperthermia 3: 307–318

Dewhirst MW, Phillips TL, Samulski TV et al. (1990) RTOG quality assurance guidelines for clinical trials using hyperthermia. Int J Radiat Oncol Biol Phys 18: 1249–1259

Dewhirst MW, Griffin TW, Smith AR, Parker RG, Hanks GE, Brady LW (1993) Intersociety Council on Radiation Oncology essay on the introduction of new medical treatments into practice. J Natl Cancer Inst 84: 951–957

Edelstein-Keshet L, Dewhirst MW, Oleson JR, Samulski TV (1989) Characterization of tumour temperature distribution in hyperthermia based on assumed mathematical forms. Int J Hyperthermia 5: 757–777

Field SB, Morris CC (1983) The relationship between heating time and temperature: its relevance to clinical hyperthermia. Radiother Oncol 1: 179–186

Gerweck LE (1977) Modification of cell lethality at elevated temperatures. The pH effect. Radiat Res 70: 224–235

Gerweck LE, Richards B, Michaels HB (1982) Influence of low pH on the development and decay of 42 degree thermotolerance in CHO cells. Int J Radiat Oncol Biol Phys 8: 1935–1941

Hahn GM, Shiu EC (1985) Protein synthesis, thermotolerance and step-down heating. Int J Radiat Oncol Biol Phys 11: 159–164

Hahn GM, Ning SC, Elizaga M, Kapp DS, Anderson RL (1989) A comparison of thermal responses of human and rodent cells. Int J Radiat Biol Phys 56: 817–825

Issels RD, Mittermüller J, Gerl A et al. (1991) Improvement of local control by regional hyperthermia combined with systemic chemotherapy (ifosfamide plus etoposide) in advanced sarcomas: updated report on 65 patients. J Cancer Res Clin Oncol 117 (Suppl): s141–s147

Kapp DS, Cox RS, Barnett TA, Ben-Yosef R (1992) Thermoradiotherapy for residual microscopic cancer: elective or post-excisional hyperthermia and radiation therapy in the management of local-regional recurrent breast cancer. Int J Radiat Oncol Biol Phys 24: 261–277

Lanks KW, Gao JP, Kasambalides EJ (1988) Nucleoside restoration of heat resistance and suppression of glucose-regulated protein synthesis by glucose-deprived L929 cells. Cancer Res 48: 1442–1445

Law MP (1979) Induced thermal resistance in the mouse ear: the relationship between heating time and temperature. Int J Radiat Biol 35: 481–485

Leopold KA, Dewhirst MW, Samulski TV et al. (1992) Relationships among tumor temperature, treatment time and histopathological outcome using preoperative hyperthermia with radiation in soft tissue sarcomas. Int J Radiat Oncol Biol Phys 22: 989–998

Leopold KA, Dewhirst MW, Samulski TV et al. (1993) Cumulative minutes with T_{90} greater than $\mathrm{Temp}_{\mathrm{index}}$ is predictive of response of superficial malignancies to hyperthermia and radiation. Int J Radiat Oncol Biol Phys 25: 841–847

Mackey M, Roti Roti JL (1992) A model of heat-induced clonogenic cell death. J Theor Biol 156: 133–146

Nielson OS, Overgaard J (1982) Importance of preheating temperature and time for the induction of thermotolerance in a solid tumour in vivo. Br J Cancer 46: 894–903

Oleson JR, Dewhirst MW, Harrelson JM, Leopold KA, Samulski TV, Tso CY (1989) Tumor temperature distributions predict hyperthermia effect. Int J Radiat Oncol Biol Phys 16: 559–570

Oleson JR, Samulski TV, Leopold KA, Clegg ST, Dewhirst MW, Dodge RK, George SL (1993) Sensitivity of hyperthermia trial outcomes to temperature and time: implications for thermal goals of treatment. Int J Radiat Oncol Biol Phys 25: 289–297

Perez CA, Gillespie B, Pajak T, Hornback NB, Emami B, Rubin P (1989) Quality assurance problems in clinical hyperthermia and their impact on therapeutic outcome: a report by the Radiation Therapy Oncology Group. Int J Radiat Oncol Biol Phys 16: 551–558

Roizin-Towle L, Pirro JP (1991) The response of human and rodent cells to hyperthermia. Int J Radiat Oncol Biol Phys 20: 751–756

Samulski TV, MacFall J, Zhang Y, Grant W, Charles C (1992) Non-invasive thermometry using magnetic resonance diffusion imaging: potential for application in hyperthermic oncology. Int J Hyperthermia 8: 819–829

Sapareto SA (1987) A workshop on thermal dose in cancer therapy: introduction. Int J Hyperthermia 3: 289–290

Sapareto SA, Dewey WC (1984) Thermal dose determination in cancer therapy. Int J Radiat Oncol Biol Phys 10: 787–800

Sapozink MD, Cetas T, Corry PM, Egger MJ, Fessenden P (1988) Introduction to hyperthermia device evaluation. Int J Hyperthermia 4: 1–15

Sneed PK, Stauffer PR, Gutin PH et al. (1991) Interstitial irradiation and hyperthermia for the treatment of recurrent malignant brain tumors. Neurosurgery 28: 206–215

Valdagni R, Liu FE, Kapp DS (1988) Important prognostic factors influencing outcome of combined radiation and hyperthermia. Int J Radiat Oncol Biol Phys 15: 959–972

Pathophysiological Mechanisms

7 Microvasculature and Perfusion in Normal Tissues and Tumors

C.W. SONG, I.B. CHOI, B.S. NAH, S.K. SAHU, and J.L. OSBORN

CONTENTS

7.1 Introduction

The tissue temperature during heating is dependent on the influx of energy and efflux of heat, mainly through the convective heat transfer between the tissue and circulating blood. It follows that the temperature in tissues with poor blood circulation will rise higher than that in tissues with good blood circulation. It has been demonstrated that a variance in temperature as small as 0.5°–1.0°C in the therapeutic range, i.e., 42°–45°C, can cause a significant difference in cell killing or tissue damage (DEWEY et al. 1977; FAJARDO 1984; FIELD et al. 1977). Indications are that such a small difference in temperature can easily be caused by a small change in blood flow (JAIN 1980; SONG et al. 1980a–c; SONG 1982a,b). It is known that the anatomical characteristics of blood vessels and blood flow in different tissues or tumors are markedly different. Furthermore, the changes in blood vessels and blood flow induced by heat are profoundly different in different tissues or tumors (DEWHIRST 1987; DUDAR and JAIN 1984; JAIN and WARD-HARTLEY 1984; REINHOLD and ENDRICH 1986; SONG 1982a–c, 1991a,b; VAUPEL 1990).

The cellular or tissue damage caused by hyperthermia increases with an increase in environmental acidity, i.e., a decrease in pH (GERWECK et al. 1983; KIM et al. 1991; SONG et al. 1993; WIKE-HOOLEY et al. 1984). The tissue acidity is dependent on the formation of acidic metabolites, such as lactic acid (LEE et al. 1986; RYU and SONG 1982; STREFFER 1984), which is closely influenced by the availability of oxygen through the blood circulation. The removal of acidic metabolites from the tissue also depends on the blood circulation. It is obvious, then, that a detailed knowledge of the blood flow, and in particular the heat-induced change in blood flow, is essential for an understanding of the hyperthermic damage in tissues and for the effective use of hyperthermia in the treatment of malignant tumors. In the present chapter, we discuss the heat-induced change in blood flow in various normal tissues and tumors and its implications for the treatment of tumors with hyperthermia alone or in combination with other modalities.

C.W. SONG, PhD, Radiation Biology Section, Department of Therapeutic Radiology, University of Minnesota, Box 494 UMHC, Minneapolis, MN 55455, USA
I.B. CHOI, MD, Radiation Biology Section, Department of Therapeutic Radiology, University of Minnesota, Box 494 UMHC, Minneapolis, MN 55455, USA
B.S. NAH, MD, Radiation Biology Section, Department of Therapeutic Radiology, University of Minnesota, Box 494 UMHC, Minneapolis, MN 55455, USA
S.K. SAHU, PhD, Radiation Biology Section, Department of Therapeutic Radiology, University of Minnesota, Box 494 UMHC, Minneapolis, MN 55455, USA
J.L. OSBORN, BS, Radiation Biology Section, Department of Therapeutic Radiology, University of Minnesota, Box 494 UMHC, Minneapolis, MN 55455, USA

7.2 Hyperthermia-Induced Vascular Changes in Normal Tissues

7.2.1 Skin and Muscle

The pathological changes in burned skin or muscle have been well studied. However, only during the last 10–15 years insights have been obtained into the effect of heating at the relatively low temperatures, 41°C–45°C, used in hyperthermic treatment of tumors, on the pathophysiological parameters, including blood flow, in the cutaneous tissues. We have studied the heat-induced changes in various vascular parameters in the skin and muscle of mice, rats, and humans. Heating the leg of Sprague-Dawley (SD) rats in a 43°C water bath for 1 h increased the intravascular volume, as measured with ^{51}Cr-labeled red blood cells, by about 2.9- and 1.6-fold in the skin and muscle, respectively (Song 1978; Song et al. 1980a–c). The vascular permeability, as measured with radioactive serum albumin, in the aforementioned skin and muscle also increased by 3.6 and 2.5 times, respectively, when heated at 43°C for 1 h. The changes in blood flow, as measured with the radioactive microsphere method, in the leg skin and muscle of SD rats have also been investigated (Song et al. 1980a). As shown in Fig. 7.1, the blood flow in the skin and muscle increased by 3.7 and 2.4 times, respectively, upon heating at 43°C for 1 h. The blood flow in the skin and muscle adjacent to the subcutaneously grown Walker tumor was about twice that in control counterparts, and it increased by 3–4 times when measured after heating at 43°C for 1 h. Figure 7.1 also shows the changes in the blood flow in the Walker tumor (to be discussed later). The results of a more comprehensive investigation into the changes in blood flow in the skin and muscle of SD rats are shown in Figs. 7.2 and 7.3 (Lokshina et al. 1985). The blood flow in the skin before heating was 7.14 ml/100 g/min. During heating at 42°C or 43°C for 120 min, the blood flow in the skin continuously increased, reaching about twofold and sixfold the control value, respectively, at the end of heating. The blood flow in the skin heated at 43.5°C or 44°C increased more than 12-fold in 30 min and then began to decline. At 45°C, the skin blood flow had increased about 14-fold at 15 min and then decreased. An important feature that should be pointed out is the marked difference between the effects of heating at 43.0°C and 43.5°C: the skin blood flow steadily increased to 6 times the original value during heating at 43.0°C for 120 min, while it increased to as much as 12 times the original value at 30 min and then declined when the heating temperature was raised by merely 0.5°C to 43.5°C.

The blood flow in the muscle of SD rats before heating was 4.61 ml/100 g/min. Upon heating at 42°C, 43°C, or 43.5°C for 120 min, the muscle blood flow slowly increased by 3–5 times. When heated at 44°C, the muscle blood flow increased sixfold during the first 30 min and remained at the same level thereafter. At 45°C, the muscle blood flow increased about ninefold in 30 min and then declined to almost the original level at the end of 120 min of heating. The results shown in Figs. 7.2 and 7.3 demonstrate that the higher the temperature applied to the skin or muscle, the faster

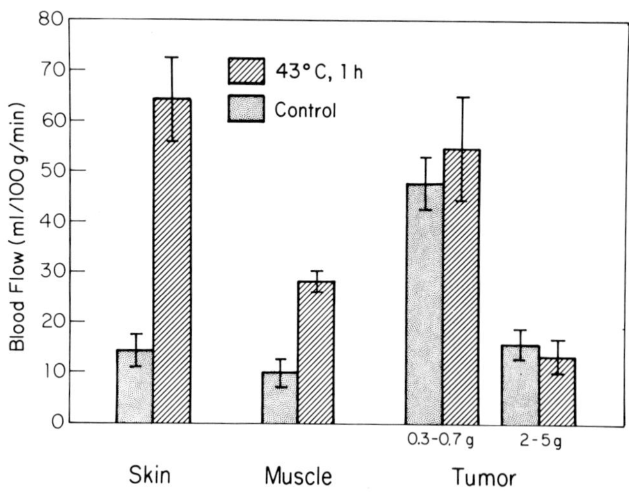

Fig. 7.1. Effects of heating at 43°C for 1 h on the blood flow in Walker tumors of different sizes and in the skin and muscle adjacent to the tumors in SD rats

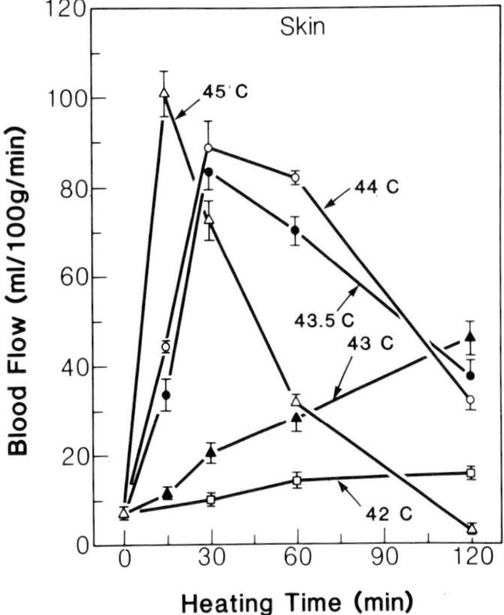

Fig. 7.2. Blood flow in the skin of SD rats measured at the end of heating for varying lengths of time at different temperatures

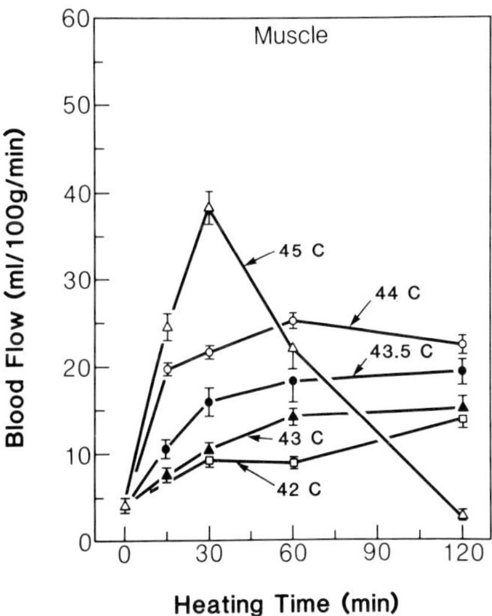

Fig. 7.3. Blood flow in the muscle of SD rats measured at the end of heating for varying lengths of time at different temperatures

and greater the increase in blood flow. When the temperature is raised above the critical temperature, the blood flow increases only briefly and declines during heating. In another investigation (RAPPAPORT and SONG 1983), we observed that the blood flow values in the skin and muscle adjacent to the mammary adenocarcinoma 13762A grown subcutaneously in the leg of Fischer F344 rats were about twofold greater than those in the normal skin and muscle. The blood flow increased by about 7.5-fold in the skin and 3.4-fold in the muscle adjacent to the tumors when heated at 43.5°C for 1 h (Fig. 7.4). These results of our own studies are in good agreement with the reports by other investigators. DICKSON and CALDERWOOD (1980) reported that the blood flow in the skin and residual tissues in the foot of Wister rats increased by as much as 20 times and 10 times, respectively, upon heating at 42°C for 1 h. Somewhat smaller increases in the blood flow in the skin or muscle of rats have been reported by SHRIVASTAV et al. (1983) and VAUPEL (1990).

The heat-induced changes in blood flow in the skin and muscle of mice have also been extensively investigated by us. Heating the legs of C3H mice for 1 h caused temperature-dependent changes in the blood flow, as measured with the ^{86}Rb uptake method, in the skin and muscle of the legs (SONG et al. 1987a). At 44.5°C, the skin blood flow had increased by about 2 times at 30 min, but declined to almost the original value at the end of 1 h heating, and then further decreased after heating. Upon heating at 43.5°C for 1 h, the skin blood flow increased by 5 times and then slowly declined after heating. The blood flow in the skin heated at 41.5°C or 42.5°C increased during the 1 h of heating and the increase continued even after heating. The blood flow in the mouse muscle

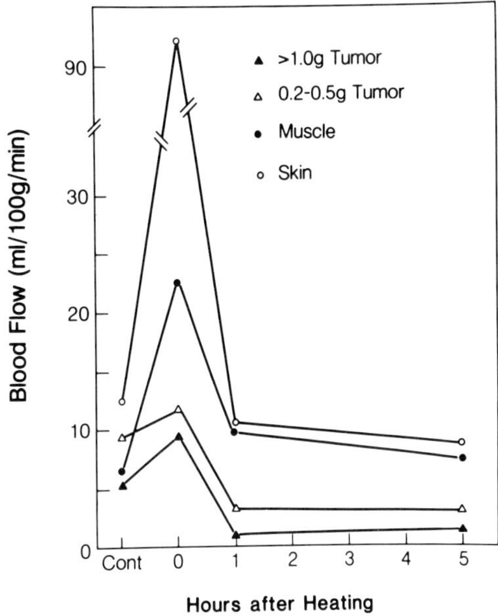

Fig. 7.4. Blood flow in 13762A mammary adenocarcinomas of Fischer rats at 0–5 h after heating at 43.5°C for 1 h

heated at 44.5°C for 1 h had increased by about 4 times at 30 min and then began to decline. During the 1 h of heating at 43.5°C, the muscle blood flow increased by more than 5 times and slowly declined after the heating. The blood flow increased by 2–3 times in the muscle during heating for 1 h at 41.5°C or 42.5°C and slowly declined after the heating. STEWART and BEGG (1983) also observed that the ^{86}Rb uptake in mouse skin increased about threefold upon heating at 42.5°C for 1 h and remained elevated for 24 h after heating. Using the newly developed laser Doppler flow (LDF) method, we continuously and noninvasively monitored the red cell flow in the mouse skin during heating (SONG et al. 1987b). The LDF in the skin of C3H mice increased upon heating, which was very similar to the increase in the ^{86}Rb uptake. MILLIGAN (1987) reported that the blood flow in the muslce of dogs was 7.5 ml/100 g/min, and it increased about fivefold in 20 min as a result of heating at 45°C. Although the muscle blood flow then began to decline after the peak increase, it was still threefold the original value at the end of 40 min of heating. DUDAR and JAIN (1984) studied the function of blood vessels in the granulation tissue formed in transplantable chambers of rabbit ear. The blood flow increased up to sevenfold compared with the control value upon heating at 45.7°C for 1 h, but it declined when the heating was continued longer than 1 h or the heating temperature was raised to 47°C.

The pathophysiological changes in human skin induced by heat have been extensively studied. Since the skin is the outermost tissue of the human body and its function is vital, it is not surprising that the thermal effect on skin has attracted such a high degree of attention. In the early studies, the blood flow in the human skin was estimated indirectly from other physiological parameters investigated using various methods and devices (ALLWOOD and BURRY 1954; BARCROFT and EDHOLM 1943; NAGASAKA et al. 1987). We have used the LDF method to reveal the effect of heat on the blood flow in human skin (SONG et al. 1989a, 1990a). The human forearm skin surface temperature before heating was about 32°C. Upon heating at 40°–43°C, the LDF abruptly increased several fold, declined for several minutes, and then gradually rose during the next 15–20 min, reaching 10–15 times the original value. The LDF then stayed elevated until the 1 h heating was terminated. When the heating was stopped, the LDF began to decline, but bounced back and then rapidly returned to the preheating level (Fig. 7.5). The relationship between the maximum increases in LDF and temperatures is shown in Fig. 7.6. The LDF gradually increased when the skin temperature was increased from 32°C to 37°C and then sharply increased with the further increase in the temperature. The LDF increased as much as 15-fold as a result of heating at 43°C for 30 min. An analysis of LDF signals indicated that the increase in LDF in the heated human skin was due to an increase in both the blood cell number and the velocity of the blood cells. The increase in the blood cell number indicated that heating caused dilation of arterioles and recruitment of capillaries. The increase in the blood cell velocity implied opening of arteriovenous anastomoses.

7.2.2 Liver

In heating deep-seated tumors, the adjacent normal tissue is inevitably also heated. Thus, the heat-induced changes in the blood flow of the internal organs have attracted the attention of investigators. HUGANDER et al. (1983) reported that the blood flow in the rat liver, as measured with the ^{133}Xe clearance method, decreased during

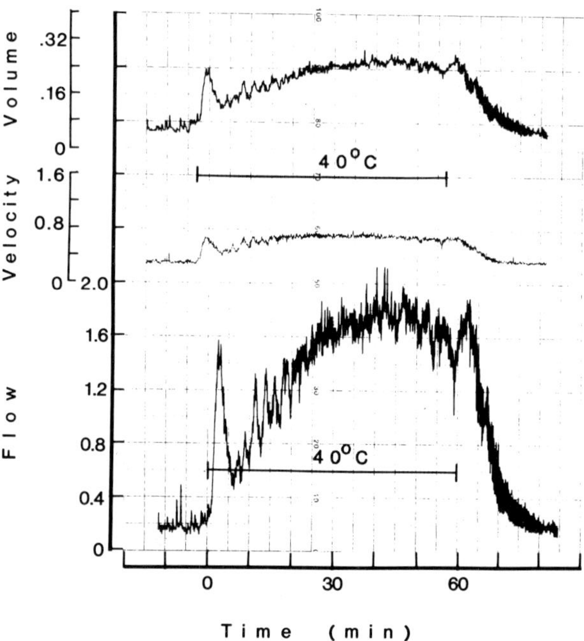

Fig. 7.5. Effect of heating on the laser Doppler flowmetric tracing of the RBC flux (blood flow), the velocity of RBCs, and the volume (number) of RBCs in human forearm skin during heating at 40°C

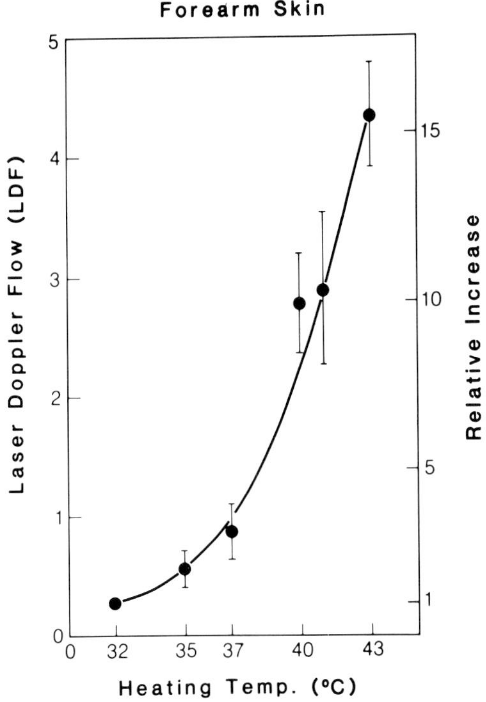

Fig. 7.6. Relative increase in LDF in human forearm skin as a function of heating temperature

1 h of heating at 42°C, but returned to the original level within 30 min after heating. The blood flow in rabbit liver, as measured with the hydrogen clearance method, decreased to 80% of the control value 2 h after heating at 42.5°C or 43°C for 20 min, but eventually recovered to its original value (MATSUDA 1989). In the rabbit liver, 50% of the arterioles were found to be damaged 24 h after local heating with RF current at 44°–45°C, while 50% of the central and portal veins were found to be damaged after heating at 41.5°–42.5°C and 42.5°–43.5°C. respectively (NISHIMURA et al. 1989).

We studied the heat-induced changes in blood flow in the rat liver using the radioactive microsphere method, which enabled us to separately determine the portal venous blood flow and hepatic arterial blood flow (NAKAJIMA et al. 1990, 1992; UDA et al. 1990). The rats were anesthetized and the liver region was placed in supine position on a lower electrode 5 cm in diameter, and an upper electrode of the same diameter was coupled over the liver region (NAKAJIMA et al. 1990). The liver was capacitively heated by applying 8 MHz RF current to the electrodes. Heating at 41°C and 43°C, as measured by thermocouples placed around the liver, slightly decreased the portal venous blood flow and slightly increased the hepatic arterial blood flow. The change in total liver blood flow paralleled the change in portal venous blood flow. This was due to the fact that the portal venous blood flow accounts for almost 85% of the total liver blood flow. The decline in the portal venous flow appeared to result, at least in part, from a significant decline in the cardiac output as a result of heating the entire liver region. When a small portion of the liver, about a 1-cm-diameter circular area in the lateral lobe, was heated at 39°C or 41°C, the arterial blood flow in the heated area and in the rest of the lobe, as well as in the whole liver, initially increased during the first 30 min of heating and then declined (UDA et al. 1990). Upon heating at 43°C, the arterial blood flow in both the heated area and the whole liver slightly increased for 15 min and then significantly decreased thereafter. The increase in blood flow in the unheated liver tissue was apparently due to a rise in temperature through the blood circulation as well as heat conduction. The area heated at 43°C for 30 min showed wedge-shaped infarctions, which changed to organized scar tissue 7 days after heating.

7.2.3 Lung

We investigated the heat-induced changes in blood flow in the Fischer rat lung. The heating was done with the capacitive heating device used for heating the liver, as described above. A small incision was made on both lateral chest walls along the midaxillary line. A thermocouple was inserted through the incision and attached with chemical glue to the parietal pleural membrane. The intraluminal temperatures of the thoracic segment of the esophagus and trachea, as well as the temperatures of other adjacent organs, were also monitored during heating. The dorsal and ventral sides of the right lung of rats in the supine position were coupled with 5-cm-diameter electrodes and 4-cm-diameter electrodes, respectively. During the heating of the lung, breathing was aided with a respirator and 20°C water was circulated through the vinyl bolus bags placed under the electrode. The blood flow in the unheated control lung was 0.53 ± 0.05 ml/1 g/min and it remained unchanged when the lung was heated at 41°C for 15–30 min. The lung blood flow increased about twofold when heated at 43°C for 15 min, but it decreased to slightly less than the original value at 30 min. Upon heating at 44°C, the lung blood flow markedly declined within 15 min. The blood flow in the unheated left lung slightly increased when the right lung was heated at 43°C. It appeared that the left lung was also heated when the right lung was heated, probably due to an exchange of air between the lungs and also to direct heat conduction from the heated right lung area to the unheated left lung area. The blood flow in the esophagus and trachea did not significantly change when the right lung was heated at 41°–44°C.

7.2.4 *Stomach*

We investigated the heat-induced changes in blood flow in the stomach of Fischer rats. The gastric temperature was measured by inserting a catheter into the stomach through the esophagus and placing a three-junction thermocouple inside the catheter. In addition, the temperatures on the ventral and dorsal surfaces of the stomach were monitored with three-junction thermocouples inserted through an incision made on the ventral site about 2 cm distal to the left midcoastal margin. The stomach was capacitively heated with the same heating devices as were used for the heating of the liver and lung, as described above. Before heating, the stomach blood flow, as measured with the radioactive microsphere method, was 0.94 ± 0.05 ml/min/g. Upon heating, the intraluminal temperature, which we used as the heating temperature, was 0.5°–1.0°C higher than the temperature of the stomach surface. When the stomach temperature was raised to 42°C, the stomach blood flow continuously increased for 30 min, reaching about 1.6 times the control value, but it declined to almost the original level at the end of 45 min of heating. At 43°C, the stomach blood flow increased about 3 times in 30 min and then declined to about twofold the original value at the end of 45 min of heating. The stomach blood flow slightly increased upon heating for 15 min at 44°C and then declined to about two-thirds of the original level. It was interesting that the esophageal blood flow decreased by almost 50% when the stomach was heated for 45 min at 43°C or for 15 min at 44°C.

7.2.5 *Small Intestine*

The effect of hyperthermia on the blood flow in the small intestine of C3H mice was studied by Peck and Gibbs (1983). Using two catgut sutures 15 mm apart, these investigators apposed approximately 15 mm of the jejunum 3–5 cm distal to the Trietz ligament to the peritoneal surface of the abdominal muscle at the midline. Two weeks later, the jejunum was heated by pulling the skin and muscle with the attached jejunum between two thermally conductive metal plates immersed in a preheated water bath. The intestinal blood flow was estimated from the washout rate of ^{133}Xe injected into the intestinal lumen. The ^{133}Xe washout rate remained unchanged when measured after heating at 44°C for 20 min, but it dropped by one-half within 46 min.

Contrary to the aforementioned results, we observed a significant increase in blood flow in the heated intestine of mice. In our study, a 1.5- to 2.0-cm-long midline incision was made in the abdominal wall of Fischer rats, and approximately 50% of the small intestine, 15 cm distal to the Trietz ligament and 20 cm proximal to the ileocecal junction, was exteriorized through the incision. The exteriorized intestine was then submersed into a glass jar containing Krebs-Ringer solution and maintained at the desired temperatures. Before heating, the blood flow in the intestine was 2.70 ml/min/g. Upon heating at 42°C or 43°C, the intestinal blood flow increased about 3.3 times and 4.0 times, respectively, in 30 min and then began to decrease. Upon heating at 44°C, the intestinal blood flow increased about 4.5-fold in 15 min and then fell to 2.5 times the original value at 30 min. During the heating of the small intestine, the blood flow in the adjacent tissues, such as the spleen, pancreas, and stomach, tended to decrease, whereas the renal and hepatic arterial blood flow remained unchanged. The cardiac output was found to decrease markedly when the intestine was heated. It was apparent that the decrease in the cardiac output should be taken into account when interpreting the changes in blood flow in the heated intestine as well as in other organs.

7.3 Hyperthermia-Induced Vascular Changes in Tumors

7.3.1 *Experimental Animal Tumors*

Realizing that hyperthermia is a potentially powerful modality for the control of human tumors and that blood flow plays a cardinal role in hyperthermic tissue damage, a number of investigators have studied the effects of heating on blood flow in tumors during the past decade. Probably more than 50 different types of tumors have been investigated thus far for the thermal effect on tumor blood flow. Tumors of different origins and tumors grown in different sites, such as in the foot, leg, or flank of mice and rats, the liver of rabbits, and the cheek pouch of hamsters, have been used. Transplantable dog tumors and tumors grown in transparent chambers have also been used. Diverse heating methods or devices, such as water bath, microwave, RF, and ultrasound, have been used. Similarly, various methods have been used to measure the tumor blood flow, i.e., ^{86}Rb uptake, ^{133}Xe clearance, isotope-labeled microspheres, thermal clearance, H_2 clearance, ^{85}Kr clearance, LDF and electronic tracing of red cell flow in capillaries in transparent chambers.

The study by SCHEID in 1961 was perhaps the first study on the effect of heat on tumor blood flow who observed severe vascular stasis in the S2 sarcoma of mice heated at 42°C for 30 min. More importantly, this investigator also observed that the vascular damage in the tumor was greater than that in the supporting mesenterium. SUTTON (1976) then reported that blood flow in the ependymoblastoma of mice increased slightly during the first 30 min of heating at 40°C, but it declined when the heating was continued. In 1978, JOHNSON (1978) reported that heating the subcutaneous adenocarcinoma of mice at 41°C initially induced a small increase in blood flow, which soon decreased markedly. REINHOLD et al. (1978) also reported that, upon heating at 42.5°C, the blood flow in the rat rhabdomyosarcoma BA1112 grown in a transparent chamber briefly increased, albeit slightly, and then decreased. In 1980, EDDY (1980) observed that 42°–43°C heating of a cervical carcinoma grown in the transparent cheek pouch chamber of Syrian hamsters induced vascular stasis, petechiae, thrombosis, endothelial degeneration, and hyperemia. VAUPEL et al. (1980) reported in 1980 that the blood flow in DS carcinoma implanted into the kidney of rats increased when the tumor temperature was raised from 37°C to 39.5°C, but decreased to a level somewhat below the initial flow rate when the tumor temperature was raised to 42°C. A feature common to all the aforementioned early investigations is that the tumor vascular beds were unable to endure heating at 41°–43°C. However, a somewhat different observation was made by us in 1978. No significant vascular change occurred in the Walker carcinoma of SD rats heated at temperatures as high as 43°C, while a marked increase in blood flow in the skin and muscle occurred at the same temperature, as discussed in the previous section. When the Walker tumors were heated at 45°C, the blood flow decreased after heating, but not during heating (SONG et al. 1980a). This observation was in agreement with the report by GULLINO (1980), who observed that the vascular beds in the Walker carcinoma were resistant to heating. However, subsequent studies by us as well as other investigators using divergent rodent tumor models and methods indicated that the Walker tumor may be an exceptionally heat-resistant rodent tumor.

When the mammary adenocarcinoma 13762A grown subcutaneously in the leg of Fischer 344 rats was heated at 43.5°C for 1 h with a water bath, the tumor blood flow increased by 1.5–2.0 times, but it rapidly decreased to a negligible level after heating (Fig. 7.4) (RAPPAPORT and SONG 1983). Histological examination demonstrated widespread and diffuse hemorrhage, vasodilation, and hyperemia. Figure 7.7 shows the effect of heat on the blood flow, as measured with the ^{86}Rb uptake method, in RIF-1 tumors grown subcutaneously in the leg of C3H mice (SONG et al. 1987a). Heating at 41.5°C or 42.5°C for 1 h caused almost no change in blood flow either during or after the heating. The blood flow continuously increased during 1 h of heating at 43.5°C, reaching about 1.8-fold the original value, and then decreased during 3 h following heating. Upon heating at 44.5°C, the blood flow increased slightly at first but then began to decrease, reaching about one-third the original value at the end of 1 h of heating. Note that the earliest time when the blood flow was measured during the 44.5°C heating was 15 min, and it is possible that a peak increase in blood flow may have occurred prior to the determination at 15 min.

The heat-induced change in blood flow in SCK mammary carcinoma of A/J mice (Fig. 7.8) (SONG et al. 1989b) was slightly different from that in RIF-1 tumors. Whereas the blood flow in RIF-1 tumors remained unchanged during and after heating at 42.5°C for 1 h, the blood flow in the SCK tumor increased during 1 h of heating at 42.5°C and decreased after the heating. Note that the pattern of blood flow change in SCK tumors heated at 42.5°C for 1 h (Fig. 7.8) was similar to that in the RIF-1 tumors heated at 43.5°C for 1 h (Fig. 7.12). When the SCK tumors were heated at 43.5°C for 1 h, there was an initial increase in

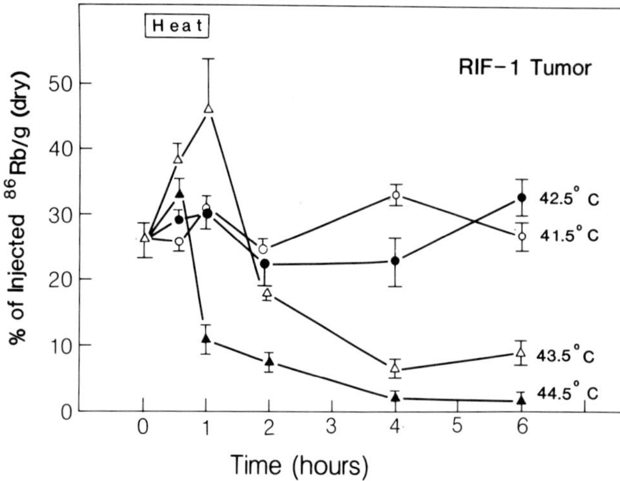

Fig. 7.7. ^{86}Rb uptake in RIF-1 tumors during and after heating at different temperatures for 1 h

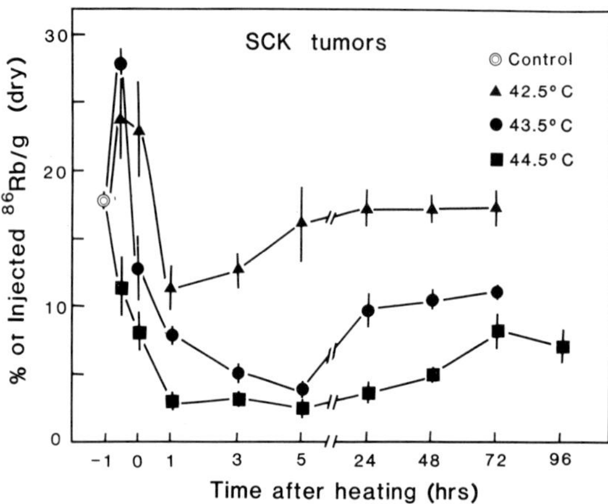

Fig. 7.8. ^{86}Rb uptake in SCK tumors during and after heating a different temperatures for 1 h

blood flow during the first 30 min, followed by a decrease which continued for several hours after heating. The SCK tumor blood flow began to decline immediately upon heating at 44.5°C. It is not surprising that the magnitude and length of decline in tumor blood flow after heating were dependent on the temperature applied. The changes in blood flow in SCK tumors during continuous heating at different temperatures were studied (LIN and SONG 1993). At 41.5°C, the blood flow remained unchanged for as long as 3 h; it then began to decrease, and almost completely stopped after heating for 7 h. At 42.5°C, the blood flow increased about 1.3-fold in 30 min, began to decline from 1 h, and stopped after 3 h of heating. A slightly greater increase in blood flow occurred when the tumors were heated at 43.5°C rather than at 42.5°C, but the blood flow began to decline sooner at 43.5°C than at 42.5°C. At 43.5°C, the blood flow slightly increased initially and then began to decline from 30 min, while at 44.5°C and 45.5°C, the blood flow rapidly declined without any increase.

As mentioned above, there have been numerous studies on heat-induced changes in blood flow using divergent experimental tumors. These studies have shown unequivocally that the tumor vascular beds are vulnerable to heat. This was also observed by us in RIF-1 tumors in C3H mice (Fig. 7.7), SCK tumors in A/J mice (Fig. 7.8), and 13762A tumors in Fischer rats (Fig. 7.4), although the temperature and length of heating for the induction of vascular damage varied somewhat depending on many factors, including the tumor type. In some tumors, the blood flow decreased when heated at temperatures as low as 41°C for 30–60 min, whereas in other types of tumors heating at 42°–43°C for 30–60 min was needed to induce a considerable decline in tumor blood flow. Obviously, the temperature and the length of heating required to induce the vascular changes were interrelated. For the same temperature, e.g., 43°C, the length of heating needed to induce a decrease in blood flow varied depending on tumor type. Likewise, for the same length of heating, the temperature at which the vascular damage was induced varied depending on the tumor type. As shown in Fig. 7.7, the blood flow in RIF-1 tumors continuously increased during 1 h of heating at 43.5°C, reaching about twice the original value and declining when the heating was terminated, while that in the SCK tumors began to decrease after heating for only 30 min at 43.5°C, as shown in Fig. 7.8. In many rodent tumors, the blood flow begins to decline almost immediately upon heating at temperatures higher than 44°C. A slight and temporary increase in blood flow prior to a rapid decline upon heating at such high temperatures may or may not be seen depending on the tumor type and the method of blood flow measurement employed. One of the important factors in the heat-induced vascular damage in tumors is the rate of tumor growth. HILL et al. (1989) reported that higher temperatures may be needed to cause a vascular shutdown in slowly growing tumors than in rapidly growing tumors, probably because rapid vascular expansion in the rapidly growing tumors resulted in a fragile and thermosensitive capillary network. Even in the slowly growing mouse tumors, however, complete vascular shutdown occurred upon heating at 43°C for 1 h. The possible relationship between the vascular structure and vascular thermosensitivity was investigated by NISHIMURA et al. (1988). In mouse tumors, the vasculature supported by perivascular connective tissue bands and/or dense endothelial cells was more heat resistant than that supported by only sparse endothelial cells.

7.3.2 *Human Tumors*

Xenografts of human tumors in immunosuppressed rodents have been used to study the heat-induced vascular changes in human tumors by VAUPEL and his colleagues (1988a) and VAN DEN BERG-BLOK and REINHOLD (1987). The thermal response of the vessels in the human tumor xenografts was similar to that in rodent tumors. It should be emphasized, however, that the vascular changes which occur in heated human tumor xenografts may not represent the vascular changes in heated human tumors since the vasculature in the xenografts does not originate from the xenografted cells but from the host tissues.

Attempts have been made to reveal the heat-induced vascular changes in human tumors in situ. SUGAAR and LEVEEN (1979) examined histopathological changes in human tumors after hyperthermic treatment and observed thrombosis and obliteration of blood vessels in part of the tumors. LYNG et al. (1991) investigated the relationship among vascular function, tissue temperature attained, and histopathological damage in locally advanced breast carcinoma and surrounding normal tissues of humans. The biopsies taken before the first heat treatment and those taken shortly after the last heat treatment were considerably different, reflecting a marked effect of the therapy. The tumor tissue vessels were apparently more sensitive to heat than the normal tissue vessels (Fig. 7.9) and the tumor vasculature was more sensitive to heat than the tumor tissue. The blood flow in human tumors during heating was measured by OLCH et al. (1983) with the ^{133}Xe clearance method. Out of 12 tumors studied, eight showed an appreciable increase in blood flow during heating. In this study, the temperature of the tumors could be raised to 42°C in only six of the 12 cases. The authors attributed the failure to heat the tumors to an increase in tumor blood flow.

WATERMAN et al. (1986) used the thermal clearance method to determine the blood flow in 15 superficial human tumors during heating with 915-MHz microwaves. The mean blood flow rates in the human tumors studied ranged between 0 and 34 ml/100 g/min, with an average value of 15 ml/100 g/min. The mean blood flow rate increased by 10%–15% at between 15 and 30 min and remained nearly constant thereafter until the end of 60 min of heating. The blood flow, however, did not always increase and a reduction in blood flow was observed in one tumor when the temperature reached above 44°C. The response of tumor blood flow was independent of temperature in the range of 40°–44°C and no evidence of

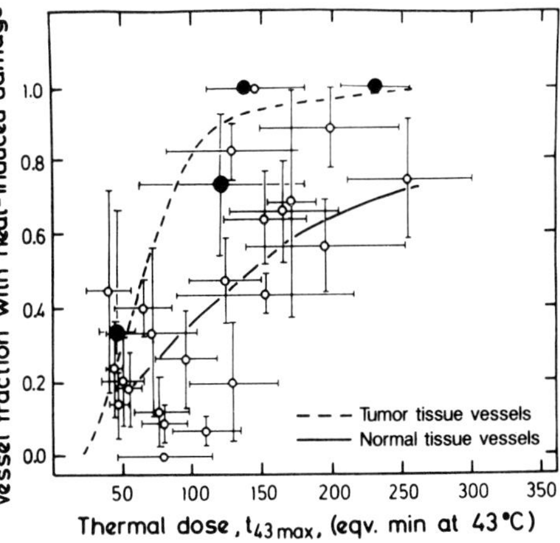

Fig. 7.9. The fraction of damaged tumor tissues vessels (●) and the fraction of damaged normal tissue vessels (○) versus the largest thermal dose achieved in one heat fraction (LYNG et al. 1991)

a sharp reduction in flow was observed. This observation is in apparent contrast to the observations made in numerous animal tumors in which the vascular changes are temperature dependent, at least in the same type of tumor, and the blood flow starts to decline during or after heating at 42°–44°C. It must be pointed out that in the study by WATERMAN and his colleagues (1986) only 40 thermal washout measurements were made in 15 tumors, i.e., fewer than three measurements per tumor. Perhaps the numbers of measurements for each tumor were too small to observe real vascular changes during heating.

Using a newly developed LDF probe, ACKER et al. (1990) monitored the blood flow in human tumors during hyperthermia treatments in combination with radiotherapy. Blood flow differences within individual tumors were found to be as large as 55-fold, and there was a greater than 100-fold difference between different tumor types. There were four general patterns of vascular changes in the tumor during heating: (a) an initial increase was followed by a plateau in 27% of the tumors; (b) no change occurred during heating in 36% of the tumors; (c) an abrupt or a steady decline occurred in 23% of the tumors; and (d) an initial increase was followed by a drop in 14% of the tumors. The magnitude of the increase in LDF or blood flow was in the range of 25%–250%, which was in general agreement with the results from the animal model studies performed by other investigators.

The observations on heat-induced changes in blood flow in human tumors described above suggest that the vascular beds in human tumors might be heat-resistant as compared to those in rodent tumors. The vascular beds in human tumors may be more mature than those in rodent tumors, and thus they may be heat-resistant relative to the rodent tumor vascular beds. It is possible, however, that the small changes in blood flow or vascular damage caused by hyperthermia in human tumors were due in part to inadequate heating. It is a wellknown fact that achieving a therapeutic temperature throughout the entire tumor volume in human tumors, particularly bulky and deep-seated tumors, is rather difficult with the currently available heating devices. It may be concluded that the data on heat-induced blood flow in human tumors are still too scarce to draw any definite conclusion and further studies with better heating methods and blood flow measurement methods are needed.

7.3.3 Mechanisms of Hyperthermia-Induced Vascular Changes in Tumors

The different effects of heat on the vasculature and blood flow in tumors and normal tissues may be attributed to the intrinsic nature of vascular structures in malignant tumors. The newly formed tumor vasculature, composed of single-layered endothelium, is usually devoid of basement membrane and neural junction. In rapidly growing tumors or rapidly growing parts in individual tumors, the capillary-like vessels are often made of a mixture of tumor cells and endothelial cells. It is natural that such immature tumor vessels are damaged and lose their functional integrity as a result of a thermal dose which is innocuous to the mature normal tissue vessels. It is well known that the tumor vessels are leaky (SONG 1978), probably because of the immature structure. When the components of the vessel wall, such as endothelial cells, and tumors undergo configurational changes, the gap between the cells may widen, the vessels become more leaky, and the circulatory blood extravasate, resulting in vascular stasis. An increase in the adhesion of lymphocytes and platelets to endothelial cells, thrombosis, and hardening of red blood cells have also been suggested to cause a decline in tumor blood flow during and after heating. A detailed discussion on the mechanism of induction of vascular changes by hyperthermia is beyond the scope of this chapter, and it is suggested that readers refer to other reviews on this subject (JAIN and WARD-HARTLEY 1984; REINHOLD and ENDRICH 1986; SONG 1984, 1991; VAUPEL 1990).

7.4 Effects of Multiple Heatings on Blood Flow

In clinical hyperthermia, tumors are usually treated with multiple heatings. Therefore, we investigated the response of blood vessels in tumors and normal tissues to repeated heatings (LOKSHINA et al. 1985; LIN and SONG 1993; NAKAJIMA et al. 1992; SONG 1991; SONG et al. 1987a, 1989a, 1990b). As shown in Fig. 7.10, the ^{86}Rb uptake or blood flow in RIF-1 tumors of C3H mice increased during 1 h of heating at 43.5°C, but declined to an almost negligible level after heating (SONG et al. 1990). The blood flow 24 h after heating at 42.5°C was slightly less than that in the unheated control tumors, and the magnitude of the increase in blood flow during

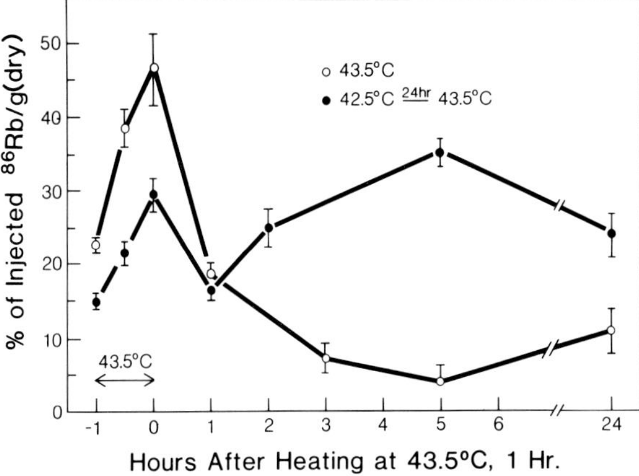

Fig. 7.10. Changes in ^{86}Rb uptake RIF-1 tumors as a function of time after 1 h of heating at 43.5°C. The tumors were heated only once at 43.5°C for 1 h (○) or preheated at 42.5°C for 1 h and then reheated 24 h later at 43.5°C for 1 h (●)

reheating at 43.5°C was significantly less than that induced by 43.5° heating without preheating. Moreover, the blood flow 5 h after the reheating was more than twice the control value while that at 5 h after a single heating at the same temperature, i.e., 43.5°C, was less than one-third of the control value. These results demonstrated that preheating at 42.5°C for 1 h rendered the tumor vessels resistant to reheating applied 24 h later indicating thermotolerance developed in the blood vessels.

To further delineate the kinetics of vascular thermotolerance, we preheated the RIF-1 tumors at 42.5°C and reheated them at different times thereafter at 43.5°C or 44.5°C for 1 h. The blood flow was measured 5 h after the reheating since that is the time the vascular damage in RIF-1 tumors is fully manifested. Figure 7.11 shows that when the tumors were preheated at 42.5°C for 1 h and then immediately reheated at 43.5°C or 44.5°C for 1 h, the blood flow measured 5 h after the reheating was negligible, indicating that the tumor vasculature was severely damaged by the two heatings applied. However, when the time interval between the preheating and the reheating was increased, the reheating increased the tumor blood flow. The maximum increase in blood flow due to the reheating was observed when the preheating and reheating were separated by 36 h. Thus, it was concluded that the vascular thermotolerance in RIF-1 tumors as a consequence of preheating at 42.5°C for 1 h peaked 36 h after the preheating and decayed thereafter. The vascular thermotolerance appeared to have decayed completely 96 h after preheating at 42.5°C.

The development of vascular thermotolerance in SCK tumors of A/J mice was also elucidated by preheating the tumors for 1 h at 41.5°C, 42.5°C, or 43.5°C and then reheating (test-heating) the tumors at 43.5°C for 1 h at different times after the preheating (LIN and SONG 1993). Figure 7.12 shows that preheating at 41.5°C or 42.5°C induced vascular thermotolerance, which peaked at 5 h and 18 h, respectively, after the preheating. The vascular thermotolerance gradually decayed over the following 2–3 days. The vascular thermotolerance which appeared 48 h after preheating at 43.5°C was rather small. Severe vascular damage induced by the 43.5°C preheating may be incriminated in the failure to develop significant vascular thermotolerance. It should be noted that the rate of development of vascular thermotolerance after preheating at 42.5°C in the SCK tumors was slower than that after preheating at 41.5°C, while the magnitude of the vascular thermotolerance induced by 42.5°C preheating

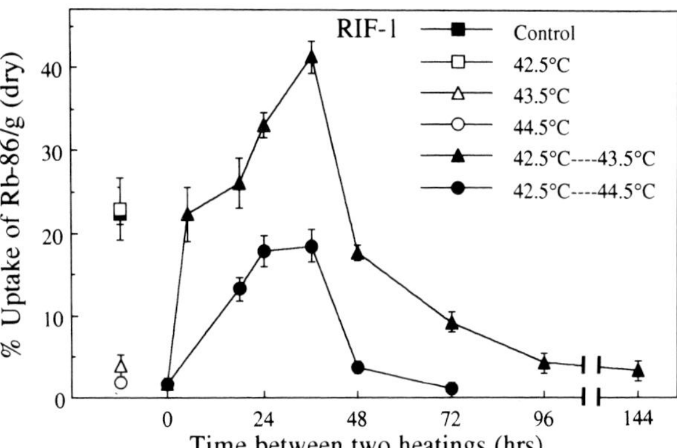

Fig. 7.11. Kinetics of vascular thermotolerance in RIF-1 tumors. Tumors were preheated at 42.5°C for 1 h and then reheated 0–144 h later at 43.5°C or 44.5°C for 1 h

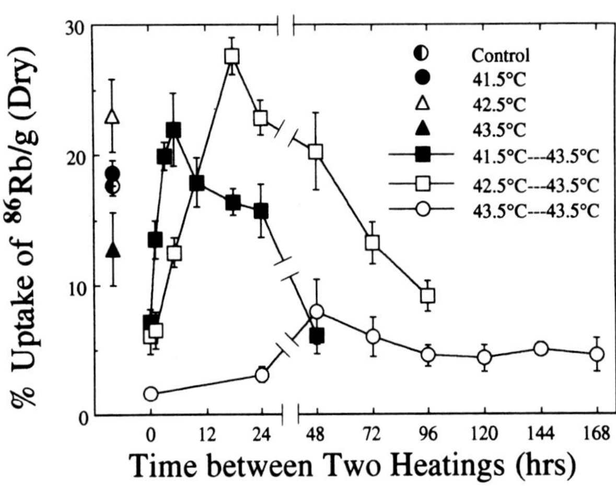

Fig. 7.12. Kinetics of vascular thermotolerance in SCK tumors. The tumors were preheated at 41.5°C, 42.5°C, or 43.5°C for 1 h and reheated 0–168 h later at 43.5°C for 1 h. The ^{86}Rb uptake was measured at the end of reheating

was greater than that induced by 41.5°C preheating. These phenomena are in agreement with the observation in other biological systems that the magnitude of thermotolerance and the time required to reach peak tolerance increase with an increase in heat dose. As expected, the rate of development of vascular thermotolerance was tumor type dependent. As shown in Fig. 7.11, the peak vascular thermotolerance after preheating at 42.5°C appeared at 36 h in RIF-1 tumors whereas it appeared at 18 h in SCK tumors, as mentioned above. Figure 7.13 shows that when SCK tumors were continuously heated at 42.5°C without preheating, the ^{86}Rb uptake slightly increased during the first hour and then rapidly declined. On the other hand, reheating was rather ineffective in reducing the ^{86}Rb uptake in preheated tumors. The ^{86}Rb uptake declined by 50% in 2.5 h when the tumors were heated at 42.5°C for the first time, but such a reduction required 7 h when the tumors were heated for the second time. The rate of decrease in ^{86}Rb uptake caused by reheating at 42.5°C, shown in Fig. 7.13, was slower than that caused by heating at 41.5°C without preheating, as described above.

The implication of vascular thermotolerance in the changes in blood flow that are induced by multiple heatings in RIF-1 tumors is evident from Fig. 7.14 (Song et al. 1987a). The blood flow was measured after one to five repeated heatings at 43.5°C for 1 h each, separated by 1–3 days. The blood flow in the RIF-1 tumors increased by about twofold upon heating at 43.5°C for 1 h and decreased 1 day or 3 days later. The second heating, applied 1 or 3 days after the first heating, neither increased nor decreased the blood flow. Likewise, the blood flow was changed little by the third, fourth, and fifth heatings applied at 1- or 3-day intervals. Such a lack of change in the blood flow as a result of the second to fifth heatings was

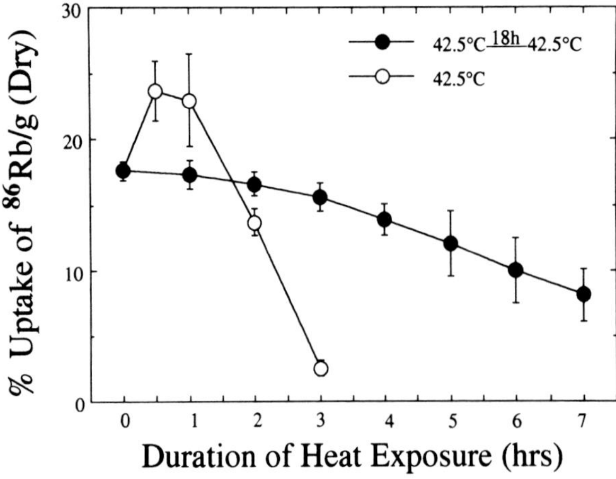

Fig. 7.13. Effects of heating at 42.5°C for varying lengths of time on ^{86}Rb uptake with or without preheating for 1 h at 42.5°C in SCK tumors. The reheating was carried out 18 h after the preheating

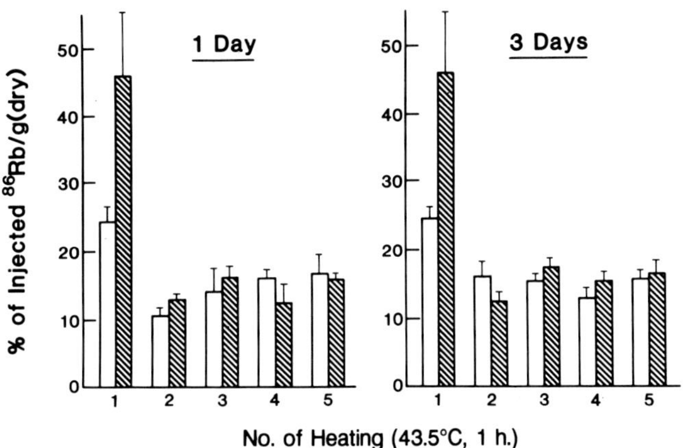

Fig. 7.14. Effects of multiple heatings on the ^{86}Rb uptake in RIF-1 tumors. The tumors were heated one to five times at 43.5°C for 1 h each, with 1-day or 3-day intervals between the heatings. The ^{86}Rb uptake was measured immediately before (*open bars*) and at the end (*shaded bars*) of each heating

apparently due to the development of vascular thermotolerance.

A series of investigations conducted in our laboratory have revealed that the development of vascular thermotolerance is not unique to tumors, but also occurs in normal tissues, as shown in Fig. 7.15 (SONG et al. 1987a). The blood flow in the leg skin of C3H mice was increased by a factor of about 5 by the first heating at 43.5°C for 1 h and returned to slightly higher than the original value 1 day later. The second heating, applied 1 day after the first, caused little change in the blood flow, which, however, was found to be slightly increased on the third day. The third, fourth, and fifth heatings applied at 1-day intervals caused virtually no change in the blood flow. There was a twofold increase in the blood flow 3 days after the first heating at 43.5°C for 1 h. The second to fifth heatings applied at 3-day intervals were slightly more effective in increasing the blood flow than those applied at 1-day intervals, implying that the vascular thermotolerance may decay slightly within 3 days in the skin. Essentially the same results were obtained in the leg muscle of C3H mice. We also demonstrated the development of vascular thermotolerance in the skin and muscle of rat (LOKSHINA et al. 1985). The second heating at 43.5°C for 1 h, applied 1–3 days after the first heating at the same temperature, was less effective than the first heating in increasing blood flow, as measured with radioactive microspheres. The vascular thermotolerance in the skin or muscle of rat appeared to decay in 3–4 days since repeated heating at 5-day intervals was more or less as effective as a single heating in increasing the blood flow. Other investigators have reported that when the second heating was applied several hours to several days after the first heating, it was less effective than the first heating in causing vascular damage in tumors (EDDY and

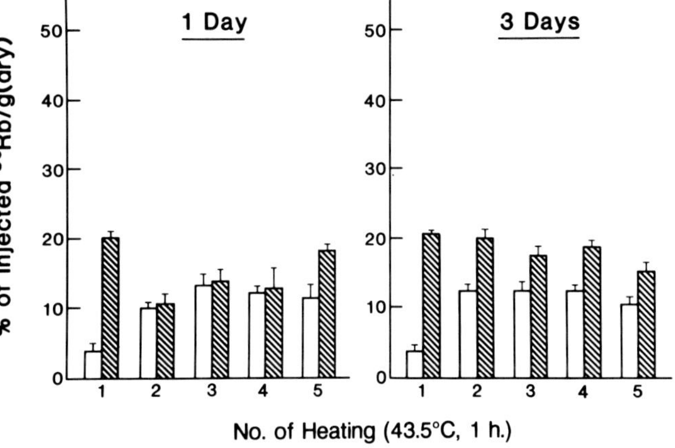

Fig. 7.15. Effects of multiple heatings on the ^{86}Rb uptake in the leg skin of C3H mice. The legs were heated one to five times at 43.5°C for 1 h for each heating with 1-day or 3-day intervals between the heatings. The ^{86}Rb uptake was measured immediately before (*open bars*) and at the end (*shaded bars*) of each heating

Chmielewski 1982), increasing blood flow in canine muscle (Milligan 1987), or reducing canine liver blood flow (Prionas et al. 1985).

7.5 Implications of Vascular Changes for the Clinical Use of Hyperthermia

The role of blood perfusion in hyperthermic tissue damage may also be discussed from both biophysical and biochemical points of view.

The biophysical significance of blood flow in the hyperthermic treatment of tumors is its role in heart transfer. When normal tissue is heated or even cooled by external factors, homeostatic control mechanisms increase the blood flow either to deliver heat to the cooled tissue or to remove heat from the heated tissue (Song et al. 1989a, 1990a). The most desirable condition in the hyperthermic treatment of tumors is to raise the temperature only in the tumor. Unfortunately, no external heating devices currently used in clinical hyperthermia are able to selectively deliver heat energy only to the target tumor. However, indications are that, in experimental or clinical hyperthermia, tumors are quite often preferentially heated relative to adjacent normal tissues. It is believed that such a preferential heating is due largely to the different response of blood vessels in tumors and normal tissues to heating, as discussed above and summarized in Fig. 7.16 (Song 1984). In most rodent tumors studied thus far, the blood flow markedly declines or stops during heating at 41°–43°C for 30–60 min. On the other hand, the blood flow in the skin or muscle of rodents increases by 5–15 times upon heating. The critical temperature for vascular damage and decline in blood flow in rodent skin and muscle has been demonstrated to be 1.0°–2.0°C higher than that in the tumors. Therefore, the tumor blood flow tends to decrease while the normal tissue blood flow remains elevated. Consequently, the tumors are preferentially heated relative to normal tissues.

It should be noted that it is not how many fold the blood flow in normal tissues or tumors increases or decreases, but the difference in the absolute blood flow rate in tumors and normal tissues which determines whether the tumors will be preferentially heated. The blood flow markedly varies with the tumor type, the site of tumor growth, and the size of the tumor. Table 7.1 shows the blood flow values in R3230 Ac tumors, 4–7 mm in diameter, grown in various sites in Fischer rats, and the blood flow values in the tissues in which the tumors grew (Hasegawa and Song 1991). The ratio of blood flow value in the tumors to that in the normal tissues (T/N) is also shown. At normal temperatures, the T/N ratio was smaller than 1.0 in all cases except for the tumors grown in the flank muscle of the rats. Note that the smaller the T/N ratio, the greater the preferential heating of tumors. The T/N ratio of 2.41 for the R3230 Ac tumors grown in the muscle

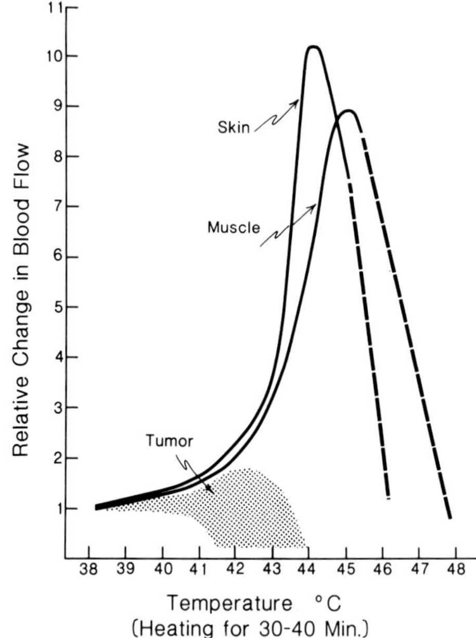

Fig. 7.16. Relative change in blood flow in the skin and muscle and in various experimental rodent tumors upon heating at various temperatures

Table 7.1. Blood flow in R3230 Ac tumors and host tissues

	Blood Flow (ml/g/min)	T/N[a]
Kidney	4.785 ± 0.095 (30)[b]	0.08
Tumor	0.400 ± 0.068 (6)	
Liver	1.263 ± 0.039 (30)	0.12
Tumor	0.155 ± 0.024 (5)	
Small intestine	3.455 ± 0.151 (30)	0.06
Tumor	0.203 ± 0.061 (12)	
Mesentery	0.279 ± 0.015 (24)	0.78
Tumor	0.217 ± 0.049 (12)	
Cecum	2.469 ± 0.141 (29)	0.15
Tumor	0.375 ± 0.080 (4)	
Muscle	0.064 ± 0.004 (14)	2.41
Tumor	0.154 ± 0.016 (16)	

[a] Ratio of blood flow in tumors to that in host tissues
[b] Number of samples shown within parentheses

may appear to indicate that tumors grown in the muscle may not be preferentially heated. However, because the muscle blood flow increases several times while the blood flow in the R3230 Ac tumor increases only slightly upon heating, the T/N ratio may become less than 1.0 during heating, and thus the tumor temperature may rise higher than that in the muscle. This relationship in the skin or muscle of Walker tumors in Sprague-Dawley (SD) rats can be seen in Fig. 7.1. At ambient temperature (control), the blood flow in small Walker tumors was several times greater than that in the skin or muscle near the tumors. At 43°C, the blood flow in skin near the tumors increased and became greater than that in the small tumors. Because the increase in the muscle blood flow was relatively small at 43°C, the muscle blood flow was still smaller than the tumor blood flow. The blood flow in large tumors was considerably smaller than that in the small tumors before heating. Upon heating, the tumor blood flow was smaller than that in the skin or muscle or the T/N ratio was smaller than 1.0, a desirable condition for the preferential heating of tumors.

VAUPEL (1992) discussed a hypothetical situation in which the blood flow in tumors was compared with that in the skin, and concluded that preferential heating of the tumor may be difficult because the tumor blood flow exceeds that in the skin. The hypothetical tumor blood flow used by Vaupel in his discussion was as high as 1.0 ml/g/min. Based on the reports of blood flow in various animal and human tumors, JAIN and Ward-HARTLEY (1984) concluded that the blood flow rate was 0.01–0.2 ml/g/min in 50% of tumors, 0.2–0.5 ml/g/min in 30%, and >0.5 ml/g/min in 20%. As described in Sect. 7.3.2, WATERMAN et al. (1986) found that the blood flow in superficial human tumors was 0–34 ml/100 g/min, with an average of 15 ml/100 g/min (0.15 ml/g/min). The blood flow cited by Vaupel in his discussion, 1.0 ml/g/min, appears to be much higher than the blood flow in most human tumors and it may be unrealistic to compare such a high tumor blood flow with that of the skin, which has the lowest blood flow among the normal tissues. Although the magnitude of the increase in blood flow in most normal tissues as a result of hyperthermia may not be as great as that in the skin or muscle, the normal tissue blood flow may increase by 2–4 times, as we observed in the lung, stomach, and intestine. On the other hand, the blood flow in most tumors may either increase by less than about twofold or decrease at therapeutic temperatures, i.e., 42°–45°C. It would then be reasonable to conclude that the T/N ratio would remain smaller than 1.0, and thus preferential tumor heating may be expected.

The biochemical role of blood flow in the hyperthermic treatment of tumors concerns its influence on the interstitial environment, such as pH, pO_2, and nutritional condition, which affect the thermosensitivity of tissues. It is a well-established fact that a low pH environment potentiates the cytotoxicity of hyperthermia and that the interstitial environment in the tumor is acidic relative to that in normal tissues. We, as well as other investigators, have unequivocally demonstrated that the intratumoral pH further declines when tumors are heated (LILLY et al. 1984; SONG et al. 1980c; RHEE et al. 1985; VAUPEL et al. 1988a; WIKE-HOOLEY et al. 1984). Such a decline in the tumor pH upon heating may be attributed to an increase in the formation of lactic acid as a result of vascular damage and the ensuing hypoxia. It has been suggested that the decrease in intratumoral pH induced by heat may not necessarily enhance the thermal damage in tumors since tumor cells chronically exposed to a low pH environment are not thermosensitized by a further increase in acidity. However, it must be noted that not all the tumor cells are surrounded by an acidic environment, and thus such cells may become thermosensitive when their environment becomes acidic during heating. This possibility is supported by the experimental evidence that tumor cells in vivo are far more thermosensitive than tumor cells maintained in vitro (KANG et al. 1980). The vascular damage and decline in blood flow accompanied by an increase in acidity, hypoxia, and deterioration of nutritional conditions may account for the different heat sensitivity in vivo and in vitro. The possibility that a reduction in tumor blood flow and an increase in acidity may increase the thermal damage in tumors has led investigators to apply a number of different approaches to perturb tumor blood flow. These have included use of high doses of glucose (hyperglycemia), hydralazine, and cytokines, such as TNF-α and interleukin-1a (HASEGAWA and SONG 1991; JAIN and WARD-HARTLEY 1984; SONG et al. 1993; VAUPEL 1990). Although these approaches have been reported to be useful for enhancing the thermal response of experimental tumors, clinical usefulness for human tumors has not been established.

7.6 Summary

- The vascular supply and blood flow in tumors are markedly different from those in normal tissues. In general, the blood perfusion in tomors is poorer than that in the host's normal organs or tissues.
- Vascular beds in tumors are poorly organized and the blood perfusion throughout the tumor is heterogeneous, resulting in an insufficient blood supply to parts of the tumor mass. Consequently, varying fractions of tumor cells are in a hypoxic environment, thus increasing anaerobic glycolytic metabolism and the concomitant formation of lactic acid.
- Little is unknown about the effects of hyperthermia on the vasculature and blood flow in human tumors, but the hyperthermic effect on blood flow in rodent tumors has been extensively investigated. It has been unequivocally demonstrated that the vasculature in these tumors are more vulnerable than that in normal tissues. Upon heating at 42°–44°C, the vasculature in tumors tends to break down and the blood flow decreases, whereas the blood flow in normal tissues increases significantly.
- The blood flow in the skin and muscle in rodents, as well as in humans, is known to increase as much as 20-fold.
- Limited experimental results indicate that the blood flow in internal organs, such as the lung, stomach, liver, and small intestine, does not increase as much as that in the skin or muscle. However, the blood flow in the internal organs is far greater than that in the skin or muscle and usually exceeds that in the tumors growing in the organs. Therefore, normal tissue blood flow in these organs tends to remain higher than that in tumors during heating. Consequently, heat dissipation through blood flow is much more effective in normal tissues than in tumors, resulting in a preferential heating of tumors.
- As a consequence of the breakdown of blood flow, the intratumoral environment becomes more acidic, hypoxic, and nutritionally deprived, which enhances the thermal killing of tumor cells.
- The preferential damage in tumors that is induced by hyperthermia may be enhanced by agents which selectively decrease the tumor blood flow, increase the intratumoral acidity, and increase the intracellular acidity.
- Recently, the response of vasculatures in normal tissues as well as those in tumors to reheatings has been found to be less than that to a single heating. Such vascular adaptation or vascular thermotolerance may have significant implications for the repeated heatings in the clinical use of hyperthermia.

Acknowledgements. The authors would like to thank Ms. Peggy Evans for her assistance in the preparation of the manuscript. This work was supported by NCI grant numbers CA13353 and CA44114.

References

Acker JC, Dewhirst MW, Honore GM, Samulski TV, Tucker JA, Oleson JR (1990) Blood perfusion measurements in human tumors: evaluation of laser Doppler methods. Int J Hyperthermia 6: 287–304

Allwood MJ, Burry HS (1954) The effect of local temperature on blood flow in the human foot. J Physiol 124: 345–347

Barcroft H, Edholm OG (1943) The effect of temperature on blood flow and deep temperature in the human forearm. J Physiol 102: 5–20

Dewey WC, Hopwood LE, Sapareto SA, Gerweck LF (1977) Cellular responses to combination of hyperthermia and rediation. Radiology 123: 463–474

Dewhirst MW (1987) Physiological effects of hyperthermia. In: Paliwal BR, Hetzel FW, Dewhrist MW (eds) Biological, physical and clinical aspects of hyperthermia. American Institute of Physics, New York, pp 16–56

Dickson JA, Calderwood SK (1980) Temperature range and selective sensitivity of tumors to hyperthermia: a critical review. Ann NY Acad Sci 335: 180–205

Dudar TE, Jain RK (1984) Differential response of normal and tumor microenvironment to hyperthermia. Cancer Res 44: 605–612

Eddy HA (1980) Alteration in tumor microvasculature during hyperthermia. Radiology 137: 515–521

Eddy HA, Chmielewski G (1982) Effect of hyperthermia, radiation and adriamycin combinations on tumor vascular function. Int J Radiat Oncol Biol Phys 8: 1167–1175

Fajardo LF (1984) Pathological effects of hyperthermia in normal tissues. Cancer Res (Suppl) 44: 4826s–4835s

Field SB, Hume SP, Law MP, Myers R (1977) The response of tissues to combined hyperthermia and x-rays. Br J Radiol 50: 129–134

Gerweck LE, Dahlberg WK, Greco B (1983) Effects of pH on single or fractionated heat treatment at 42°–45°C. Cancer Res 43: 1163–1167

Gullino PH (1980) Influence of blood supply on thermal properties and metabolism of mammary carcinomas. Ann NY Acad Sci 335: 1–21

Hasegawa T, Song CW (1991) Effect of hydralazine on the blood flow in tumors and normal tissues in rats. Int J Radiat Oncol Biol Phys 20: 1001–1007

Hill SA, Smith KA, Denekamp J (1989) Reduced thermal sensitivity of the vasculature in a showly growing tumor. Int J Hyperthermia 2: 379–387

Hugander A, Golmsjo M, Hafstrom L, Persson B (1983) Liver blood flow studies during local hyperthermia. An experimental study in rats. J Clin Oncol 9: 303–310

Jain RK (1980) Temperature distributions in normal and neoplastic tissues during normothermia and hyperthermia. Ann NY Acad Sci 335: 48–66

Jain RK, Ward-Hartley K (1984) Tumor blood flow: characterization, modifications and role in hyperthermia. IEEE Trans Sonics Ultrasonics SU-31: 504–526

Johnson RJR (1978) Radiation and hyperthermia. In: Streffer C, van Beuningen D, Dietzel F et al. (eds) Cancer therapy by hyperthermia and radiation. Urban and Schwarzenberg, Baltimore, pp 89–95

Kang MS, Song CW, Levitt SH (1980) Role of vascular function in response of tumors in vivo to hyperthermia. Cancer Res 40: 1130–1135

Kim GE, Lyons JC, Levitt SH, Song CW (1991) Effects of amiloride on intracellular pH and thermosensitivity. Int J Radiat Oncol Biol Phys 20: 541–549

Lee SY, Ryu KH, Kang MS, Song CW (1986) Effect of hyperthermia on the lactic acid and β-hydroxybutyric acid contact in tumors. Int J Hyperthermia 2: 213–222

Lilly MB, Ng TC, Evanochko WT et al. (1984) Loss of high-energy phosphate following hyperthermia demonstrated by in vivo ^{31}P-nuclear magnetic resonance spectroscopy. Cancer Res 44: 633–638

Lin JC, Song CW (1993) Influence of vascular thermotolerance on the heat-induced changes in blood flow, pO_2 and cell survival in tumors. Cancer Res 53: 2076–2080

Lokshina AM, Song CW, Rhee JG, Levitt SH (1985) Effect of fractionated heating on the blood flow in normal tissues. Int J Hyperthermia 1: 117–129

Lyng H, Monge OR, Bohler PJ, Rofstad EK (1991) The relevance of tumour and surrounding normal tissue vascular density in clinical hyperthermia of locally advanced breast carcinoma. Int J Radiat Biol 50: 189–193

Matsuda H, Sugimachi K, Kuwano H, Mora M (1989) Hyperthermia, tissue, microcirculation, and temporarily increased thermosensitivity in VX2 carcinoma in rabbit liver. Cancer Res 49: 2777–2782

Milligan AJ (1987) Canine muscle blood flow during fractionated hyperthermia. Int J Hyperthermia 3: 353–359

Nagasaka T, Hirata K, Nunomura T, Cabanac M (1987) The effect of local heating on blood flow in the finger and the forearm skin. Can J Physiol Pharmacol 65: 1329–1332

Nakajima T, Osborn J, Rhee JG, Song CW (1990) Effect of regional heating of upper body on the liver blood flow in rats. Int J Hyperthermia 6: 1–14

Nakajima T, Rhee JG, Song CW, Onoyama Y (1992) Effects of a second heating on the rat liver blood flow. Int J Hyperthermia 8: 679–687

Nishimura Y, Shibamoto Y, Jo S, Akuta K, Hiraoka M, Takashi M, Abe M (1988) Relationship between heat-induced vascular damage and thermosensitivity in four mouse tumors. Cancer Res 48: 7224–7230

Nishimura Y, Jo S, Akuta K et al. (1989) Histological analysis of the effect of hyperthermia on normal rabbit hepatic vasculature. Cancer Res 49: 4295–4297

Olch A, Kaiser L, Silberman A, Storm F, Graham L, Morton D (1983) Blood flow in human tumors during hyperthermia therapy: demonstration of vasoregulation and an applicable physiological model. J Surg Oncol 23: 125–132

Peck JW, Gibbs FA (1983) Capillary blood flow in murine tumors, feet and intestines during localized hyperthermia. Radiat Res 96: 65–81

Prionas SD, Taylor MK, Fajardo LF, Kelly NJ, Nelson TS, Hahn GM (1985) Thermal sensitivity to single and double heat treatments in normal canine liver. Cancer Res 45: 4791–4797

Rappaport DS, Song CW (1983) Blood flow and intravascular volume of mammary adenocarcinoma 13762A and normal tissues of rat during and following hyperthermia. Int J Radiat Oncol Biol Phys 9: 539–547

Reinhold HS, Endrich B (1986) Tumor microcirculation as a target for hyperthermia. Int J Hyperthermia 2: 111–137

Reinhold HS, Blachiewicz B, van den Berg-Blok AE (1978) Decrease in tumor microcirculation during hyperthermia. In: Streffer C, van Beuningen D, Dietzel F et al. (eds) Cancer therapy by hyperthermia and radiation. Urban and Schwarzenberg, Baltimore, pp 231–232

Rhee JG, Kim TH, Levitt SH, Song CW (1985) Changes in acidity of mouse tumor by hyperthermia. Int J Radiat Oncol Biol Phys 10: 393–399

Ryu KH, Song CW (1982) Changes in lactic acid content in tumors by hyperthermia. Radiat Res 91: 319–320

Scheid P (1961) Funktionelle Besonderheiten der Mikrozirkulation im Karzinom. Bibliotheca Anatomica 1: 327–335

Shrivastav S, Kaelin WG, Joines WT, Jirtle R (1983) Microwave hyperthermia and its effect on tumor blood flow in rats. Cancer Res 43: 4665–4669

Song CW (1978) Effect of hyperthermia on vascular function of normal tissues and experimental tumors: brief communication. J Natl Cancer Inst 60: 711–713

Song CW (1982a) Blood flow in tumors and normal tissues in hyperthermia. In: Storm K (ed) Hyperthermia in cancer therapy. G.K. Hall, Boston, pp 187–206

Song CW (1982b) Physiological factors in hyperthermia. Natl Cancer Inst Monogr 61: 169–176

Song CW (1982c) Physiological factors in hyperthermia of tumors. In: Nussbaum GH (ed) Physical aspects of hyperthermia. American Institute of Physics, New York, pp 43–62

Song CW (1984) Effect of local hyperthermia in blood flow and microenvironment: a review. Cancer Res 44: 4721s–4730s

Song CW (1991a) Role of blood flow in hyperthermia. In: Urano M, Douple EB (eds) Hyperthermia and oncology, vol 3. VSP, Utrecht, pp 275–315

Song CW (1991b) Tumor blood flow response to heat. In: Vaupel P, Jain RK (eds) Tumor blood supply and metabolic microenvironment, characterization and implications for therapy. Funktionsanalyse Biologischer System 20: 123–141

Song CW, Kang MS, Rhee JG, Levitt SH (1980a) Effect of hyperthermia on vascular function in normal and neoplastic tissues. Ann NY Acad Sci 335: 35–47

Song CW, Kang MS, Rhee JG, Levitt SH (1980b) Effect of hyperthermia on vascular function, pH and cell survival. Radiology 137: 795–803

Song CW, Rhee JG, Levitt SH (1980c) Blood flow in normal tissues and tumors during hyperthermia. J Natl Cancer Inst 64: 119–124

Song CW Patten MS, Rhee JG, Levitt SH (1987a) Effect of multiple heating on the blood flow in RIF-1 tumors, skin and muscle of C3H mice. Int J Hyperthermia 3: 535–545

Song CW, Rhee JG, Haumschild DJ (1987b) Continuous and noninvasive quantitation of heat-induced changes in blood flow in the skin and RIF-1 tumor of mice by laser Doppler flowmetry. Int J Hyperthermia 3: 71–77

Song CW, Chelstrom LM, Levitt SH, Haumschild DJ (1989a) Effects of temperature on blood circulation measured with the laser Doppler method. Int J Radiat Oncol Biol Phys 17: 1041–1047

Song CW, Lin JC, Chelstrom LM, Levitt SH (1989b) The kinetics of vascular thermotolerance in SCK tumors of A/J mice. Int J Radiat Oncol Biol Phys 17: 799–802

Song CW, Chelstrom LM, Haumschild DJ (1990a) Changes in human skin blood flow by hyperthermia. Int J Radiat Oncol Biol Phys 18: 903–907

Song CW, Chelstrom LM, Sung JH (1990b) Effect of second heating on the tumor blood flow. Radiat Res 122: 66–71

Song CW, Lin JC, Lyons JC (1993) Antitumor effect of Interleukin-1a in combination with hyperthermia. Cancer Res 53: 324–328

Stewart F, Begg A (1983) Blood flow changes in transplanted mouse tumours and skin after mild hyperthermia. Br J Radiol 56: 477–482

Streffer C (1984) Mechanism of heat injury. In: Overgaard J (ed) Hyperthermic oncology 1984, vol 2. Taylor & Francis, London, pp 213–222

Sugaar S, Leveen HH (1979) A histopathologic study on the effects of radiofrequency thermotherapy on malignant tumors of the lung. Cancer 43: 767–783

Sutton CH (1976) Necrosis and altered blood flow produced by microwave-induced tumor hyperthermia in murine glioma. In: Weinhouse S (ed) Proc. 12th Annual Meeting of the American Society for Clinical Oncology Williams & Wilkins Co., Baltimore, MD, 17: 63

Uda M, Osborn JL, Lee CKK, Nakhleh RE, Song CW (1990) Pathophysiological changes after local heating of rat liver. Int J Radiat Oncol Biol Phys 18: 903–907

van den Berg-Blok AE, Reinhold HS (1987) Experimental hyperthermic treatment of human colon carcinoma xenografts. The thermal sensitivity of the tumor microcirculation. Eur J Cancer Clin Oncol 23: 1177–1180

Vaupel P (1990) Pathophysiological mechanisms of hyperthermia in cancer therapy. In: Gautherie M (ed) Biological basis of oncologic thermotherapy. Springer, Berlin Heidelberg New York, pp 73–134

Vaupel P (1992) Effect of physiological parameters on tissue response to hyperthermia: new experimental facts and their relevance to clinical problems. In: Gerner EW, Cetas TC (eds) Proceedings of the 6th International Congress on Hyperthermic Oncology, Tucson Avizona, April. Arizona Bourd of Rejents 2: 17–24

Vaupel P, Ostheimer K, Mueller-Klieser W (1980) Circulatory and metabolic response of malignant tumors during localized hyperthermia. J Cancer Res Clin Oncol 98: 15–29

Vaupel P, Kallinowski F, Kluge M, Egelhof E, Fortmeyer HP (1988a) Microcirculatory and pH alterations in isotransplanted rat and xenotransplanted human tumors associated with hyperthermia. Recent Results Cancer Res 109: 173–182

Vaupel P, Kluge M, Ambroz MD (1988b) Laser doppler flowmetry in subepidermal tumors and in normal skin of rats during localized ultrasound hyperthermia. Int J Hyperthermia 4: 307–321

Vaupel P, Okunieff P, Kluge M (1989) Response of tumor red blood cell flux to hyperthermia and/or hyperglycemia. Int J Hyperthermia 5: 199–210

Waterman FM, Nerlinger RE, Moylan DJ III, Leeper DB (1986) Response of human tumor blood flow to local hyperthermia. Int J Radiat Oncol Biol Phys 13: 75–82

Wike-Hooley JL, Haveman J, Reinhold HS (1984) The relevance of tumor pH to the treatment of malignant disease. Radiother Oncol 2: 343–366

8 Metabolic Status and Reaction to Heat of Normal and Tumor Tissue

P.W. VAUPEL and D.K. KELLEHER

CONTENTS

8.1 Introduction

The occurrence of differential heating and differential thermal sensitivity between malignant tumors and normal tissues is thought to be due to limited heat dissipation and energy depletion in many solid tumors which in turn results from an inadequately functioning tumor microcirculation (JAIN and WARD-HARTLEY 1984; SONG 1984, 1991; VAUPEL and KALLINOWSKI 1987; REINHOLD 1988; VAUPEL et al. 1988a; VAUPEL 1990). As a consequence of the latter pathophysiological condition, supply and drainage function are restricted in many solid tumors or, at least, in some tumor areas, thus creating a hostile metabolic microenvironment characterized by tissue hypoxia, acidosis, and energy depletion. Thermal sensitivity has been shown to depend greatly on tumor pH, and on energy and nutritional status of the tumors treated. Although no conclusive evidence is so far available concerning the ranking of these pivotal factors, there is no doubt that the rate and homogeneity of blood perfusion plays a paramount role in determining the metabolic and energy status.

In *low-flow tumors* or tumor regions, the bioenergetic status and the limited convective heat dissipation are often worsened upon heating by a shutdown of blood flow, an intensified tissue acidosis, an enlargement of hypoxic tissue areas, and an inhibition of glucose oxidation (VAUPEL 1993a).

In *high-flow tumors* or tissue areas, heat dissipation can be so efficient that therapeutically relevant temperatures may not be achieved, and a hostile metabolic microenvironment may initially not exist or may not develop during therapeutic hyperthermia, thus limiting the therapeutic efficiency of this treatment modality.

In this chapter, the complex physiological effects which accompany tissue heating will be reviewed. Particular attention will be focused on the metabolic status, i.e., supply of the major substrate(s), tissue oxygenation, formation and removal of acidic waste products, and bioenergetic status. Besides actual substrate turnover rates, the metabolic status of tumors is greatly dependent on microcirculatory function. For this reason, tumor blood flow upon heating will be discussed throughout this chapter as appropriate.

8.2 Tissue Oxygenation upon Hyperthermia

Tissue oxygenation, which reflects the distribution of O_2 partial pressures or concentrations

P.W. VAUPEL, Dr. MD, Professor, Institute of Physiology and Pathophysiology, Universität Mainz, Duesbergweg 6, D-55099 Mainz, FRG

D.K. KELLEHER, PhD, Institute of Physiology and Pathophysiology, Universität Mainz, Duesbergweg 6, D-55099 Mainz, FRG

within a given tissue, results from O_2 supply (or O_2 availability) to the tissue and the respiration rate of the (parenchymal and stromal) cells composing the tissue (VAUPEL et al. 1989a; VAUPEL 1993b). Figure 8.1 shows how various factors, including temperature, can affect pO_2 distribution in any given tissue. Respiration rate and O_2 availability can be greatly modulated by the actual tissue temperature, the latter parameter being strongly influenced by the efficiency of blood flow and microcirculatory function (Fig. 8.2). This explains the experimental finding that changes in tumor tissue oxygenation, as a rule, more or less merely reflect changes in blood flow.

8.2.1 Blood Flow and Oxygen Availability

The increase in blood flow rate upon heating in *normal tissues* (e.g., skin, subcutis, resting skeletal muscle) is due to thermoregulatory mechanisms and is accompanied by a balanced enhancement of heat dissipation by convection, which counteracts a deleterious heat load in these tissues as long as tissue temperature levels of 45°C, exposure times of 30–60 min, and heating-up rates of 0.7°C/min are not exceeded (response of blood flow through normal tissues to single and multiple heatings has been reviewed by VAUPEL 1990). As a result, O_2 supply to the heated tissue is significantly improved, as shown by the data depicted in Fig. 8.3.

Recent data on blood perfusion in human *tumors* clearly show that flow rates exhibit a pronounced variability, ranging from 0.01 to $1.0\,ml \cdot g^{-1} \cdot min^{-1}$ (VAUPEL et al. 1989a, 1991) despite similar histology and primary site. Flow data from multiple locations within a tumor show marked heterogeneity, and no association could be found between tumor size and flow rate. Because the arterial O_2 concentration is the same for all tumors (approx. 0.2 ml O_2/ml blood), the O_2 availability is expected to show similar intra- and intertumor variabilities.

Changes in blood flow in human tumors upon heating are minor and, as yet, studies investigating patterns of change in these tumors have proven to be inconclusive (for a review see VAUPEL 1993a). Flow patterns seen during and after heating could not be correlated with the average temperature recorded at the site of measurement.

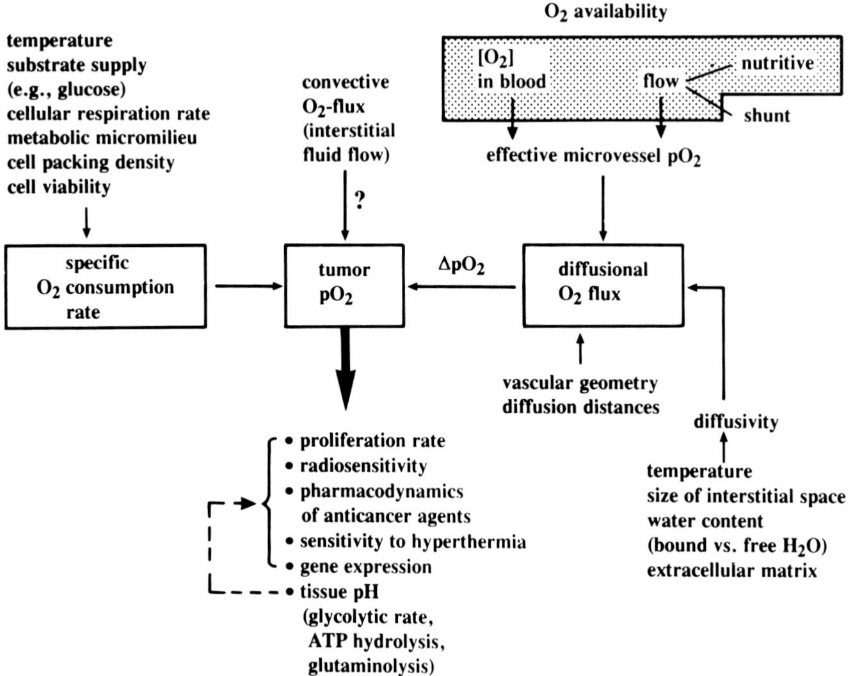

Fig. 8.1. Diagram showing factors which can critically determine the actual pO_2 distribution in any tissue, the role of temperature in modifying several relevant parameters, and mechanisms that can be modulated by tissue oxygenation

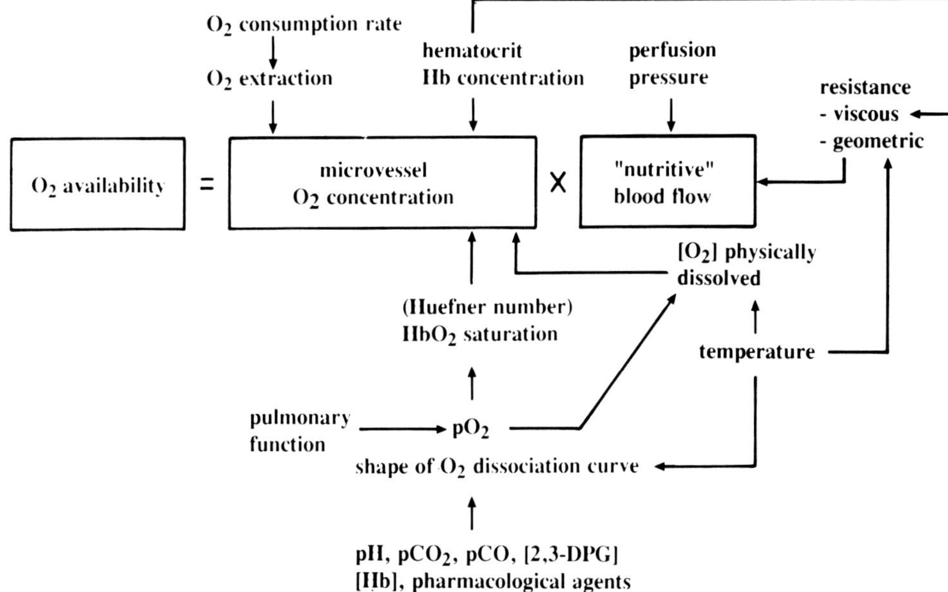

Fig. 8.2. Diagram with parameters determining the O_2 availability to any given tissue, and the impact of the temperature on some of the factors listed

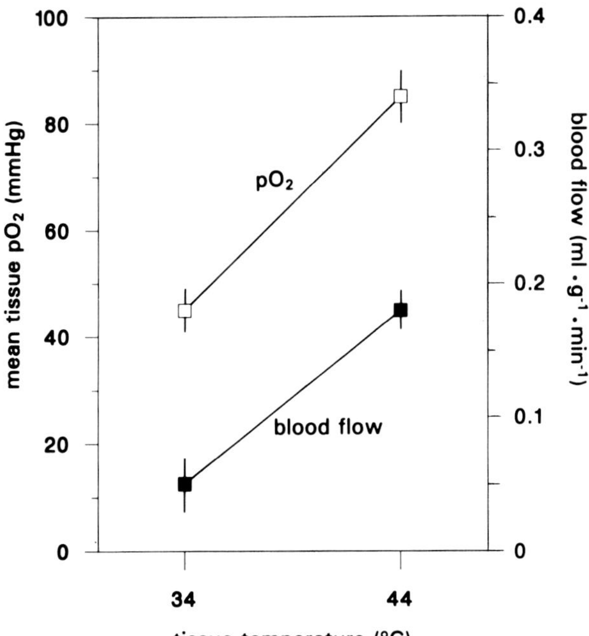

Fig. 8.3. Blood flow and mean O_2 partial pressure (pO_2) in the rat skin (hind foot dorsum) before and during 44°C hyperthermia at t = 30 min (values are means ± SEM)

Experiments on rodent tumors of varying volumes and thus, quite different flow rates before heating (0.3–1.1 ml · g^{-1} · min^{-1}, with the larger tumors exhibiting the lower flow values) can provide a more detailed insight into the blood flow behavior of tumors upon heat treatment. Results clearly show that heat-induced flow changes (or changes in O_2 availabilities) not only depend on the heat dose applied and on the tumor cell line investigated but also on the absolute blood flow rate of the tumors before treatment. In experimental tumor models, blood flow and O_2 availability are also dependent on the tumor volume and the site of implantation.

Therefore, these latter parameters can also modulate the response of tumors to heat.

Tumor O_2 supply is mainly determined by the red blood cell flux (RBC flux), which can experimentally be assessed by laser Doppler flowmetry (LDF) (VAUPEL et al. 1988b, 1989c). RBC flux critically influences the amount of O_2 reaching the tumor cells, whereas plasma flow is of minor importance in this respect [LDF in normal tissues and tumors during localized hyperthermia has been reviewed by VAUPEL (1990)].

KELLEHER et al. (1995) have measured RBC fluxes simultaneously in s.c. rat tumors (DS-sarcoma) at multiple sites using invasive laser Doppler flow probes. From these measurements the following conclusions could be drawn:

1. The response of the tumor to heat was dependent on tumor volume: the smaller the tumor (i.e., the higher the initial blood flow values) the less pronounced (and/or less often) the shutdown of microcirculatory function following a slight, initial increase in flow (Fig. 8.4).
2. The extent and direction of flow changes observed within a tumor did not correlate with the tumor site (peripheral vs central regions) or with the actual tissue temperature at the site of measurement (42.4° vs 44.5°C).
3. Variability in flux responses to heat were similar in small (0.7 ml) and large tumors (2.5 ml).
4. Whereas flux substantially increased by a factor of 2.3 in some tumor areas during the heating period, in others it steadily decreased by 75% upon hyperthermia; biphasic changes in flux could often be observed with an initial flow increase in many cases.

Flow increases reported in experimental tumor systems (e.g., AUSMUS et al. 1992) may help to explain the responsiveness of many human tumors to heat when the clinical situation is critically evaluated (WATERMAN et al. 1991; LAMMERTSMA et al. 1991; MOLLS and FELDMANN 1991; BOWMAN et al. 1992). Heat dissipation in small, high-flow experimental and human tumors (or at least in some tumor areas) can be so efficient that therapeutically relevant temperatures may not be achieved, and the metabolic status may be as adequate as in normal tissues and may even improve during therapeutic heating.

At least in experimental tumor models, the techniques of heating may have an additional

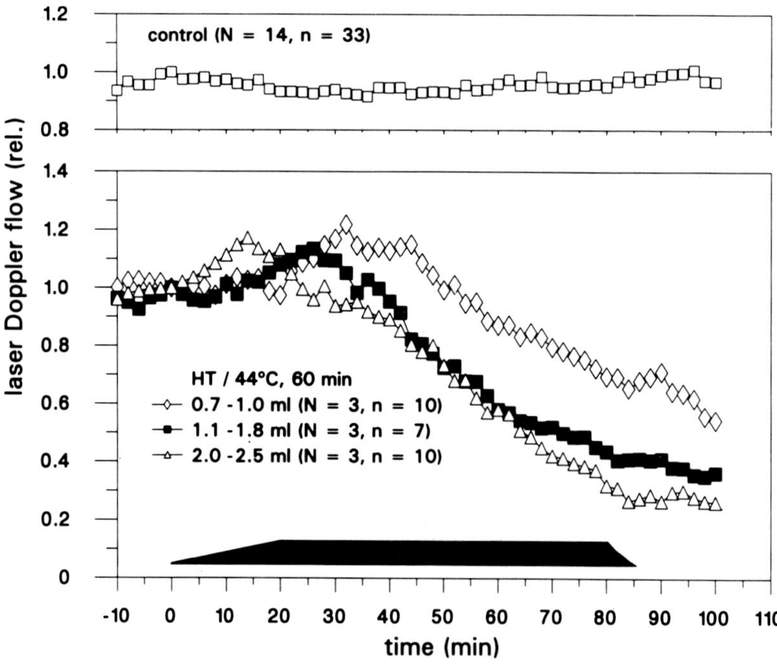

Fig. 8.4. Laser Doppler flow in subcutaneous DS-sarcomas in sham-treated tumors (control, *upper panel*) and in malignancies of different volume ranges upon 44°C hyperthermia for 60 min (*lower panel*). Values are means; *N*, number of tumors; *n*, number of intratumor locations observed. The *black area* indicates the heating period

impact on the biological behavior. In the case of water-bath hyperthermia, the highest temperatures are to be found in the tumor shell, which in many experimental systems exhibits the highest flow rates before treatment. In contrast, other heating devices lead to a maximum energy deposition in more central parts of the tumors which are often characterized by lower perfusion rates. This difference may explain the importance of the localisation of maximum heat deposition with respect to high- and low-flow regions, despite comparable mean tissue temperatures.

8.2.2 Cellular Oxygen Consumption at Elevated Temperatures

In general, the actual uptake of O_2 and nutrients by a tissue is determined by the respective availabilities in the microcirculation, the diffusional flux in the interstitial compartment, and the metabolic requirements of the cells. This holds true for both normal tissue and solid tumors during normothermia and hyperthermia. Whereas under in vitro conditions where no supply limitations are present, the capacity of the cells to consume oxygen is the limiting factor, the in vivo O_2 availability (i.e., microcirculatory function at normoxemia) is the paramount limiting parameter for many solid tumors. This means that changes in the in vivo O_2 uptake during hyperthermia only occur when tumor heating is accompanied by changes in nutritive blood flow (VAUPEL 1990). In other words, O_2 uptake rates in vivo will parallel changes in nutritive flow in either direction.

Temperature dependency of cellular oxygen consumption rates has been reviewed by VAUPEL (1990). On average, isolated tumor cells (exponentially) increase their O_2 consumption rate following temperature elevation, to maximum values at 41°–42.5°C. DS-sarcoma cells suspended in native ascitic fluid exhibit a maximum O_2 consumption rate of $42\,\mu l \cdot g^{-1} \cdot min^{-1}$ at 42°C. This consumption rate is comparable to that of the brain at 37°C (VAUPEL et al. 1989a).

8.2.3 Tissue Oxygenation at Elevated Temperatures

Prolonged tissue hypoxia can substantially increase the thermal sensitivity of cancer cells. Whether hypoxia has a direct effect or whether the sensitization effect is mediated through indirect mechanisms (e.g., acidification of the tissue, energy deprivation; GERWECK 1988) is still a matter of dispute. Since tumor tissue oxygenation is closely related to the efficiency of tumor microcirculation, changes in perfusion rate upon localized heating are followed by parallel changes in oxygenation. Alterations in tumor tissue oxygenation upon hyperthermia, like changes in blood flow, are of particular importance when considering the sequencing and timing of multifraction heat therapy or of combination treatment with standard irradiation or anticancer drugs.

In the normal *subcutis* of the rat, heat-induced increases in flow are accompanied by improvements of tissue oxygenation (see Fig. 8.3). During heating at 44°C, tissue pO_2 can reach values which are typical for arterial blood. This behavior is utilized in the monitoring of the arterial blood O_2 status in newborns (HUCH and HUCH 1985). In contrast, the application of large thermal doses in experimental *tumor systems* (isotransplanted rodent tumors and xenografted human malignancies in immune-deficient animals) which lead to flow declines are accompanied by increasing hypoxia (for a review of changes in tumor tissue oxygenation upon heating see VAUPEL 1990). Low thermal doses can, in some instances, increase tissue oxygenation provided that improvements in tumor microcirculation occur under these conditions.

The oxygenation of high-flow tumors may substantially ameliorate during heating. Upon 43°C hyperthermia for 60 min, an increased median pO_2 value in human breast cancer and sarcoma xenografted into nude mice was observed (ROSZINSKI et al. 1991; WIEDEMANN et al. 1992). Higher median pO_2 values during heating were accompanied by smaller numbers of pO_2 readings in the lowest pO_2 class (0–5 mmHg). After heating, median pO_2 values decreased, returning to baseline values 45 min after the end of heating. Similar results were observed in small and medium-sized DS-sarcomas when the average tumor pO_2 was measured by miniaturized catheter electrodes (STOHRER et al. 1992). In these experiments, average pO_2 values in tumors with volumes less than 1 ml significantly increased during the first hour of heating (42.6°–44.5°C) and then declined, reaching initial pO_2 levels 2 h after commencement of heating. In tumors with volumes between 1 and 2 ml, average pO_2 values were significantly higher for approximately 30 min upon heating. Afterwards they returned to values which were not significantly different from starting levels. In "bulky" tumors with volumes between 2 and 2.5 ml, biphasic changes were commonly seen, with a reduction of the average O_2 tension to below starting levels after an initial increase.

When considering the effects of hyperthermia (or other treatment modalities) on tissue oxygenation, mean and/or median pO_2 values need to be treated with caution. Upon heating for 2 h at 42.6°–44.5°C, the mean and median pO_2 values in DS-sarcomas changed only slightly (Fig. 8.5). In the same experiments, however, this hyperthermia treatment led to a drastic increase in the (therapeutically relevant) fraction of pO_2 readings in the range between 0 and 2.5 mmHg (Mayer et al. 1992). This finding may be explained by a heterogeneous flow response upon hyperthermia with a decrease in perfusion in low-flow areas occurring together with a flow increase in the well-perfused tissue areas.

The oxygen response in a mouse mammary adenocarcinoma at two different transplantation sites (leg and flank) was found to be remarkably different even though the tumor cure rate was identical for a given hyperthermia dose in terms of time and temperature (Hetzel et al. 1992). In leg tumors, all measured pO_2 values were $\leq$5 mmHg following doses leading to 10% or 60% tumor cures at 30 days. In flank tumors, tissue oxygenation improved after heating, reaching maximum values 1 day after treatment in the low-dose group, and 2 days after hyperthermia in the high-dose group.

8.3 Glucose and Lactate Levels upon Hyperthermia

The paramount parameter governing nutrient supply to solid tumors (and drainage of waste products) is the microcirculatory function. In the case of the substrates essential for growth, nutritive blood flow to cancer cells is the major factor as long as the supply is not compromised by a decrease in the respective arterial concentrations.

8.3.1 Glucose Levels During Heat Treatment

Glucose has become the most extensively studied "thermosensitizer" of experimental tumors. To assess the influence of hyperthermia on the glucose supply to tumors, glucose concentrations were determined in tumor tissue samples immediately after termination of treatment (44°C for 60 or 120 min). Data were compared with those obtained from skeletal muscle specimens of the same animals. During local hyperthermia, the temperature of the muscle tissue was approximately 1°C lower than that of the tumors (42.7°–43.5°C), thus closely resembling the clinical situation. Global glucose concentrations were compared with glucose microdistributions in representative tissue slices using single-photon counting and quantitative bioluminescence

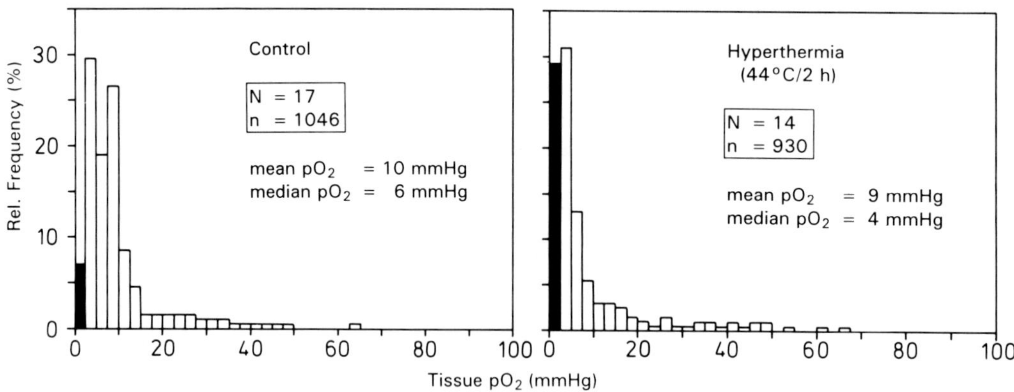

Fig. 8.5. Frequency distributions of measured intratumor O_2 tensions (pO_2 histograms) in s.c. DS-sarcomas in the rat. Data obtained in sham-treated tumors are shown in the *left panel*, whereas the respective values measured immediately following hyperthermia at 44°C for 2 h are depicted in the *right panel*. The proportions of pO_2 readings falling into the lowest pO_2 class (0–2.5 mmHg) are marked by *black columns*. *N*, number of tumors investigated; *n*, number of pO_2 measurements performed. (From Mayer et al. 1992)

(SCHAEFER et al. 1993) since metabolite distributions in malignant tumors can be quite heterogeneous (VAUPEL et al. 1989a), a property which cannot be detected when global concentrations are determined.

Cellular energy depletion resulting from a reduced nutrient supply can sensitize tumor cells to hyperthermia. Because some experimental *tumors* exhibited decreased glucose (and glucose-6-phosphate) levels after hyperthermic treatment (STREFFER and VAN BEUNINGEN 1987), it has been hypothesized that tumor cells may experience a thermal sensitization upon heat treatment in the sense of a positive feedback. However, these metabolic changes vary greatly between individual cell lines and are apparently closely related to heat-induced changes in blood flow and the development of an interstitial edema during heating. Glucose levels decreased in a mouse adenocarcinoma and in one melanoma xenograft line while they remained almost constant in two other melanoma cell lines (STREFFER 1988). In DS-sarcomas, global concentrations of glucose were found to decrease with enlarging tumor size (2.4 ± 0.2 to 1.4 ± 0.1 μmol/g), with levels being higher in heat-treated tumors (44°C, 60 min), irrespective of tumor size (Fig. 8.6; KELLEHER et al. 1995). Measurement of glucose microdistributions by single-photon imaging and quantitative bioluminescence confirmed these findings (Fig. 8.7).

The higher intratumor glucose concentrations upon heating may be the result of different pathogenetic mechanisms: (a) an (at least temporarily) increased blood flow and a 20% higher glucose concentration in arterial blood (MAYER et al. 1992), which together result in a higher glucose availability to the tumor cells and a somewhat more homogeneous glucose distribution (SCHAEFER et al. 1993); (b) an expansion of the interstitial compartment (where the glucose concentration is higher than within the cells) as a result of edema formation (increase in tissue water content of 4% w/w).

During local heating of the tumor, the temperature of the adjacent *muscle tissue* was raised as already described. As was the case with tumor tissue, this elevated temperature in muscle was also accompanied by an increase in glucose levels. Since significant interstitial edema does not occur in skeletal muscle during heating (KRÜGER et al. 1993), this higher glucose level is most probably due to a substantial hyperemia in skeletal muscle upon heating (KRÜGER et al. 1991).

8.3.2 *Lactate Levels During Heat Treatment*

In DS-sarcomas, global concentrations of lactate were found to increase with enlarging tumor size (9.4 ± 0.8 to 13.7 ± 0.9 μmol/g). Upon therapeutic heating (44°C, 60 min), tumor lactic acid concentrations increased significantly, with the differences between concentrations in control and heat-treated tumors increasing as a function of tumor size (Fig. 8.8). The bioluminescence

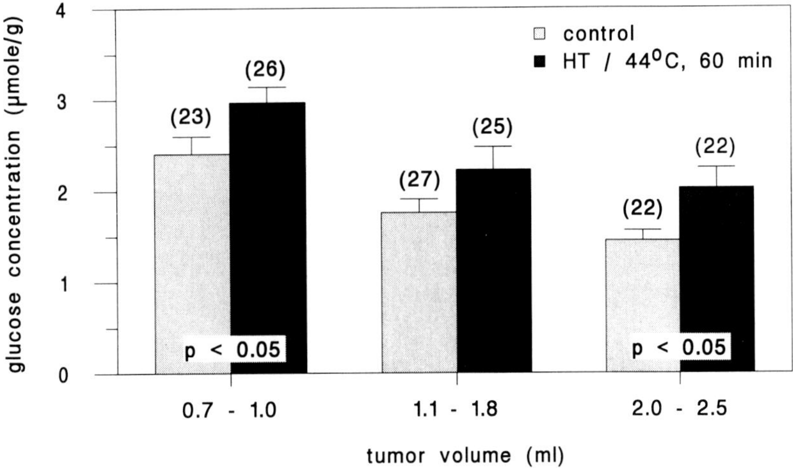

Fig. 8.6. Global glucose concentrations in control (*left columns*) and heat-treated (44°C/60 min) tumors (*right columns*) of three different size ranges (DS-sarcomas heated with water-filtered infrared-A radiation). Values are means ± SEM; the number of tumors investigated is shown in parentheses

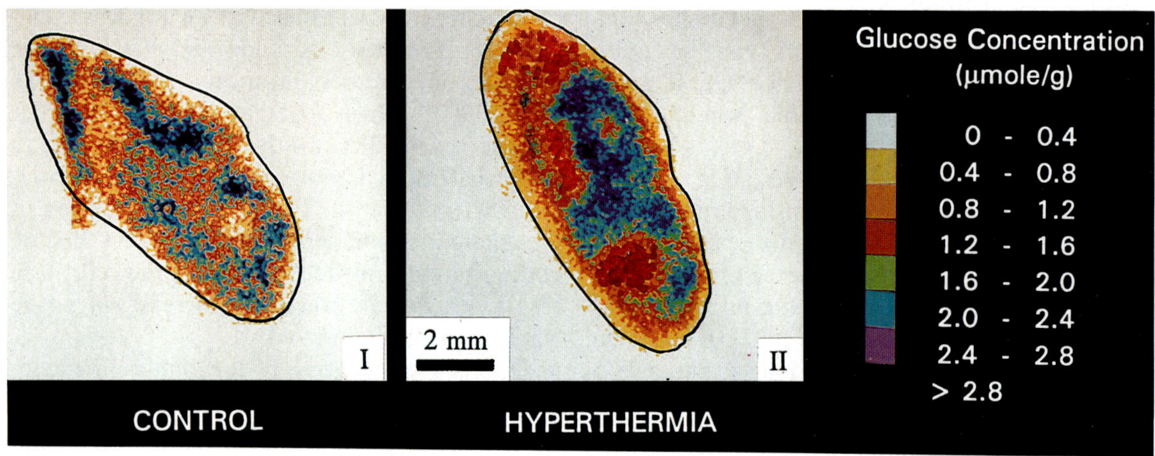

Fig. 8.7. Representative color-coded distributions of glucose concentrations measured in cryosections of control and heat-treated (44°C/60 min) DS-sarcomas (tumor volume ≈ 1 ml)

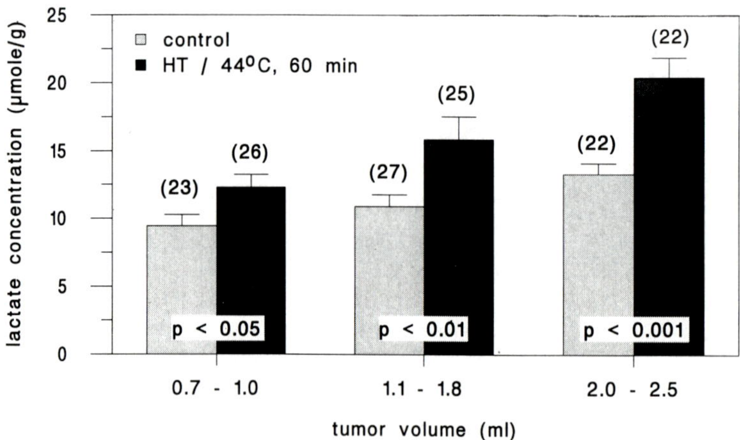

Fig. 8.8. Global lactate concentrations in control (*left columns*) and heated (44°C/60 min) tumors (*right columns*) of three different size classes. For further details see legend to Fig. 8.6

pictures in Fig. 8.9 showing the microregional lactate distribution confirmed these findings. The histogram for the lactate concentrations in the control tumors is left-shifted with a median of 11 μmol/g (Fig. 8.10, left panel). Following hyperthermia, the lactate distribution curve becomes more or less Gaussian with a median lactate level of 19 μmol/g (Fig. 8.10, right panel).

In normoxic tumor areas, lactic acid can be the catabolite of aerobic glycolysis and glutaminolysis. Lactate accumulation in tumors upon heating is the result of an intensified glycolytic breakdown of glucose with an 18-times poorer ATP yield than that occurring with glucose oxidation (Streffer 1990). The degradation of pyruvate to acetyl-CoA and the following oxidative pathway are impaired in hyperthermia (Streffer 1984). These heat-induced metabolic changes lead to an enhanced production of lactic acid, β-hydroxybutyric acid, and acetoacetic acid (Streffer 1982). From these latter acidic waste products, lactic acid is the paramount factor determining tumor tissue pH upon heat treatment (Schaefer et al. 1993).

8.4 Tumor pH During Heat Treatment

Low intracellular pH can increase the cellular *sensitivity to heat* by reducing the stability of proteins (Dewey 1989). This has been shown in a series of experimental systems (Gerweck

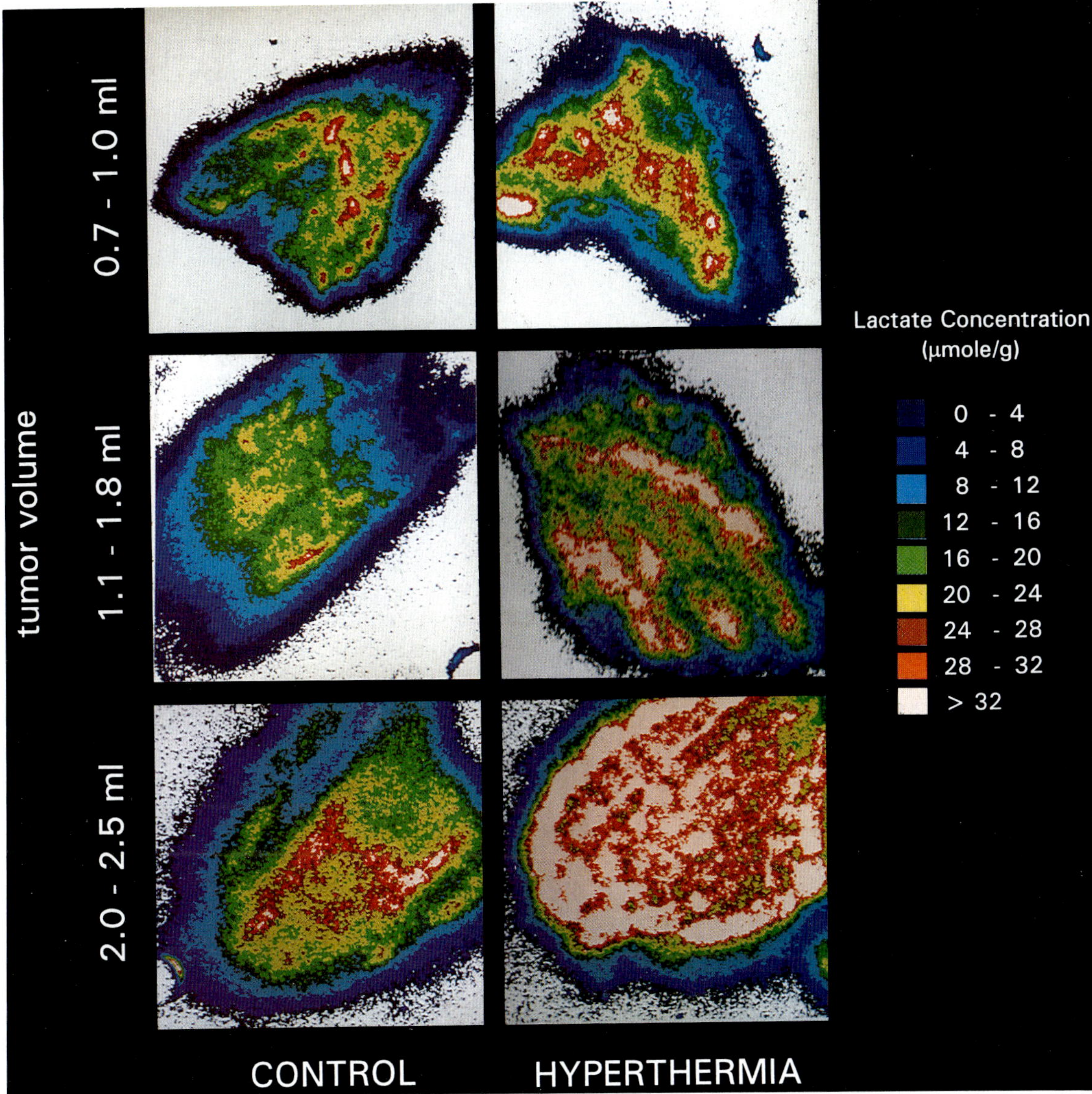

Fig. 8.9. Representative color-coded distributions of lactate concentrations measured in cryosections of control (*left panels*) and heat-treated (44°C/60 min) DS-sarcomas of three different volume ranges

1988) and can be observed both with single heat treatment and during fractionated hyperthermia. Response to heat is decreased in cells that are adapted to low pH values. Acidosis in tumors may contribute to cell death even in the absence of therapy. Most probably, acidosis does not greatly contribute to *radioresistance* in hypoxic tumor areas. It may influence, at least under in vitro conditions, cellular uptake and activation of a series of *anticancer drugs* (Wike-Hooley et al. 1984).

The notion of tissue acidosis in tumors is based on experiments with invasive *pH electrodes* (Vaupel et al. 1989a, Vaupel 1992). With this technique, measured pH values preferentially reflect the acid-base status of the extracellular space, which occupies approx. 50% of the total tissue volume in malignant tumors (Vaupel and Müller-Klieser 1983). This is in strong contrast to most normal tissues, where, on average, the extracellular compartment encompasses only 15–25%. The pH values measured in experimental rodent and human malignancies with electrodes are shifted to more acidic values with respect to normal tissues (0.3–0.5 pH units; Vaupel et al. 1989a; Vaupel 1992).

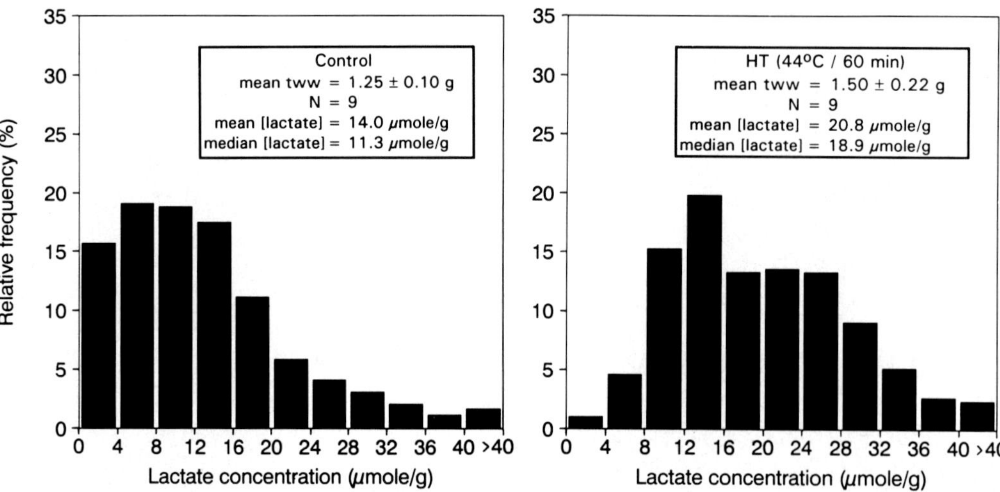

Fig. 8.10. Frequency distributions of lactate concentrations measured by quantitative bioluminescence in sham-treated DS-sarcomas (*left panel*) and upon hyperthermia at 44°C for 60 min (*right panel*). *tww*, tumor wet weight; *N*, number of cryosections investigated

pH measurements using *^{31}P-NMR spectroscopy* yield quite a different picture. The data obtained mainly reflect intracellular pH values and appear to be very similar to those found in normal tissues (VAUPEL et al. 1989a; GRIFFITHS 1991; VAUPEL 1992). This would suggest that tumor cells can maintain their internal pH (pH_i) at a relatively constant level (pH_i is near neutrality or slightly alkaline) despite a significant production of protons predominantly through glycolysis, ATP hydrolysis, and glutaminolysis (Fig. 8.11). At the very least, tumor cells keep their internal pH above the extracellular level over a considerable range of pH_e values. When pH_i values of murine tumors were measured using ^{31}P-MRS, acid pH_i values were found only in bulky, poorly oxygenated, energy- and nutrient-deprived tumors (e.g., in FSaII mouse sarcomas when tumor volumes exceeded 1.5% of body weight; VAUPEL et al. 1989b).

The difference between intra- and extracellular pH is most probably due to the fact that tumor cells, like normal cells, have efficient mechanisms for intracellular pH homeostasis. These include intracellular buffer systems and several efficient mechanisms for exporting protons into the extracellular space and importing HCO_3^- into the intracellular compartment (TANNOCK and ROTIN 1989; NEWELL and TANNOCK 1991). The subsequent inadequate removal of H^+ ions from the enlarged extracellular space in low-flow areas may result in an extracellular acidosis, as has often been demonstrated by electrode measurements in solid tumors. Another possible mechanism contributing to intracellular pH homeostasis may be the formation of ammonium ions (NH_4^+) from H^+ and ammonia (NH_3), the latter being liberated during amino acid turnover.

8.4.1 pH Measurements Using ^{31}P-MRS upon Hyperthermia

Upon localized hyperthermia, pH values derived from the PCr-P_i chemical shift in ^{31}P-MRS (pH_{NMR}, nominal intracellular pH) drop in a dose-dependent manner as long as temperatures higher than 42°C and exposure times of 30 min or longer are employed (VAUPEL et al. 1990; for a recent review see VAUPEL 1990). Besides increasing the thermosensitivity of cancer cells (GERWECK et al. 1980; LYONS et al. 1992), lowering the (intracellular) pH of tumors is known to inhibit the development of thermotolerance (LIN et al. 1991) and the repair of thermal damage, and may influence the interaction between drugs and heat.

Relevant pathogenetic mechanisms leading to acidification are:

1. Accumulation of lactic acid, β-hydroxybutyric acid, and acetoacetic acid
2. Changes in chemical equilibria of the intra- and extracellular buffer systems ($\Delta pH/\Delta T = -0.016$ pH units/°C)
3. An intensified ATP hydrolysis during tissue heating
4. An increase in CO_2 partial pressures (VAUPEL 1990)

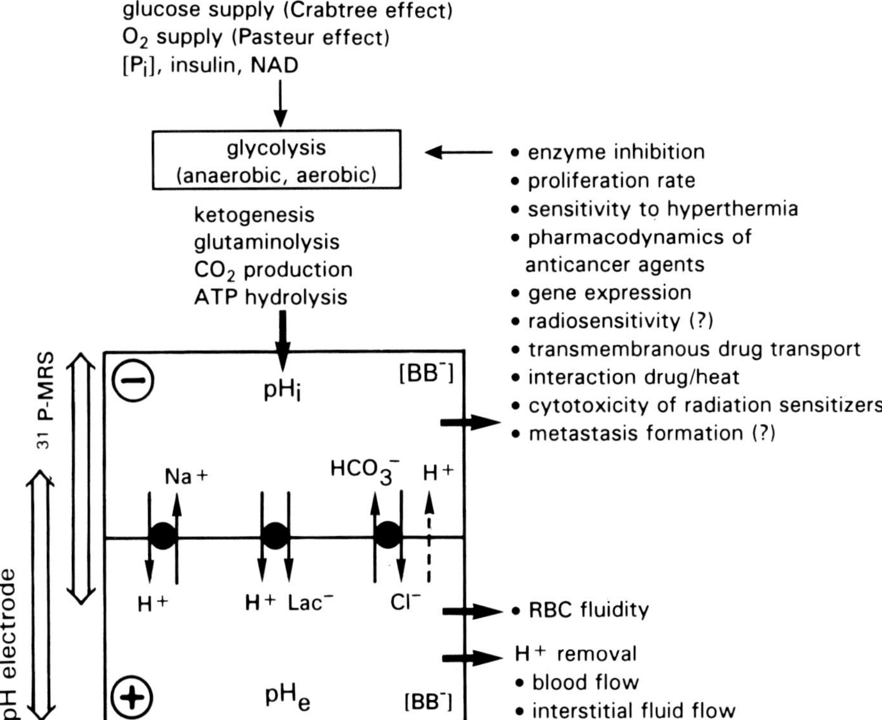

Fig. 8.11. Diagram showing parameters that are involved in intracellular pH homeostasis, mechanisms that can be modulated by intra- (*pH_i*) and extracellular pH (*pH_e, right part of the diagram*), and the tissue compartments which are investigated by different techniques (pH electrode vs ^{31}P-MRS). *Lac*⁻, lactate; *BB*⁻, buffer bases; *RBC*, red blood cell

5. An inhibition of the Na^+/H^+ antiport function in the cell membrane (Liu et al. 1992).

On average, pH_{NMR} in FSaII tumors was 7.18 before treatment. Following hyperthermia at 43.5°C for 15 min, pH_{NMR} declined only marginally during the first hour after heating ($\Delta pH = -0.14$ pH units, NS) and recovered thereafter (Fig. 8.12). pH_{NMR} returned to pre-heating values over the subsequent 6 h (Vaupel et al. 1990). Upon hyperthermia for 30 min, the mean pH_{NMR} significantly dropped during the first 90 min following heating ($\Delta pH = -0.30$ pH units, $2P < 0.01$) and partially recovered thereafter. Following heating for 60 min, pH_{NMR} values declined and attained a steady state which was 0.43 pH units below baseline pH ($2P < 0.001$).

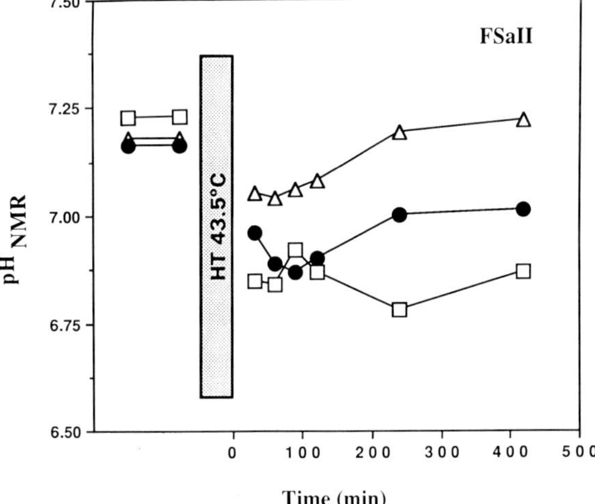

Fig. 8.12. Changes in the mean pH_{NMR} in FSaII tumors following heating at 43.5°C for 15 min (*triangles*), 30 min (*closed circles*), and 60 min (*squares*). Heating as indicated by the *vertical bar* was completed at $t = 0$ min

8.4.2 pH Measurements Using Invasive Electrodes upon Hyperthermia

Dose-dependent changes in *intratumor pH* values have also been observed by Hetzel et al. (1989) with invasive pH-sensitive microelectrodes. In these experiments, higher heat doses were associated with greater pH drops, longer time periods of intensified acidosis, and higher local cure rates. These findings further implicate that the extracellular pH may also be related to hyperthermic sensitization, perhaps through indirect measures, but is most probably less important than pH_i. One of these measures may be a decrease in the deformability of red blood cells and thus an increased viscous resistance to flow. Low extracellular pH, tissue hypoxia, and lactate accumulation together are known to cause this unfavorable condition (KAVANAGH et al. 1993).

Only minor post-treatment changes in *skeletal muscle pH* were observed by HETZEL and CHOPP (1990). Unlike the response observed in tumors, no hyperthermia dose-dependency was observed in the muscle response. No heat-induced pH changes were seen in the rat *subcutis* following localized hyperthermia at 44°C for 60 min (pH = 7.32 before heating vs 7.35 1 h after heating; KALLINOWSKI and VAUPEL 1989).

Various other factors besides heat dose can modulate the acidification of tumor tissue upon localized hyperthermia. pH reduction may be dependent on tumor size, heating-up rates, the location within a given tumor, actual blood flow rate, glucose availability, and the extent of the heat-induced interstitial edema (KALLINOWSKI and VAUPEL 1989).

In contrast to many investigators who have demonstrated a pH drop in experimental tumors during and generally up to 1 day following hyperthermia (Fig. 8.13; for a review see VAUPEL 1990), ROSZINSKI et al. (1991) and WIEDEMANN et al. (1992) failed to show heat-induced decreases in tumor pH upon 43°C hyperthermia for 60 min in two xenografted human cell lines (breast cancer, sarcoma), which are characterized by a relatively high blood flow rate and thus a physiological oxygenation status. Under these conditions, one has to expect a significant flow increase upon heating with an improved clearance of acidic catabolites from the interstitial compartment.

The significance of the baseline pH and changes occurring during hyperthermia in clinical studies remains unclear, since results obtained generally solely reflect the mandatory changes in physicochemical equilibria which are instantly reversed upon cooling (VAN DE MERWE et al. 1990). Other mechanisms may therefore have contributed

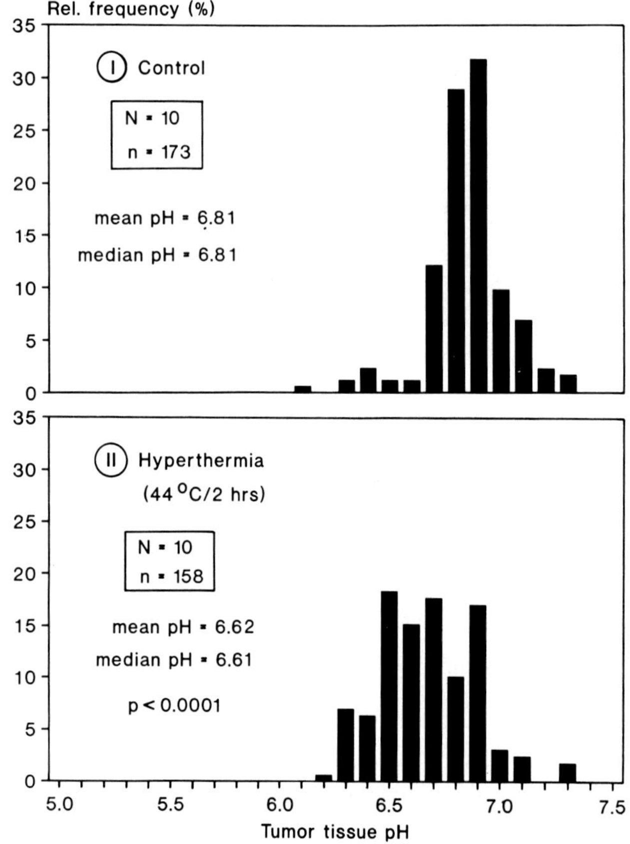

Fig. 8.13. Frequency distributions of tissue pH values (pH histograms) of DS-sarcomas. Measurements in sham-treated (*upper panel*) and heated umors (*lower panel*) were performed immediately after termination of treatment using pH-sensitive electrodes. *N*, number of tumors investigated; *n*, number of pH values measured

to the remarkable pH drop (and tumor regression) observed in some tumors, e.g., induced hypoperfusion or ischemia (VAN DER ZEE et al. 1989). Although data are still fragmentary, clinical results strongly suggest that acutely induced pH drops can contribute to the effect of hyperthermia (VAN DEN BERG et al. 1991). This notion is not contradicted by the experimental finding that tumors with high intracellular pH values before treatment show a favorable response to combined radiotherapy and hyperthermia (VAN DEN BERG et al. 1989; DEWHIRST et al. 1991) since the therapeutic response may preferentially reflect the effect of radiotherapy on well-oxygenated tumors, which usually exhibit neutral or alkaline intracellular pH values (VAUPEL et al. 1989b).

8.5 Bioenergetic Status

Cellular ATP depletion (e.g., through a reduced substrate supply) is thought to sensitize tumor cells to hyperthermia (GERWECK et al. 1984, 1989; KOUTCHER et al. 1990), although in a recently published investigation, OSINSKY et al. (1993) found no correlation between preheating energy charge [(ATP + 0.5 ADP)/(AMP + ADP + ATP)] in the tumor and the extent of the antitumor effect of hyperthermia (43°C, 60 min).

8.5.1 ^{31}P-MRS in Tumors

High-resolution ^{31}P nuclear magnetic resonance spectroscopy (^{31}P-MRS, ^{31}P-NMR) allows for non-invasive, non-destructive, serial and painless monitoring of tumor metabolic status and intracellular pH. In recent years using in vivo ^{31}P-MRS, researchers have gained important and new insights into human and animal tumors, and have confirmed or rejected some postulated characteristics of tumors. Several comprehensive studies of the effect of therapeutic heating on tumor energy metabolism have been performed (for a review see VAUPEL 1990). The results of these investigations are qualitatively quite similar, with only small differences being found accountable to the heat dose, the heating technique, the tumor volumes employed, and the use or absence of general anesthesia.

In vivo ^{31}P-NMR spectroscopy was used to monitor the bioenergetic status, pH_{NMR}, and membrane phospholipid turnover in subcutaneously growing murine fibrosarcomas (FSaII) and mammary carcinomas (MCaIV) treated at 43.5°C for 15, 30, or 60 min. Experiments were performed on conscious mice with biologically relevant tumor volumes (VAUPEL et al. 1990). The study focused on *acute* heat-induced bioenergetic changes (up to 7 h post-heating). ^{31}P-NMR spectra of both murine tumors were characterized by relatively high pretreatment levels of phosphomonoesters (PME), inorganic phosphate (P_i), and nucleoside triphosphates (NTP), and lower levels of phosphodiesters (PDE), phosphocreatine (PCr), and diphosphodiesters (DPDE) (Fig. 8.14). Following hyperthermia, NTP and PCr levels decreased (Figs. 8.15, 8.16). This drop was accompanied by a prompt and substantial increase in P_i. After heating for 15 min, the limited spectral changes observed for the high-energy phosphates

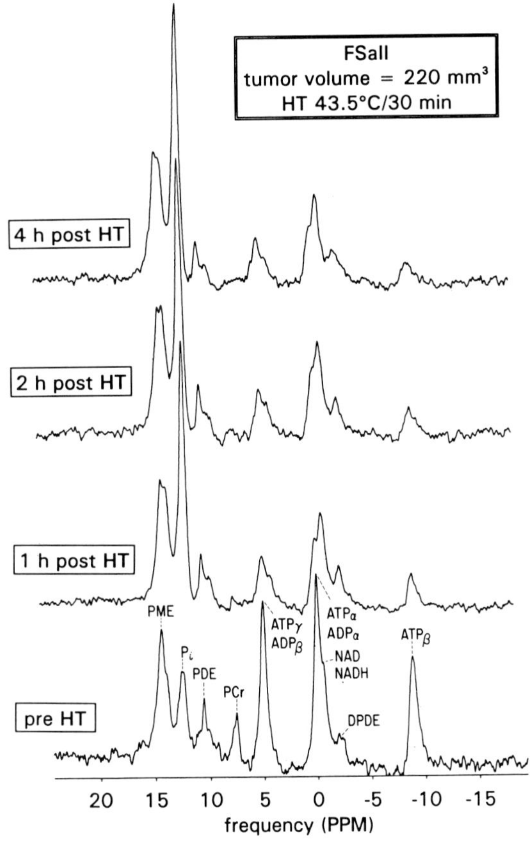

Fig. 8.14. Serial ^{31}P-NMR spectra of a 220 mm^3 FSaII tumor before (*lower spectrum*) and at different time intervals after hyperthermia (*HT*) at 43.5°C for 30 min. The assignment of the resonances is in accordance with literature data

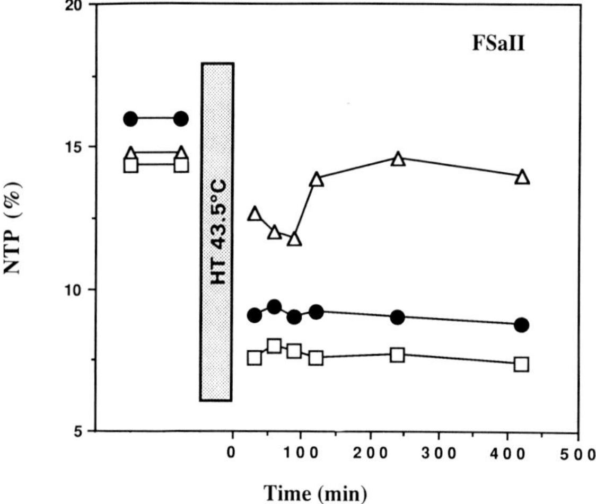

Fig. 8.15. Mean relative concentrations of nucleoside triphosphate (*NTP*, in percentage of total tumor phosphate compounds) in FSaII tumors before and after hyperthermia at 43.5°C for 15 min (*triangles*), 30 min (*closed circles*), and 60 min (*squares*). Heating was completed at $t = 0$ min

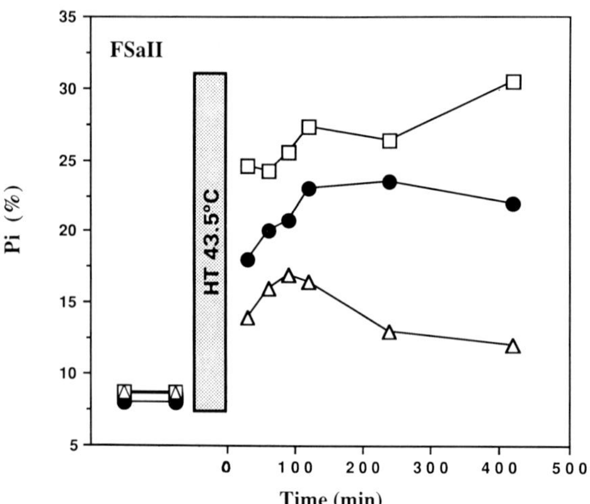

Fig. 8.16. Mean relative concentrations of inorganic phosphate (P_i, in percentage of total tumor phosphate compounds) in FSaII tumors before and after hyperthermia at 43.5°C for 15, 30, and 60 min. For further explanation see legend to Fig. 8.15

were nullified within 7 h, whereas P_i remained significantly elevated. Metabolic ratios (PCr/P_i and NTP/P_i) decreased after heating and did not recover thereafter (Figs. 8.17, 8.18). Upon longer heat exposure times (30 and 60 min) the high-energy phosphates, PCr/P_i, and NTP/P_i all decreased in a dose-dependent manner and remained at the respective lower levels.

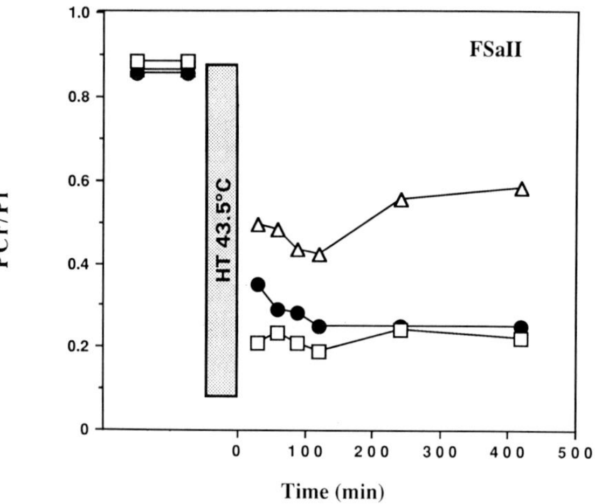

Fig. 8.17. Mean phosphocreatine/inorganic phosphate ratio (PCr/P_i) in FSaII tumors before and after hyperthermia at 43.5°C for 15, 30, and 60 min. For further explanation see legend to Fig. 8.15

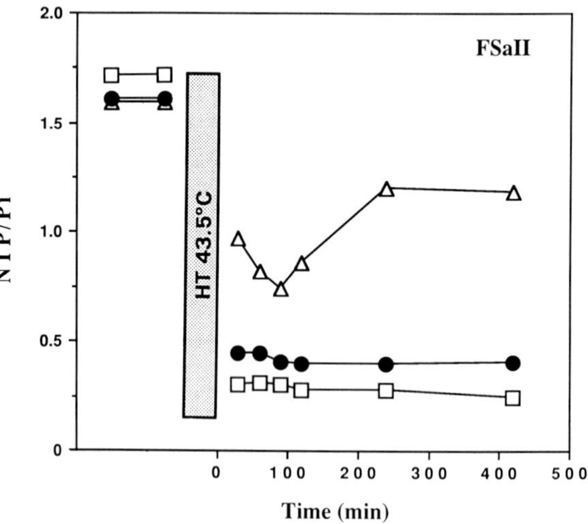

Fig. 8.18. Mean nucleoside triphosphate/inorganic phosphate ratio (NTP/P_i) in FSaII tumors before and after heating at 43.5°C for 15, 30, and 60 min. For further explanation see legend to Fig. 8.15

The remaining NTP resonances after "subcurative" heat doses had chemical shifts suggesting that high concentrations of nucleoside diphosphates (NDP) are present (Vaupel et al. 1990). Concomitantly PME levels often increase, consistent with the accumulation of glycolytic intermediates and perhaps of nucleoside monophosphates (NMP). As a rule, all of these changes can reverse within 24–36 h after hyperthermia.

No analysis has yet been undertaken to evaluate the adenylate kinase kinetics during the low-NTP/

high-NDP state. This would be of great interest since it would help to clarify whether or not the pH sensitivity of hyperthermia may ultimately be due to pH-induced changes of the kinetics of the adenylate kinase reaction, e.g., heat-treated cells may be killed because ATP cannot be synthesized at the necessary pace.

8.5.2. Analysis of Bioenergetic Status Using High-Pressure Liquid Chromatography and Acid Tissue Extracts

In DS-sarcomas, global concentrations of ATP (HPLC), inorganic phosphate, and phosphocreatine (enzymatic tests) were measured before and immediately after 44°C hyperthermia for 60 min using water-filtered infrared-A radiation (VAUPEL et al. 1992) or saline-bath heating (KRÜGER et al. 1991; SCHAEFER et al. 1993). Mean preheating ATP levels were found to range from 1.0 to 1.6 μmol/g. Upon hyperthermia, global ATP concentrations significantly decreased, this change being accompanied by a significant increase in the fraction of tumor tissue exhibiting cellular damage (SCHAEFER et al. 1993). The extent of these heat-induced changes was not related to tumor size (Fig. 8.19).

The ATP decline observed upon hyperthermia is most probably due to several mechanisms. Most relevant in this context are:

1. An increased ATP turnover rate (intensified ATP hydrolysis) during heating
2. A poorer ATP yield (on a molar basis) during hyperthermia because there is a shift from oxidative glucose breakdown to glycolysis
3. A restriction of the microcirculatory function and thus of relevant substrates for energy metabolism (in some tumor lines)
4. Hypothetically, an inhibition of the adenylate kinase reaction due to tissue acidosis (a so far unproven notion)

As a result of an intensified ATP degradation, an accumulation of purine catabolites has to be expected together with a formation of protons at several stages during degradation to the final product uric acid. Proton formation in turn can contribute to the development of heat-induced acidosis. Furthermore, oxidation of hypoxanthine and xanthine may result in the formation of active oxygen species, which may lead to DNA damage, lipid peroxidation and protein denaturation, thus also contributing to heat-induced cytotoxicity. In hyperthermia experiments a tumor-size dependent, significant increase in the levels of the following catabolites has been demonstrated: Σ[IMP + GMP], inosine, hypoxanthine, xanthine and uric acid, together with a drop in ATP and GTP levels (BUSSE and VAUPEL 1994). Thus, the formation of active oxygen species and protons during purine degradation may play a significant role in the antitumor effect of hyperthermia (see also SKIBBA et al. 1986; ANDERSTAM et al. 1992; YOSHIKAWA et al. 1993).

Mean inorganic phosphate concentrations increased (from 6.5 ± 0.9 to 9.9 ± 1.0 μmol/g) and phosphocreatine levels decreased (from 1.2 ± 0.1 to 0.2 ± 0.1 μmol/g) with increasing tumor size. Upon hyperthermia, the former tended to increase and the latter to decrease. The extent of these heat-induced changes was not related to tumor size, a finding that was also observed with ATP.

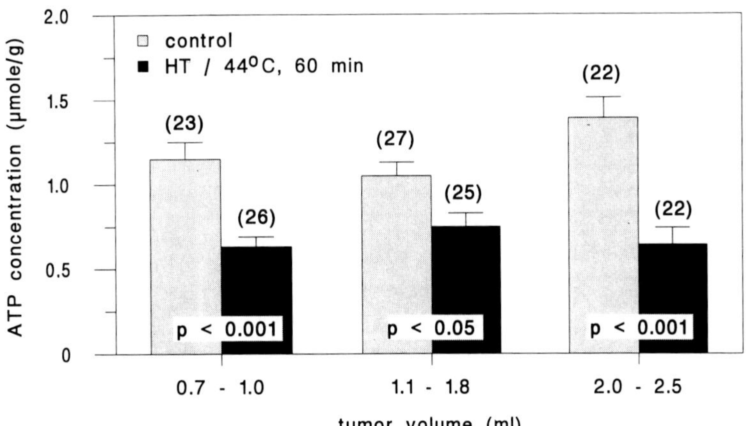

Fig. 8.19. Global ATP concentrations in control (*left columns*) and heated (44°C/60 min) DS-sarcomas (*right columns*) of three different volume classes. For further details see legend to Fig. 8.6

ADP ($0.4 \pm 0.04\,\mu$mol/g) and AMP levels ($0.3 \pm 0.04\,\mu$mol/g) and adenylate energy charge (0.75 ± 0.03) remained relatively constant with increasing tumor volume. Following hyperthermia, energy charge decreased significantly, ADP slightly decreased, but no changes were observed in AMP concentrations.

Traditionally, adenylate energy charge and other energy indices (e.g., phosphorylation potential) have been used to give an indication of the energy status under varying conditions. P_i and ADP levels measured using acid tissue extracts of HPLC, however, yield total compound concentrations, including free and bound substances. Such indices are only meaningful if calculated from concentrations of free compounds.

8.5.3 Microregional ATP Distribution

In general, measurement of microregional ATP concentration distributions by single-photon imaging and quantitative bioluminescence confirmed data described in Sect. 8.5.2. Mean ATP

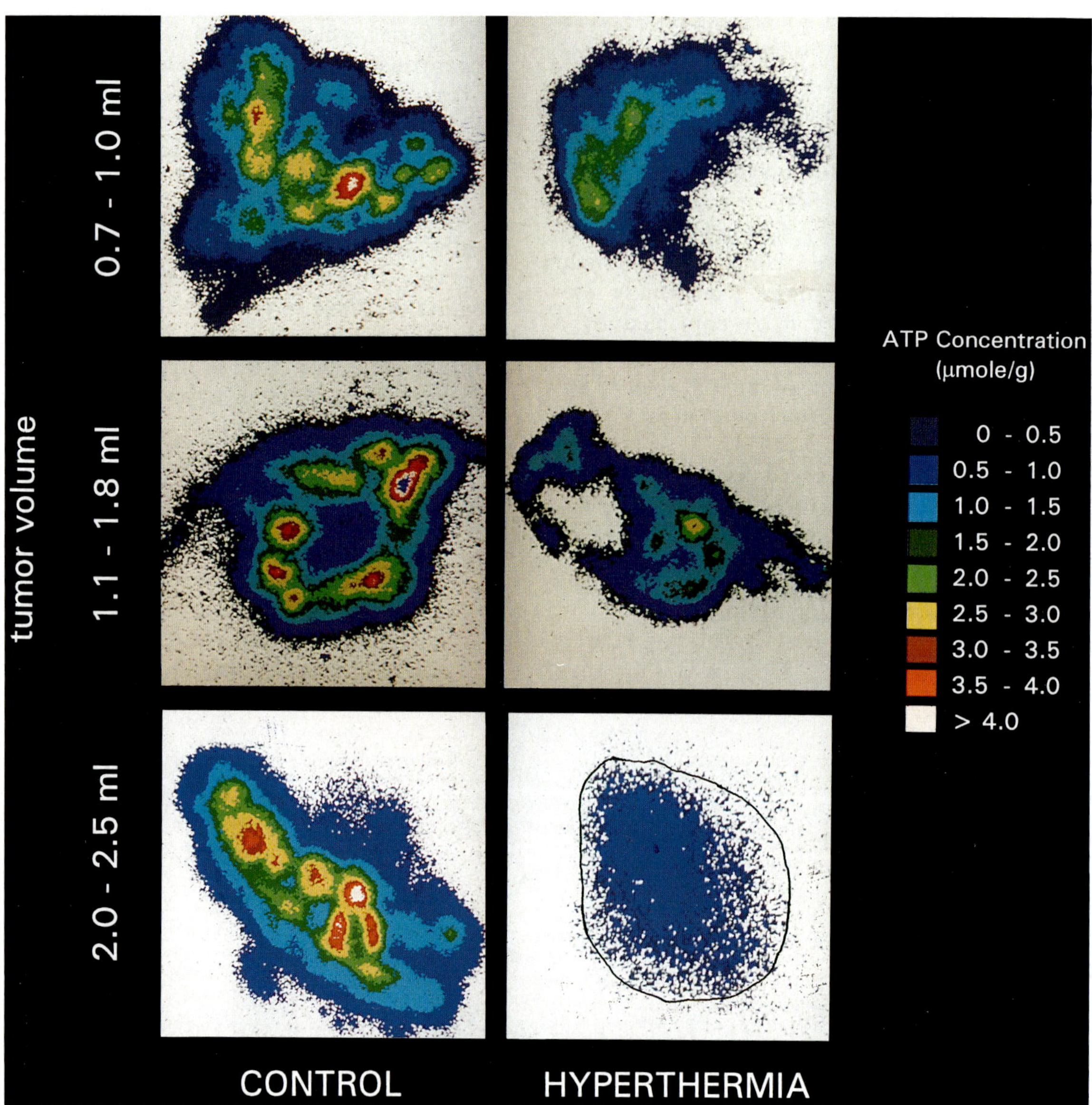

Fig. 8.20. Representative color-coded distributions of ATP concentrations measured in cryosections of sham-treated (*left panels*) and heat-treated (*right panels*) DS-sarcomas of three different volume ranges

levels in control tumors obtained with this technique are approximately 1.0 μmol/g (KRÜGER et al. 1991; DELLIAN et al. 1993; SCHAEFER et al. 1993). Following hyperthermia, an immediate, significant drop is observed in the tumor lines investigated with nadir ATP concentrations 12 h following treatment (DELLIAN et al. 1993). In contrast, in the latter study lowest values of blood flow were measured 3 h after treatment. Thus, no time-dependent correlation between the decrease in blood flow and ATP levels upon hyperthermia could be detected.

Control tumors revealed a wide intertumor variability, with ATP levels falling mainly into the range from 0.1 to 3.5 μmol/g (DELLIAN et al. 1993; SCHAEFER et al. 1993). In DS-sarcomas, ATP concentrations above 2.2 μmol/g could no longer be detected upon heating. The heat-induced decrease in ATP levels was greatest in the larger tumors (Figs. 8.20, 8.21). In amelanotic hamster melanomas (A-Mel-3) no values >1.0 μmol/g could be found following water-bath hyperthermia at 43.3°C for 30 min. In the majority of control tumors a high degree of correlation between the microregional distribution of blood flow and ATP concentration was found. This relationship between these parameters was no longer evident following hyperthermia treatment (DELLIAN et al. 1993). In the latter study, blood flow and ATP levels in normal tissues (muscle, subcutaneous fat, skin) did not change significantly upon heat treatment, indicating that heat treatment can sensitize tumor cells (but not normal tissues) in the sense of a positive feedback.

8.6 Conclusions and Prospective View

Thermal sensitivity has been shown to depend greatly on the efficacy of tumor blood flow and parameters defining the metabolic microenvironment, which is often characterized by hypoxia, acidosis, substrate restriction, accumulation of metabolic waste products, and energy depletion. If recent experimental data are critically evaluated, there is evidence that, besides microcirculatory function, intracellular pH and the bioenergetic status may be *the* decisive factors ultimately modulating the thermosensitivity of cancer cells (Fig. 8.22).

Results recently obtained from *high-flow* experimental tumors and patient malignancies suggest that therapeutically relevant changes in these physiological parameters may be quite different from those seen in fast-growing, *low-flow* rodent tumors upon heat treatment. Thus, biological principles that seem favorable in experimental rodent tumors may not hold in tumors with high perfusion rates or, at least, in well-perfused tumor regions. Further studies on small tumors with high flow rates may advance our knowledge of the pathophysiological mechanisms that may determine and/or modulate the sensitivity of malignant tumors to hyperthermia.

A further understanding of the role of physiological factors may help to identify possible predictors of the heat sensitivity of individual tumors and may help to "fine-tune" (individualize) therapy. This individualization is urgently needed to overcome the pronounced heterogeneity

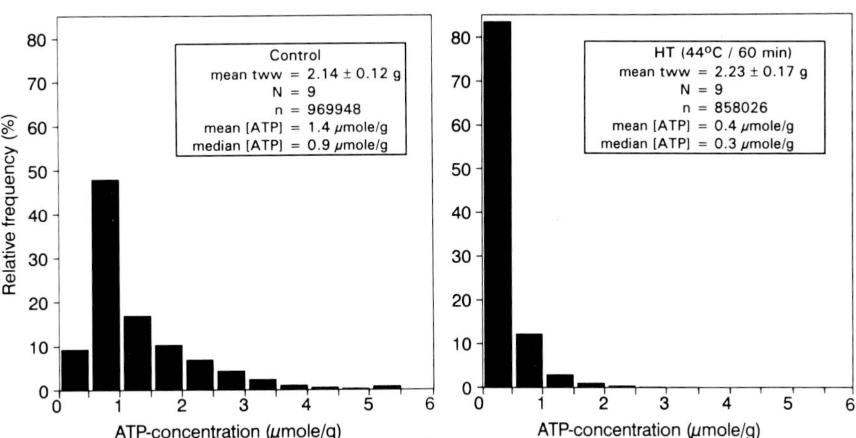

Fig. 8.21. Frequency distributions of ATP concentrations measured by quantitative bioluminescence in sham-treated DS-sarcomas (*left panel*) and immediately following hyperthermia at 44°C for 60 min (*right panel*). *tww*, tumor wet weight; *N*, number of cryosections investigated; *n*, number of pixels evaluated

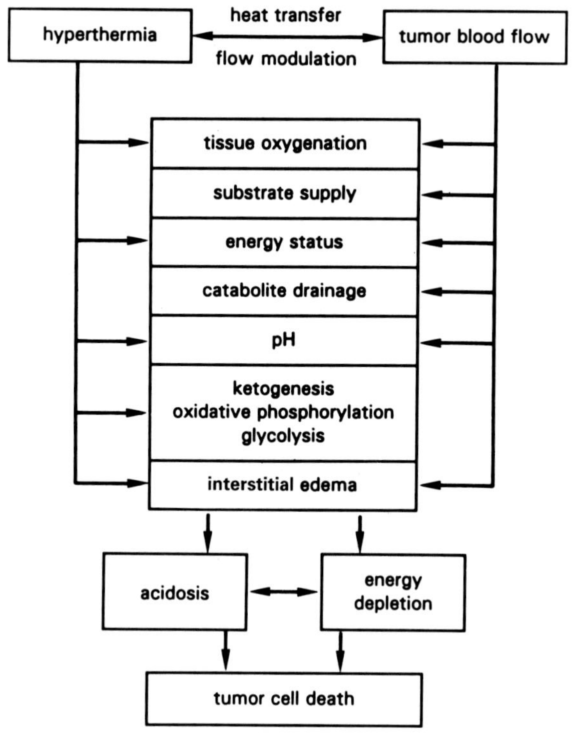

Fig. 8.22. Simplified diagram showing the role of physiological factors in heat-induced tumor cell destruction under in vivo conditions

apparent between tumors even of the same grade and stage. In addition, the substantial heterogeneity occurring within any given solid tumor may lead to a non-uniform response to heat treatment. As a result of this and other properties of tumor tissue, hyperthermia using therapeutically relevant temperatures is likely to be most effective when complementary treatment modalities are combined. Timing and sequencing of the latter needs further critical evaluation in clinically relevant tumor models.

8.7 Summary

- Rates of blood flow in human tumors exhibit pronounced heterogeneity and flow changes upon heating are unpredictable and variable both spatially and temporally. Flow increases in some experimental and human tumors may result in an improved heat dissipation to the extent that therapeutically relevant temperatures may not be achieved.
- Changes in tumor oxygenation tend to reflect changes in blood flow during hyperthermia. An increase in oxygenation followed by a return to baseline levels has been reported for some human and experimental tumors.
- Changes in tumor glucose levels upon hyperthermia vary greatly, but appear to be related to heat-induced changes in blood flow and the development of interstitial edema.
- Lactate levels increase upon hyperthermia due to intensified glycolysis.
- Both intra- and extracellular pH decrease upon hyperthermia. Subsequent recovery to baseline levels seems to depend on the dose of hyperthermia delivered.
- Tumor bioenergetic status worsens during HT, as seen by decreases in ATP and phosphocreatine and increases in inorganic phosphate levels. ATP hydrolysis results in an accumulation of purine catabolites and proton formation, which may in turn contribute to a heat-induced acidosis. Additionally, the formation of active oxygen species may contribute to heat-induced cytotoxicity.
- Microcirculatory function, intracellular pH and bioenergetic status appear to be pivotal factors for the modulation of thermosensitivity in tumors.

References

Anderstam B, Vaca C, Harms-Ringdahl M (1992) Lipid peroxide levels in a murine adenocarcinoma exposed to hyperthermia: the role of glutathione depletion. Radiat Res 132: 296–300

Ausmus PL, Wilke AV, Frazier DL (1992) Effects of hyperthermia on blood flow and cis-diamminedichloroplatinum (II) pharmacokinetics in murine mammary adenocarcinomas. Cancer Res 52: 4965–4968

Bowman HF, Martin GT, Newman WH, Kumar S, Welch C, Bornstein B, Herman TS (1992) Human tumor perfusion measurements during hyperthermia therapy. In: Gerner EW (ed) Hyperthermic oncology 1992, vol 1. Arizona Board of Regents, Tucson, p A17

Busse M, Vaupel P (1994) Accumulation of purine catabolites in rat tumors exposed to hyperthermia. 14th Conf Europ Soc Hyperthermic Oncol, Amsterdam, Book of Abstracts

Dellian M, Walenta S, Kuhnle GEH, Gamarra F, Mueller-Klieser W, Goetz AE (1993) Relation between autoradiographically measured blood flow and ATP concentrations obtained from imaging bioluminescence in tumors following hyperthermia. Int J Cancer 53: 785–791

Dewey WC (1989) The search for critical cellular targets damaged by heat. Radiat Res 120: 191–204

Dewhirst MW, Charles HC, Sostman HD, Leopold KA, Oleson JR (1991) MRI and MRS for prognostic evaluation and therapy monitoring in soft tissue sarcomas treated with hyperthermia and radiotherapy. In: Dewey

WC, Edington M, Fry RJM, Hall EJ, Whitmore GF (eds) Radiation research: a twentieth century perspective, vol II. Academic Press, San Diego, pp 957–961

Gerweck LE (1988) Modifiers of thermal effects: environmental factors. In: Urano M, Douple E (eds) Hyperthermia and oncology, vol I. VSP, Utrecht, pp 83–98

Gerweck LE, Jennings M, Richards B (1980) Influence of pH on the response of cells to single and split dose of hyperthermia. Cancer Res 40: 4019–4024

Gerweck LE, Dahlberg WK, Epstein LF, Shimm D (1984) Influence of nutrient and energy deprivation on cellular response to single and fractionated heat treatments. Radiat Res 99: 573–581

Gerweck LE, Urano M, Koutcher J, Fellenz MP, Kahn J (1989) Relationship between energy status, hypoxic cell fraction, and hyperthermic sensitivity in a murine fibrosarcoma. Radiat Res 117: 448–458

Griffiths JR (1991) Are cancer cells acidic? Br J Cancer 64: 425–427

Hetzel FW, Chopp M (1990) Changes in muscle pH following hyperthermia. Radiat Res 122: 229–233

Hetzel FW, Avery K, Chopp M (1989) Hyperthermic "dose" dependent changes in intralesional pH. Int J Radiat Oncol Biol Phys 16: 183–186

Hetzel FW, Chopp M, Dereski MO (1992) Variations in pO_2 and pH response to hyperthermia: dependence on transplant site and duration of treatment. Radiat Res 131: 152–156

Huch R, Huch A (1985) Transkutaner pO_2. Prinzip, Handhabung, klinische Erfahrung und Grenzen der Methode. In: Ehrly AM, Hauss J, Huch R (eds) Klinische Sauerstoffdruckmessung: Gewebesauerstoffdruck und transkutaner Sauerstoffdruck bei Erwachsenen. Münchner Wissenschaftliche Publikationen, München, pp 53–59

Jain RK, Ward-Hartley K (1984) Tumor blood flow – characterization, modifications, and role in hyperthermia. IEEE Trans Sonics Ultrasonics SU-31: 504–526

Kallinowski F, Vaupel P (1989) Factors governing hyperthermia-induced pH changes in Yoshida sarcoma. Int J Hyperthermia 5: 641–652

Kavanagh BD, Coffey BE, Needham D, Hochmuth RM, Dewhirst MW (1993) The effect of flunarizine on erythrocyte suspension viscosity under conditions of extreme hypoxia, low pH, and lactate treatment. Br J Cancer 67: 734–741

Kelleher DK, Engel T, Vaupel P (1995) Changes in microregional perfusion, oxygenation, ATP and lactate distribution in subcutaneous rat tumours upon water-filtered IR-A hyperthermia. Int J Hyperthermia 11: 241–255

Koutcher JA, Barnett D, Kornblith AB, Cowburn D, Brady TJ, Gerweck LE (1990) Relationship of changes in pH and energy status to hypoxic cell fraction and hyperthermia sensitivity. Int J Radiat Oncol Biol Phys 18: 1429–1435

Krüger W, Mayer WK, Schaefer C, Stohrer M, Vaupel P (1991) Acute changes of systemic parameters in tumour-bearing rats, and of tumour glucose, lactate, and ATP levels upon local hyperthermia and/or hyperglycaemia. J Cancer Res Clin Oncol 117: 409–415

Krüger W, Gersing E, Vaupel P (1993) Electrical impedance spectroscopy (1 Hz–10 MHz) of experimental tumors in vivo upon local hyperthermia. 13th Conf Europ Soc Hyperthermic Oncol, Brüssel, Book of Abstracts

Lammertsma AA, Wilson CB, Jones T (1991) In vivo physiological studies in human tumors using positron emission tomography. Funktionsanalyse biologischer Systeme 20: 319–325

Lin JC, Levitt SH, Song CW (1991) Relationship between vascular thermotolerance and intratumor pH. Int J Radiat Oncol Biol Phys 22: 123–129

Liu FF, Diep K, Hill RP (1992) Intracellular pH regulation and heat sensitivity in vitro. In: Gerner EW (ed) Hyperthermic oncology 1992, vol 1. Arizona Board of Regents, Tucson, p 132

Lyons JC, Kim GE, Song CW (1992) Modification of intracellular pH and thermosensitivity. Radiat Res 129: 79–87

Mayer WK, Stohrer M, Krüger W, Vaupel P (1992) Laser Doppler flux and tissue oxygenation of experimental tumours upon local hyperthermia and/or hyperglycaemia. J Cancer Res Clin Oncol 118: 523–528

Molls M, Feldmann HJ (1991) Clinical investigations of blood flow in malignant tumors of the pelvis and the abdomen in patients undergoing thermoradiotherapy. Funktionsanalyse biologischer Systeme 20: 143–153

Newell K, Tannock I (1991) Regulation of intracellular pH and viability of tumor cells. Funktionsanalyse biologischer Systeme 20: 219–234

Osinsky SP, Bubnovskaja LN, Ganusevich II (1993) Tumor energy status upon induced hyperglycemia and antitumor effect of local hyperthermia. Exp Oncol 15: 60–65

Reinhold HS (1988) Physiological effects of hyperthermia. Recent Results Cancer Res 107: 32–43

Roszinski S, Wiedemann G, Jiang SZ, Baretton G, Wagner T, Weiss C (1991) Effects of hyperthermia and/or hyperglycemia on pH and pO_2 in well oxygenated xenotransplanted human sarcoma. Int J Radiat Oncol Biol Phys 20: 1273–1280

Schaefer C, Mayer WK, Krüger W, Vaupel P (1993) Microregional distributions of glucose, lactate, ATP and tissue pH in experimental tumours upon local hyperthermia and/or hyperglycaemia. J Cancer Res Clin Oncol 119: 599–608

Skibba JL, Quebbeman EJ, Kalbafleisch JH (1986) Nitrogen metabolism and lipid peroxidation during hyperthermic perfusion of human livers with cancer. Cancer Res 46: 6000–6003

Song CW (1984) Effect of hyperthermia on blood flow and microenvironment. Cancer Res (Suppl) 44: 4721s–4730s

Song CW (1991) Tumor blood flow response to heat. Funktionsanalyse biologischer Systeme 20: 123–141

Stohrer M, Fleckenstein W, Vaupel P (1992) Effect of localized hyperthermia on tissue oxygen tension in superficial tumours. In: Ehrly AM, Fleckenstein W, Landgraf M (eds) Clinical oxygen pressure measurement III. Blackwell Wissenschaft, Berlin, pp 121–128

Streffer C (1982) Aspects of biochemical effects by hyperthermia. Natl Cancer Inst Monogr 61: 11–17

Streffer C (1984) Mechanisms of heat injury. In: Overgaard J (ed) Hyperthermic oncology, 1984, vol 2. Taylor and Francis, London, pp 213–222

Streffer C (1988) Aspects of metabolic change after hyperthermia. Recent Results Cancer Res 107: 7–16

Streffer C (1990) Biological basis of thermotherapy. In: Gautherie M (ed) Biological basis of oncologic thermotherapy. Springer, Berlin Heidelberg New York, pp 1–71

Streffer C, van Beuningen D (1987) The biological basis

for tumour therapy by hyperthermia and radiation. Recent Results Cancer Res 104: 24–70

Tannock IF, Rotin D (1989) Acid pH in tumors and its potential for therapeutic exploitation. Cancer Res 49: 4373–4384

Van den Berg AP, Wike-Hooley JL, Broekmeyer-Reurink P, van der Zee J, Reinhold HS (1989) The relationship between the unmodified initial tissue pH of human tumours and the response to combined radiotherapy and local hyperthermia treatment. Eur J Cancer Clin Oncol 25: 73–78

Van den Berg AP, van de Merwe SA, van der Zee J (1991) Prognostic value of tumor tissue pH for tumor response to hyperthermia. In: Dewey WC, Edington M, Fry RJM, Hall EJ, Whitmore GF (eds) Radiation research: a twentieth century perspective, vol II. Academic Press, San Diego, pp 951–956

Van de Merwe S, van den Berg AP, van der Zee J, Reinhold HS (1990) Measurement of tumor pH during microwave induced experimental and clinical hyperthermia with a fiber optic pH measurement system. Int J Radiat Oncol Biol Phys 18: 51–57

Van der Zee J, Broekmeyer-Reurink MP, van den Berg AP, van Geel BN, Jansen RFM, Kroon BBR, van Wjik J, Hagenbeek A (1989) Temperature distribution and pH changes during hyperthermic regional isolation perfusion. Eur J Cancer Clin Oncol 25: 1157–1163

Vaupel P (1990) Pathophysiological mechanisms of hyperthermia in cancer therapy. In: Gautherie M (ed) Biological basis of oncologic thermotherapy. Springer, Berlin Heidelberg New York, pp 73–134

Vaupel P (1992) Physiological properties of malignant tumours. NMR Biomed 5: 220–225

Vaupel PW (1993a) Effects of physiological parameters on tissue response to hyperthermia: new experimental facts and their relevance to clinical problems. In: Gerner EW, Cetas TC (eds) Hyperthermic oncology, 1992, vol 2. Arizona Board of Regents, Tucson, pp 17–23

Vaupel P (1993b) Oxygenation of solid tumors. In: Teicher BA (ed) Drug resistance in oncology. Marcel Dekker, New York, pp 53–85

Vaupel P, Kallinowski F (1987) Physiological effects of hyperthermia. Recent Results Cancer Res 104: 71–109

Vaupel P, Mueller-Klieser W (1983) Interstitieller Raum und Mikromilieu in malignen Tumoren. Mikrozirk Forsch Klin 2: 78–90

Vaupel P, Kallinowski F, Kluge M (1988a) Pathophysiology of tumors in hyperthermia. Recent Results Cancer Res 107: 65–75

Vaupel P, Kluge M, Ambroz MC (1988b) Laser Doppler flowmetry in subepidermal tumours and in normal skin of rats during localized ultrasound hyperthermia. Int J Hyperthermia 4: 307–321

Vaupel P, Kallinowski F, Okunieff P (1989a) Blood flow, oxygen and nutrient supply, and metabolic microenvironment of human tumors: a review. Cancer Res 49: 6449–6465

Vaupel P, Okunieff P, Kallinowski F, Neuringer LJ (1989b) Correlation between ^{31}P-NMR spectroscopy and tissue O_2 tension measurements in a murine fibrosarcoma. Radiat Res 120: 477–493

Vaupel P, Okunieff P, Kluge M (1989c) Response of tumour red blood cell flux to hyperthermia and/or hyperglycaemia. Int J Hyperthermia 5: 199–210

Vaupel P, Okunieff P, Neuringer LJ (1990) In vivo ^{31}P-NMR spectroscopy of murine tumors before and after localized hyperthermia. Int J Hyperthermia 6: 15–31

Vaupel P, Schlenger K, Höckel M (1991) Blood flow and oxygenation of human tumors. Funktionsanalyse biologischer Systeme 20: 165–185

Vaupel P, Kelleher DK, Krüger W (1992) Water-filtered infrared-A radiation: a novel technique to heat superficial tumors. Strahlenther Onkol 168: 633–639

Waterman FM, Tupchong L, Nerlinger RE, Matthews J (1991) Blood flow in human tumors during local hyperthermia. Int J Radiat Oncol Biol Phys 20: 1255–1262

Wiedemann G, Roszinski S, Biersack A, Weiss C, Wagner T (1992) Local hyperthermia enhances cyclophosphamide, ifosfamide and cis-diamminedichloroplatinum cytotoxicity on human-derived breast carcinoma and sarcoma xenografts in nude mice. J Cancer Res Clin Oncol 118: 129–135

Wike-Hooley JL, van der Zee J, van Rhoon GC, van den Berg AP, Reinhold HS (1984) Human tumour pH changes following hyperthermia and radiation therapy. Eur J Cancer Clin Oncol 20: 619–623

Yoshikawa T, Kokura S, Tainaka K, Itani K, Oyamada H, Kaneko T, Naito Y, Kondo M (1993) The role of active oxygen species and lipid peroxidation in the antitumor effect of hyperthermia. Cancer Res 53: 2326–2329

9 Manipulation of Physiological Parameters During Hyperthermia

D.M. PRESCOTT

CONTENTS

9.1 Introduction

Thermal sensitivity of tumors depends on a number of physiological parameters such as tumor pH and metabolic status. Therefore, efforts to improve the efficacy of hyperthermia treatments have led to attempts to manipulate these various physiological factors either directly or indirectly. The parameters most often studied have been tumor pH and tumor blood flow. Tumor blood flow will influence tumor temperatures achieved during the treatment, as well as oxygen and nutrient delivery to the tumor and waste by-product removal from the tumor that can ultimately impact on tumor pH. Thus, manipulation of tumor blood flow can affect many physiological parameters in the tumor. This chapter will cover some of the methods and results used to manipulate these physiological parameters.

Murines with transplantable tumors have been used in the majority of in vivo studies investigating the manipulation of physiological parameters to enhance tumor thermal sensitivity. It is very important to remember the large step necessary to get these experimental techniques which appear to work in rodents into the human cancer clinic. Although spontaneous tumors in privately owned dogs appear to be a useful intermediate animal model between murines and humans, the ultimate validation of the efficacy of any method must be achieved in the human clinic, and information from human studies is currently very limited to nonexistent.

D.M. PRESCOTT, DVM, PhD, Assistant Professor, Department of Radiation Oncology, Duke University Medical Center, P.O. Box 3455, Durham, NC 27710, USA

9.2 Tumor pH

In the mid 1970s, several investigators showed that decreasing extracellular pH enhanced cellular thermal sensitivity and inhibited thermotolerance development for in vitro preparations, particularly for pH values <7.0 (GERWECK and ROTTINGER 1976; GERWECK 1977; NIELSON and OVERGAARD 1979). However, cells allowed to chronically adapt to the acidic extracellular pH are not as sensitive to hyperthermia as cells acutely exposed to low extracellular pH conditions (HAHN and SHIU 1986; CHU and DEWEY 1988; COOK and FOX 1988). Cells chronically exposed to low extracellular pH conditions are able to adjust their intracellular pH back to a normal range (COOK and FOX 1988; CHU et al. 1990; GRIFFITHS 1991). Acute decreases in intracellular rather than extracellular pH are better at enhancing thermal responses (HOFER and MIVECHI 1980; CHU et al. 1990). Therefore, methods to acutely decrease tumor pH, and in particular intracellular pH, immediately before or during hyperthermia treatments have been investigated. These techniques include induction of hyperglycemia, use of various ion channel blockers, and inhibition of mitochondrial respiration. Although partial or complete obstruction of blood flow will also result in acidification of tumors indirectly, this technique will be discussed in Sect. 9.3, addressing tumor blood flow.

9.2.1 Cellular pH Regulation

The major mechanisms by which mammalian cells regulate intracellular pH are: (a) the sodium-hydrogen (Na^+/H^+) exchange system, (b) the Na^+-dependent chloride-bicarbonate (Cl^-/HCO_{3^-}) exchange system, and (c) the Na^+-independent Cl^-/HCO_{3^-} exchange system (for reviews see Roos and Boron 1981; Mahnensmith and Aronson 1985; Tannock and Rotin 1989). The first two mechanisms involve primarily the removal of excess H^+ in acid-loaded cells while the last mechanism participates in decreasing the intracellular pH in alkaline-loaded cells. The Na^+/H^+ exchanger uses the energy of the Na^+ gradient that exists across the cell membrane to transport H^+ out of the cells. The Na^+-dependent Cl^-/HCO_{3^-} exchanger moves HCO_{3^-} into the cell to prevent intracellular pH from severe acidification. The Na^+/H^+ exchange system has been detected in every mammalian cell line examined but the activity of the Na^+-dependent Cl^-/HCO_{3^-} exchanger differs considerably in different cell lines. The Na^+/H^+ exchange system and the Cl^-/HCO_{3^-} exchange system clearly account for almost all the intracellular pH regulating ability in mammalian cells (Roos and Boron 1981).

To acidify intracellular tumor pH, the mechanisms by which a cell regulates its intracellular pH must be overcome. This may sound like an easy task but cells have a tremendous ability to maintain homeostasis (i.e., pH neutrality) in their environment.

9.2.2 Hyperglycemia

Since tumor cells have a high glycolytic capacity, stimulation of glycolysis with glucose administration to increase production of acidic metabolites is one way of reducing pH in the tumor tissue. Therefore, hyperglycemia has been studied extensively to decrease tumor pH. Figure 9.1 is a

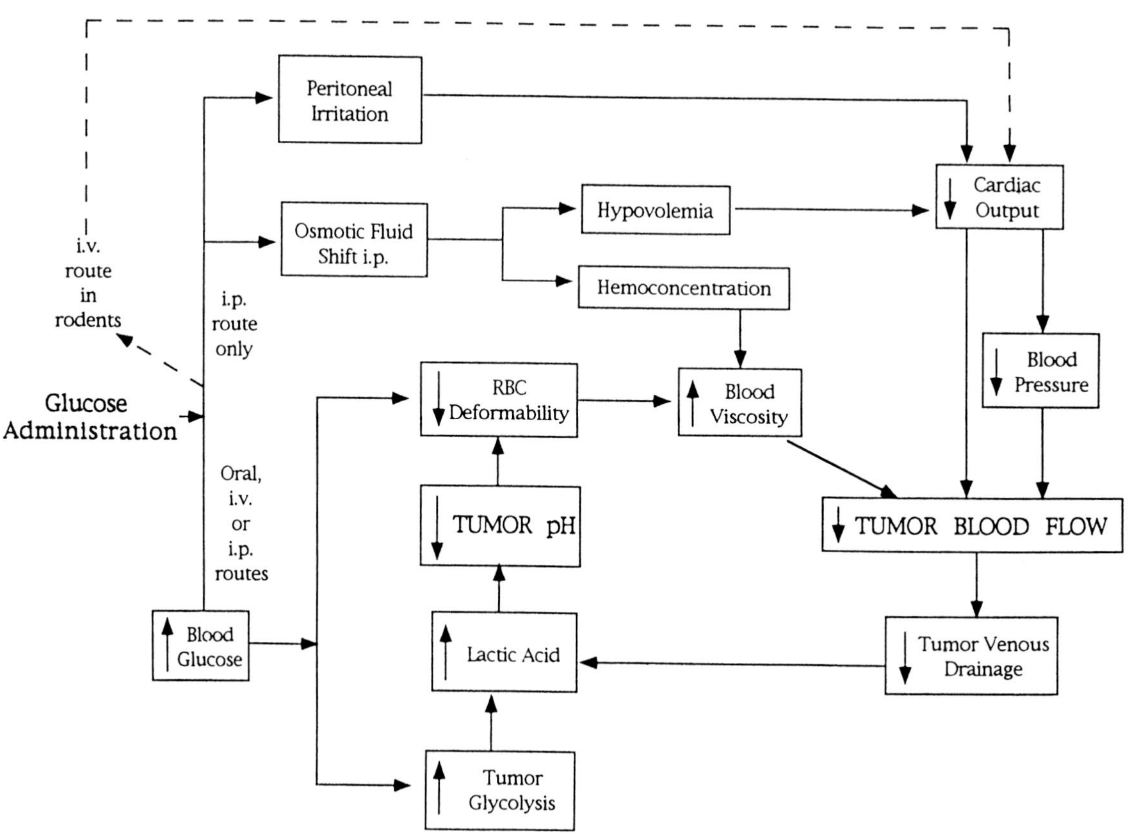

Fig. 9.1. Proposed mechanisms responsible for decreases in tumor blood flow and tumor pH following induction of hyperglycemia. (Modified from Vaupel and Okunieff 1988)

schematic of the various proposed local and systemic mechanisms associated with tumor acidification due to elevated blood glucose levels.

Hyperglycemia has been induced by intraperitoneal (i.p.), intravenous (i.v.), and oral administration of glucose and the effects of induced hyperglycemia on tumor pH have been reviewed elsewhere (WARD and JAIN 1988). The majority of the work using hyperglycemia in vivo has been done in murine systems where glucose leads to significant decreases in tumor pH (ranging from 0.3 to 1.1 pH units) following i.p. or i.v. administration (WARD and JAIN 1988). However, i.p. glucose administration in murines causes significant osmotic water shifts from the extracellular (primarily intravascular) compartment into the peritoneal cavity, resulting in hypovolemic hemoconcentration (VAUPEL and OKUNIEFF 1988). Systemic effects have also been reported following i.v. glucose administration (DIPETTE et al. 1986). Therefore, tumor pH reductions associated with i.p. and i.v. administration of glucose in murines appears to be primarily the result of systemic effects leading to reduction and redistribution of cardiac output (DIPETTE et al. 1986; WARD et al. 1991). Although local mechanisms (Fig. 9.1) were thought to be the primary mode by which high blood glucose levels acidified tumors, it appears, at least in rodents, that systemic effects leading to a decrease in tumor blood flow are the primary mechanism. This has a large impact on the use of hyperglycemia in a clinical situation. Will hyperglycemia induced in a clinically rational way result in tumor acidification similar in magnitude to the changes seen in rodent models?

Intracellular and extracellular tumor pH was measured before and during glucose administration in dogs with spontaneous tumors (PRESCOTT et al. 1993). Hyperglycemia was induced with a bolus injection of 20% glucose (0.6 mg/kg) and maintained with a drip infusion of 20% glucose (0.14–0.27 ml/kg/min) for approximately 90 min. The extracellular and intracellular tumor pH were measured using interstitial pH microelectrodes and phosphorus-31 magnetic resonance spectroscopy (^{31}P-MRS), respectively. Although blood glucose levels were increased to greater than 250 mg/dl in the dogs, no significant change was seen in extracellular (Table 9.1) or intracellular tumor pH (Fig. 9.2).

A 0.6 g/kg bolus of glucose was given i.v. to induce hyperglycemia in the dogs while the majority of studies evaluating the i.v. administration of glucose in rodents used a dose of 5.0–6.0 g/kg (WARD and JAIN 1988). In rodents the rapid blood volume expansion resulting from a bolus injection of this magnitude likely results in deleterious cardiovascular systemic effects. In dogs, the glucose dose did not create any detectable changes in systemic cardiovascular function (i.e., heart rate, blood pressure) (PRESCOTT et al. 1993). Therefore, the difference in cardiovascular effects created by the different doses used in canines and rodents probably accounts for the different response to hyperglycemia in the two species.

In human cancer patients, i.v. glucose infusions have been used to raise and maintain blood glucose levels to 400 mg/dl for 3 h with no side-effects (KRAG et al. 1990). However, attempts to maintain blood glucose levels above 700 mg/dl

Table 9.1. Mean tumor pH_e during normo- and hyperglycemic conditions (from PRESCOTT et al. 1993)

Dog	Treatment	No. of positions measured[a]	Preglucose pH_e mean (± SE)	Glucose pH_e mean (± SE)
BH	Glucose	4/8	7.10 (± 0.02)	7.13 (± 0.03)
BN	Glucose	7/10	7.35 (± 0.01)	7.40 (± 0.02)
OP	Glucose	4/4	7.04 (± 0.03)	7.05 (± 0.02)
PR	Glucose	6/6	6.92 (± 0.02)	6.87 (± 0.02)
SB	Glucose	8/8	7.33 (± 0.04)	7.29 (± 0.02)
ID	Control	5/5	7.18 (± 0.03)	7.21 (± 0.02)
RC	Control	4/4	6.83 (± 0.02)	6.78 (± 0.07)
SS	Control	5/5	7.33 (± 0.01)	7.29 (± 0.02)

pH_e, extracellular pH

[a] Preglucose/glucose conditions

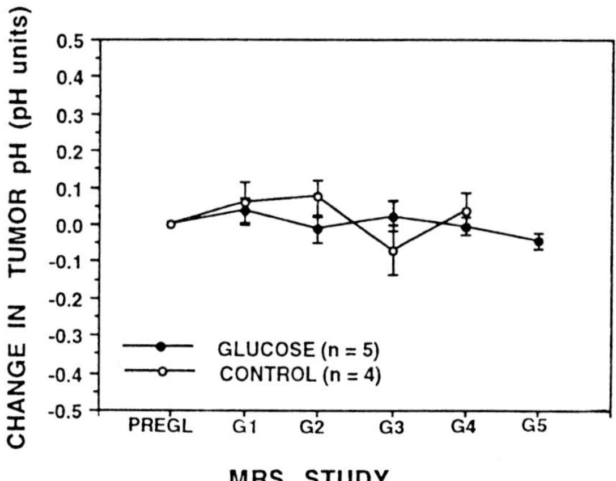

Fig. 9.2. Mean intracellular tumour pH (pH_i) change from baseline values (preglucose pH_i) measured with five consecutive ^{31}P-MRS scans during control and hyperglycemic conditions (glucose pH_i-1 to 5). *PREGL*, baseline values; *G1*, first ^{31}P-MRS scan during hyperglycemia; *G2*, second ^{31}P-MRS scan during hyperglycemia; *G3*, third ^{31}P-MRS scan during hyperglycemia; *G4*, fourth ^{31}P-MRS scan during hyperglycemia; *G5*, fifth ^{31}P-MRS scan during hyperglycemia. (From PRESCOTT et al. 1993)

were unsuccessful in these patients because of a commensurate increase in the urinary glucose excretion.

ASHBY et al. (1966) infused intravenously 100 g glucose to nine patients with malignant melanomas and carcinomas. Tumor pH was measured with a 5-mm electrode. Of these patients, one demonstrated a slight increase in tumor pH while eight developed decreases in tumor pH (range 0.08–0.56 pH units; mean = 0.2 pH units). THISTLETHWAITE et al. (1987) administered 100 g oral glucose to nine patients with metastatic or recurrent tumors and measured tumor pH for 50–80 min with an interstitial electrode. Of these patients, one demonstrated no change in tumor pH, three developed increases in tumor pH (attributed to abnormal glucose responses), and five developed decreases in tumor pH ranging from 0.05 to 0.47 pH units (mean = 0.2 pH units). Although 13 of these 18 patients exhibited a decrease in tumor pH, only eight (44%) had a decreäse of 0.2 pH units or greater. Tumor pH was measured at only one to two tumor sites per patient in these studies. Neither study had a control group.

In a recent study, LEEPER et al. (1994) stratified 25 patients into three groups based on their response to oral glucose (100 g) administration. These groups were: (a) transient hyperglycemic responders (blood glucose rises transiently to a peak value less than 200 mg/dl; $n = 14$ patients), (b) persistently hyperglycemic responders (blood glucose rises and persists above 200 mg/dl; $n = 8$ patients), and (c) hypoglycemic responders (blood glucose it less than 60 mg/dl; $n = 3$ patients). Extracellular tumor pH decreased or remained stable in the transient hyperglycemic population and did not change or increased in the persistent hyperglycemic population. In the transient hyperglycemic group, the greatest decrease in tumor pH occurred when there was the smallest change in blood glucose (Fig. 9.3). Of the 25 patients, only 5 of the 14 (36%) transient hyperglycemic responders had a decrease in extracellular tumor pH of 0.2 pH units or greater. Categorizing patients prior to therapy could increase the likelihood of selecting patients who will exhibit decreases in tumor pH when given oral glucose. Further work needs to be done to further characterize this relationship between oral glucose

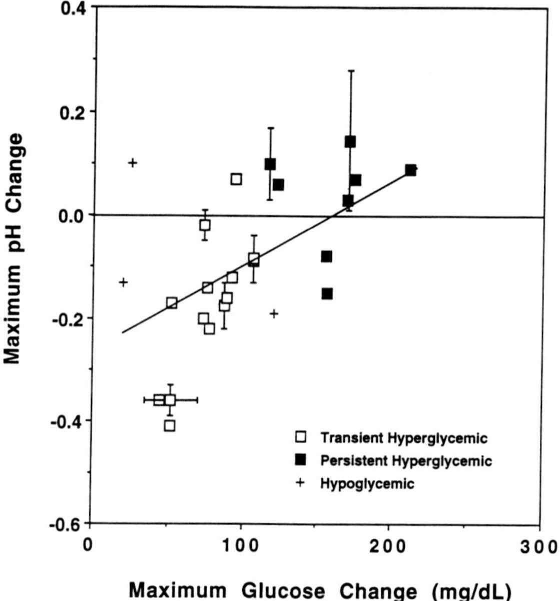

Fig. 9.3. The maximum change in tumor extracellular pH is plotted for a given patient's maximum change in blood glucose. Although some tumor pH responses had not peaked since blood glucose was still rising at the end of observation, sufficient time had elapsed (at least 35–40 min) for an estimate of effect. The line through both transient hyperglycemic and persistent hyperglycemic patients was calculated by least squares, 0.0017 ± 0.0005 pH units/mg/dl ($P < 0.0005$, $r = 0.55$). In seven patients duplicate extracellular pH determinations were averaged. *Vertical error bars* indicate range between pH determinations, and *horizontal error bars* indicate range between blood glucose determinations on separate days (From LEEPER et al. 1994)

response and the effect on extracellular tumor pH.

Are decreases in tumor pH of less than 0.2 pH units clinically significant in human tumors? How will decreases in extracellular tumor pH of 0.2 pH units impact on thermal sensitivity in the human clinic? With these small changes in extracellular tumor pH, will the intracellular tumor pH be maintained at normal values? How much of the tumor develops a decrease in pH? These are some of the questions which are unanswered currently and require further investigation.

9.2.3 Ion Channel Blockers and Related Agents

Amiloride (3,5-diamino-6-chloro-*N*-(diaminomethylene) pyrazine carboxamide) is a diuretic agent known to inhibit the Na^+/H^+ transport protein on the plasma membrane surfaces of mammalian cells (MAHNENSMITH and ARONSON 1985). Because amiloride and Na^+ compete for the external transport site of the exchanger, when Na^+ is at physiological levels, amiloride is not an effective inhibitor of Na^+/H^+ exchange unless relatively high concentrations of the drug are used. However, several analogs of amiloride have been found which are up to 100 times more potent than amiloride in inhibiting Na^+/H^+ exchange (VIGNE et al. 1984; ZHUANG et al. 1984). Since Na^+/H^+ exchange is one of the major mechanisms by which mammalian cells transport hydrogen out of the cells to regulate intracellular pH, manipulation of this ion channel with amiloride and its various analogs has received much attention in recent years.

Other approaches to lowering intracellular pH are the use of DIDS (4,4-diisothiocyanatostilbene-2,2′-disulfonic acid) or B-3(+) (*R*(+)-[(5,6-dichloro, -2,3,9,9a-tetrahydro-3-oxo-9a-propyl-

Table 9.2. Effect of ion channel agents on thermosensitivity and tumor pH

Reference	Cell line	Assay	Agent	Temp. (°C)	Results
HAVEMAN (1979)	M8013S	CSF	C	43	↓ Survival > at pH_e 6.5 than 8.0
HAVEMAN and HAHN (1981)	HA-1	CSF	C	43	↓ Survival > at pH_e 6.5 than 8.0
KIM et al. (1984)	HeLa	CSF	Q	41, 42	↓ Survival: > at pH_e 6.7 than 7.4; > at 42° than 41°C
MIYAKOSHI et al. (1986)	V-79	CSF	A	42	↓ Survival > at pH_e 6.6 than 7.3
RUIFROK and KONINGS (1987)	LM fibroblast	CSF	A	44	↓ Survival: = at pH_e 6.8 and 7.4; > in TT cells than non-TT cells
VARNES et al. (1989)	CHO	CSF	N	42.1	↓ Survival > at pH_e 6.4 than 7.4
KIM et al. (1991)	SCK	CSF	A	42, 43	↓ Survival of thermotolerant cells > at 6.6 pH_e than 7.2; pH_i ↓ approx. 0.1 pH units with drug
LYONS et al. (1992)	SCK	CSF	A, D, N	43	A + D + N: pH_i ↓ by 0.3 and 0.4 pH units at pH_e 7.2 and 6.6, respectively; > thermosensitization at pH_e 6.6 than 7.2; see text for results from other drug combinations
LYONS et al. (1993)	SCK	TGD	A, D	42.5, 43.5	A + D: ↑ TGD 4 days and survival 2.5 days; >effect on hypoxic than oxic cells; ↓ pH_i 0.6 pH units; see text for results with A and D alone
SONG et al. (1993a)	SCK	CSF	E	43	>Thermosensitization and ↓ pH_i at pH_e 6.6 than 7.2; 10 μM E = 500 μM A for ↑ thermosensitization and ↓ pH_i
SONG et al. (1993b)	SCK	CSF	H, B	43	H + B: > thermosensitization at pH_e 6.6 than 7.5; see text for results with H and B alone
SONG et al. (1994)	SCK	TGD	H	42.5, 43, 43.5	↑ TGD 3–4 days; ↓ pH_i in vitro 0.15 and 0.3 pH units at pH_e 7.5 and 6.6, respectively

CSF, clonogenic surviving fraction; TGD, tumor growth delay; C, CCCP; Q, quercetin; A, amiloride; N, nigericin; D, DIDS; E, EIPA; H, HMA; B, B-3(+); TT = thermotolerant; pH_e, extracellular pH; pH_i, intracellular pH

1H-fluoren-7-yl)oxy]acetic acid), both of which inhibit the Cl^-/HCO_3^- exchanger. Nigericin, which is a K^+/H^+ ionophore, carbonyl cyanide *m*-chlorophenylhydrazone (CCCP), which is a H^+ ionophore, and quercetin, which inhibits lactate transport from the cell, are agents which have been explored for their ability to enhance thermal damage. The results with respect to these various ion channel blockers and related agents are summarized below and in Table 9.2.

In studies designed to investigate the mechanisms for hyperthermia-induced cell death, CCCP (10 μM) significantly increased thermosensitivity of normal and tumor cells in vitro (HAVEMAN 1979; HAVEMAN and HAHN 1981). This effect was greater when extracellular pH was 6.5 compared to 8.0. In 1984, KIM et al. reported the effects of quercetin on HeLa cell survival following hyperthermia. KIM et al. used both 41° and 42°C treatments with the cell medium at pH 6.7 and 7.4. Although the potentiating effect of quercetin on thermal-induced cell killing was present at 41°C and pH 7.4, the thermosensitization was far more pronounced at 42°C and pH 6.7 (KIM et al. 1984). VARNES et al. (1989) reported that nigericin enhanced thermal killing of CHO cells preferentially under acidic conditions. Cell survival following 30 min of heating at 42.1°C in the presence of nigericin (1.0 μg/ml) at extracellular pH 7.4, 6.8, 6.6, and 6.4 was 0.6, 0.08, 0.003, and 0.00003, respectively, relative to a survival of 1.0 for control cultures (Fig. 9.4) (VARNES et al. 1989). In the mid 1980s, amiloride was shown to enhance the thermal sensitivity of mammalian cells and to inhibit the development of thermotolerance (MIYAKOSHI et al. 1986; RUIFROK and KONINGS 1987). None of these previous studies measured the intracellular pH of the cells being studied, so the mechanism for the thermal enhancement could only be conjectured. Using SCK tumor cells, KIM et al. recently showed that the effect of amiloride on thermal sensitivity and thermotolerance is due at least partially to decreases in intracellular pH created by amiloride (KIM et al. 1991).

In further in vitro studies, the thermosensitization by amiloride was enhanced by the addition of nigericin and DIDS (Table 9.3) (LYONS et al. 1992). This enhanced thermal sensitization was more pronounced at an extracellular pH of 6.6 rather than 7.2, suggesting that these drugs may preferentially thermosensitize tissues in an acidic environment (i.e., tumor versus normal

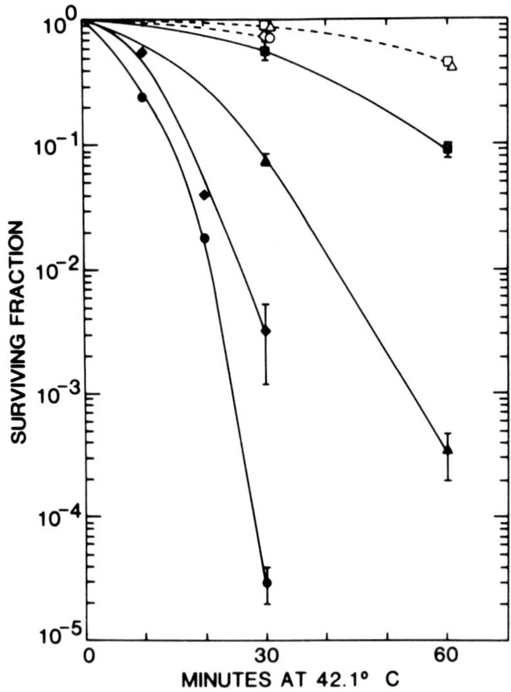

Fig. 9.4. Effect of nigericin on heat sensitivity of CHO cells at various extracellular pH (pH_e) values. Log-phase monolayer cultures were incubated in Hanks' buffered saline solution containing 1.0 mg/ml nigericin during the time of heating and were plated for survival immediately after heating. □, △, ◇, ○: control cells at pH_e 7.4, 6.8, 6.6, and 6.4, respectively; ■, ▲, ◆, ●: nigericin-treated cells at pH_e 7.4, 6.8, 6.6, and 6.4, respectively Values represent averages of duplicate flasks from a representative experiment. (From VARNES et al. 1989)

tissues). Figure 9.5 shows the linear relationship between the thermosensitivity of SCK cells (closed circles: extracellular pH = 6.6; opened circles: extracellular pH = 7.2) and the final intracellular pH achieved after various combinations of amiloride, DIDS, and nigericin (LYONS et al. 1992).

In 1993, LYONS et al. reported the effects of amiloride and DIDS alone and in combination on intracellular pH and thermal sensitivity of SCK tumors grown in vivo. Intracellular pH and energy status of the tumors were measured using ^{31}P MRS. Tumor growth delay curves and cell survival curves from in vivo–in vitro excision assays were used to study the effects on tumor thermal sensitivity. The combination of amiloride (10 mg/kg) and DIDS (25 mg/kg) with hyperthermia (60 min at 43.5°C) resulted in an additional growth delay of approximately 4 days beyond that observed with heat alone. Figure 9.6 shows the effect of hyperthermia with amiloride and DIDS on

Table 9.3. Effects of drugs on sensitivity of SCK cells to heat (from LYONS et al. 1992)

Drug conditions	pH_e 7.2		pH_e 6.6		
	D_0 (min)	DER[a]	D_0 (min)	DER	pH ER[b]
Control	32.6 ± 1.0	–	19.4 ± 0.3	–	1.68
0.5 m*M* amiloride	30.2 ± 1.2	1.08	15.7 ± 0.7	1.22	1.91
0.1 m*M* DIDS	31.2 ± 1.4	1.04	17.4 ± 0.7	1.11	1.79
0.1 μg/ml nigericin	28.7 ± 2.4	1.14	13.0 ± 0.4	1.49	2.21
0.25 μg/ml nigericin	23.2 ± 2.3	1.40	12.0 ± 0.6	1.60	1.91
1.0 μg/ml nigericin	22.9 ± 1.4	1.42	11.8 ± 0.6	1.63	1.93
Amiloride + DIDS	23.6 ± 1.2	1.37	12.1 ± 0.3	1.61	1.97
Amiloride + 0.1 μg/ml nigericin	26.4 ± 1.4	1.23	12.5 ± 0.7	1.55	2.11
Amiloride + 1.0 μg/ml nigericin	19.2 ± 0.7	1.69	9.8 ± 0.2	1.96	1.94
Amiloride + DIDS + 0.1 μg/ml nigericin	20.1 ± 1.6	1.62	11.8 ± 0.5	1.64	1.70
Amiloride + DIDS + 1.0 μg/ml nigericin	16.9 ± 1.3	1.93	7.3 ± 0.3	2.70	2.31

[a] DER (drug enhancement ratio) = D_0 without drug(s)/D_0 with drug(s)
[b] pH ER (pH enhancement ratio) = D_0 at pH 7.2/D_o at pH 6.6

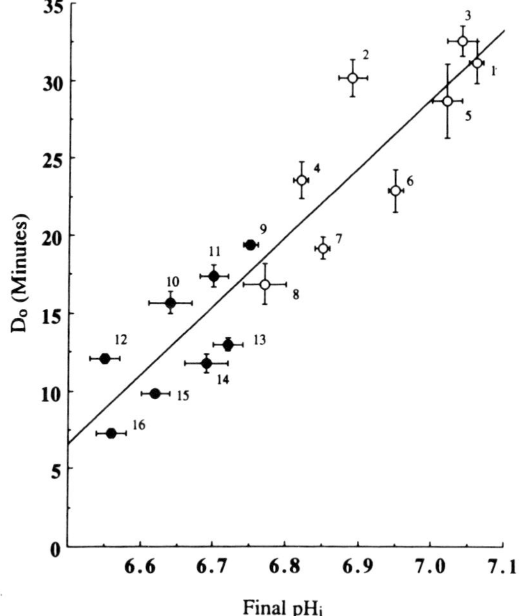

Fig. 9.5. Relationship between thermosensitivity (D_o) and final intracellular pH after heating at 43°C for 120 min. The *open circles* are from experiments performed at extracellular pH 7.2 and the *closed circles* are from experiments performed at extracellular pH 6.6. The *number next to each symbol* indicates the following drug conditions: *1* and *9*, control; *2* and *10*, 0.5 m*M* amiloride; *3* and *11*, 0.1 m*M* DIDS; *4* and *12*, amiloride + DIDS; *5* and *13*, 0.1 mg/ml nigericin; *6* and *14*, 1.0 mg/ml nigericin; *7* and *15*, amiloride + DIDS + 0.1 mg/ml nigericin; *8* and *16*, amiloride + DIDS + 1.0 mg/ml nigericin. (From LYONS et al. 1992)

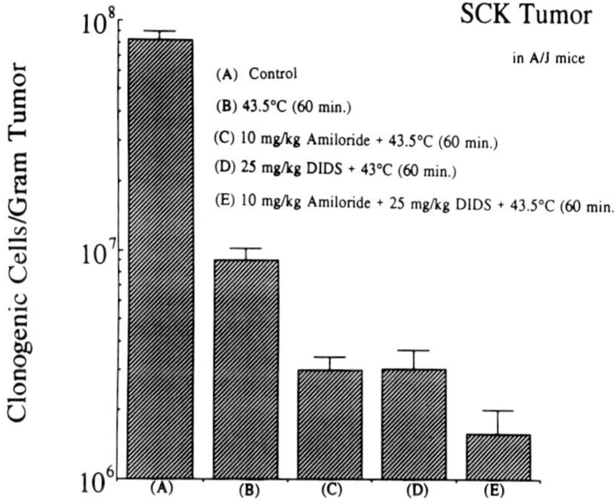

Fig. 9.6. Effect of hyperthermia treatment in combination with 10 mg/kg of amiloride and/or 25 mg/kg of DIDS on the number of clonogenic cells/gram tumor. (From LYONS et al. 1993)

survival of clonogenic cells. The effect of amiloride and DIDS is greater on cells growing in both acidic and hypoxic conditions, as seen in Fig. 9.7. Hyperthermia (42.5°C for 1 h) alone significantly lowered intracellular pH (0.2 pH units) in vivo while the administration of amiloride (10 mg/kg) and DIDS (25 mg/kg) in combination at normothermia did not change intracellular tumor pH from baseline values. However, when amiloride (25 mg/kg) and DIDS (25 mg/kg) were given 1 h before the heat treatment, intracellular pH decreased by 0.6 pH units (LYONS et al. 1993).

Two analogs of amiloride which have been investigated as thermosensitizers are EIPA (3-amino-6-chloro-5-(*N*-ethyl-*N*-isopropylamino)-*N*-(diaminomethylene) pyrazine carboxamide) and HMA (3-amino-6-chloro-5-(1-homopiperidyl)-*N*-(diaminomethylene) pyrazine carboxamide). SONG et al. (1993a,b) have demonstrated that

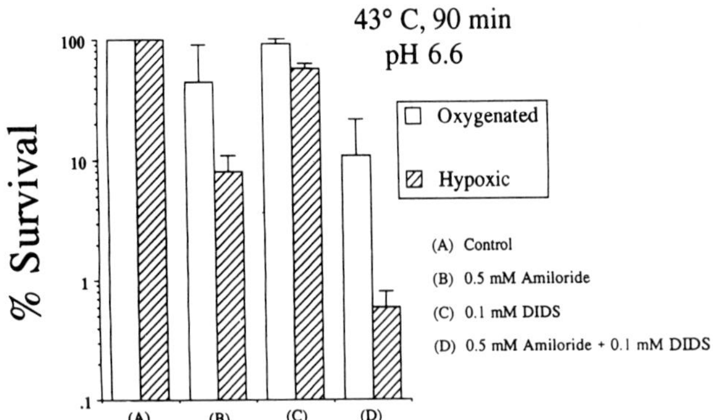

Fig. 9.7. Effect of amiloride and/or DIDS combined with hyperthermia at 43°C for 90 min on SCK cells in vitro under oxygenated and hypoxic conditions. All cell survival data were normalized using the cell survival under oxygenated or hypoxic conditions without drugs as 100%. (From LYONS et al. 1993)

both EIPA and HMA are more powerful than amiloride at increasing the thermosensitivity of SCK tumor cells in vitro and EIPA is more potent than amiloride at decreasing intracellular pH. For both EIPA and HMA, a dose of $10\,\mu M$ was as effective as $500\,\mu M$ amiloride at decreasing intracellular pH and increasing the thermal sensitivity of SCK cells grown in an acidic environment, indicating these analogs are at least 50-fold more potent than amiloride (SONG et al. 1993a,b). Just as the efficacy of amiloride was enhanced when it was used in combination with DIDS (LYONS et al. 1992, 1993), the thermosensitization of HMA was enhanced by an inhibitor of Cl^-/HCO_{3^-} exchange, B-3(+) (SONG et al. 1993b).

Recently, HMA was used to enhance the thermosensitivity of tumors in vivo (SONG et al. 1994). SCK tumors grown subcutaneously in the legs of A/J mice were heated at 42.5° or 43.5°C for 1 h with and without prior administration of HMA. The administration of HMA (0.1 mg/kg, i.v.) 20 min before heating the tumors at 43.5°C increased the tumor growth delay by 4 days as compared with heat alone. Using heat treatments of 42.5°C, HMA administration (1–10 mg/kg) increased the tumor growth delay by approximately 2–2.5 days. Amiloride (5 mg/kg, i.p.) given before heating at 43.5°C increased the tumor growth delay by only 2 days (LYONS et al. 1993). Direct comparison of the tumor thermosensitization of amiloride and HMA in vivo from these two studies is not possible as different routes of drug administration were used.

In vivo data on the use of various ion channel blockers during hyperthermia treatments are very limited. Although the few in vivo studies cited above are promising, as are the in vitro data, more in vivo information is needed. Use of the various drugs described above in clinical trials will depend largely on the safety of their administration to humans. Amiloride is currently used clinically as a diuretic agent in humans at an oral dose of 5–20 mg/day. However, amiloride's more potent analogs, EIPA and HMA, are not approved for use in humans and detailed information on their pharmacokinetics is unavailable. On the other hand, the pharmacokinetics of B-3(+) have been studied extensively and clinical trials are underway to determine the usefulness of B-3(+) in reducing brain edema (CRAGOE 1987).

9.2.4 Other Methods

m-Iodobenzylguanidine (MIBG) is an inhibitor of mitochondrial respiration which has been used to increase the H^+ ion activity in both transplanted rat tumors and human tumor xenografts (JAHDE et al. 1992). MIBG alone reduced the mean pH from 6.90 to 6.70 in a human mesothelioma xenograft 5 h after administration, and when MIBG was combined with a low-dose i.v. glucose infusion (plasma glucose concentration, 14 ± 3 m*M*) the tumor pH was reduced by an addition 0.5 pH units. However, the pH response to MIBG alone in the four tumors investigated was not uniform, with pH shifts of 0.05–0.30 units (mean = 0.2 units). The acidosis induced by MIBG was tumor specific. The usefulness of MIBG during hyperthermia has yet to be demonstrated.

9.3 Tumor Blood Flow

Although decreasing tumor blood flow during hyperthermia is often attempted to decrease heat loss from the tumor and thereby increase tumor temperatures, it can also lead to changes in other physiological parameters such as tumor pH (Fig. 9.1). The effects of hyperglycemia on blood flow in tumor and normal tissues have been reviewed by WARD and JAIN (1991). In rodents, the size of the tumor blood flow reduction is greatly dependent on the route of administration, with the i.p. route leading to greater reductions than the i.v. route (93% vs 72%, respectively: WARD et al. 1991). In dog tumor studies where tumor blood flow measurements were obtained using the laser Doppler flow probe, no significant change was observed during hyperglycemia (PRESCOTT et al. 1993).

9.3.1 Hydralazine

The use of vasoactive agents as a preferred method to decrease tumor blood flow has been discussed previously (JIRTLE 1988). Vasodilatory agents that act upon smooth muscle of normal blood vessel walls are relatively ineffective on tumor vessels because of their lack of smooth muscle (CHAN et al. 1984). Nevertheless, vasodilating agents could manipulate the distribution of blood flow between tumor and normal tissue by selectively dilating normal tissue vessels (VOORHEES and BABBS 1982). Using transplanted transmissible venereal tumors in canines, VOORHEES and BABBS were the first to demonstrate that hydralazine (0.5 mg/kg i.v.) resulted in a decrease in tumor blood flow and an increase in tumor temperatures during hyperthermia. However, because of its prolonged action, the use of hydralazine at this dose in normotensive human patients can lead to side-effects such as postural hypotension, nausea, and headaches. To avoid these potential problems in human cancer patients, lower hydralazine doses (0.125 mg/kg i.v.) were studied in normal dogs. The lower hydralazine dose effectively increased muscle blood flow, but blood pressure effects were not reported (ROEMER et al. 1988).

Recently, Dewhirst et al. evaluated the effect of hydralazine on tumor temperature distributions in both human and canine patients receiving hyperthermia. Hydralazine at 0.125 mg/kg i.v. resulted in a slight reduction in blood pressure in humans but was ineffective in increasing tumor temperatures. In canines, the same dose of hydralazine was effective in reducing blood pressure and increasing median tumor temperature by 0.8°C. In addition, there was a direct relationship between the degree of hypotension and the magnitude of temperature elevation in the tumor (DEWHIRST et al. 1990). Therefore, investigation of other vasodilating agents, such as sodium nitroprusside (Nitropress, Abbott Laboratories, Pharmaceutical Product Division, North Chicago, IL 60064, USA) or calcitonin gene-related peptide, which have shorter half lives and temporally are more controllable, thus avoiding side effects of hydralazine, are currently underway.

9.3.2 Nitroprusside

Sodium nitropursside is an immediate acting hypotensive agent which causes peripheral vasodilation by direct action on vascular smooth muscle (WALKER and GENITON 1989). It is administered as an intravenous infusion (1–10 μg/kg/min) to effect while monitoring arterial blood pressure. When the infusion is stopped, the hypotensive effect resolves within minutes. Although this drug can result in cyanide toxicity with prolonged continuous use, administration of nitroprusside during hyperthermia treatments ranging from 30 to 90 min should not result in toxicities if dosage directions are followed (SCHULZ 1984).

Use of nitroprusside to create controlled reductions in systemic blood pressure with resultant increased tumor temperatures during hyperthermia has been proposed previously by VON ARDENNE and co-workers (VON ARDENNE and KELL 1970; VON ARDENNE and REITNAUER 1980). Recently, PRESCOTT et al. (1992) demonstrated that nitroprusside-induced hypotension (60% of baseline) can be carried out safely and successfully during local hyperthermia in tumor-bearing dogs. Figure 9.8 shows a significant increase in the tumor temperature distribution when nitroprusside was used during hyperthermia. The average tumor temperature increased by 1.6°C while the minimum tumor temperatures increased by an average of 0.9°C (Table 9.4). Although the maximum normal tissue temperatures increased significantly as well, no toxicities were noted in these dogs (PRESCOTT et al. 1992). These initial results on use of nitropursside to manipulate tumor temperatures during local hyperthermia appear very promising but further work needs to be done before use of nitroprusside during local hyperthermia is attempted in human patients.

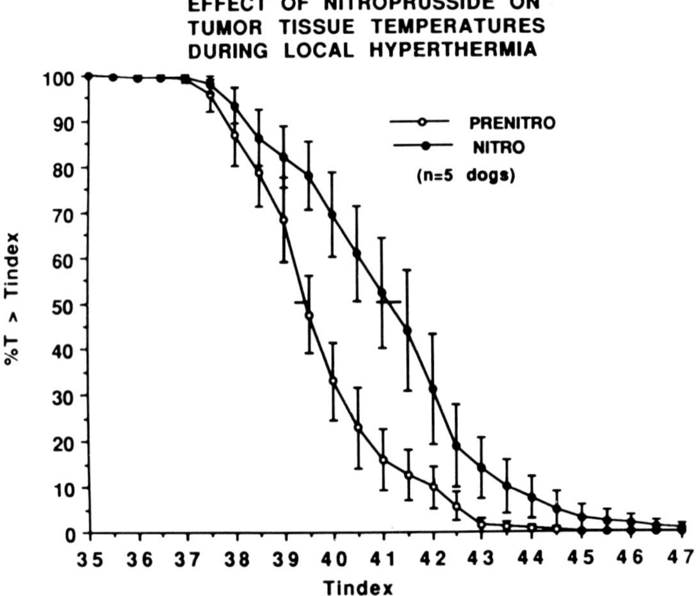

Fig. 9.8. Mean integral temperature distribution for tumor tissue during the prenitroprusside (○) and nitroprusside (●) periods in five tumor-bearing dogs. The *horizontal bars* are standard error of the mean for the estimated median temperatures (T_{50}). *Vertical error bars* are standard error of the mean %T > T_{index} (From PRESCOTT et al. 1992)

Table 9.4. Mean change in T% descriptors due to nitroprusside (from PRESCOTT et al. 1992)

T%	Tumor tissue		Normal tissue	
	ΔT mean ± SE	*P* value	ΔT mean ± SE	*P* value
T_{10}	1.8 ± 0.2	0.001	1.8 ± 0.6	0.045
T_{50}	1.6 ± 0.3	0.009	1.2 ± 0.7	0.164
T_{90}	0.9 ± 0.4	0.114	0.4 ± 0.2	0.118

9.3.3 Other Methods

Calcitonin gene-related peptide is an endogenous neuropeptide which is the most potent vasodilator described in man (STRUTHERS et al. 1986). In humans the plasma and biological half-life of calcitonin gene-related peptide are 9 min and 19 min, respectively (BURNEY et al. 1991). Using phosphorus MRS, BURNEY et al. (1991) evaluated the effects of calcitonin gene-related peptide on mean arterial pressure and tumor bioenergetics. Calcitonin gene-related peptide was given intravenously in rats with a transplanted fibrosarcoma in the flank. As the dose of calcitonin gene-related peptide increased from 300 to 2000 pmol, mean arterial pressure decreased and the ratio of tumor inorganic phosphorus to total phosphorus content increased. The changes in the phosphorus spectra indicate decreases in tumor blood flow, although no direct measurements of blood flow were made. When compared to hydralazine, calcitonin gene-related peptide was far more effective at decreasing tumor blood flow, as measured by changes in tumor bioenergetics, at clinically acceptable reductions in blood pressure. In later studies, a continuous infusion of calcitonin gene-related peptide resulted in a blood flow reduction to 30% of baseline with only a 15%–20% decrease in systemic blood pressure (FIELD et al. 1994).

9.4 Summary

Manipulation of tumor pH and tumor blood flow during hyperthermia should enhance tumor thermosensitivity in human patients. Below are some major points summarized regarding physiologic manipulations which have been emphasized in this chapter:

- Tumor pH and tumor blood flow are the physiologic parameters most often manipulated in an attempt to enhance thermal sensitivity.
- The majority of in vivo studies investigating the manipulation of tumor physiology have

been done in murines with transplantable tumors.
- Cells chronically exposed to low extracellular pH conditions are able to adjust their intracellular pH back to a normal range and acute decreases in intracellular pH are better at enhancing thermal responses than acute decreases in extracellular pH.
- Tumor pH reductions associated with i.p. and i.v. administration of glucose in murines appears to be primarily the result of systemic effects leading to reduction and redistribution of cardiac output.
- Although oral glucose reduces extracellular tumor pH by ⩾0.2 pH units in a subpopulation of human patients, the effect of this treatment on intracellular pH has not been documented.
- Several ion channel blockers have been investigated for their effect on thermal response and development of thermotolerance. Recently, amiloride and its more potent analogs, HMA and EIPA, have been shown to enhance thermal sensitivity in vitro and in vivo and is due at least partially to decreases in intracellular pH.
- Combinations of agents which affect different ion channels (such as amiloride and DIDS) enhance thermosensitization more than the single agents alone.
- The enhanced thermal sensitization from the ion channel blockers is more pronounced at an acidic extracellular pH suggesting that these drugs may preferentially thermosensitize tumor versus normal tissue.
- Several vasoactive agents have been used to decrease tumor blood flow and increase temperatures during hyperthermia. However, the magnitude of tumor temperature elevation appears to be directly related to the degree of hypotension induced by some vasoactive agents such as hydralazine or nitroprusside.
- Newer vasoactive agents such as calcitonin gene-related peptide may effectively increase tumor temperatures during hyperthermia with clinically acceptable reductions in blood pressure.
- The ultimate validation of any tumor physiologic manipulation must be obtained in human patients.

Extending these manipulation studies into the human clinic is necessary but very difficult. Many of the drugs discussed in this chapter are not approved for use in humans. Extrapolating drug dosages from rodents to humans is complicated. Will the effects observed in rodents be seen in humans when safe drug doses are given? Will tumor heterogeneity complicate the therapeutic efficacy of these perturbations in the human clinic? Will nonuniform temperature distributions during hyperthermia treatments in human patients impact on the results of these perturbations? Will normal tissues be spared from enhanced thermal damage when these techniques are used? These are just a few of the quesions which can be asked when these techniques are moved into the human clinic.

References

Ashby BS (1966) pH studies in human malignant tumors. Lancet II: 312–315

Burney IA, Maxwell RJ, Griffiths JR, Field SB (1991) The potential for prazosin and calcitonin gene-related peptide (CGRP) in causing hypoxia in tumours. Br J Cancer 64: 683–688

Chan RC, Babbs CF, Vetter RJ, Lamar CH (1984) Abnormal response of tumor vasculature to vasoactive drugs. J Natl Cancer Inst 72: 145–150

Chu GL, Dewey WC (1988) The role of low intracellular pH or extracellular pH in sensitization to hyperthermia. Radiat Res 114: 154–167

Chu GL, Wang Z, Hyun WC, Pershadshigh HA, Fulwyler JJ, Dewey WC (1990) The role of intracellular pH and its variance in low pH sensitization of killing by hyperthermia. Radiat Res 122: 288–293

Cook JA, Fox MH (1988) Effects of chronic pH 6.6 on growth, intracellular pH, and response to 42.0°C hyperthermia of Chinese Hamster Ovary cells. Cancer Res 48: 2417–2420

Cragoe EJ Jr (1987) Drugs for the treatment of traumatic brain injury. Med Res Rev 7: 271–305

Dewhirst MW, Prescott DM, Clegg S et al. (1990) The use of hydralazine to manipulate tumor temperatures during hyperthermia. Int J Hyperthermia 6: 971–983

Dipette DJ, Ward-Hartley KA, Jain RK (1986) Effect of glucose on systemic hemodynamics and blood flow rate in normal and tumor tissues in rats. Cancer Res 46: 6299–6304

Field SB, Burney IA, Needham S, Maxwell RJ, Griffiths JR (1994) From hydralazine to CGRP to man? Int J Hyperthermia 10: 451–455

Hahn GM, Shiu EC (1986) Adaptation to low pH modifies thermal and thermochemical responses to mammalian cells. Int J Hyperthermia 2: 379–387

Haveman J (1979) The pH of the cytoplasm as an important factor in the survival of in vitro cultured malignant cells after hyperthermia. Effects of carbonylcyanide 3-chlorophenylhydrazone. Eur J Cancer 15: 1281–1288

Haveman J, Hahn GM (1981) The role of energy in hyperthermia-induced mammalian cell inactivation: a study of the effects of glucose starvation and an un-

coupler of oxidative phosphorylation. J Cell Physiol 107: 237–241
Hofer KG, Mivechi NF (1980) Tumor cell sensitivity to hyperthermia as a function of extracellular and intracellular pH. J Natl Cancer Inst 65: 621–625
Gerweck LE (1977) Modification of cell lethalilty at elevated temperatures: the pH effect. Radiat Res 70: 224–235
Gerweck LE, Rottinger E (1976) Enhancement of mammalian cell sensitivity to hyperthermia by pH alteration. Radiat Res 67: 508–511
Griffiths JR (1991) Are cancer cells acidic? Br J Cancer 64: 425–427
Jahde E, Volk T, Atema A, Smets LA, Glusenkamp KH, Rajewsky MF (1992) pH in human tumor xenografts and transplanted rat tumors: effect of insulin, inorganic phosphate, and *m*-iodobenzylguanidine. Cancer Res 52: 6209–6215
Jirtle RL (1988) Chemical modification of tumour blood flow. Int J Hyperthermia 4: 355–371
Kim JH, Kim SH, Alfievi AA, Young CW (1984) Quercetin, an inhibitor of lactate transport and a hyperthermic sensitizer of HeLa cells. Cancer Res 44: 102–106
Kim GE, Lyons JC, Song CW (1991) Effects of amiloride on intracellular pH and thermosensitivity. Int J Radiat Oncol Biol Phys 20: 541–549
Krag DN, Storm FK, Morton DL (1990) Induction of transient hyperglycaemia in cancer patients. Int J Hyperthermia 6: 741–744
Leeper DB, Engin K, Thistlethwaite AJ, Hitchon HD, Dover JD, Li D-J, Tupchong L (1994) Human tumor extracellular pH as a function of blood glucose concentration. Int J Radiat Oncol Biol Phys 28: 935–943
Lyons JC, Kim GE, Song CW (1992) Modification of intracellular pH and thermosensitivity. Radiat Res 129: 79–87
Lyons JC, Ross BD, Song CW (1993) Enhancement of hyperthermia effect in vivo by amiloride and DIDS. Int J Radiat Oncol Biol Phys 25: 95–103
Mahnensmith RL, Aronson PS (1985) The plasma membrane sodium-hydrogen exchange and its role in physiological and pathophysiological processes. Circ Res 56: 773–788
Miyakoshi J, Oda W, Hirata M, Fukuhori N, Inagaki C (1986) Effects of amiloride on thermosensitivity of Chinese hamster cells under neutral and acidic pH. Cancer Res 46: 1840–1843
Nielson OS, Overgaard J (1979) Effect of extracellular pH on thermotolerance and recovery of hyperthermic damage in vitro. Cancer Res 39: 2772–2778
Prescott DM, Samulski TV, Dewhirst MW, Page RL, Thrall DE, Dodge RK, Oleson JR (1992) Use of nitroprusside to increase tissue temperature during local hyperthermia in normal and tumor-bearing dogs. Int J Radiat Oncol Biol Phys 23: 377–385
Prescott DM, Charles HC, Sostman HD et al. (1993) Manipulation of intra- and extracellular pH in spontaneous canine tumours by use of hyperglycaemia. Int J Hyperthermia 9: 745–754
Roemer RB, Forsyth K, Oleson JR, Clegg ST, Sim DA (1988) The effect of hydralazine dose on blood perfusion changes during hyperthermia. Int J Hyperthermia 4: 401–415
Roos A, Boron WF (1981) Intracellular pH. Physiol Rev 61: 296–434
Ruifrok ACC, Konings AWT (1987) Effects of amiloride on hyperthermic cell killing of normal and thermotolerant mouse fibroblast LM cells. Int J Radiat Biol 52: 385–392
Schulz V (1984) Clinical pharmacokinetics of nitroprusside, cyanide, thiosulphate, and thiocyanate. Clin Pharmacokinet 9: 239–251
Song CW, Lyons JC, Griffin RJ, Makepeace CM (1993a) Thermosensitization by lowering intracellular pH with EIPA. Radiother Oncol 27: 252–258
Song CW, Lyons JC, Griffin RJ, Makepeace CM, Cragoe EJ Jr (1993b) Increase in thermosensitivity of tumor cells by lowering intracellular pH. Cancer Res 53: 1599–1601
Song CW, Lyons JC, Makepeace CM, Griffin RJ, Cragoe EJ Jr (1994) Effects of HMA, an analog of amiloride, on the thermosensitivity of tumors in vivo. Int J Radiat Oncol Biol Phys 30: 133–139
Struthers AD, Brown MJ, MacDonald DWR, Beacham JL, Stevenson JC, Morris HR, MacIntyre I (1986) Human calcitonin gene related peptide: a potent endogenous vasodilator in man. Clin Sci 70: 389–393
Tannock IF, Rotin D (1989) Acid pH in tumors and its potential for therapeutic exploitation. Cancer Res 49: 4373–4384
Thistlethwaite AJ, Alexander GA, Moylan DJ, Leeper DB (1987) Modification of human tumor pH by elevation of blood glucose. Int J Radiate Oncol Biol Phys 13: 603–610
Varnes ME, Glazier KG, Gray C (1989) pH-dependent effects of the ionophore nigericin on response of mammalian cells to radiation and heat treatment. Radiat Res 117: 282–292
Vaupel PW, Okunieff PG (1988) Role of hypovolemic hemoconcentration in dose-dependent flow decline observed in murine tumors after intraperitoneal administration of glucose or mannitol. Cancer Res 48: 7102–7106
Vigne P, Felin C, Audinot M, Borsotto M, Cragoe EJ Jr, Lazdunski M (1984) [^{3}H]Ethylpropylamiloride, a radiolabelled diuretic for the analysis of the Na^+/H^+ exchange system. Its use with kidney cell membranes. EMBO J 3: 2647–2651
von Ardenne M, Kell E (1979) Berechnung des dynamischen Aufheizprozesses in mehrschichtigen Modellgeweben bei Lokalhyperthermie nach dem CMT-Selectotherm-Verfahren. Arch Geschwulstforsch 49: 590–612
von Ardenne M, Reitnauer PG (1980) Selective occlusion of cancer tissue capillaries as the central mechanism of the cancer multistep therapy. Jpn J Clin Oncol 10: 31–48
Voorhees WD, Babbs CF (1982) Hydralazine-enhanced selective heating of transmissible venereal tumor implants in dogs. Eur J Cancer Clin Oncol 18: 1027–1034
Walker HJ, Geniton DJ (1989) Vasodilator therapy and the anesthetist: a review of nitroprusside, labetalol, hydralazine and nitroglycerin. J Am Assoc Nurse Anesthetists 57: 435–444
Ward KA, Jain PK (1988) Response of tumours to hyperglycaemia: characterization, significance and role in hyperthermia. Int J Hyperthermia 4: 223–250
Ward KA, Jain RK (1991) Blood flow response to hyperglycemia. In: Vaupel P, Jain RK (eds) Tumor blood supply and metabolic microenvironment: characterization and implications for therapy. Gustav Fischer, Stuttgart, pp 87–107

Ward KA, Dipette DJ, Held TN, Jain RK (1991) Effect of i.v. versus i.p. glucose injection on systemic hemodynamics and blood flow rate in normal and tumor tissue in rats. Cancer Res 51: 3612–3616

Zhuang YX, Cragoe EJ Jr, Glaser JS, Cassel D (1984) Characterization of potent Na^+/H^+ exchange inhibitors from the amiloride series in A431 cells. Biochemistry 23: 4481–4488

Physical Principles and Engineering

10 Electromagnetic Superficial Heating Technology

E.R. LEE

CONTENTS

10.1 Clinical Requirements

The clinical studies done on superficial depth malignancies during the last two decades have highlighted the promise of hyperthermia as an effectively adjuvant treatment modality (KAPP and KAPP 1993), as well as the need to improve the ability of heating devices to treat effectively the anatomically diverse diseased tissue sites encountered in clinical practice.

Increasing the surface area that the devices are able to heat was found to be necessary. While some cancers are confined to small localized nodules, metastatic breast cancer can involve superficial depth regions encompassing the entire upper torso, including the arms and the head and neck. In addition, mathematical simulations have shown that in order to uniformly heat even small tumors, if the local blood perfusion rate is high it may be necessary to preheat the inflowing blood at and beyond the tumor margins. If verified by clinical testing, this may require large area heating patterns even for small tumor nodules.

Tumor-bearing tissue regions can also be highly heterogeneous both electrically and thermally, requiring that applicators have the ability to locally alter their power deposition pattern in real time in order to produce uniform temperatures. Compound curvature of the surface areas to be treated must also be accommodated, especially in the head and neck, and in axillary regions in movement-impaired patients.

Patient tolerance of the treatment and thermometry procedures also introduces heating system design constraints. Hyperthermia treatments usually involve heating intervals on the order of an hour, during which the applicator must remain accurately positioned on the patient. Because few patients can remain totally immobile for this period, the applicator system should not be excessively sensitive to patient movements.

The limitations of current clinical thermometry systems must be accounted for in the design of applicator power control procedures. No commercially available high-resolution noninvasive thermometry devices exist at this time. Both setup time constraints and patient tolerance preclude large numbers of invasive catheter insertions into the areas to be treated.

Applicator designers have attempted to meet these challenges with a new generation of highly refined basic radiating elements as well as their integration into mechanically scanned, conformal array, and phased array heating devices. Site-specific applicators have been developed to heat sensitive or highly contoured body regions. This chapter is intended as a brief survey of the current state of electromagnetic superficial depth applicator development as well as a review of the current unsolved engineering and clinical problems.

E.R. LEE, BSEE, Physical Science Research, SLAC-Mail Stop 61, Stanford, CA 94305, USA

10.2 Electromagnetic Properties of Biological Tissue

The physical mechanisms responsible for the heating of biological tissue by electromagnetic waves have been dealt with extensively in previous literature (JOHNSON and GUY 1972; FOSTER and SCHEPPS 1981; DURNEY et al. 1986; HAND 1990; ISKANDAR 1982). Only a summary will be presented here of the results relevant to the design of hyperthermia applicators. The important tissue parameters for the design of electromagnetic heating devices are the measured tissue dielectric constants and conductivities. A summary of these tissue parameters is given in Table 10.1.

The dielectric constant of the tissue determines the coefficient of reflection at tissue interfaces and the wavelength in tissue of the electromagnetic waves utilized for heating. The wavelength in tissue is important in that it determines the spatial resolution of the power control possible by manipulations of the applicator's amplitude or phase. The ratio of wavelength in tissue to applicator aperture size can also affect the depth of heating of a given antenna design independent of operating frequency effects. Effective penetration depth was found to be compromised if the lateral dimension of the radiating aperture is less than one to two wavelengths in tissue (GUY 1971b; HAND and HIND 1986). The maximum (plane wave) penetration depth is calculable from the measured real and complex permittivities (Table 10.1). The attenuation mechanism in tissue is from ohmic losses resulting from the conduction of free charges or ions, as well as from the rotation of polar molecules at the frequency of the applied electric field (E Field). This molecular rotation or ionic motion is converted to heat due to the viscous losses in the dielectric. The strong dependence on frequency below 150 MHz arises from the dispersion associated with the intracellular membrane capacitance. The slight increase in attenuation with frequency from 200 MHz to 1 GHz is due to the progressive excitation of different polar intracellular macromolecules. There is a strong dispersion past 2 GHz associated with the excitation of molecular H_2O. The current consensus among applicator designers is to utilize frequencies below 1 GHz except for devices intended to treat very specialized sites (GUY and LEHMANN 1966; TURNER 1983; GUY 1990).

Note from Fig. 10.1 that in the frequency range most often used for superficial depth hyperthermia, 300 MHz to 1 GHz, the effective penetration depth changes by only 20%. The wavelength in tissue, however, changes by a factor of 3. Stationary single-aperture applicators are often designed to operate at the lowest practical frequency to maximize penetration depth. In designing array and mechanically scanned applicators capable of local alterations in deposited power one must consider that small tissue regions such as scars can preferentially heat and act as power-limiting points. Operating at low frequencies, which enhances penetration depth, forces one to accept having large wavelengths, which results in very poor spatial resolution in the applicator's power control. Utilizing an applicator array with a very low operating frequency may result in a small high-conductivity or low-perfusion spot (i.e., scar), forcing the power down to subtherapeutic levels over very large surface areas. Since maximizing depth of penetration requires decreasing the operating frequency and maximizing spatial resolution requires increasing the operating frequency, it is clear that the choice of operating frequency is a compromise with optimization being dependent upon the degree of tissue heterogeneity in the treated regions. The weak dependence of penetration depth on changes in frequency between 300 MHz and 1 GHz would probably make operation at

Table 10.1. Dielectric properties of biological tissue (data from JOHNSON and GUY 1972)

Frequency (MHz)	ε'	ε''	Conductivity (S/W)	−3 dB penetration depth (cm)
a) Electrical characteristics of high water content tissue				
27	113	399	0.602	5.0
100	72	159	0.885	2.3
200	57	90	1.00	1.7
300	54	69	1.15	1.3
433	53	49	1.18	1.2
915	51	25	1.28	1.1
2450	47	16	2.17	0.6
b) Electrical characteristics of low water content tissue				
27	20	7.2–28.6	10.9–43.2	55
100	7.5	3.4–13.6	19.1–75.9	21
200	6.0	2.3–8.5	25.8–94.2	14
300	5.7	1.9–6.4	31.6–107	11
433	5.6	1.6–4.9	37.9–118	9.1
915	5.6	1.1–2.9	55.6–147	6.1
2450	5.5	0.7–1.6	96.4–213	3.9

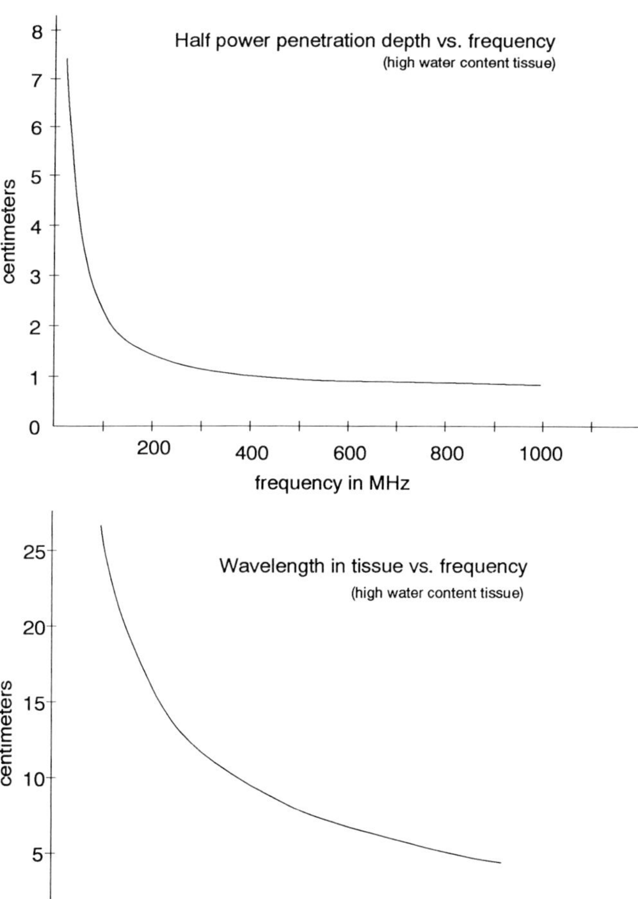

Fig. 10.1. Plane wave penetration depth and wavelength in muscle, skin, and other high water content tissues. (Data from JOHNSON and GUY 1972)

higher frequencies more likely to optimize this spatial resolution versus penetration trade-off.

Tissue heterogeneity, in addition to affecting what temperatures are produced by a given SAR distribution, can also act to directly alter the qualitative shape of an applicator's power deposition pattern in tissue. Specific examples of changes which can occur in an applicator's power deposition pattern with changes in fat thickness, frequency, E-field orientation, and bolus type are given in SCOTT et al. (1986), CHOU et al. (1990a,b), and CHOU (1992). The most dramatic results in these studies of commercial waveguide applicators showed that small changes in the thickness of an overlying fat layer can cause a frequency-dependent shift from a centrally peaked distribution of power in tissue to a heating pattern with dual hot spots at the applicator edge. Tests in layered inhomogeneous cylindrical phantoms showed hot spot production at interfaces at depth that varied in relative magnitude with each other with changes in E-field orientation. Different applicators were shown to have different changes in their heating patterns with changes in the geometry and composition of the heating target. The thermometry probes placed in the heating field have also been shown to alter applicator power deposition patterns (CHAN et al. 1988).

10.3 A Survey of Major Antenna Types

The 300-MHz to 1-GHz frequency range over which most superficial depth hyperthermia applicators operate is normally defined as being in the VHF/UHF portion of the electromagnetic spectrum. The biological tissues into which hyperthermia applicators radiate have a dielectric constant in the range of 5–60 which reduces the wavelength such that antennas and techniques more typically utilized in microwave engineering are employed, hence the common reference to superficial EM applicators as microwave devices despite the actual frequency of operation.

10.3.1 Waveguides

The design theory for waveguide applicators is well established and will not be repeated in detail here. As a short summary of the general characteristics of waveguide hyperthermia applicators, this class of radiator is constructed from a section of a hollow rectangular or circular waveguide transmission line, open at one end, excited with a coupling antenna consisting of a loop or a linear short extension of the coax feed line into the cavity. The distance from the feed point to the closed end of the waveguide is chosen to optimize the impedance match of the coupling antenna. The minimum physical dimensions of these waveguide applicators are constrained by operation in the TEM 1,0 mode, with dielectric loading and the placement of ridges in the cavity utilized to reduce the dimensions of the applicator so that physical placement of the applicator on a patient is more clinically practical. The output power deposition pattern has a theoretical $\cos^2$ cross-section for a uniformly loaded waveguide cavity. Waveguide applicators in general have the advantage over other radiator types in more easily producing high ratios of parallel versus perpendicular E fields near the radiating aperture.

Proper bolusing or air gap spacing is still required. Tests of experimental and commercial designs for waveguide hyperthermia applicators used in direct contact with tissue or phantom have been found to produce localized hot spots near the edges of the aperture (GUY 1971a,b; SCOTT et al. 1986; CHOU et al. 1990a).

Waveguide applicators have been the most extensively utilized design for performing clinical oncological hyperthermia. There have been large amounts of work done to optimize waveguide applicators for bandwidth, penetration depth, efficiency, SAR pattern size, and symmetry. Examples of some widely utilized commercial devices are shown in Fig. 10.2.

The frequency of operation for which hyperthermia waveguide applicators have been designed to operate has ranged from 27 MHz (STERZER et al. 1980; PAGLIONE 1982) to 2450 MHz. The requirement that hyperthermia applicators be as small and light as possible, both for ease of clinical setup and for potential assembling of the waveguides into applicator arrays, has stimulated much work into miniaturizing these applicators while retaining penetration depth and near-field quality. Common engineering methods used alone and in combination to alter and optimize the performance of these devices have included dielectric loading of the waveguide cavity, reconfiguring the geometry of the cavity by the addition of ridges, tapering the cavity, utilizing multiple feeds, the incorporation of electromagnetic lensing structures, and the utilization of special coupling boluses (KANTOR 1981; VAGUINE et al. 1982; KANTOR and WITTERS 1983; TURNER 1983; NUSSBAUM and LEYBOVICH 1984; REBOLLAR and

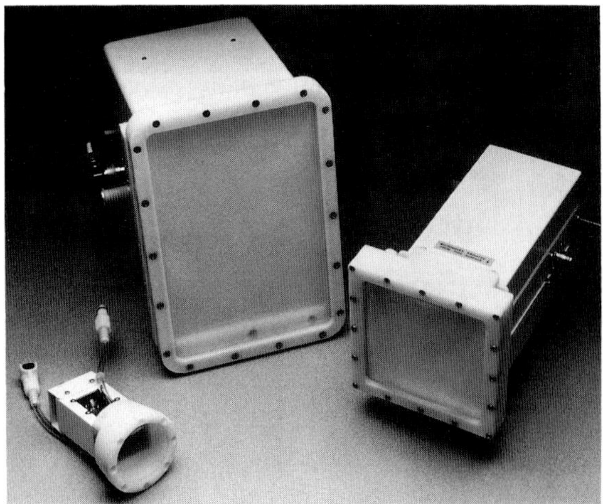

Fig. 10.2. Small and large treatment area waveguide hyperthermia applicators. *Photograph, from left*: MA-151 620- to 1000-MHz water-coupled applicator, MA-120 680- and 915-MHz (optional 434 MHz tuning available) air- or water-coupled applicator, MA-100 600- and 915-MHz air- or water-coupled applicator. *Power deposition graphs in phantom from top*: MA-151, MA-100, MA-120. Actual power deposition patterns in tissue will vary with operating frequency, bolusing, tissue type, and surface geometry. Sample SAR patterns are shown to illustrate the changes in heating pattern size possible within a given frequency range by innovative applicator design. All applicators manufactured by BSD Medical Corporation, Salt Lake City, Utah, USA. (Photograph and applicator data by courtesy of BSD Medical Corporation)

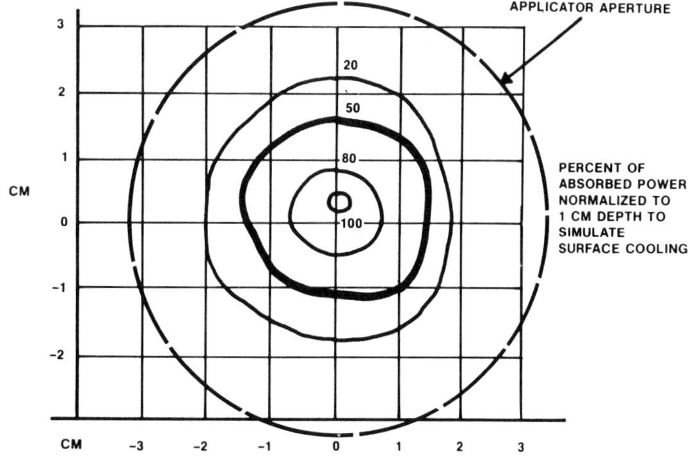

• TOP VIEW AT 1 CM DEPTH IN PHANTOM

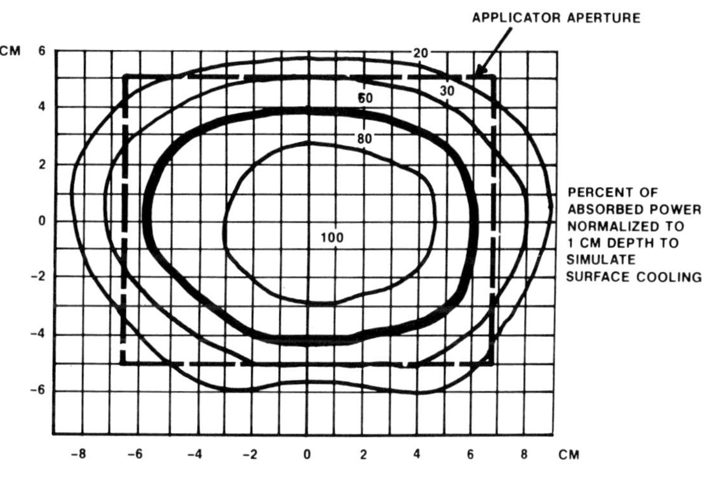

• TOP VIEW AT 1 CM DEPTH IN PHANTOM

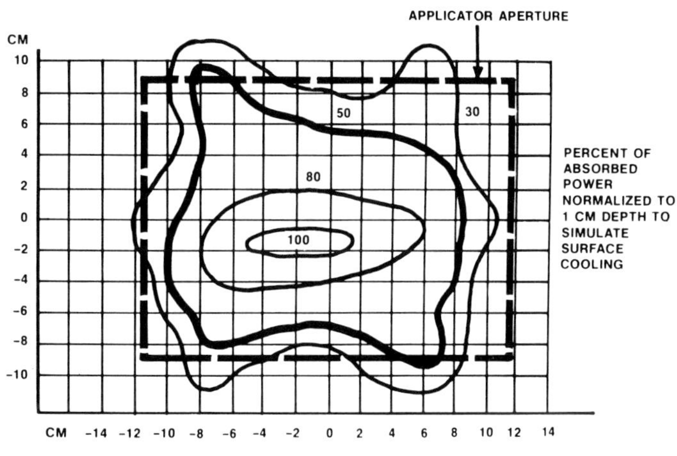

• TOP VIEW AT 1 CM DEPTH IN PHANTOM

ENCINAR 1984; LOVISOLO et al. 1984; NIKAWA et al. 1986a,b; MATSUDA et al. 1990; LEYBOVICH et al. 1991).

The primary drawback to the majority of waveguide applicator designs, because of the minimum cut-off frequency associated with aperture dimensions, has been the small effective heating pattern diameter compared with the physical size and weight of the applicator.

10.3.2 Horn Applicators

Hyperthermia applicators referred to as horns in the literature (TURNER 1983; LOVISOLO et al. 1984), while having superficially similar external contours, may have significantly different design origins. The most common type is the "waveguide horn," which is an applicator utilizing a loop or short linear probe driving a section of waveguide open at one end. The waveguide, however, is tapered, expanding in dimensions towards its radiating aperture, usually with the intent of obtaining a superior radiative impedance match with the tissue to be heated. This design has been utilized in both liquid-coupled and air-coupled applicators and from a design standpoint is a variation of the standard waveguide applicator.

A second type of horn applicator of fundamentally different design is represented by the MA-201 applicator manufactured by BSD Medical Corporation (Fig. 10.3). This applicator is based upon a tapered, centrally dielectrically loaded, directly excited, parallel plate transmission line with no electrical connection between the two conducting strips past the coaxial connector feed point. Since there is no conductive material between the conductive strips it can operate in the TEM mode with no lower cut-off frequency, making it an extremely versatile wideband applicator. The MA-201 has been used clinically both as a superficial depth applicator operating in the 200- to 400-MHz range and as a deep heating device when operated near 90 MHz as part of a coherent two-element phased array.

The water-filled Lucite Cone Applicator (RIETVELD and VAN RHOON 1992; VAN RHOON et al. 1992) is a horn-configured applicator designed for use in applicator arrays which has characteristics of both the waveguide horn and the MA-201, and in addition utilizes variable dielectric loading to shape and increase the effective heating area. This applicator design launches its field

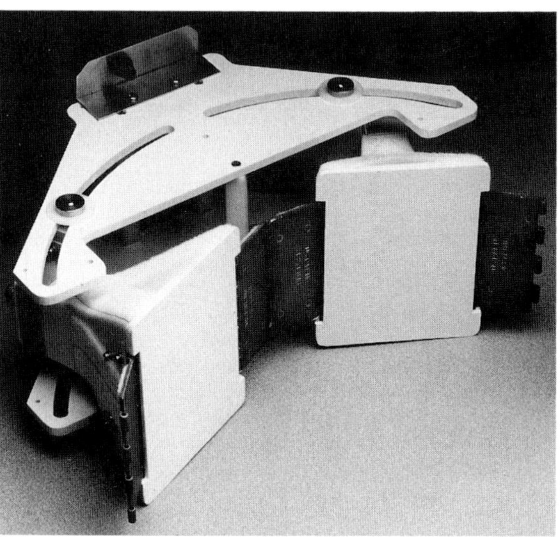

Fig. 10.3. MA-201 dual-horn hyperthermia applicator manufactured by BSD Medical Corporation. The horn applicators can be dismounted from the array configuration and used individually (MA-200). Recommended operating frequencies are 87 MHz to 95 MHz low range and 175 MHz to 190 MHz high range. A 4-cm to 5-cm-thick deionized water coupling bolus (not shown) is used as the patient coupling interface. (Photograph by courtesy of BSD Medical Corporation)

from a standard TEM 1,0 rectangular guide excited by an inserted probe. The flared horn section differs from conventional designs in that the walls parallel to the direction of the E-field are a nonconductive dielectric rather than metal. The applicator is dielectrically loaded using deionized water. Within the horn, immersed in the deionized water, is a polyvinylchloride (PVC) cone positioned centrally in the aperture. This combination of water loading, nonconductive side walls, and a central conical dielectric insert has been shown to significantly increase the heating pattern area over a conventional waveguide horn of the same physical size.

10.3.3 Dipoles

The use of dipole radiating elements to heat tissue therapeutically dates back to early diathermy devices (GUY 1990). These early devices were typically reflector-backed air-coupled high-frequency (2450 MHz) radiators. More recent experimental devices utilize lower operating frequencies and fluid dielectric coupling. TURNER et al. (1989) describe a large surface area applicator consisting of an array of coaxial dipole antennas commonly utilized for interstitial hyperthermia, mounted parallel to each other on the back of a transparent water bolus. Interelement cross-talk is suppressed by optimizing the proximity of the element to the patient and operating in coherent mode, matching the interelement spacing to the frequency of operation. LEE et al. (1988) describe an applicator utilizing an array of eight reflector-backed coaxial dipole antennas, mechanically scanned in parallel tubes built within a body conformal coupling bolus. The applicator operated in noncoherent mode with interelement cross-talk suppressed by the internal reflectors. The power to each of the scanned dipoles could be controlled individually as a function of scan position to locally alter the SAR pattern. The utilization of coaxial dipoles as surface applicator antenna elements requires careful design to minimize cross-talk between adjacent antennas and variations in the longitudinal SAR pattern of the coaxial dipole with insertion distance into the coupling bolus.

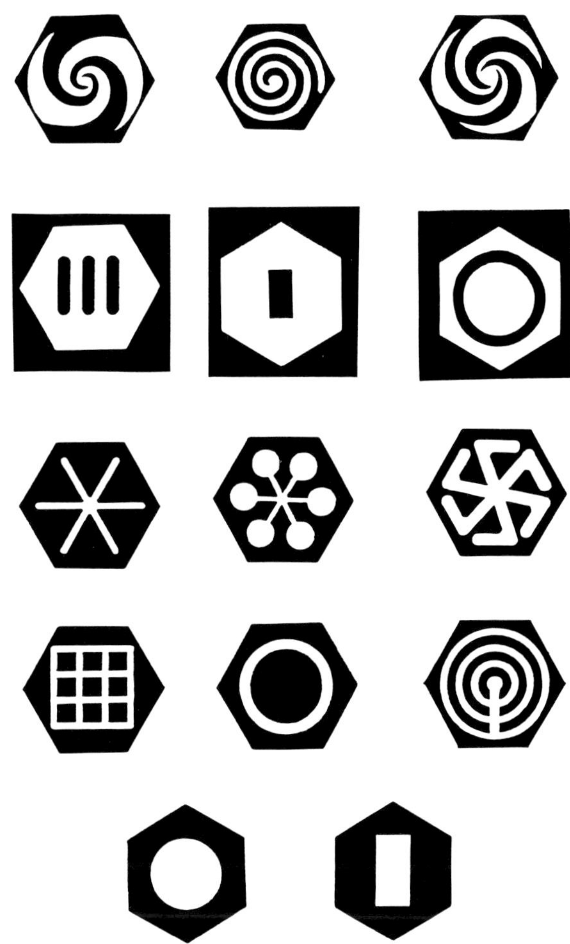

Fig. 10.4. A partial sample of the microstrip antenna patterns fabricated and tested by Varian Associates (Varian Associates, Palo Alto, Calif., USA) in collaboration with Stanford University Medical Center for potential use in hyperthermia applicators. *Top row*, microstrip spiral antennas; *second row*, microstrip slot antennas; *third row*, multiarm microstrip antennas; *fourth row*, microstrip loop antennas; *bottom row*, microstrip patch antennas. The Archimedean spiral microstrip antenna (*top row center*) proved to have the best balance of bandwidth, efficiency, and SAR pattern quality of the patterns tested, and was used in subsequently designed mechanically scanned antenna and conformal antenna array applicators. One potential disadvantage of the microstrip spiral antenna, however, is circular polarization, which makes its utilization as an array element in focused phased arrays more difficult than with linearly polarized antennas

10.3.4 Microstrip Antennas

Microstrip antenna applicators encompass that class of applicator in which the radiating element is constructed from a planar dielectric on which are etched or attached conductive metallic patterns designed to radiate electromagnetic waves. This definition is general because of the large varieties of microstrip antenna types in the literature intended for use in hyperthermia applicators (Fig. 10.4). Microstrip patch antennas, consisting of a resonant rectangular, circular, or elliptical metallic pattern backed by a continuous metallic back plane, were among the earliest and most studied types of microstrip radiators (JOHNSON et al. 1984; AUDONE et al. 1985; SANDHU and KOLOZSVARY 1985; JAMES et al. 1986; UNDERWOOD and MAGIN 1988; UNDERWOOD et al. 1989, 1992; MONTECCHIA 1992). Other microstrip configurations studied included multiple dipoles (MENDECKI et al. 1979; STERZER et al. 1980), microstrip-microslot (CHIVE et al. 1984), loop (BAHL et al. 1982; AUDONE et al. 1985), dual-arm spiral (TUMEH et al. 1989; DE LEO et al. 1989), and single-arm spiral (TANABE et al. 1983, 1985; KAPP et al. 1988; SAMULSKI et al. 1990; RYAN and COUGHLIN 1992; LEE et al. 1992; MONTECCHIA 1992). Early suggested approaches to utilizing microstrip antennas attempted to maximize their compactness by using them in direct contact with the tissue to be treated. This produced problems due to the intense quasi-static nonradiative electric fields near the edges of the conductive microstrip patterns. The near fields were often irregular in shape and contained large perpendicular E-field components which can cause overheating in superficial fat. Utilizing microstrips in direct contact with tissue also limits the power which can be applied to the antenna element since the dielectric losses will heat the antenna element and hence, the skin by direct conduction. The beam pattern in the near field can also be highly divergent (LEE et al. 1992), reducing the effective penetration depth. The early simple patch antennas also had problems with low efficiency. Refinements in microstrip antenna applicator design have subsequently solved these problems. The ratio of the normal versus tangential component of the near field has been found to vary with microstrip design (UNDERWOOD et al. 1992), implying that high near-field perpendicular E-field components are not intrinsic to the technology and that optimization of microstrip geometry to maximize the tangential E-field components is possible. The most important design concept was to sacrifice some compactness and efficiency with existing antenna designs to obtain an electric field distribution at the patient with more desirable characteristics by interposing a liquid coupling bolus of adequate thickness between the microstrip antenna and the tissue to be heated. Attenuation of the normal E-field component in microstrip patch and spiral antennas operating in the 400–900 MHz range to levels low enough for clinical use has been found experimentally to require at least a 2-cm to 3-cm bolus thickness (JOHNSON et al. 1984; HENDERSON et al. 1985; UNDERWOOD et al. 1992; SANDHU and KOLOZSVARY 1985; SAMULSKI et al. 1990). SANDHU and KOLOZSVARY (1985) and HAND (1987) also pointed out that the presence of an external coupling bolus has the benefit of reducing the effect of changes in the external loading on the resonance frequency of the microstrip antenna. By circulating the coupling fluid, usually deionized water, through a heat exchanger, conductive heating or cooling of the skin surface can be utilized to help optimize the effective depth of heating. The circulating liquid also acts as a heat sink for the antenna element, allowing sustained operation at high power. Some microstrip designs actually utilize deionized water as the microstrip dielectric (MONTECCHIA 1992; KOBAYASHI et al. 1989). It was found that the radiative efficiency of microstrip antennas could be enhanced by reducing the impedance mismatch between the solid dielectric–metallic strip microstrip antennas and the deionized water coupling bolus by the addition of a dielectric cover layer, or superstrate, between the microstrip pattern and the coupling bolus (JOHNSON et al. 1984; JAMES et al. 1986; UNDERWOOD and MAGIN 1988; UNDERWOOD et al. 1992; LEE et al. 1992). Appropriate designs utilizing these techniques have been demonstrated to be capable of producing clinically proven antennas with a wide bandwidth impedance match to a 50-ohm power amplifier system without external matching components (TANABE et al. 1985; SAMULSKI et al. 1990; LEE et al. 1992).

10.3.5 Magnetically Coupled Applicators

Magnetic fields in themselves are not useful for tissue heating since the magnetic permeability of the human body is approximately that of free space. However, Maxwell's equations state that a changing magnetic field gives rise to an associated electric field which can dissipate energy in tissue. Flat Magnetic induction coils tuned for operation at the 13.56-MHz and 27.12-MHz ISM frequencies, which generate a magnetic dipole perpendicular to the body surface, have long been used for medical diathermy (LERCH and KOHN 1983; HAND et al. 1982; GUY 1990). Due to a theoretical power deposition null in the center of simple single-turn coils and an irregular near field for multiturn coils (HAND and TER HAAR 1981; HAND et al. 1982), the heating patterns are far from optimal for superficial depth clinical hyperthermia, where temperatures must be more precisely controlled. These devices have seen little use in current superficial depth hyperthermic clinical practice. However, CORRY and BARLOGIE (1982) have described the effective use of a dual solenoidal magnetic induction system for bulky deep tumors.

More recent devices utilizing magnetic inductive coupling (BACH ANDERSEN et al. 1984; FRANCONI et al. 1986; HAND 1990; JOHNSON et al. 1990; LUMORI et al. 1990; GOPAL et al. 1992) generate the magnetic dipole parallel to the body surface with a current sheet produced by a wide conductive rectangular loop or loops with the long axis running parallel to the surface to be treated (Fig. 10.5). The power deposition patterns produced by these devices have a centrally peaked Gaussian shape similar to those produced by waveguides. Unlike waveguide applicators, resonant current sheet applicators have no intrinsic cut-off frequency associated with applicator physical dimensions. In principle the capacitive load on the flat current sheet conducting coil can

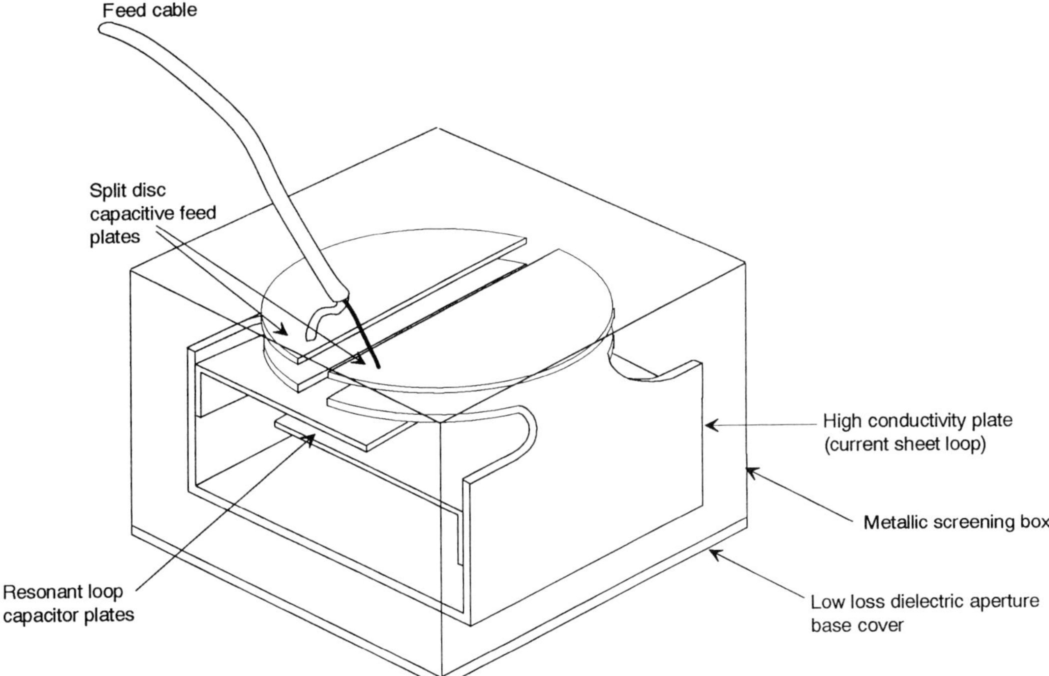

Fig. 10.5. Current sheet applicator (after JOHNSON et al. 1987; HAND 1990). A "U"-shaped high-conductivity metallic strip in series with a flat plate capacitor form a resonant loop, excited with a capacitively coupled split disc. The loop design and construction of the screening box concentrate the radiated field towards the base of the applicator. By changing the number of resonant loop capacitor plates or the plate spacing, the frequency of the applicator can be changed while retaining the same loop dimensions. This applicator design has no cut-off frequency associated with applicator dimensions, making possible very large ratios of heating pattern size versus applicator size. Fine tuning of frequency can be implemented by altering the spacing between the split disc capacitive feed plates and the corresponding resonant loop half plates

be tuned to resonate the coil at any specified frequency. This technology can potentially be used to design applicators with very large ratios of heating pattern size versus applicator size (JOHNSON et al. 1987). Engineering problems associated with these devices are very narrow theoretical bandwidths with center frequencies which shift with loading, and residual quasi-static near-field hot spots caused by near-field effects associated with the electric field components of the current loop (BACH ANDERSEN et al. 1984). Nevertheless, careful design has produced compact magnetically coupled applicators reliable and practical enough for routine clinical use (JOHNSON et al. 1987; GOPAL et al. 1992).

10.4 Techniques for Heating Large Surface Areas

Milignancies can occur in any region of the body and often involve surface areas of hundreds of square centimeters or more. Since patchwork treatment regimes requiring dozens of heat fields for a single patient are clinically impractical in many combined modality protocols, much effort has gone into developing techniques to enable electromagnetic applicators to treat large surface areas.

10.4.1 Single Large Aperture Devices

One conceptually simple approach to synthesizing large heating areas is to scale the applicator design to operate at lower frequencies, increasing the wavelength and hence the size of the heating pattern. It is also possible at a given fixed frequency range through appropriate design techniques to enlarge an applicator's effective heating area (Fig. 10.2). However, there are several problems associated with this simple approach to increasing effective heating pattern size.

The most basic problem encountered in clinical practice is that tissue electrical and thermal heterogeneities and the complex external contours of the human body act to produce differential heating within the treated volume. The larger the heated area, the more likely that there will be a tissue region included in the heated volume that will limit applied power due to pain or local high temperatures. Large volumes of tissue can thereby be fixed at subtherapeutic temperatures by a single hot point.

The power deposition contours of single aperture devices typically have a centrally peaked $\cos^2$ or Gaussian cross-section. The tumor/normal tissue boundary at the tumor periphery, however, has been observed to have the highest blood perfusion, indicating that a centrally peaked nonalterable power deposition pattern is geometrically suboptimal in that it will underheat the rapidly growing outer portions of the tumor as compared with the center. Single-aperture devices scaled to operate at low frequencies also tend to be large and heavy, making clinical setups difficult, particularly near areas such as the head and neck where physical access is limited.

Despite these potential disadvantages, the practical utility of well-designed stationary single-aperture applicators should not be minimized. Relatively homogeneous tissue regions containing tumors with low perfusion rates can and have been successfully heated by large-field single-aperture devices. Because of the intrinsic penetration depth–wavelength characteristics of propagating electromagnetic waves in tissue, even sophisticated phased arrays and scanning antenna applicators will not be able to compensate fully for the measured temperature variations encountered in practice. The low system cost and simplicity of utilization of single-aperture stationary heating devices are positive factors which should not be overlooked in selecting heating systems for sites and tumor types where more complex devices may not be needed.

10.4.2 Antenna Array Applicators

One approach to the problem of generating large heating patterns that also has some potential for accommodating tissue heterogeneity is to utilize arrays of standard single-source radiators. Advantages in the use of array applicators over that of single-source applicators are the potential to controllably vary the power deposition pattern in real time and to shape and enlarge the area of the heating pattern by simply adding additional antenna elements. Also some designs for hyperthermia applicator arrays were constructed with sufficient mechanical flexibility to be able to conform to body curvature.

Most of the hyperthermia engineering literature on applicator arrays refers to theoretical studies and computer models. The following summary lists only those tests in which actual hardware was constructed or evaluated. Tests of microstrip patch applicator arrays are reported by Sandhu and Kolozsvary (1985), Underwood et al. (1989), and Gee et al. (1984). Tests in phantom and clinical use of microstrip spiral arrays are described by Tanabe et al. (1983), Tanabe (1985), Wilsey et al. (1988), Kapp et al. (1989), Tumeh et al. (1989), Samulski et al. (1990), Lee et al. (1992; Fig. 10.6), and Ryan and Coughlin (1992).

Testing and use of arrays of waveguide applicators have been described by Loane et al. (1986), Wyslouzil et al. (1987), and Diederich and Stauffer (1992). An example of a commercially available 915-MHz waveguide array applicator hyperthermia system is shown in Fig. 10.7.

Other antenna array types intended for large-area superficial depth heating which have been constructed and tested have been based on: microstrip dipoles (Sterzer et al. 1980; Mendecki et al. 1979), dielectrically loaded parallel plate horns (Turner 1983; Fig. 10.3), microstrip-slot (Chive et al. 1984), helical antennas (Kawabata et al. 1984), coaxial dipole antennas (Lee et al. 1988; Turner et al. 1989), concentric ring antennas (Stauffer and Diederich 1993), Lucite-cone wave guide applicators (Rietveld and van Rhoon 1992; van Rhoon et al. 1992; Fig. 10.8), and current sheet devices (Hand 1990; Lumori et al. 1990; Gopal et al. 1992; Fig. 10.9). Single-cavity applicators which have local power deposition control are described in Leybovich et al. (1991), where the applicator design consists of a shortened waveguide cavity with multiple-probe antennas capable of generating locally controllable power deposition patterns with a large ratio of heating area to aperture size. Rappaport and Morgenthaler (1986) describe the theory and engineering design behind a leaky-wave troughguide applicator capable of local power control.

Constructing a clinically usable antenna array applicator involves more than simply adjoining multiple antennas. The problems which must

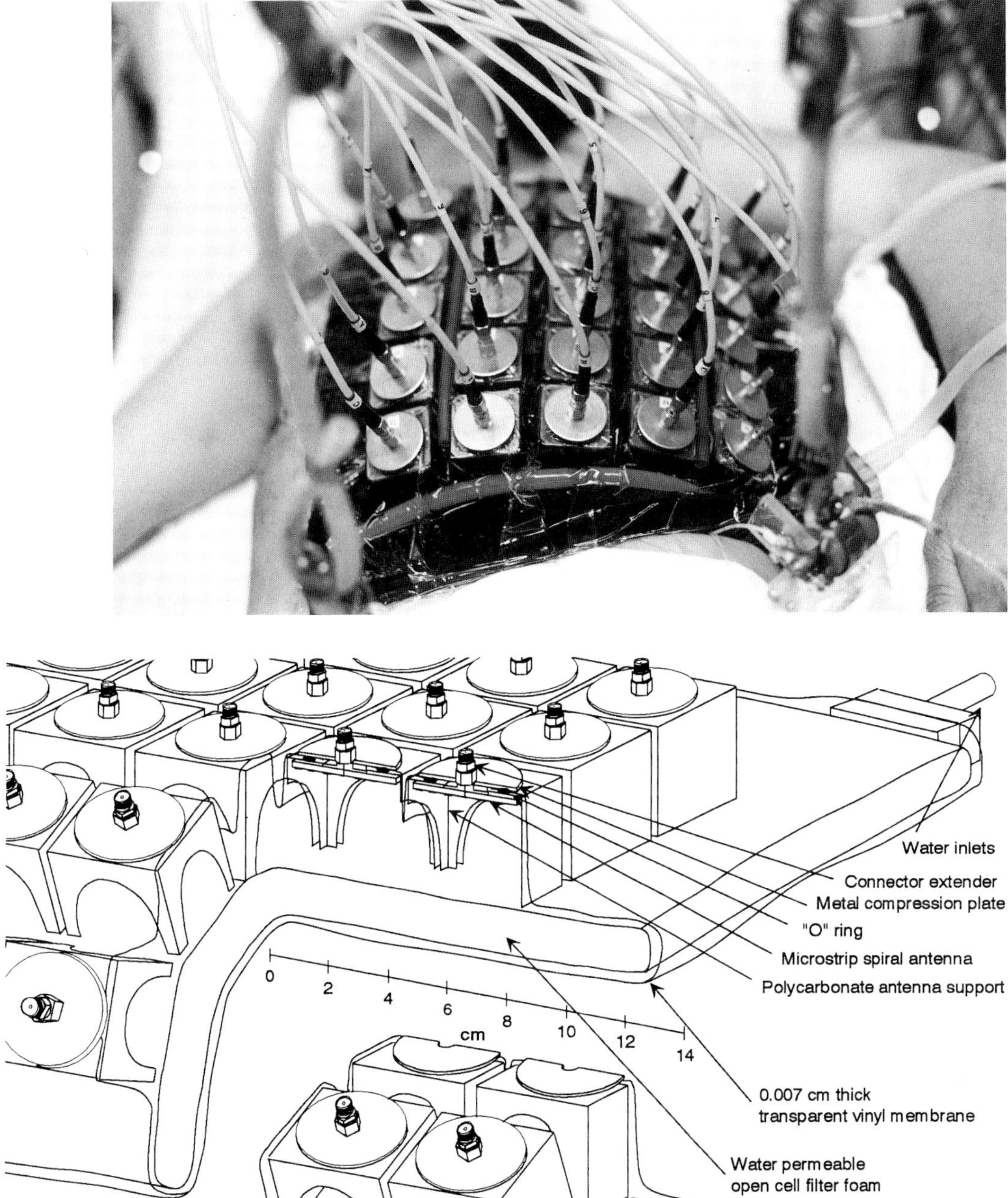

Fig. 10.6. Body conformal microstrip spiral antenna array applicator. This design for a large surface area applicator operates noncoherently at 915 MHz with circularly polarized microstrip antenna elements. Mounting the antenna elements on independent plastic support frames which are attached at their base to a flexible sheet of open cell fluid permeable filter foam allows the array to conform to convex surfaces while maintaining for each antenna a constant spacing from the heated tissue, and a constant illuminated surface area. This structure is sealed in transparent plastic through which is circulated temperature-controlled deionized water. This type of applicator has been constructed with 6, 12, 16, and 25 antenna elements (LEE et al. 1992). *Top*: 25-element array in place during a patient treatment; *bottom*: applicator design details

be addressed are: the combining of individual antenna radiation patterns to form a uniform net power deposition pattern, minimization of inter-antenna cross-talk, proper phasing for coherent arrays, allowing conformation to body contours while retaining predictable SAR patterns, and economically powering, monitoring, and individually controlling large numbers of elements.

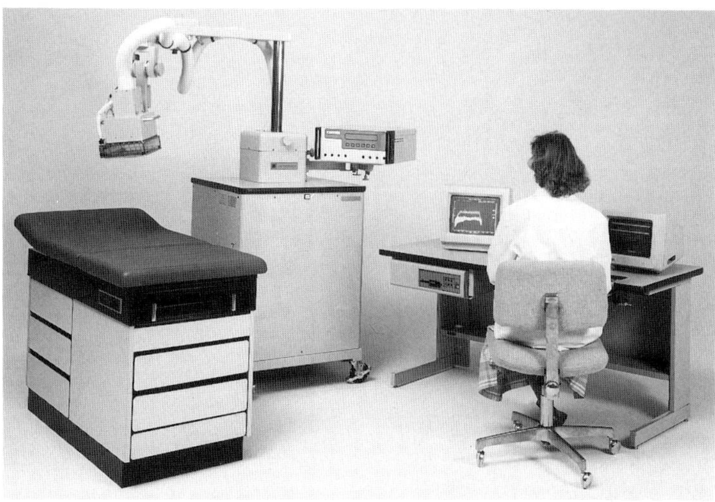

Fig. 10.7. Microtherm 1000, 915-MHz superficial depth hyperthermia treatment system, manufactured by Labthermics Technologies (Champaign Ill., USA). This treatment system is designed to power 4- and 16-element planar waveguide arrays at up to 60 W per antenna with an independent solid state amplifier for each array element. The arrays operate in noncoherent mode with an upgrade to operation as a coherent phased array (Microtherm 2000) undergoing laboratory testing. The basic radiating antenna in these applicator arrays is a 3.8 cm by 3.8 cm aperture dielectrically loaded waveguide antenna. The electromagnetic energy is coupled through a temperature-controlled deionized water bolus. Power to each array element can be independently varied under computer control or operator manual control. (Photograph by courtesy of Labthermics Technologies, Inc.)

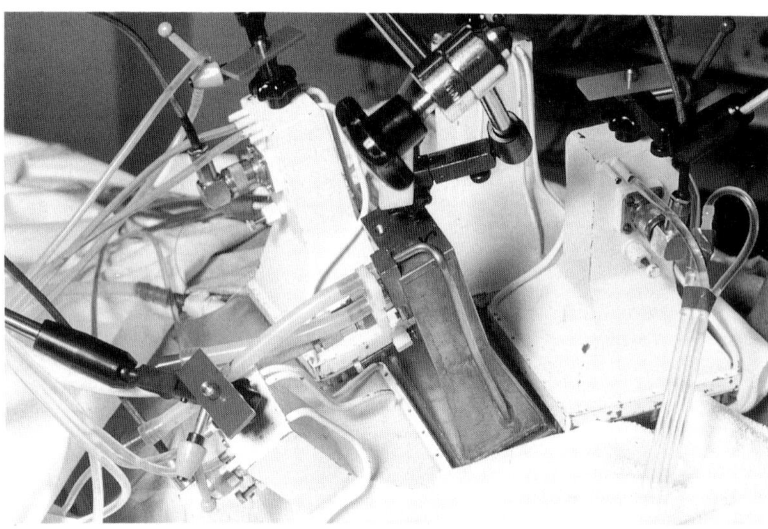

Fig. 10.8. Five-element Lucite Cone applicator array in place on a patient under treatment (Rietveld and van Rhoon 1992; van Rhoon et al. 1992). Each applicator can be independently positioned and power controlled. A temperature-controlled water coupling bolus is used as the patient to applicator array interface. (Photograph by courtesy by G.C. van Rhoon, Dr. Daniel den Hoed Cancer Center, Rotterdam)

Combining the SAR patterns of stationary antennas together to obtain a uniform heating pattern without cold regions between antenna elements requires that the radiating elements comprising the array have heating patterns that are large compared with their physical outlines. Lee et al. (1992) performed a two-dimensional summation of Gaussian SAR patterns for a simulated 25-element noncoherent close packed array for different interelement spacings and concluded that in order to obtain less than 10% drops in power deposition between antenna

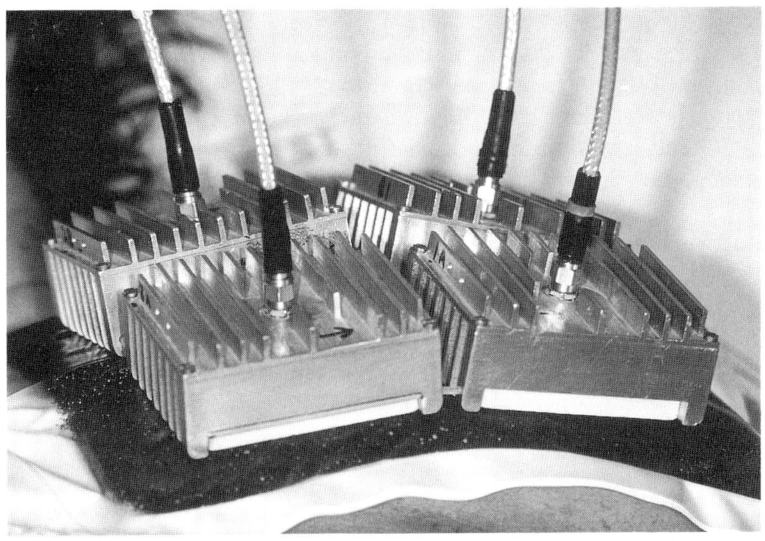

Fig. 10.9. Current sheet applicator array in place on a patient. This array is operated in noncoherent mode by two independent, multiplexed 434-MHz generators (HAND et al. 1992). The individual array elements are jointed to each other with thin, flexible polyethylene pins to maintain constant interelement spacing while allowing conformation to body curvature. A 2-cm-thick water bolus containing low-density plastic foam is used to couple the antenna elements to the patient. (Photograph by courtesy of J.W. Hand, Hammersmith Hospital, London)

elements, the −3 dB diameter must be greater than the center to center inter-antenna element spacing. This was confirmed by the construction of prototype arrays with different interelement spacings. GOPAL et al. (1992), similarly describe theoretical and experimental work done with a four-element coherent current sheet applicator array demonstrating that coherent operation can produce an enhanced uniformity of the power deposition pattern over noncoherent operation when the interelement spacing does not allow this −3 dB radius condition to be met. An alternative to antenna miniaturization has been described by RYAN and COUGHLIN (1993), who demonstrated a successful technique for physically overlapping simultaneously radiating spiral microstrip antenna patterns, with the spiral elements retaining their ability to be independently powered.

Coherent operation of applicator arrays offers the advantage, as previously mentioned, of allowing greater interelement separation for an equivalent degree of power deposition uniformity. It was also demonstrated by theoretical analysis (HAND et al. 1986; HAND and HIND 1986; MAGIN and PETERSON 1989) and tests in phantoms (GEE et al. 1984; LOANE et al. 1986; FENN et al. 1993) that planar coherent arrays can be phased to produce a convergent beam, yielding a local enhancement in penetration depth. Anatomical considerations and limitations in current sensor technology, however, may make this potential advantage in penetration depth difficult in clinical practice to actually utilize. Metastatic breast cancer, for instance, can involve the tissue from the skin surface down to a depth of 2–3 cm over an area which can extend over hundreds of square centimeters. The area at depth is nearly equal to the area at the surface, hence tissue geometry does not allow for a power deposition gain at depth by phased focusing without sacrificing heating efficacy in the tissue outside the converging beam. The differences in the dielectric constants of high and low water content tissue are sufficiently large that calculations of the proper drive phase for each array element require precise knowledge of the anatomy of the treated region. At the frequencies commonly used for superficial depth heating, phase shifts caused by alterations in tissue geometry are not negligible. At 915 MHz in high water content tissue, a 1-cm change in effective path length will cause an 80° phase shift. Reflections from multiple tissue interfaces, refraction, and scattering in the direct beam paths, as well as changes in the path lengths caused by motions of the patient, make direct calculation of the proper amplitudes and phases difficult. In addition to the lengths of the effective beam paths, differential heating of the near-surface tissue through which the beams pass must be taken into account in calculating the overall drive phases and amplitudes. While obtaining proper phasing for heating a single point at depth has been demonstrated in phantoms, what is required for performing clinical hyperthermia treatments is optimization of heating at all points throughout a volume. Until breakthroughs are made in sensor technology or combined electromagnetic and thermal modeling, it is unlikely that heating systems based on radiative electromagnetic phased arrays can operate at their full theoretical potential in heterogeneous living tissue.

Noncoherent operation of arrays, while inferior to coherent operation in degrees of freedom for shaping the power deposition pattern, can offer several practical advantages. HAND et al. (1992) reported theoretical and experimental results which showed that noncoherent operation of an applicator array can result in larger effective heating patterns than the operation of the same array in coherent mode.

It is far easier with the limited thermometry available with current technology hyperthermia systems to implement control algorithms for noncoherent arrays. The SAR pattern of a noncoherent array is the linear sum of amplitudes of the SAR patterns of the individual elements. The absence of wave interference effects with adjacent antennas makes predicting the resultant changes in local power deposition in nonhomogeneous tissue after changes are made in the drive amplitudes of the antenna elements far less complicated. Noncoherent operation precludes, for instance, the possibility of a decrease in amplitude of one element, causing a local increase in the deposited power near a neighboring element by a reduction of local E-field cancellation. This monotonic overall power deposition response is especially important when attempting to respond to complaints of pain by reducing power locally by trial and error to individual elements. As a consequence of this lack of need to calculate relative phase between adjacent elements, the complication of controlling a body conformal noncoherent applicator array is less than with a coherent conformal array. A flexible body conformal applicator with movable pivoting antenna elements, if implemented with coherent array technology, will require the proper initial setting and real time readjustment of drive phase for antennas whose relative physical orientation will vary between treatment sites and during a given treatment if the patient moves. As mentioned previously, knowledge of relative path lengths accurate to 1 cm or less may be required, depending upon the operating frequency. While adjustment of phase by retrofocusing has been demonstrated in an inhomogeneous phantom for optimizing heating at a single point at depth (LOANE et al. 1986), optimizing the heating throughout a large surface area treatment field will require more invasive sensing points than current clinical practice and sensor technology allow.

10.4.3 Mechanically Scanned Antenna Applicators

Generating a large effective electromagnetic field by physically moving a directional antenna is a very old practice in radio and radar technology. Physically moving a radiative energy device (usually ultrasound) over a region to be heated has long been standard practice in physical diathermy. It was expected, then, that moving antenna techniques would eventually find use in generating large-area heating patterns with electromagnetic hyperthermia applicators.

There are multiple engineering advantages to generating large-area heating patterns by mechanically scanning individual or groups of antennas. Antennas utilized in mechanically scanned systems, unlike those intended for use in static arrays, are not required to have heating patterns large compared with their physical outline in order to be usable for producing a uniform power deposition pattern. Analyses by GUY (1971b) and HAND and HIND (1986) show that reduction of the aperture size to a width of less than approximately 1 to 2 wavelengths in tissue impairs the penetration depth of radiative electromagnetic applicators. In mechanically static arrays, apertures large compared with their wavelength in tissue will yield cold interelement zones. In scanning antenna systems, however, varying the scan line spacing in principle can produce a uniform power deposition pattern with any applicator power deposition half-width diameter. Scanned antenna applicators utilizing machine-controlled positioning can, by varying duration over each point, or power as a function of position, controllably customize the distribution of energy delivered to tissue in real time. Finally, the uniformity of the antenna's power deposition pattern is less critical in scanned antenna systems than in mechanically static arrays. The averaging over the scan path of small singular cold or hot regions within an applicator's near field can eliminate the local nulls or hot points which in a stationary device would cause unacceptable local heating heterogeneities (HAND and TER HAAR 1981).

Moving applicator diathermy treatments were implemented by scanning the applicator by hand with patient feedback of the resultant heating sensations determining the relative duration over a point and the overall power level. The greater precision required in oncological hyperthermia in quantifying the energy deposition and the resultant temperatures produced has placed the emphasis on designing systems with machine-controlled mechanical scanning of the applicator antennas with multipoint thermometry providing power control information. The experimental systems mentioned in the literature vary greatly in their degree of sophistication. In their review of heating techniques, HAND and TER HAAR (1981) describe a mathematical simulation of a mechanically scanned "pancake coil" magnetic induction applicator where the central null common to flat coil applicators was eliminated. PALIWAL et al. (1985) describe a system tested in animals and phantom utilizing an air-coupled waveguide applicator mounted on a pivoting arm, scanned in an arc with the motion of the arm actuated by a cammed variable speed motor. SAMULSKI et al. (1990) reported on the experimental and clinical use of applicators comprising an integral water bolus and a computer-controlled stepper motor scanning a single- or dual-element microstrip spiral antenna in a fixed reciprocating circular path over the internal water bolus. These scanning microstrip spiral applicators have the ability to control applied power as a function of antenna position (Fig. 10.10). LEE et al. (1988) describe an applicator array consisting of coaxial dipole antennas, mechanically scanned in parallel tubes embedded in a conformal, water-filled plastic foam and metal reflector structure. Power could be controlled as a function of linear scan position for each of the eight scanned coaxial antennas. The eight-element array has been tested only in phantom. A two-element scanned coaxial antenna array has been tested for a site-specific application on one patient in a location that conventional applicators could not physically access. Scanning antenna heating systems utilizing antennas moved by robotic arms are described in STERZER et al. (1985, 1986), LEE et al. (1986), and TENNANT et al. (1990). Only the system described by STERZER et al. (1985, 1986) had been tested on humans (Fig. 10.11). At the time of this writing none of these experimental robotic applicators is in use treating patients.

10.5 Site-Specific Applicators

Tissue heterogeneity and highly contoured surfaces can produce difficult to heat regions requiring applicators custom designed for these specific body areas. An example of an applicator intended specifically to accommodate extreme cylindrical curvature is the Varian designed spiral (microstrip antenna) arm cuff applicator. This two- by eight-element array is flexible enough in one dimension to be able to fit around the circumference of a limb of radius greater than 8 cm in diameter (WILSEY et al. 1988). Conversely, body regions with extreme negative (concave) curvature such as the axilla on patients with an impaired range of arm movement require an applicator able to radiate a nearly cylindrical outwardly propagating power deposition pattern. Such an applicator, utilizing coaxial dipole antennas longitudinally scanned in tubes mounted in a deionized water-saturated plastic foam-filled coupling bolus, contoured to fit against the axilla, was designed and clinically tested (LEE et al. 1988).

An applicator constructed to treat superficial disease over the facial region near the eyes and the bridge of the nose had to be designed to solve multiple engineering problems not normally encountered in applicators intended to treat extremities and chest walls. Electromagnetic applicators tend to preferentially heat structures proximal to the radiating aperture. Tests in a facial contour phantom showed preferential power deposition in the nose with conventional applicators. The proximity of the eyes is an important factor in designing heating devices for this particular treatment site because of the risk of microwave-induced cataracts. An applicator was designed for this task utilizing ten independently powered 915-MHz microstrip spiral antenna elements mounted on a semirigid water permeable foam base, contoured to the outlines of the central facial area. The eyes were protected by a separate pair of 1-cm-thick local conformal boluses circulating cooled isotonic saline. This

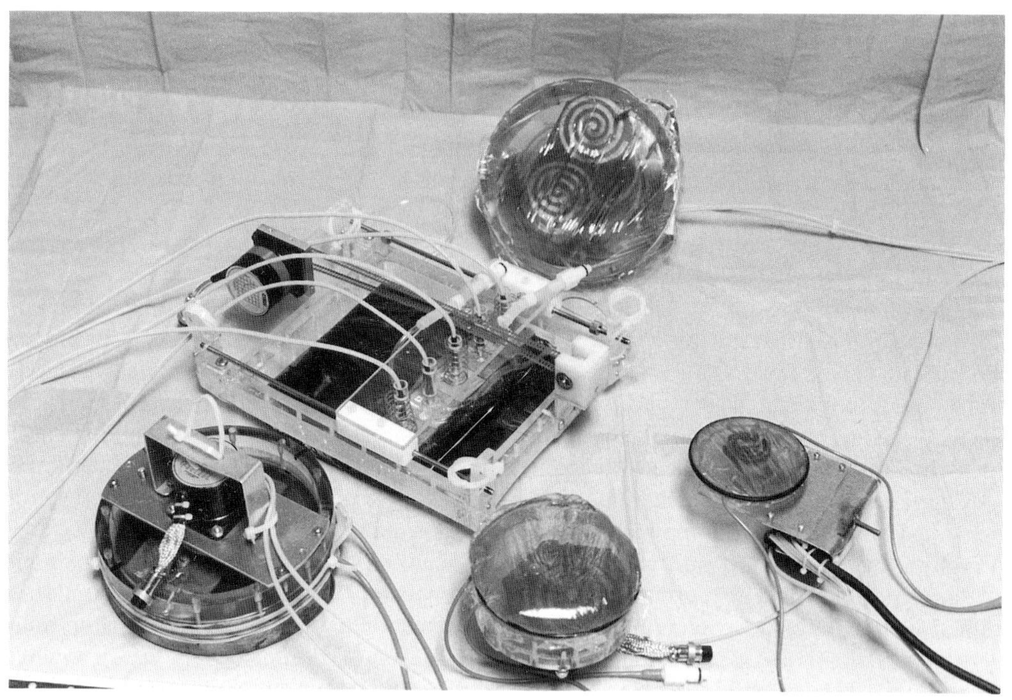

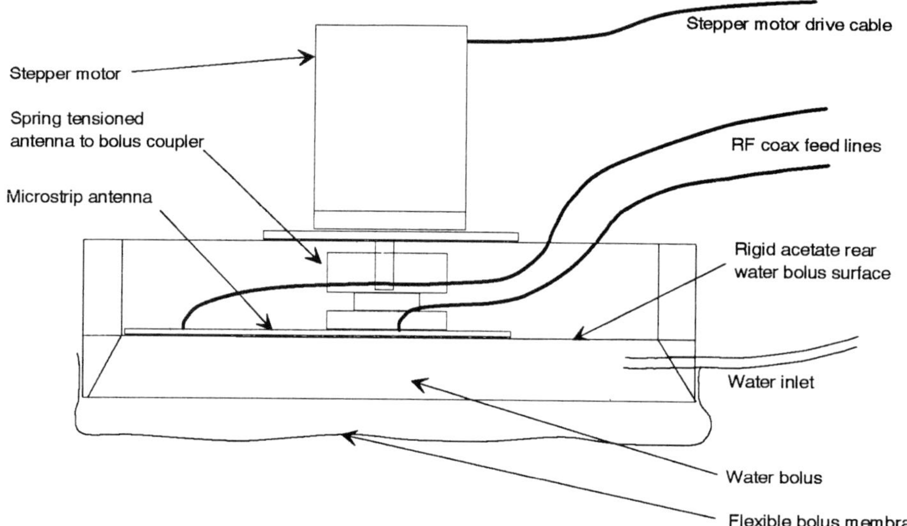

Fig. 10.10. *Top*: Mechanically scanned microstrip spiral antenna applicators (SAMULSKI et al. 1990). *From the top clockwise*: Two-element 390-MHz scanning antenna applicator (*bottom view*), 915-MHz scanning antenna applicator, 390-MHz single-element scanning antenna applicator, two-element 390-MHz scanning antenna applicator (*top view*), five-element 915-MHz linear array scanning antenna applicator. All applicators except for the five-element 915-MHz scanning linear array have been used on patients. *Bottom*: Design details for the mechanically scanned two-element microstrip spiral antenna applicator. This applicator utilizes a rectangular printed circuit board on which are etched two 7.5-cm-diameter center driven Archimedean spiral, antenna patterns. This two-element rectangular microstrip antenna array is scanned in a reciprocating circular path with the radii of rotation of the antennas at 2.8 cm and 5.8 cm. Power to each antenna is controlled synchronously with the stepper motor position. The applicator operating software allows control of output amplitude independently to each antenna at 45° scan intervals. The antennas are operated noncoherently at 390 MHz. Over a thousand treatments have been performed at Stanford University Medical Center with this scanning antenna applicator design

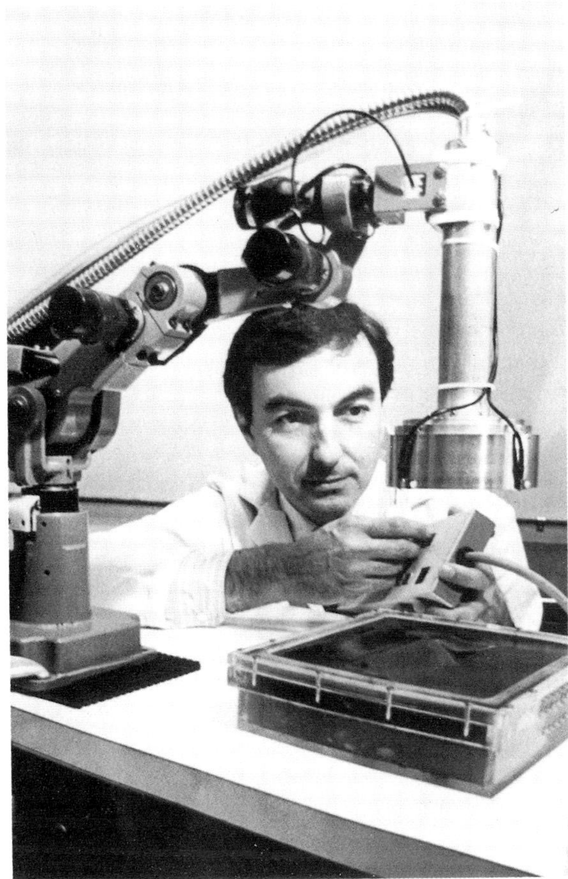

Fig. 10.11. Experimental robotic arm hyperthermia applicator developed at RCA Laboratories (STERZER et al. 1986). The applicator is air coupled, operating at 2450 MHz. The applicator head contains a compressed air fitting for blowing cold air to cool the skin surface when needed, and an infrared noncontacting thermometer to provide data for real time feedback power control. Mechanical proximity sensors protect the patient from accidental contact with the scanning robotic arm. Lead through programming is used to input the scan path into the five-axis arm. The automatic power control system is capable of acquiring a temperature value and altering the applied power in less than a second, allowing continuous contouring of the applied power along the scan path. (Photograph by courtesy of F. Sterzer)

secondary bolus, placed over the eyes, absorbed microwave energy and cooled the eyes by conduction without perturbing the field patterns of the antennas as would metal introduced into the field. Successful heating was accomplished with this device of the patient for whom it was designed and constructed (KAPP et al. 1989).

Other applicators conversely were designed to treat malignancies of the eye itself (FINGER et al. 1983; LAGENDIJK 1982a; SCHIPPER and LAGENDIJK 1986; STAUFFER et al. 1988). The applicator described by FINGER et al. is hemispherical and contoured to fit against the outer surface of the eye. A microstrip antenna consisting of a spiral wound, flat strip transmission line shorted at the end is etched into the inner surface of the applicator and tuned for operation at 5.8 GHz.

The ophthalmic applicator designed by J.J.W. Lagendijk is constructed of flexible silicone rubber which conforms to the eye and can form a liquid-tight seal allowing the circulation of cooling water against the surface of the cornea. The radiating element is a single-turn stripline antenna built into this silicone rubber structure, tuned to operate at 2450 MHz. An ultrasound ranging transducer is built into the body of the applicator for positive indexing of position.

The applicator described in STAUFFER et al. (1988) utilizes a 2450-MHz ring antenna. This ring antenna is constructed from copper tubing through which temperature-controlled fluid can be circulated to conductively regulate the surface temperature of the treated tissue. This temperature-controlled antenna is built into a plaque applicator into which radioactive seeds can be placed. This allows for simultaneous heating and irradiation with a single device.

10.6 Thermometry and Control

Successful design of hardware and software for controlling the power to hyperthermia applicators, particularly for those applicators capable of real time local alterations of their power deposition patterns, is dependent upon being able to characterize accurately in real time the temperatures induced in the object one wishes to heat controllably. The complexity of the system required to perform this task adequately varies greatly with the degree of heterogeneity in the heated object. As extreme examples, a homogeneous heating target, such as a well-characterized phantom, can have its temperature distribution pattern under certain microwave irradiation predicted by mathematical simulations without any applied thermometry. A large surface area radiation therapy treatment field containing normal tissue, multiple discrete nodules, surgical scars, and necrotic regions, on a body region such as the head and neck which has surface contours that change with patient motion, may require subcentimeter real time temperature monitoring to map out the resultant variations in temperatures when undergoing external heating.

The magnitudes of the variation in heating caused by blood perfusion and tissue heterogeneity has been the topic of both mathematical simulations (ROEMER 1991) and clinical thermometry studies. LAGENDIJK (1982b), LAGENDIJK et al. (1984), and CREEZE and LAGENDIJK (1992) describe research utilizing computer models and experimental work done with perfused gel and tissue phantoms to establish the magnitude of local cooling caused by the presence of large vessels in the heated tissue. Using the assumptions of homogeneous tissue with uniform energy deposition, temperature drops on the order of 4°C per cm were predicted near large vessels. GIBBS et al. (1985) and OLESON et al. (1985) presented high-resolution linear temperature maps taken in tumor and normal tissue in human patients heated by both local and regional electromagnetic hyperthermia devices. These measurements showed temperature gradients that in extreme cases exceeded 7°C per cm in tissue heated by superficial external microwave applicators (Fig. 10.12). These variations were interpreted by the authors to be caused by variations in tissue properties, blood perfusion, and reflections from tissue interfaces. Even with electromagnetic regional heating devices, measured temperature gradients on the order of 4–5°C per cm were recorded with absolute temperature variations within treated tissue of up to 10°C. These variations manifested themselves as local maxima as well as minima. The spatial frequency of these observed variations were rapid enough in extreme cases that power deposition resolution on the order of 1 cm or less would be required to compensate. CREEZE and LAGENDIJK (1992) predicted on the basis of their modeling and experimental testing that subcentimeter power deposition control resolution is needed to compensate for temperature variations caused by perfusion differentials.

There are currently no thermometry systems available for routine clinical treatments which can provide real time subcentimeter spatial resolution throughout realistic treatment volumes. Research into techniques which in theory can be used to perform high-resolution noninvasive thermometry, however, is ongoing (BOLOMEY and HAWLEY 1990). In addition, subcentimeter spatial power resolution in tissue would require applicator

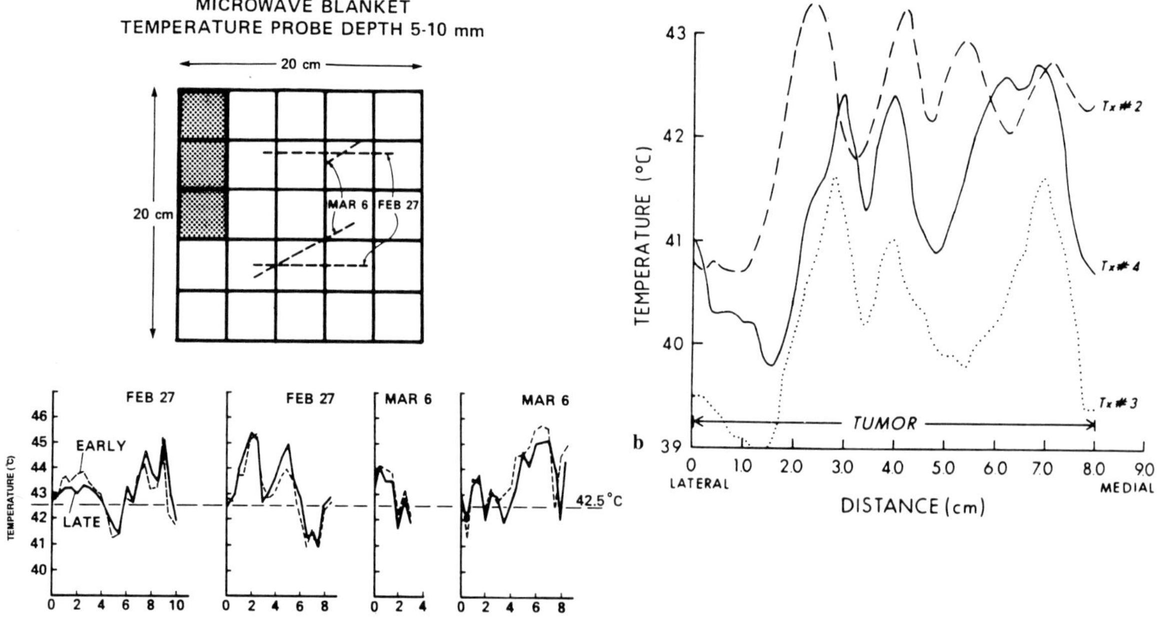

Fig. 10.12a,b. Interstitial temperature maps taken during microwave superficial depth hyperthermia treatments. **a** Temperature maps taken at Stanford University Medical Center during two chest wall treatments in the same patient. A 915-MHz, 25-element microstrip array applicator was the heating device. **b** Temperature maps taken at Duke University Medical Center during three successive chest wall treatments. The heating device was a waveguide applicator. The catheter remained in place for all three treatments. (From OLESON et al. 1985)

operating frequencies in excess of 5 GHz. Operation in this frequency range is not clinically feasible due to the excessive loss in penetration depth. If the goal of superficial depth hyperthermia is to uniformly heat the upper 2–3 cm of large surface area diseased tissue, the physics of propagating electromagnetic waves in tissue combined with the theoretical and observed scale of tissue heterogeneity prevents radiative electromagnetic applicators from being able to accomplish this task reliably even if knowledge of temperature at every tissue point were available. Because the spatial resolution of the ability to deposit energy is larger by an order of magnitude than the currently measured dimensional scale of physiological caused heating variations, successful heating depends as much upon favorable blood flow rates and tissue electrical properties as upon the capabilities of the heating device. Still, the higher the spatial resolution, the better. This treatment methodology, where one deposits energy and hopes that the tissue properties allow for effective heating, has been termed "reliance on thermal opportunism" (ROEMER 1990), and more derisively as "dump and pray" (STROHBEHN 1984). Questions concerning the quality of heating actually required in combined modality therapy to yield a significant clinical gain and the possible physiological manipulations suggested to enhance uniformity of heating are beyond the scope of this presentation.

Current superficial depth electromagnetic hyperthermia systems suffer, then, from both incomplete thermometry and inadequate spatial resolution of power control. Taking both of these factors into account, the optimization goal for power control can be more realistically redefined from achieving a uniform specified temperature throughout the treatment volume to maximizing the amount of applied power from each array element, or scan path segment, without causing unacceptable amounts of treatment-related complications. This will maximize the thermal dose that can be safely administered to the diseased tissue despite the limitations in spatial power resolution. This only requires knowledge of the highest temperature point in each control zone, as opposed to complete knowledge of all temperatures, since it is the time averaged T_{max} which has been shown to correlate with heat related complications (KAPP et al. 1992). Orthogonal placement of multiple invasive temperature-mapping catheters through the center of the treatment field where the Gaussian shaped power deposition pattern has its maximum amplitude can give treatment systems utilizing single aperture devices an excellent chance of sampling the maximum induced temperature.

Optimized control of large surface area array or scanning antenna applicators is more difficult and is currently an unsolved problem. The treatment areas can extend over hundreds of square centimeters, with current systems having up to 25 degrees of freedom for local power control. Inserting sufficient catheters to produce an interstitial thermometry density comparable to that utilized during treatments with small single-aperture applicators would not be tolerated by most patients. If continuous thermal mapping (GIBBS 1983) is utilized, the few interstitial sensors that are inserted cannot be utilized as data sources for power control due to inadequate retrace time.

One reported clinical power control protocol (LEE et al. 1992) for a 25-element noncoherent array utilizes probes placed on the skin surface as the primary source of control information. These skin surface sensors are placed in locations such as scars, discrete nodules, and necrotic regions that are likely to preferentially heat. At least one sensor must be under each array element regardless of anatomy. Two interstitial catheters with automatically mapped single junction sensors are placed at depth between 0.5 and 2.0 cm within the tumor-bearing region, primarily for the purpose of assessing heating efficacy. These sensors are used for control only if temperatures in excess of 50°C are sensed, in which case thermal mapping is stopped at the hot spot and array power is reallocated. Reports by the patient of pain in the heating field are assumed to be caused by unmeasured high temperatures, and power is locally or globally reduced to stay below the patient's pain tolerance. No analgesic agents are employed for the purpose of masking treatment-related pain. Despite the use of up to 40 thermometry probes in the treatment field, 74% of the treatments produced pain, not correlated with measured high temperatures, which required reductions in applied power. Power control is done manually with mouse-controlled graphical interfaces for both the thermometry and power control computers. An automated power control interface has been developed and tested successfully in dynamic perfused phantoms but has not yet been proven clinically (ZHOU and FESSENDEN 1993).

This type of control scheme is common in practice for large surface area devices but has significant shortcomings. There is no way to assure that the skin surface sensors are actually at the local highest temperature points at the skin surface or that higher temperatures are not being produced at depth. The existence of unmeasured high temperature points is strongly implied by the high incidence of pain during treatment and the lesser occurrences of post-treatment blisters. The temperatures measured by the skin surface thermometry sensors may not be accurate. There is evidence that temperatures measured by sensors placed between the skin and a temperature-regulated coupling bolus may be skewed away from the true skin temperature towards the temperature of the circulating bolus fluid (LEE et al. 1994). Also, regulating power by maintaining the patient at the edge of the patient's pain threshold for the duration of the treatment in order to maximize thermal dose is psychologically stressful on both the patient and the medical staff. In addition, the temperature pain threshold has been experimentally found to vary between individuals and vary with time within the same individual (JAMES et al. 1988). The requirement that the patient be able to inform the operator of unmeasured hot spots precludes utilizing general or local anesthesia. This again illustrates that optimized clinical use and control of hyperthermia applicators will not be achieved until some form of practical high-resolution noninvasive thermometry is developed.

10.7 Conclusion

The basic engineering aspects of radiative electromagnetic hyperthermia applicators have progressed considerably since the initial days of oncological hyperthermia, where adaptations of physical diathermy heating devices were used. Large amounts of basic research into waveguide, horn, dipole, microstrip, and magnetic inductive radiating elements have produced clinically tested basic building blocks for advanced heating systems.

Numerous research institutions have reported assembling these antennas into array applicators and mechanically scanned antenna systems. Clinically operational arrays utilized primarily for large surface area chest wall treatments have been assembled from waveguide, microstrip, and current sheet radiating elements. Far less work has gone into mechanically scanned antenna applicators, though a design for a scanning microstrip spiral antenna applicator has been extensively clinically utilized and a robotic arm applicator has undergone limited clinical testing.

Lack of adequate thermometry is a serious problem that is currently handicapping treatments performed with hyperthermia applicators in general and applicators with multiple power control degrees of freedom in particular.

Developments are being made in the field of noninvasive thermometry that have the theoretical potential to produce subcentimeter spatial resolution thermometry with temperature resolution in tenths of degrees. The potential problems here are as much economic as technical, particularly for the magnetic resonance imaging thermometry methods. No solution is probably possible for the mismatch between the available power deposition spatial resolution and the observed scale of tissue heating heterogeneities. Subcentimeter control over power deposition is not possible with radiative electromagnetic heating devices if penetration depths of more than a few millimeters are required. Without external manipulations of perfusion, body baseline temperature, and tissue conductivity, it is generally not possible for radiative electromagnetic heating modalities even in theory to reliably raise all tumor points to the therapeutic range given the theoretical and observed temperature variations in tumors and normal tissue.

Despite these limitations of current and future equipment, a randomized and retrospective comparison of radiation versus radiation plus hyperthermia studies showed an enhancement of response rate by a factor of 2 (KAPP and KAPP 1993). One surprising aspect of these data (Fig. 10.13) is the similarity of response rates among institutions with large variations in the type and sophistication of heating equipment. It will require further clinical studies to determine where the point of diminishing returns sets in for the trade-off between clinical efficacy versus hyperthermia system complexity in combined modality treatments and which hyperthermia applicator performance parameters and utilization protocols correlate with tumor response. For instance, it has been suggested that cold spots caused solely by local high blood perfusion, and not by lack of deposited power, are not important in combined radiation plus hyperthermia therapy because the enhancement in local radiation effect

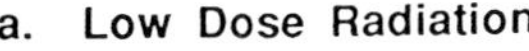

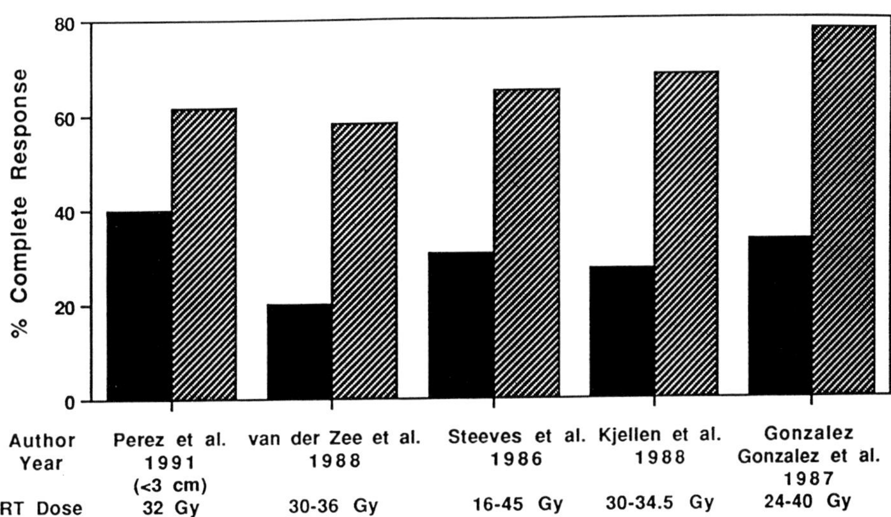

b. Full Dose Radiation

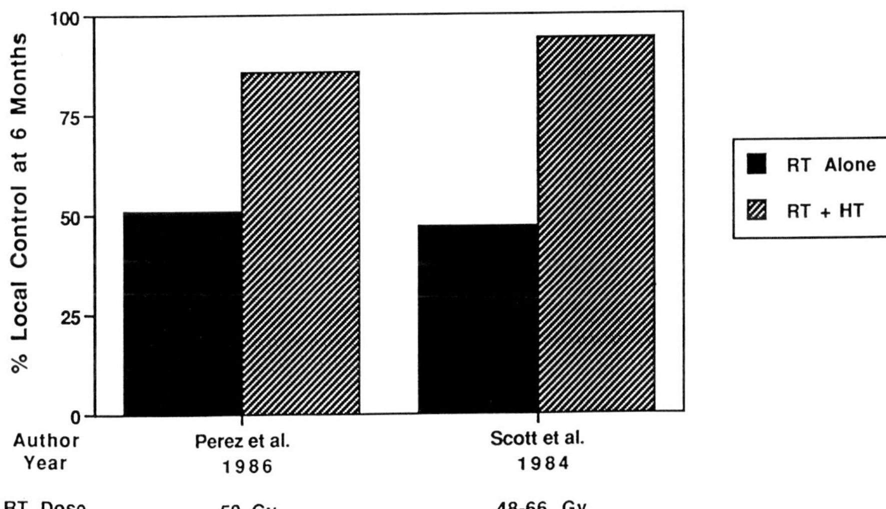

Fig. 10.13. Randomized and retrospective comparison studies of local response rates for radiation alone versus radiation plus hyperthermia therapies for local-regional breast cancer. (From KAPP and KAPP 1993)

by the increased oxygenation compensates for the reduced thermal dose. This is speculative, but if true would make the ability of an applicator to locally enhance power deposition over small areas a less important design parameter. Conversely, some clinical groups view localized burns as an acceptable consequence of a hyperthermia treatment, e.g., "If there is no choice, it would be more beneficial for the patient to have an effective treatment with a few blisters rather than a safe but ineffective treatment. It is easier to treat the burns than the cancer." (CHOU 1992). Following this aggressive treatment philosophy, the ability to locally reduce an applicator's deposited power is potentially counterproductive if the applicator power control cannot resolve down to the local hot spot size, since reduction of power to the region near a small hot spot may compromise the thermal dose administered to the diseased tissue surrounding that localized hot spot. Most current clinicians, however, will not knowingly and deliberately allow a burn to be produced in the course of a routine treatment and will try to perform as effective a treatment as possible commensurate with zero intended complications.

These examples emphasize that the design of clinical equipment should not be undertaken by engineers without imput from practicing clinicians and radiobiologists. The type of enhancements in the capabilities of future heating devices, along with the resultant higher level of cost and complexity, must be matched to actual clinical needs and the magnitude of the anticipated improvements in tumor response.

10.8 Summary

- There exist a large body of theory, experimental studies and clinical data on radiative electromagnetic devices intended for heating shallow depth diseased tissue. The basic technology is fairly mature.
- Advanced applicators capable of local power control have been constructed and clinically tested. Both array and mechanically scanned antenna applicators have been utilized on a routine basis for clinical treatments.
- Currently available thermometry systems are inadequate for providing sufficient information to properly control power steerable applicators.
- The maximum theoretical resolution of spatial power control for radiative electromagnetic applicators is too large by a factor of ten to compensate for the currently measured thermal variations in human patients undergoing hyperthermia treatments. Because of this, there may be a limit on the efficacy of heating possible with applicators based on radiative electromagnetic devices.
- What optimized design means for advanced radiative electromagnetic applicators depends strongly upon radiobiological factors and medical treatment protocols. Seriously suboptimal heating systems can result from attempts to design applicators without this source of input.

References

Audone B, Bolla L, Marone G, Gabriele P (1985) Hyperthermic thermology by waveguide and microstrip applicators. In: Overgaard J (ed) Hyperthermic oncology 1984, vol 1. Taylor and Francis, London, pp 655–658

Bahl IJ, Stuchly SS, Lagendijk JJW, Stuchly MA (1982) Microstrip loop radiators for medical applications. IEEE Trans Microwave Theory Tech 30: 1090–1093

Bach Andersen J, Baurn A, Harmark K, Heinzl L, Raskmark P, Overgaard J (1984) A hyperthermia system utilizing a new type of inductive applicator. IEEE Trans Biomed Eng 31: 21–27

Bolomey JC, Hawley MS (1990) Noninvasive control of hyperthermia. In: Bautherie H (ed) Methods of hyperthermia control. Springer, Berlin Heidelberg New York, pp 35–111

Chan KW, Chou CK, McDougall JA, Luk KH (1988) Changes in heating patterns due to perturbations by thermometer probes at 915 and 434 MHz. Int J Hyperthermia 4: 447–456

Chive M, Plancot M, Giaux G, Prevost B (1984) Microwave hyperthermia controlled by microwave radiometry: technical aspects and first clinical results. J Microw Power 19: 233–241

Chou CK (1992) Evaluation of microwave applicators. Bioelectromagnetics 13: 581–597

Chou CK, McDougall JA, Chan KW, Luk KH (1990a) Evaluation of captive bolus applicators. Med Phys 17: 705–709

Chou CK, McDougall JA, Chan KW, Luk KH (1990b) Effects of fat thickness on heating patterns of the microwave applicator MA-150 at 631 and 915 MHz. Int J Radiat Oncol Biol Phys 19: 1067–1070

Chou CK, McDougall JA, Chan KW, Luk KH (1991) Heating patterns of microwave applicators in inhomogeneous arm and thigh phantoms. Med Phys 18: 1164–1170

Corry PM, Barlogie B (1982) Clinical application of high frequency methods for local hyperthermia. In: Nussbaum G (ed) Physical aspects of hyperthermia. AAPM Press, New York, pp 307–328

Crezee J, Lagendijk JJW (1992) Temperature uniformity during hyperthermia: the impact of large vessels. Phys Med Biol 37: 1321–1337

De Leo R, Cerri G, Moglie F (1989) Microstrip patch applicators. IEEE 1989 International Symposium on Antennas and Propagation. IEEE, New York, pp 524–527

Diederich CJ, Stauffer PR (1993) Pre-clinical evaluation of a microwave planar array applicator for superficial hyperthermia. Int J Hyperthermia 9: 227–246

Durney CH, Massoudi H, Iskandar MF (1986) Radiofrequency radiation dosimetry handbook 4th edn. US Government publication National Technical Information Service, pp 4.1–4.22

Fenn AJ, Diederich CJ, Stauffer PR (1993) Experimental evaluation of an adaptive focusing algorithm for a microwave planar phased-array hyperthermia system at UCSF. Technical report 977, Lincoln Laboratory, Massachusetts Institute of Technology

Finger PT, Packer S, Svitra P, Paglione RW, Albert DM, Chess J (1983) A 5.8 GHz optithalmic microwave applicator for treatment of choroidal melanoma 1983 IEEE MTT-S International Microwave Symposium Digest. IEEE, New York, pp 177–179

Foster KR, Schepps JL (1981) Dielectric properties of tumor and normal tissues at radio through microwave frequencies. J Microwave Power 16: 107–119

Franconi C, Tiberio CA, Raganella L, Begnozzi L (1986) Low-frequency twin-dipole applicator for intermediate depth hyperthermia. IEEE Trans Microwave Theory Tech 34: 612–619

Gee W, Lee SW, Bong NK, Cain CA, Mittra R, Magin RL (1984) Focused array hyperthermia applicator: theory and experiment. IEEE Trans Biomed Eng 31: 38–46

Gibbs FA Jr (1983) "Thermal mapping" in experimental cancer treatment with hyperthermia: description and use of a semi-automatic system. Int J Radiat Oncol Biol Phys 9: 1057–1063

Gibbs FA Jr, Sapozink MD, Stewart JR (1985) Clinical thermal dosimetry: why and how. In: Overgaard J (ed) Hyperthermic oncology 1984, vol 2. Taylor and Francis, London, pp 155–167

Gopal MK, Hand JW, Lumori MLD, Alkhairi S, Paulsen KD, Cetas TC (1992) Current sheet applicator arrays for superficial hyperthermia of chest wall lesions. Int J Hyperthermia 8: 227–240

Guy AW (1971a) Analysis of electromagnetic fields induced in biological tissues by thermographic studies on equivalent phantom models. IEEE Trans Microwave Theory Tech 19: 205–214

Guy AW (1971b) Electromagnetic fields and relative heating patterns due to a rectangular aperture source in direct contact with bilayered biological tissue. IEEE Trans Microwave Theory Tech 19: 214–223

Guy AW (1990) Biophysics of high-frequency currents and electromagnetic radiation. In: Lehmann JF (ed) Therapeutic heat and cold, 4th edn. William & Wilkins, Baltimore, pp 179–361

Guy AW, Lehmann JF (1966) On the determination of an optimum microwave diathermy frequency for a direct contact applicator. IEEE Trans Biomed Eng 13: 76–87

Hand JW (1987) Electromagnetic applicators for non-invasive local hyperthermia. In: Field SB, Franconi C (eds) Physics and technology of hyperthermia. Martinus Nijhoff, Dordrecht, pp 189–210

Hand JW (1990) Biophysics and technology of electromagnetic hyperthermia. In: Gautherie M (ed) Methods of external hyperthermic heating. Springer Berlin Heidelbery New York, pp 1–59

Hand JW, ter Haar G (1981) Heating techniques in hyperthermia. Br J Radiol 54: 443–466

Hand JW, Hind AJ (1986) A review of microwave and RF applicators for localized hyperthermia. In: Hand JW, James JR (eds) Physical techniques in clinical hyperthermia. Research Studies Press, Letchworth, Herts., England, pp 98–140

Hand JW, Ledda JL, Evans NTS (1982) Considerations of radiofrequency induction heating for localized hyperthermia. Phys Med Biol 27: 1–16

Hand JW, Cheetham JL, Hind AJ (1986) Absorbed power distributions from coherent microwave arrays for localized hyperthermia. IEEE Trans Microwave Theory Tech 34: 484–489

Hand JW, Vernon CC, Prior MV, Forse GR (1992) Current sheet applicator arrays for superficial hyperthermia. In: Gerner EW (ed) Hyperthermic oncology 1992, vol 2. Arizona Board of Regents

Henderson A, James JR (1985) Near-field power transfer effects in small electromagnetic applicators for inducing hyperthermia. IEE Proc 132: 189–197

Iskandar MF (1982) Physical aspects and methods of hyperthermia production by rf currents and microwaves. In: Nussbaum GH (ed) Physical aspects of hyperthermia. American Institute of Physics, New York, pp 151–191

James JR, Henderson A, Johnson RH (1986) Compact electromagnetic applicators. In: Hand JW, James JR (eds) Physical techniques in clinical hyperthermia. Research Studies Press, Letchworth Herts., England, pp 149–207

James RD, Williams P, Jones A, Nelis P, Farrow N, Lukka H, Pye DW (1988) Determination of human skin pain threshold using 27 MHz radiofrequency heating (correspondence). Br J Radiol 61: 344–345

Johnson CC, Guy AW (1972) Nonionizing electromagnetic wave effects in biological materials and systems. Proc IEEE 60: 692–718

Johnson RH, James JR, Hand JW, Hopewell JW, Dunlop PRC, Dickinson RJ (1984) New low-profile applicators for local heating of tissue. IEEE Trans Biomed Eng 31: 28–37

Johnson RH, Preece AW, Hand JW, James JR (1987) A new type of lightweight low-frequency electromagnetic hyperthermia applicator. IEEE Trans Microwave Theory Tech 35: 1317–1321

Johnson RH, Preece AW, Green JL (1990) Theoretical and experimental comparison of three types of electromagnetic hyperthermia applicator. Phys Med Biol 35: 761–779

Kantor G (1981) Evaluation and survey of microwave and radiofrequency applicators. J Microw Power 16: 135–150

Kantor G, Witters DM (1983) The performance of a new 915 MHz direct contact applicator with reduced leakage. J Microw Power 18: 133–142

Kapp DS, Fessenden P, Samulski TV et al. (1988) Stanford University institutional report. Phase I evaluation of equipment for hyperthermia treatment of cancer. Int J Hyperthermia 4: 75–115

Kapp DS, Lee ER, Tarczy-Hornoch P, Fessenden P (1989) Specially designed applicators for hyperthermia (HT) treatment of facial tumors (Abstract Ad-2). In: Abstracts of the 9th NAHG Meeting, Seattle, Washington, March 1989. Radiation Research Society, Philadelphia, p 8

Kapp DS, Cox RS, Fessenden PF, Meyer JL, Prionas SD, Lee ER, Bagshaw MA (1992) Parameters predictive for complications of treatments with combined hyperthermia and radiation therapy. Int J Radiat Oncol Biol Phys 22: 999–1008

Kapp KS, Kapp DS (1993) Hyperthermia's emerging role in cancer therapy. Contemp Oncol 3(6): 19–30

Kawabata K, Jo S, Hiroka M, Nohara H, Takahashi M, Abe M (1984) A helical array applicator system of a microwave for the extension of the homogeneous heat area. In: Matsuda T, Kikuchi M (eds) Hyperthermic oncology. Proceedings of the Sixth Annual Meeting of Hyperthermia Group of Japan. Japan Society of Hyperthermic Oncology, Tokyo, pp 96–97

Kobayashi H, Nikawa Y, Okada F, Mori S (1989) Flexible microstrip patch antenna for hyperthermia. IEEE 1989 International Symposium on Antennas and Propagation, IEEE, New York, pp 536–539

Lagendijk JJW (1982a) Microwave applicator for hyperthermic treatment of retinoblastoma. In: Dethlefsen LA, Dewey WC (eds) Third international symposium: cancer therapy by hyperthermia, drugs, and radiation. National Institute of Health Publication No. 82-2437 Bethesda, Maryland, pp 469–471

Lagendijk JJW (1982b) The influence of blood flow in large vessels on the temperature distribution in hyperthermia. Phys Med Biol 27: 17–23

Lagendijk JJW, Schellenkens M, Schipper J, van der Linden PM (1984) A three-dimensional description of heating patterns in vascularised tissue during hyperthermia treatment. Phys Med Biol 29: 495–507

Lagendijk JJW, Hofman P, Schipper J (1985) A computer-controlled microwave hyperthermia system. In: Overgaard J (ed) Hyperthermic oncology 1984, vol 1. Taylor and Francis, London, pp 699–702

Lee ER, Samulski TV, Fessenden P (1986) Controlled scan surface heating (Abstract Ce-6). In: Abstract of Papers for the 34th Annual Meeting of the Radiation Research Society, April 1986. Radiation Research Society, Philadelphia, p 31

Lee ER, Tarczy-Hornoch P, Fessenden P, Kapp DS, Prionas S (1988) Scanning dipole antenna array applicator (abstract Bc-6). In: Abstracts of the 8th NAHG meeting, April 1988. Radiation Research Society, Philadelphia, p 15

Lee ER, Wilsey TR, Tarczy-Hornoch P, Kapp DS, Fessenden P, Lohrbach A, Prionas SD (1992) Body conformable 915 MHz microstrip array applicators for large surface area hyperthermia. IEEE Trans Biomed Eng 39: 470–483

Lee ER, Kapp DS, Lohrbach AW, Sokol J (1994) The influence of water bolus temperature on measured skin surface and intradermal temperatures. Int J Hyperthermia 10(1): 59–72

Lerch IA, Kohn S (1983) Radiofrequency hyperthermia: the design of coil transducers for local heating. Int J Radiat Oncol Biol Phys 9: 939–948

Leybovich LB, Nussbaum GH, Straube WL, Emami BN (1991) Theory and design of "shortened" multiantenna microwave applicators with controllable SAR patterns. Med Phys 18: 178–183

Loane J, Ling H, Wang BF, Lee SW (1986) Experimental Investigation of a Retro-Focusing Microwave Hyperthermia Applicator. Conjugate-Field Matching Scheme. IEEE Trans Microwave Theory Tech 34(5): 490–494

Lovisolo GA, Adami M, Arcangeli G, Borrani A, Calamai G, Cividalli A, Mauro F (1984) A multifrequency water-filled waveguide applicator: thermal dosimetry in vivo. IEEE Trans Microwave Theory Tech 32: 893–896

Lumori MLD, Hand JW, Gopal MK, Cetas TC (1990) Use of Gaussian beam model in predicting SAR distributions from current sheet applicators. Phys Med Biol 35: 387–397

Magin RL, Peterson AF (1989) Invited review noninvasive microwave phased arrays for local hyperthermia: a review. Int J Hyperthermia 5: 429–450

Matsuda T, Takasuka S, Nikawa Y, Kikuchi M (1990) Heating characteristics of a 430 MHz microwave heating system with a lens applicator in phantoms and miniature pigs. Int J Hyperthermia 6: 685–696

Mendecki J, Friedenthal E, Botstein C, Sterzer F, Paglione R (1979) Therapeutic potential of conformal applicators for induction of hyperthermia. J Microw Power 14: 139–144

Montecchia F (1992) Microstrip antenna design for hyperthermia treatment of superficial tumors. IEEE Trans Biomed Eng 39: 580–588

Nikawa Y, Watanabe H, Kikuchi M, Mori S (1986a) A direct-contact microwave lens applicator with a computer-controlled heating system for local hyperthermia. IEEE Trans Microwave Theory Tech 34: 626–630

Nikawa Y, Katsumata T, Kikuchi M, Mori S (1986b) An electric field converging applicator with heating pattern controller for microwave hyperthermia. IEEE Trans Microwave Theory Tech 34: 631–635

Nussbaum GH, Leybovich LB (1984) Multiple-antenna applicators for microwave-induced local hyperthermia (Abstract Aa-8). In: Abstracts of Papers for the 32nd Annual Meeting of the Radiation Research Society, March 1984. Radiation Research Society, Philadelphia, p 4

Oleson JR, Dewhirst MW, Duncan D, Engler M, Thrall D (1985) Temperature gradients: prognostic and dosimetric implications. In: Proceedings of the 7th Annual Conference of the IEEE Engineering in Medicine and Biology Society, Chicago, September 1985, vol 1. IEEE, New York, pp 355–360

Paglione RW (1982) Power deposition with microwaves. In: Nussbaum GH (ed) Physical aspects of hyperthermia. American Institute of Physics, New York, pp 192–208

Paliwal B, Higgins P, Steeves R, Sandhu T, Severson S (1985) A moving microwave beam hyperthermia induction system. In: Overgaard J (ed) Hyperthermic oncology 1984, vol 1. Taylor and Francis, London, pp 723–726

Rappaport CM, Morgenthaler FR (1986) Localized hyperthermia with electromagnetic arrays and the leaky-wave troughguide applicator. IEEE Trans Microwave Theory Tech 34: 636–643

Rebollar JM, Encinar JA (1984) Design and optimization of multi-stepped applicators for medical applications. J Microw Power 19: 259–267

Rietveld P JM, van Rhoon GC (1992) Coherent and non-coherent 2/4 array applications of the 433 MHz water filled lucite-cone applicator. In: Gerner EW (ed) Hyperthermic oncology 1992, vol 1. Arizona Board of Regents, p 330

Roemer RB (1990) Thermal dosimetry. In: Gautherie M (ed) Thermal dosimetry and treatment planning. Springer, Berlin Heidelberg New York, pp 119–216

Roemer RB (1991) Optimal power deposition in hyperthermia. I. The treatment goal: the ideal temperature distribution: the role of large blood vessels. Int J Hyperthermia 7: 317–341

Ryan TP, Coughlin CT (1993) Non-moving microstrip applicators to conform to large superficial treatment areas with 433 MHz microwave hyperthermia (Abstract P-03-12). In: Abstracts of the 13th NAHG meeting, March 1993. Radiation Research Society, Philadelphia, p 13

Samulski TV, Fessenden P, Lee ER, Kapp DS, Tanabe E, McEuen A (1990) Spiral microstrip hyperthermia applicators: technical details and clinical performance. Int J Radiat Oncol Biol Phys 18: 233–242

Sandhu TJ, Kolozsvary AJ (1985) Conformal hyperthermia applicators. In: Overgaard J (ed) Hyperthermic oncology 1984, vol 1. Taylor and Francis, London, pp 675–678

Schipper J, Lagendijk JJW (1986) The treatment of retinoblastoma by fractionated radiotherapy combined with hyperthermia. In: Anghileri LJ, Robert J (eds) Hyperthermia in cancer therapy, vol III. CRC Press, Boca Raton, Florida, pp 79–87

Scott RS, Chou CK, McCumber M, McDougall, J, Luk KH (1986) Complications resulting from spurious fields produced by a microwave applicator used for hyperthermia. Int J Radiat Oncol Biol Phys 12: 1883–1886

Stauffer PR, Diederich CJ (1992) 915 MHz conformal array microwave applicator (abstract P-03-11). In: Abstracts of the 13th NAHG meeting, March 1993. Radiation Research Society, Philadelphia, p 13

Stauffer PR, Swift PS, Sneed PK, Char DH, Phillips TL (1988) Temperature controlled microwave ring radiator for hyperthermia therapy. IEEE Eng Med Biol Soc 10th Annual Int Conference, pp 1273–1274

Sterzer F, Paglione RW, Mendecki J, Friedenthal E, Botstein C (1980) RF therapy for malignancy. IEEE Spectrum, December 1980, pp 32–37

Sterzer F, Paglione RW, Friedenthal E, Mendecki J (1985) A microwave apparatus for producing uniform hyperthermic temperatures over large surfaces. 1985 IEEE MTT-S International Microwave Symposium Digest, IEEE, New York, pp 90–92

Sterzer F, Paglione RW, Wozniak FJ, Friedenthal E, Mendecki J (1986) A robot-operated microwave hyperthermia system for treating large malignant surface lesions. Microw J 29: 7: 147–151

Strohbehn JS (1984) Summary of physical and technical studies. In: Overgaard J (ed) Hyperthermic oncology 1984, vol 2. Review Lectures, Symposium Summaries and Workshop Summaries. Taylor and Francis, London, pp 353–369

Tanabe E, McEuen AH, Norris CS, Fessenden P, Samulski TV (1983) A multielement microstrip antenna for local hyperthermia. In: IEEE MTT-S 1983 International Microwave Symposium Digest. IEEE New York, pp 183–185

Tanabe E, Harris S, McEuen A, Samulski T, Fessenden P (1985) Microstrip antenna applicators – design and clinical experience. In: Abe M, Takahashi M, Sugahara T (eds) Hyperthermia in cancer therapy. Proceedings of the First Annual Meeting of the Japanese Society of Hyperthermic Oncology November 19–20, 1984, Mag Bros, Tokyo, pp 151–153

Tennant A, Conway J, Anderson AP (1990) A robot-controlled microwave antenna system for uniform hyperthermia treatment of superficial tumours with arbitrary shape. Int J Hyperthermia 6: 193–202

Tumeh AM, Turner PF, Schaefermeyer TN, Nguyen T (1989) Variable frequency spiral applicator for EM hyperthermia (Abstract Cr-1). In: Abstracts of the 9th NAHG meeting, April 1989. Radiation Research Society, Philadelphia, p 15

Turner PF (1983) Electromagnetic hyperthermia devices and methods. MS Thesis, University of Utah, Salt Lake City

Turner PF, Tumeh AM, Schaefermeyer TN, Nguyen T (1989) Interstitial antenna arrays with central destructive interference (Abstract Bg-1). In: Abstracts of the 9th NAHG meeting, April 1989. Radiation Research Society, Philadelphia, p 47

Underwood HR, Magin RL (1988) Rectangular microstrip radiator for a multielement local hyperthermia applicator. Proc IEEE Engineering in Medicine & Biology Society 10th Annual International Conference, IEEE, New York, pp 864–865

Underwood HR, Petersen AF, Magin RL (1989) Analysis and measurement of a microstrip array applicator for hyperthermia therapy. Proc IEEE Engineering in Medicine & Biology Society 11th Annual International Conference, IEEE, New York, pp 1145–1146

Underwood HR, Petersen AF, Magin RL (1992) Electric field distribution near rectangular microstrip radiators for hyperthermia heating: theory versus experiment in water. IEEE Trans Biomed Eng 39: 146–153

Vaguine VA, Tanabe E, Giebeler RH, McEuen AH, Hahn GM (1982) Microwave direct-contact applicator system for hyperthermia therapy research. In: Dethlefsen LA, Dewey WC (eds) Third International Symposium: Cancer therapy by hyperthermia, drugs, and radiation. National Institute of Health Publication No. 82-2437 Bethesda Maryland, pp 461–464

van Rhoon GC, Rietveld PJM, Broekmeyer-Reurink MP, Verloop-van't Hof EM, van den Berg AP, van der Ploeg SK, van der Zee J (1992) A 433 MHz waveguide applicator system with an improved effective field size for hyperthermia treatment of superficial tumors on the chest wall. In: Gerner EW (ed) Hyperthermic oncology 1992, vol 2. Arizona Board of Regents

Wilsey TR, McEuen AH, Fessenden P, Lee ER, Tanabe E, Nelson LV, Schlitter RC, Kapp DS (1988) Arm cuff microwave microstrip array applicator (abstract bc-5). In: Abstracts of the 8th NAHG meeting, April 1988. Radiation Research Society, Philadelphia, p 15

Wyslouzil W, Kashyap S, Daien DM (1987) Heating patterns for an array of 915 MHz Rectangular waveguide applicators. J Microw Power 22: 213–220

Zhou L, Fessenden P (1993) Automation of temperature control for large-array microwave surface applicators. Int J Hyperthermia 9: 479–490

11 Electromagnetic Deep Heating Technology

P. WUST, M. SEEBASS, J. NADOBNY, and R. FELIX

CONTENTS

11.1 Physical Considerations

Deep heating represents an attempt to achieve effective temperatures in and around large extended tumors of the pelvis and abdomen. The term *regional hyperthermia* is used for heat treatments of such extensive volumes. It is important to realize that tumor lesions considered for regional hyperthermia are typically nonresectable, i.e., they infiltrate surrounding tissues, are not clearly delimited, and are adherent to neighboring tissues and organs such as bone and bladder wall. Consequently, an effective heat treatment should generously cover a larger volume (known as the biological or clinical target volume in radiotherapy) containing a macroscopic tumor and tumor boundaries as well as parts of the suspicious vicinity. The target volume can also include different types of tissues, e.g., tumor, infiltrated fatty tissue, and infiltrated bone. Typical depths of tumors (absorption lengths) as derived from human cross-sections are in the range of 10–15 cm. Disagreement persists as to whether electromagnetic radiation is suitable for heating deep-seated tumors. Several issues will be discussed in this chapter.

Every kind of electromagnetic heating technology generates an alternating electric field of amplitude $\underline{\mathbf{E}}$ in human tissue. The initial assumption is that the excitation of frequency ω is time-harmonic, i.e., sinusoidal. In this case $\underline{\mathbf{E}}$ can be represented as a *phasor*, i.e., vector with length and direction (indicated by a bold letter) and a complex number (indicated by underlining) contributing a phase ϕ with respect to a reference point (e.g., the exciting generator). One specific feature of this representation is the additivity of $\underline{\mathbf{E}}_j$ at every point if several sources j with a fixed phase relation generate $\underline{\mathbf{E}}_j$. That means that the final electric field is simply $\underline{\mathbf{E}} = \Sigma\underline{\mathbf{E}}_j$. The electric field (V/m) deposits a power density measured in mW/g in the exposed tissue, the so-called specific absorption rate, SAR $= (\sigma/2\rho)E^2$. Here, σ is the *electrical conductivity* of the absorbing tissue in S/m, which together with the *relative dielectric constant* ε_r determines the absorption and wavelength of electromagnetic waves, and ρ in g/cm^3 is the *density*. The dielectric distribution of (σ, ε_r) in the human body is only approximately known. A quick estimation of heating capabilities is obtained by differentiating between high water

P. WUST, PhD, Department of Radiation Oncology, Universitätsklinikum Rudolf Virchow, Standort Wedding, Freie Universität Berlin, Augustenburger Platz 1, D-13353 Berlin, FRG
M. SEEBASS, PhD, Konrad Zuse Zentrum for Information Technology, Heilbronner Straße 10, D-10711 Berlin, FRG
J. NADOBNY, PhD, Department of Radiation Oncology, Universitätsklinikum Rudolf Virchow, Standort Wedding, Freie Universität Berlin, Augustenburger Platz 1, D-13353 Berlin, FRG
R. FELIX, MD, Department of Radiation Oncology, Universitätsklinikum Rudolf Virchow, Standort Wedding, Freie Universität Berlin, Augustenburger Platz 1, D-13353 Berlin, FRG

content tissue (ε_r = 70–80, σ = 0.6–0.8 S/m) and low water content tissue (ε_r = 5–10, σ = 0.05 S/m, at a frequency around 100 MHz). A 2/3-conductivity of σ = 0.55 S/m is a reasonable estimate when averaging the electrical behavior of patient cross-sections in the abdomen or pelvis. Two-dimensional calculations support this. In the interesting frequency range from 30 to 100 MHz (see below) a slight decrease in ε_r as well as a slight increase in σ with increasing frequency has been established.

The very first investigations into applying electromagnetic waves for deep heating examined the penetration of a plane wave of given frequency illuminating a homogeneous lossy medium with the propagation direction perpendicular to the medium boundary. We call this the *one-dimensional electromagnetic problem* of radiofrequency hyperthermia. The E field in the medium is an attenuated harmonic wave of the form $\exp(-\gamma z)$ in the propagation direction $\mathbf{z}^0$. The *propagation constant* $\gamma = \alpha + j\beta$ is derived from the *attenuation constant* α and the *phase constant* β which depends on frequency and electrical constants according to the formulas in Table 11.1, The 50% *depth* $d_{1/2}$ is defined as the depth where the SAR is reduced to 50% (normalized to the maximum at zero depth), and is equal to $0.346/\alpha$. According to Table 11.1, values of (σ, ε_r), the clinical 50% depth for muscle (σ = 0.8 S/m) are limited, with $d_{1/2}$ = 3.2 . . . 6.7 cm if the frequency decreases from 100 . . . 30 MHz. For a medium with lower 2/3-conductivity (σ = 0.55 S/m), the 50% depth increases slightly up to $d_{1/2}$ = 3.7 . . . 7.8 cm (same frequency range). The *wavelength* λ in the medium under consideration is derived from β and ranges from about 30 cm (for 100 MHz) to 80 cm (for 30 MHz), thus indicating the required dimensions of the applicators, which should be on the order of several λ (but at least $\lambda/2$) for appropriate radiation into the medium.

Obviously, illuminating a lossy medium from several directions to create an interference pattern in the interior should improve penetration depth as well as steering capabilities (Bach Andersen 1985). Thus the concept of annular phased arrays (APAs) came into being very early (Turner 1984b). The APA principle deals with a suitable arrangement of applicators/antennas controlled in phase and power around the volume to be heated. Several technical implementations of this concept are introduced and discussed in the next section.

It is interesting to inspect the best case of an SAR distribution which is physically possible for idealized cases of homogeneous media with given

Table 11.1. Physical behavior of a plane wave with frequency f incident perpendicularly on an infinitely extended lossy medium σ, ε_r. This is called the one-dimensional electromagnetic problem of hyperthermia

	$\varepsilon_r = 80, \sigma = 0.8$ S/m				$\varepsilon_r = 80, \sigma = 0.55$ S/m			
f [MHz]	α [1/m]	β [1/m]	$d_{1/2}$ [cm]	λ [cm]	α [1/m]	β [1/m]	$d_{1/2}$ [cm]	λ [cm]
100	10.9	21.6	3.2	29	9.3	10.9	3.7	30
70	8.7	15.8	4	40	7.5	15.1	4.5	42
50	7.1	11.7	4.9	54	6.2	11.2	5.6	56
30	5.1	7.6	6.7	83	4.5	7.2	7.8	88

$$\alpha\,[\mathrm{l/m}] = 0.0148 f \sqrt{\varepsilon_r} \sqrt{\sqrt{1 + \frac{1800\,\sigma}{\varepsilon_r f}} - 1}$$ attenuation constant

$$\beta\,[\mathrm{l/m}] = 0.0148 f \sqrt{\varepsilon_r} \sqrt{\sqrt{1 + \frac{1800\,\sigma}{\varepsilon_r f}} + 1}$$ phase constant

$\gamma = \alpha + j\beta$ propagation constant

$\gamma\,[\mathrm{l/m}] = (1.9\,10^{-7}\,\varepsilon_r^{\,2} f^4 + 62.2\,\sigma^2 f^2)^{1/4}$

$\lambda = 2\pi/\beta$ wavelength

$d_{1/2} = 0.346/\alpha$ 50% depth (for SAR/2)

f [MHz] frequency, σ [S/m] electrical conductivity, ε_r relative dielectric constant

σ, ε_r. This problem has been solved in a closed form for a conducting cylinder of infinite length and radius R (BREZOVICH et al. 1982) as well as for a conducting sphere of radius R (KLODT 1990). The highest SAR maximum in the center of a cylinder is achieved by exciting the ground mode in a cylindrical cavity. In this case the differential equation for E(ρ), where ρ is the distance from the cylinder axis, results in a ratio of Bessel functions of zero order $J_0(k\rho)$. Similarly, the highest SAR in the center of the sphere is obtained by the ground mode in a spherical resonator yielding an E_{01} spherical wave. Such calculations are useful because they permit a quick estimation of the most favorable E field or SAR which can ever be achieved in the center of a cylinder or sphere of given radius R and electrical properties σ, ε_r using a harmonic excitation of frequency ω. σ and R in particular prove to be critical for the SAR achieved in the center relative to the surface – and a particularly critical dependency lies just within the range of typical anatomical dimensions and the estimated electrical parameters of tissues. An optimum frequency for a given radius and electrical conductivity exists where the power deposition in the center and the peripheral load are balanced (e.g., 70 MHz for R = 14 cm and σ = 0.55 S/m, BREZOVICH et al. 1982). Lowering the frequency further compromises the steering capabilities more than it enhances the SAR. Higher frequencies rapidly increase the load in the periphery of the cross-section. The preconditions for electromagnetic heating are considerably better for smaller radii of around 10 cm, as are common in pediatrics. Such problems can be referred to as an idealized *two-dimensional electromagnetic problem* of hyperthermia, since all directions in a plane are used for the incident electromagnetic radiation. The basic ideas can be generalized to apply to elliptical cross-sections as well as to arbitrary inhomogeneous two-dimensional cross-sections without compromising the validity of the conclusions.

In contrast to one-dimensional estimations (Table 11.1), achieved power deposition patterns in homogeneous cross-sections show a pronounced dependency on conductivity (Fig. 11.1). For a typical elliptical cross-section (major axis 38 cm, minor axis 24 cm) a deterioration of central power deposition from 70% to 30% is seen, if conductivity is increased from σ = 0.55 S/m (2/3-conductivity) to σ = 0.8 S/m (muscle equivalent). Since the electrical parameters of heterogeneous tissues are only approximately known, a considerable uncertainty exists. However, a quite favorable SAR distribution is predicted for σ = 0.55 S/m, the averaged conductivity of human cross-sections.

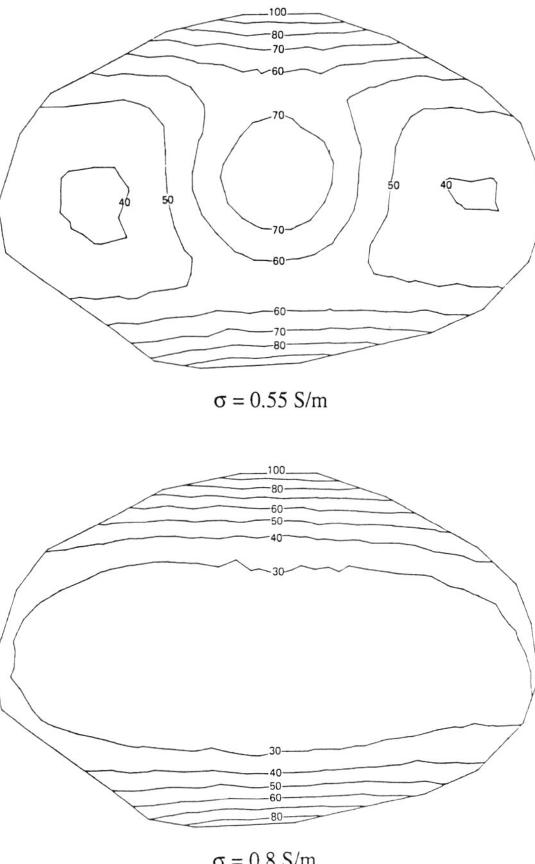

Fig. 11.1. Best-case estimations for the two-dimensional hyperthermia problem two-dimensional TM calculations (integral equation method) of iso-SAR lines in homogeneous cross-sections with typical dimensions (24 × 38 cm²). SAR is generated by eight antennas with equal phase and am-plitude, spaced equidistantly on a circle of diameter 60 cm (like in the SIGMA applicator). A strong dependency on electrical conductivity σ is shown: σ = 0.55 S/m (2/3-conductivity), σ = 0.8 S/m (muscle equivalent). Other parameters: ε_r = 78, frequency 105 MHz

In the case of *spherical* focusing in a homogeneous medium, i.e., if *more* spatial directions are exploited, the physical prerequisites for creating a focus are even better. This is referred to as an idealized *three-dimensional electromagnetic problem* for hyperthermia which necessarily yields even more optimistic predictions regarding application of electromagnetic radiation for controlled heating. However, because of tissue heterogeneities and nonspherical shapes the real electromagnetic problem (in clinical practice) is much more complicated, as will be discussed later.

Basic physics of electromagnetic radiation with consideration to hyperthermia have been reviewed by NUSSBAUM (1982), HAND and JAMES (1986), FIELD and FRANCONI (1987), and HAND (1990). However the implications of threedimensional structuration and heterogeneity of human tissues as well as its physiological behavior have not been discussed extensively by these authors.

11.2 Design of Existing Systems for Electromagnetic Deep Heating

11.2.1 Components of a Hyperthermia System

The most important components of a hyperthermia system and their linkage are shown in Fig. 11.2. The critical part of such a system is the *applicator*, which is a device for positioning a patient, arranging antennas in a suitable manner around the patient, and applying power to certain anatomical regions of the patient. Technical implementations of various applicators are described in this section; typical problems and phenomena are outlined in the next section.

It is important to note that the whole setup before the applicator, i.e., the line from the synthesizer generating a time-harmonic excitation to $i = 1 \ldots n$ power cables providing high-frequency output of amplitudes $p_{i=1 \ldots n}$ and phases $\phi_{i=1 \ldots n}$, is a standard problem of measuring and control engineering based on common components of high-frequency engineering. The actual hyperthermia-specific parts of commercially available hyperthermia systems are the thermometry equipment, applicator, and the particular E field sensors.

Controlling such a number of different electronic parts as are outlined in Fig. 11.2 requires a universal standard bus such as the IEEE bus. Synthesizer (frequency and level), phase shifter (phase), and voltage-controlled amplifier (amplitude) are adjusted by a computer. Only a gyrator circuit is suitable for a continuous phase control by a DC voltage in the low power block. Phase detectors (in the low power part) and bidirectional couplers with a power meter (behind the power amplifiers) can be used to detect the phase and power in each channel. DC voltage levels are combined in a multiplexer and digitized; a nonlinear calibration curve, preferably stored in a microprocessor, is required to obtain absolute values.

All components shown in Fig. 11.2 are standardized and commercially available. The most costly parts are preamplifiers and power amplifiers which are required for every channel. Assuming an input level of 0 dBm at 50 Ω (1.0 mW), a typical value in the low power part of the system, the preamplifier (including the preamplifier driver) must attain a total amplification of 40 dB in order to supply an input level of 10 W to the power amplifier. For a maximum power of 500 W the output amplifier needs a gain factor of 17 dB. In

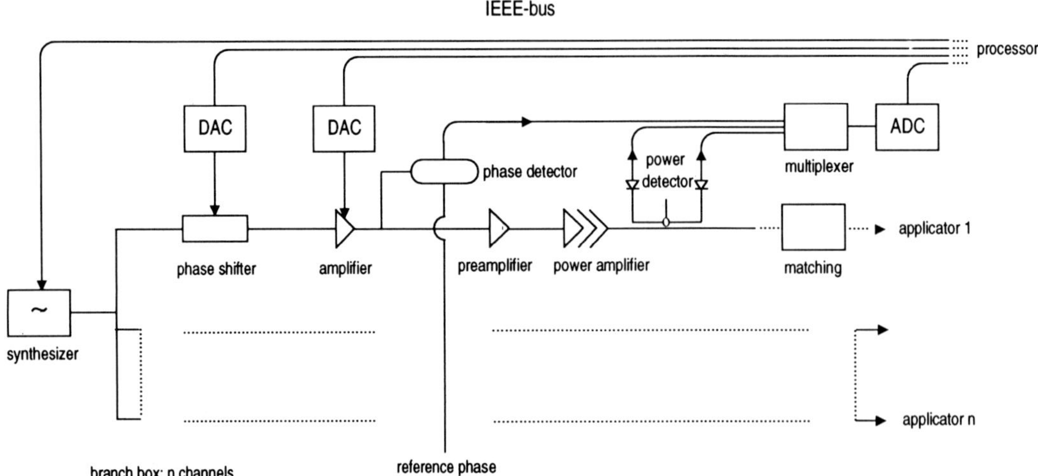

Fig. 11.2. Standard setup of a hyperthermia system with independent phase and amplitude control of *n* channels. All channels are fed by a time-harmonic synthesizer signal. Phase and amplitude are also detected and evaluated by the treatment software

the case of the BSD-2000 system (BSD Medical Corp., Salt Lake City, Utah, USA), a broadband tube amplifier with a frequency range of 300 kHz to 220 MHz is used for the output amplifier and a broadband transistor amplifier with a frequency range of 10 kHz to 500 MHz for the preamplifier. Broadband behavior and maximum power largely determine the price per channel, which can be considerably reduced by reducing the frequency range and increasing the number of channels (see Sect. 11.4). Note that transistor amplifiers with interface control are commercially available.

Various companies specialize in engineering and supply system solutions with individual components and data protocols specified by the user such as are shown on Fig. 11.2. Furthermore, user-friendly software packages are offered which permit a configuration of arbitrary components adapted to a standard bus such as the IEEE bus. Further progress in computer technology and software engineering will increase the chance of finding moderately priced commercial hardware and software packages which, even though they are not hyperthermia-specific, are already adequate or can be adapted for hyperthermia applications (at least for an initial prototype). In the following sections, we will focus on the most critical part of a hyperthermia system, the applicator.

11.2.2 Applicators for Deep Heating Systems

Various principles and applicators have been designed and evaluated theoretically and experimentally, as summarized in Fig. 11.3. The following section gives a short description and

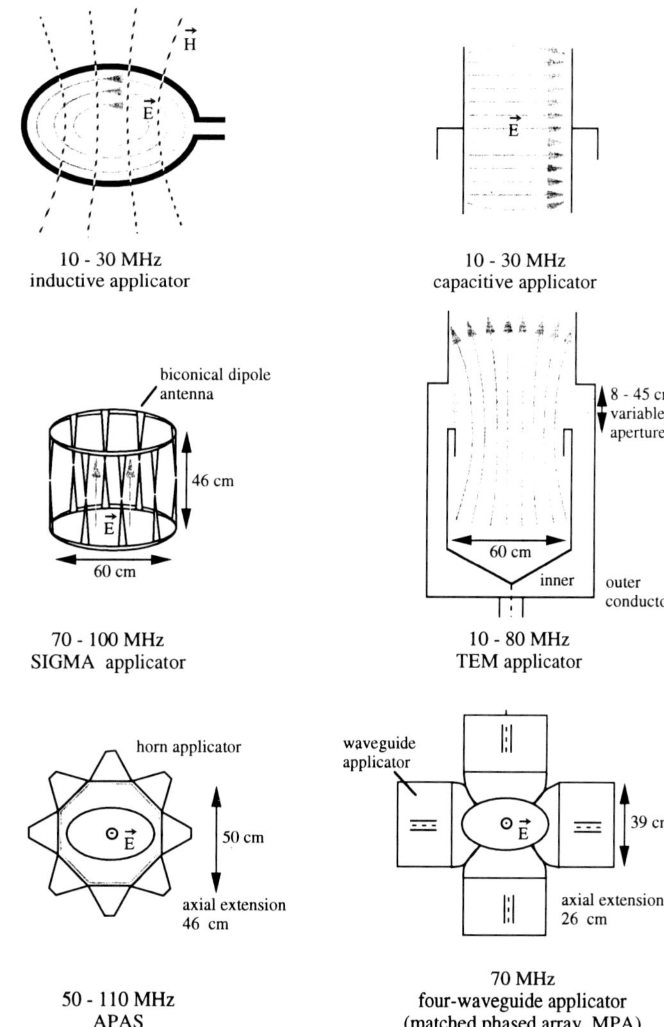

Fig. 11.3. Deep-heating devices in clinical use

estimation; for further details see HAND (1990) and the literature specified. Evaluation of equipment for hyperthermia which also includes devices for deep heating are given by KAPP et al. (1988), SAPOZINK et al. (1988), and CORRY et al. (1988). *Quasi-static* devices (i.e., with frequencies less than 30 MHz) transport power via either capacitances or inductances to a lossy medium (Fig. 11.3). Matching the 50 Ω output of the amplifier is straightforward in this frequency range. The inductive or capacitive applicator is integrated into a resonance circuit of the desired frequency using lumped circuit elements. Also a voltage transformation is required from the low 50 Ω coaxial line to the high voltage occurring at the capacitance of the resonance circuit.

In *inductive applicators* an E field is created proportional to the time rate of change of magnetic flux enclosed within the azimuth around the flux direction as per Maxwell's second equation. Specifically in the interior of the coil the E field is primarily directed toward the azimuth with respect to the coil axis and is roughly proportional to the radial distance from this axis. Therefore, deposited power in the coil center is equal to zero. Furthermore, outside the coil the magnetic field rapidly decreases, as does E or SAR, respectively. Homogeneity of the magnetic field is improved between a pair of Helmholtz coils if the distance between coils and their diameter are of the same order. Such an arrangement of coaxial coils is principally suitable to cover the part of the body located between the coils since quasi-static magnetic fields are nearly inert with respect to human tissues. Application has even been attempted in the case of endothoracic tumors (CORRY and BARLOGIE 1982). However, clinical results were disappointing and intratumoral temperatures above 42.5°C were achieved only for a small percentage of relatively superficial tumors (OLESON et al. 1983; Table 11.2).

Another inductive method uses a large concentric electrode around the cross-section, called the Magnetrode (STORM et al. 1981). It has been shown clinically as well as theoretically that this device is not suitable for heating deep-seated tumors efficiently for the same reason (zero power deposition in the center), particularly when compared with annular phased array systems (OLESON et al. 1986; PAULSEN 1990). One particular problem with this heating method is the inherent inhomogeneity of the SAR distribution even in a homogeneous medium, which causes severe local problems that limit power (OLESON et al. 1983). Obviously, electrical heterogeneities aggravate these local problems, even if the dominant E field

Table 11.2. Clinical efficiency of current systems in terms of satisfactory heat treatments (i.e., ≥42°C in the tumor)

Device	Reference	Patients/ treatments	Maximum intratumoral temperatures
Antenna arrays			
SIGMA-60	ISSELS et al. 1991	65/426	≥42°C in 74%
	FELDMANN et al. 1993	37/176	≥42°C in 64%
	WUST et al. 1995a	43/205	≥42°C in 66%
APAS	HOWARD et al. 1986	20/63	≥42°C in 78%
	SAPOZINK et al. 1986	43/175	≥42°C in 73%
TEM	DE LEEUW 1993	–/56	≥42°C in 46%
MPA	GONZÁLEZ-GONZÁLEZ et al. 1992; updated by van Dijk 1993	156/601	≥42°C in 48%
Capacitive			
Thermotron	HIRAOKA et al. 1987	60/307	≥42°C in 64%
	HISHIMURA et al. 1992	35/169	≥42°C in 53%
Inductive			
Magnetrode	OLESON et al. 1986	11/–	≥42°C in 7%
Concentric coils	OLESON et al. 1983	31/–	≥42.5°C in 19%
Ultrasonic			
Sonotherm 6500	HAND et al. 1992	9/26	≥42°C in 22%

direction is tangential with respect to superficial tissue boundaries such as fat layers. The potential of this technique is considerably enhanced if magnetic materials can be administered into the tumor or surroundings which absorb power directly from the primary magnetic field (BREZOVICH et al. 1984; JORDAN et al. 1993).

Capacitive applicators (Fig. 11.3) create E fields predominantly perpendicular to the body surface, i.e., particularly to the electrical boundary between subcutaneous fat and muscle. This E field orientation is evidently not optimal; indeed, it is possibly most unfavorable. Consequently, this technique is restricted to slim patients (thickness of fat layer less than 2 cm) and specific anatomical sites. Nevertheless, investigators using an 8-MHz or 13.56-MHz capacitive heating device achieved intratumoral temperatures of greater than or equal to 42°C in 50%–60% of sessions, which is comparable to other systems (HIRAOKA et al. 1987; NISHIMURA et al. 1992); see also Table 11.2.

All other deep-heating devices (Fig. 11.3) are based on the *APA principle* (Sect. 11.1) and generate an E field directed primarily along the patient axis (z-axis). The TEM applicator or APAS (Fig. 11.3) behave in principle like broadband resonators. The Q value is significantly decreased by the lossy medium of the patient.

In the case of the *TEM applicator* (DE LEEUW and LAGENDIJK 1987) the dominant E field occurs between the inner and outer conductor of a coaxial air line, forming on a ring a variable distance between 8 and 45 cm as aperture size (as indicated on Fig. 11.3). Matching conditions can be achieved by a tuner from 10 to 80 MHz. The operating frequency is typically 70 MHz. Coupling to the patient inside the inner conductor is carried out by tap water filling. A broad focus (for 70 MHz) is located in the center. SAR control inside a cross-section is possible by changing patient position in the transverse plane (DE LEEUW et al. 1991). Other degrees of freedom for modifying power deposition patterns are the water level in the applicator and the aperture size (DE LEEUW et al. 1990).

The ring applicator of the *APAS (annular phased array system) BSD-1000* (BSD Medical Corp., Salt Lake City, Utah, USA) consists of 16-horn (eight double-horn) applicators arranged on two octagonal rings which are fed synchronously by a power amplifier (TURNER 1984; GIBBS et al. 1984). Usually frequencies less than or equal to 70 MHz are applied which generate centrally peaked SAR distributions in homogeneous cylindrical or elliptical phantoms. Ideally, constructive interference of all radiated waves creates a relative maximum in the center. However, imbalances sensitive to frequency have been described, i.e., SAR maximums shifting to the top or bottom of the applicator (GIBBS 1987). Early clinical reports were quite optimistic in comparison to the quasistatic methods (SAPOZINK et al. 1986; HOWARD et al. 1986; Table 11.2): 70%–80% of heat treatments were considered satisfactory, i.e., temperatures greater than or equal to 42°C were achieved at least one intratumoral measurement point. For a larger group of 353 patients with abdominal and pelvic tumors, reported thermal data are less favorable, with clinically relevant thermal doses achieved in only 57% of the patients (PETROVICH et al. 1989). Other pilot studies were published by SHIMM et al. (1988) and PILEPICH et al. (1987). Clinical evaluation of the APA system BSD-1000 revealed two disadvantages: limited SAR control and suboptimum coupling by large and bothersome water boluses. Delayed access to the patient in the nontransparent overfilled ring applicator has been regarded as an additional clinical disadvantage.

To overcome these problems a second-generation system for deep regional hyperthermia has been developed: the *BSD-2000* with the ring applicator *SIGMA* (TURNER and SCHAEFERMEYER 1989, BSD Medical Corp.). Besides several mechanical improvements such as transparency, integrated bolus, and more convenient positioning, its most important innovation is independent phase and amplitude control of four antenna pairs (Fig. 11.3). These eight dipole antennas 46 cm in length are arranged equidistantly in a circle inside a Lucite cylinder. A two-dimensional theoretical and experimental approach (see Sect. 11.3) has supplied a strong rationale for this system design. However, thermal parameters of the SIGMA applicator are not in every case superior to the earlier version of the APAS applicator. For centrally located tumors (cervical cancer) SAPOZINK et al. (1990) found more satisfactory heat treatments with the APAS (77%) in comparison to the SIGMA (59%). Similarly, FELDMANN et al. (1993) report advantages of the APAS applicator in heating presacral rectal cancer.

This surprising inferiority of the more advanced SIGMA applicator in specific cases is caused by severe limitations of the SIGMA applicator with regard to coupling and three-dimensional electromagnetic phenomena (see Sect. 11.3). On the other hand, benefit of phase steering, i.e., moving a focus to a given location, has been demonstrated (Samulski et al. 1987a). Furthermore, several investigators have successfully used the BSD-2000 system for a larger number of patients (Issels et al. 1990, 1991; Feldmann et al. 1993; Wust et al. 1995a; van der Ploeg et al. 1993) with a relatively high percentage of satisfactory heat treatments (Table 11.2).

The *four-waveguide applicator* "MPA, matched phased array" (van Dijk et al. 1989) is based on a similar annular phased array principle as the SIGMA applicator and is now commercially available as VARIPHASE 5000 (Lund Science, Lund, Sweden). Reported temperatures are a bit lower than with the SIGMA or APAS, for which several reasons may be supposed (see below). However, system comparisons using an LED phantom (Schneider and van Dijk 1991) have shown all ring applicators (SIGMA, APAS, TEM, MPA) to have an equal ability to create a central focus (Schneider et al. 1994).

The *capacitive ring applicator* is another applicator with a longitudinally polarized E field (van Rhoon et al. 1988) which has been tested by phantom measurements for different frequencies from 30 to 70 MHz. Some SAR control is possible using different feeding points on the ring electrodes (van Rhoon et al. 1993). However, no clinical application has been carried out until now, and therefore a comparison with other applicators is problematic.

Table 11.2 is difficult to interpret in attempting to estimate the efficacy of available techniques. Clearly, reference to the number of satisfactory heat treatments is a very rough criterion. Sophisticated methods of thermal dosimetry and analysis have been worked out, and there is strong evidence of correlation between these deduced thermal parameters and clinical results (Oleson et al. 1989, 1993). However, as long as clinicians in practice are glad to achieve 42°C in a tumor, it is somewhat academic to inspect such complex variables for evaluation of efficacy.

It can be concluded from Table 11.2 that inductive methods without additives (e.g., ferromagnetic seeds or magnetic fluids) are unsuitable to heat deep-seated tumors for fundamental physical reasons. Capacitive methods appear to achieve intratumoral temperatures almost comparable to those yielded by APA systems. However, a strong selection of patients as well as tumor localizations must be assumed for every technique. For example, in the case of capacitive devices, patients with subcutaneous fat layers of thickness greater than or equal to 2 cm are excluded. In the case of ultrasound (US) hyperthermia, superficial and pelvic tumors are usually mixed (Harari et al. 1991). If only pelvic tumors are considered (Hand et al. 1992), temperatures achieved with US are less favorable in comparison to RF systems. For US hyperthermia an additional selection with respect to the ultrasound entrance window is performed. Clearly, supportive therapy of patients, especially analgesic and sedative premedication, has a supplementary impact on the achieved temperatures such as "*analgosedation*", which was introduced by Issels et al. (1990).

In summary, comparison of thermal parameters alone is not suitable for the evaluation of current technologies for deep heating. Specifically, thermal data must be related to anatomical localization of tumors and various other clinical variables. A combined approach involving analyses from clinical and experimental measurements and modeling considerations is given in the next section.

11.3 Evaluation of Technical Efficacy of Current Systems

11.3.1 Introduction

Only the E field oriented systems consisting of radiator groups or antenna arrays (SIGMA applicators, four-waveguide applicators) or structures similar to cavity resonators (TEM applicator, APAS) can create an SAR focus by constructive interference (see Sect. 11.2). With a two-dimensional evaluation method, using a homogeneous elliptical LED (light emitting diodes) phantom, Schneider et al. (1994) did not detect any significant differences between the systems mentioned above in creating and steering an SAR focus. Consequently, refined measurement techniques and numerical simulations have been employed and evaluations of the clinical data have been included in order to analyze the available hyperthermia technology as thoroughly as possible and to classify it accordingly.

The BSD-2000 hyperthermia system with the SIGMA applicators is the most common one in clinical use. Whereas its design is the most flexible and expandable, it appears to be the most complicated of all the systems. It is extremely suitable for use as a model system because many high-frequency effects can be demonstrated on it. Consequently, the measurements and simulation studies described below are based on the SIGMA-60 applicator.

In historical terms, two-dimensional studies (STROHBEHN et al. 1989; WUST et al. 1991a) have laid the groundwork for the radiofrequency hyperthermia technology in use today. The model calculations demonstrated significant advantages of amplitude and phase selection with respect to SAR steering, and thus hopefully the attained temperature distributions. However, it was not possible to reproduce these optimistic results in clinical practice (WUST et al. 1993b, 1995a). This discrepancy between theoretical prediction and practical experience is explained below on the basis of *coupling effects* and specific three-dimensional electromagnetic *boundary phenomena*.

Only a consistent understanding of all influences and principles limiting the effectiveness of today's clinical regional hyperthermia will permit working toward to a technological culmination in the development of these systems.

Table 11.3. Methods of evaluation for RF deep heating systems and basic references

Measurement methods
Coaxial line methods (MARSLAND and EVANS 1987; GRANT et al. 1989)
Network analysis (WUST et al. 1991b; LEYBOVICH et al. 1991; RASKMARK et al. 1994)
Visualizing phantoms (SCHNEIDER et al. 1991; WUST et al. 1994a)
Phantoms for E field scans (SCHNEIDER et al. 1992; PAULSEN and ROSS 1990)
Electro-optical E field sensor (MEIER et al. 1992, 1994; WUST et al. 1995b)

Modelling tools
Volume surface integral equation method (VSIE) (WUST et al. 1993a, NADOBNY 1993)
Finite elements method (FE) (LYNCH et al. 1985; STROHBEHN et al. 1986)
Finite integration theory method (FIT) (WEILAND 1984, 1986; DOHLUS 1992)
Finite difference time domain method (FDTD) (SULLIVAN et al. 1987, 1993; SULLIVAN 1990, 1991; SEEBASS et al. 1993b; HORNSLETH 1993)

In vivo evaluation
(ROEMER 1990a,b; SAMULSKI et al. 1987b; FELDMANN et al. 1992; WUST et al. 1995a)
Temperature/time curves
Temperature/position curves
E field sensor measurements
CT scans
Clinical observables

11.3.2 Methods of Evaluation

As indicated in Table 11.3, measurement techniques (phantoms in particular) and numerical procedures as well as information derived from clinical data are available for analyzing radiofrequency hyperthermia systems.

Network analysis is a standardized measuring technique in high-frequency engineering. This permits recording of the complex input impedance or admittance diagrams of Smith charts of antennas (the path of input reflection coefficients at the base point of the antenna in the complex plane parameterized by the frequency). Coupling coefficients between antennas have also been measured, whereby the complete information on the coupling is contained in the S matrix of an antenna ensemble (WUST et al. 1991b; LEYBOVITCH et al. 1991; RASKMARK et al. 1994).

Originally, SAR distributions were determined in elliptical phantoms performing time-consuming measurements according to the gradient of temperature rise method (ALLEN et al. 1988; MYERSON et al. 1981). An important step toward quickly registering power deposition patterns was taken with the development of *visualizing phantoms* (SCHNEIDER et al. 1991; WUST et al. 1994a, 1995c; Chap. 17 in this volume). To recreate the clinical situation free of artifacts, materials with defined electrical and mechanical properties had to be developed (σ, ε_r, durability, resistance to water, mechanical working properties, elasticity, hardness, surface behavior, etc.). This was possible using polyester resins or epoxy resins with appropriate additives (WUST et al. 1994a). A further problem was developing sensor arrays for visualizing the power deposition patterns. This can be accomplished either with light-emitting diodes (LEDs) or with suitable miniature lamps. Such visualized patterns are shown in Figs. 11.6 and 11.8. In open elliptical phantoms which are accessible from the outside additional measuring options are available such as mechanical scans with E field sensors (SCHNEIDER et al. 1992; WUST et al. 1994a, 1995b).

E field sensors can be made from visualizing sensors where the quantity of light is determined via a fiberoptic link using a photoresistor or an optical power meter. In addition to this, E field sensors with high-resistance leads were developed by several working groups (BASSEN and SMITH 1983), as well as being available commercially together with the BSD system (E field sensors EP-400 and EP-500, BSD Medical Corporation, Salt Lake City, Utah). Defined SAR profiles can be measured with single sensors for direct comparison with model calculations (see Fig. 11.7).

The development of an *electro-optical E field sensor* (MEIER et al. 1992, 1994), which can measure the phase and amplitude of the electric field, represents a further refinement in E field measuring technology. In this type of sensor, polarized light from a laser diode is conducted through a fiber that retains the polarization into a lithium niobate crystal where it is split. An appropriate electrode structure causes the electric field to act along the split path, causing phase shifts in the light. After the light paths are joined, the amplitude-modulated light signal will characterize the amplitude and phase of the modulating electric field. The signal to noise ratio of the E field measurement (in phase and amplitude) can be increased by applying the lock-in principle. Here, the antenna and laser diode are modulated with a synchronized but slightly offset operating frequency (such as 90 MHz, 90 MHz + 1 kHz) where the beat signal with the difference frequency (1 kHz) is then evaluated at the lock-in amplifier. The required reference signal for the lock-in amplifier is supplied by an electrical mixer.

Such a novel electro-optical E field sensor permits drawing conclusions about the E field distribution or SAR distribution in the interior of a medium (such as a patient) by recording E fields outside this medium (WUST et al. 1995b). To test this, a special *two-chambered phantom* was developed for the SIGMA-60 applicator. With a suitable scanning system, the interior of the elliptical phantom (filled with 0.55 S/m saline solution) is accessible as well as part of the space between the antennas and phantom wall from the outside. Here, the original bolus of the SIGMA applicator is temporally forced outside by a substitute bolus. Conducting E field scans in this substitute bolus necessitated procuring and appropriately programming a complicated four-axis steering system (Isel system, Isert-Elektronik, 36132 Eiterfeld, FRG). The substitute bolus contains either deionized water or tap water. The complicated mechanical guidance system for the electro-optical sensor was made of a nearly *water-equivalent* material ($\varepsilon_r = 50$, $\sigma = 0.02$ S/m).

Model calculations can also provide valuable insights into the function of radiofrequency hyperthermia systems (see Chap. 18 in this volume). The very first three-dimensional calculations for hyperthermia purposes were performed by PAULSEN et al. (1988), though for a homogeneous body. The initial theoretical framework had to be increasingly refined to achieve agreement between measurements and theoretical calculations. A total of four methods are available for calculating E fields (Table 11.3).

The *VSIE method* was developed by our group (WUST et al. 1993a; NADOBNY 1993). It has the advantage of physical transparency as described for the integral equation (IE) method in general by MÜLLER (1969). The calculation proceeds from the incident field of the respective antenna or applicator (Fig. 11.4). The scatter effect in the heterogeneous medium and at the boundaries in particular is represented by so-called volume currents and polarization charges. Calculation of the E field at electrical boundaries is particularly precise in comparison to difference methods (see

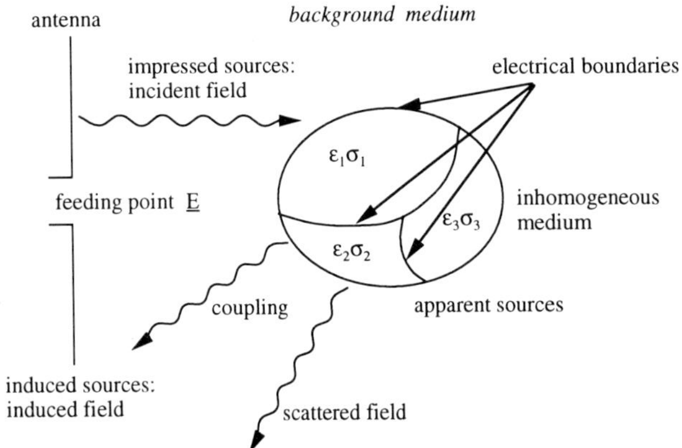

Fig. 11.4. Schematic representation of the electromagnetic problem in the theoretical framework of the VSIE method. The electric field has three parts: incident field, scattered field, and induced field.

below). Consequently, the calculation is conducted using tetrahedron grids, which can simulate boundaries better than cubic grids. The backscattering in the heterogeneous medium produces a change in the antenna currents. So-called induced sources on the antenna lead to modification of the E field to ensure the boundary condition on the metal surfaces of the antenna. However, depending on the excitation model of the antenna either the E field or current at the feeding point of the antenna (Fig. 11.4) can be used as a fixed input parameter for E field calculation. A different algorithm based on the IE method has been developed by ZWAMBORN and VAN DEN BERG (1992).

The *finite element (FE) method* is widely used (PAULSEN 1990). A two-dimensional FE code was developed in our group for calculating E fields (SEEBASS et al. 1992; NADOBNY et al. 1992). The FE method requires a complete boundary condition for the solution in the interior. This condition is not easily determined in the case of open electromagnetic problems. The hybrid method as developed by PAULSEN et al. (1988a) is an approach to provide boundary conditions for open problems. However, where a complete boundary condition is present the FE method is significantly more efficient than the VSIE method, particularly since it works with sparse matrices. This is understandable since an electromagnetic problem is better specified by stipulating a closed boundary condition (FE method) than by the input parameters of the antennas (IE method). Furthermore, for FE methods working on triangular or tetrahedron grids highly efficient numerical solvers were developed based on locally adaptive grid refining procedures (DEUFLHARD et al. 1989; BORNEMANN 1991, 1992).

The *finite integration theory (FIT) method* is a finite volume method (DOHLUS 1992; WEILAND 1986) that was originally developed for beam guiding problems encountered in constructing particle accelerators. The method works on regular grids that can also be locally modified and subdivided to adapt them to special geometries. Although at boundaries averaging over the adjacent finite volume elements is performed, in test cases this method produces results equivalent to those of the VSIE method (see WUST et al. 1993a). A particular advantage of this method is its numerical efficiency, allowing both the antennas and the outside area to be included in electromagnetic problems. Fast methods of calculating electromagnetic problems in radiofrequency hyperthermia are finite differences methods (SULLIVAN 1990, 1991). The *finite difference time domain (FDTD) method* carries out its calculations on a regular grid. This alone produces different results from methods that utilize tetrahedron grids.

Important progress in understanding hyperthermia systems has resulted from the systematic analysis of clinical data. The *temperature time curves* recorded at measuring points specified by computerized tomography (CT) contain the most important information (ROEMER et al. 1985; ROEMER 1990a,b). The SAR can be determined from the rise when switching on power and the fall when switching it off, as illustrated in Fig. 11.5. Dividing this SAR by the total power radiated in yields the relative SAR. At both the beginning and the end of therapy the effective perfusion, which accounts for both perfusion and conduction, can be determined from the transition from the temperature time curve to the plateau. The evaluation method is described in detail in WUST et al. (1995a). Temperature position curves are routinely recorded during hyperthermia with the aid of a stepping motor system. Each measuring point is then specified in the CT scans routinely conducted with the catheter in place. In this manner SAR or E field measurements can be assigned to certain geometric configurations in patients (such as bone shielding, proximity to bony structures, or other boundary areas). Precise evaluation of observable clinical data, particularly the analysis of power limiting factors, provided further information about the function of the systems (see Table 11.7).

11.3.3 Antennas and Frequency-Dependent Effects

The four antenna pairs of the SIGMA applicator (Fig. 11.3) are formed by biconical flat dipoles. The antennas are fastened to the inside of a Plexiglas cylinder, and on the side facing the interior they are covered by an extremely thin layer of silicon which is part of the bolus material. In a homogeneous medium the best frequency for operating such a dipole is the frequency corresponding to the $\lambda/2$ resonance, i.e., when the antenna length for the frequency in question is exactly half of the wavelength. The biconical shape produces an additional bandwidth around

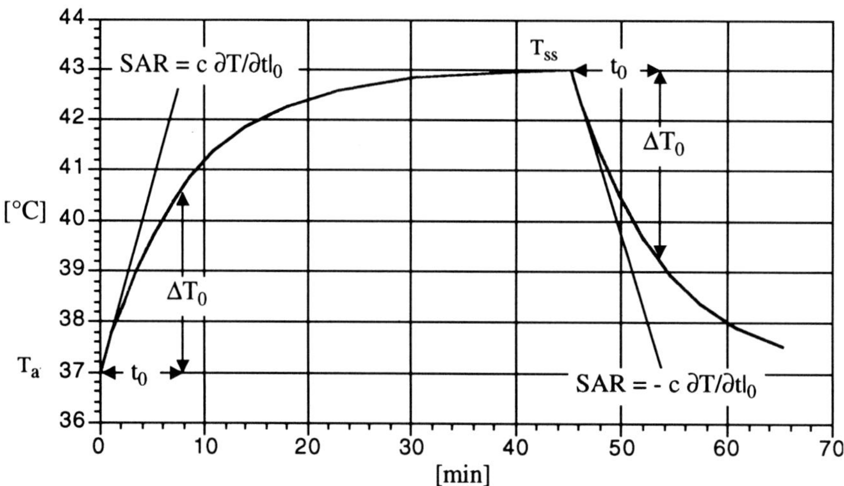

Fig. 11.5. Analysis of time/temperature curves. SAR is deduced from the gradient at the start (power on) and end (power off) of the treatment (ROEMER 1990). Effective perfusion causes a bending of the temperature curve from the straight line and can be calculated from the temperature elevation ΔT_0 at t_0 (WUST et al. 1994b). A further parameter is the temperature elevation $\Delta T = T_{ss} - T_a$ (T_a = arterial temperature, T_{ss} = steady state temperature)

the resonance frequency. On SIGMA applicators two antennas each are fed via a T-connector by the 50-Ω coaxial cable of a power amplifier. In consequence, ideal antenna matching and radiation conditions are achieved for the characteristic base point impedance of 100 Ω. This type of circuitry gives the entire antenna system a broader bandwidth.

The idealized view of such flat dipole antennas (antenna length 46 cm) at the air/water boundary in model calculations (e.g., the VSIE method) indicates that they have a $\lambda/2$ resonance at about 90 MHz. The current distribution on the antenna is then calculated as approximately cosinusoidal. The same radiation behavior is achieved if a homogeneous medium of an effective density $\varepsilon_r \approx 9$ is assumed as surrounding medium (unpublished results).

Both measurements of the Smith charts and the reflection curves in WUST et al. (1991b) and documentation of the manufacturer (BSD Medical corp.) confirm that the antenna is optimally matched at 90 MHz. However, fluctuations in these admittance or impedance curves resulted, depending on the localization of the antenna pair, the type of lossy medium (phantom or patient), and the surroundings.

In the report by WUST et al. (1991b), current distributions were measured on different antennas of the SIGMA applicator using magnetic ring antennas. Measurements revealed axial asymmetries in the current distribution on the same antenna and differences in the current distribution from antenna to antenna both on a given antenna pair and between different antenna pairs. In addition, measurements were found to be dependent on the lossy medium. Comparable fluctuations were observed when measuring coupling coefficients. Asymmetries and fluctuations were at a relative minimum at 90 MHz, and so 90 MHz was recommended as the operating frequency for the SIGMA-60 ring. It follows from this that the idealized radiation behavior of a dipole on an air/water boundary does not correspond to the behavior in a real system. Instead, in the theoretical framework of the VSIE method (Fig. 11.4), distortions in the current distribution are created by *induced sources* as a result of the radiation of the other antennas and backscattering from the heterogeneous medium. Taking these couplings into consideration in three-dimensional calculations results in modifications to the SAR distribution (see Fig. 11.7).

The FIT method assumes a *current source with an internal resistance* at the base point of the antenna, which best describes a $\lambda/2$ resonance. Significant cross-talk from antenna to antenna (coupling) will result from calculations using the FIT method (DOHLUS 1992). When the antennas are included in the overall problem (i.e., cross-talk is taken into consideration), modeling the SIGMA applicator for an elliptical phantom has consequently led to different current distributions on the antennas depending on frequency and position (DOHLUS 1992). In particular, the current distributions at frequencies greater than 100 MHz deviate significantly from the cosine form (WUST et al. 1991b). Furthermore, these calculations with the FIT method revealed frequency-dependent changes in power transmission to various reference points in the phantom which could actually be correlated with clinical observations. For example, it turned out that above 90 MHz, the transmission as evidenced by E field or SAR to the center of the phantom is at a maximum in comparison with the loads in the fat-equivalent ring. Conversely, reference points in the fat-equivalent ring (in the central plane as well as at the applicator edge) exhibit a relative maximum at 70 MHz in this model.

These calculations concur with the clinical observation that at low frequencies (i.e., less than 90 MHz) in the SIGMA applicator effective hyperthermia of deep tumors even with large cross-sections tends to be more difficult than at the resonance frequency of 90 MHz and that at these low frequencies applicator edge effects (such as musculoskeletal syndrome) are observed more frequently. Predictably, model calculations that do not allow for coupling effects between the antennas tend to favor low frequencies such as 70 MHz for large cross-sections, i.e., high absorption (see Sect. 11.1).

Calculations with FIT method also demonstrated resonance-like superimposition of the transmission curves when a closed Faraday cage was considered instead of open boundary conditions. The resonance-like structures should be regarded as idealized, since the dimensions of the shielding chamber were only estimated. In addition to this, such resonances are partially dampened away by lossy objects in the shielding chamber. Comparable effects can be observed experimentally on visualizing phantoms (such as extremely narrow-band fluctuations of light brightness at about 95 MHz) (WUST et al. 1995c). These calculations also strikingly show how strongly the SIGMA applicator's surroundings can influence SAR distribution. Therefore, the assumption of idealized applicator models, such as that shown in Fig. 11.3, does not appear suitable for a system-specific description.

Resonance-like structures resulting from the cylindrical SIGMA applicator itself due to mode excitation have also been observed in model calculations and in experiments. Such effects are particularly pronounced where a high degree of cylindrical symmetry is present, i.e., especially in cylindrical phantoms (for example in experiments with the SIGMA-60 applicator at 110 MHz). Narrow-band effects when triggering a single channel were observed between 82 and 84 MHz by SCHNEIDER et al. (1994). In our experience, the importance of frequency-dependent modes is negligible in actual patients (WUST et al. 1991b).

11.3.4 Prediction and Control of SAR Distributions in Two-Dimensional Phantoms

The first comparison of systems by SCHNEIDER et al. (1994) with an LED phantom revealed no significant differences among the four field-oriented systems (APAS, SIGMA applicator, TEM applicator, and four-waveguide applicator) in creating a central focus. However, the SIGMA applicator in particular was tested under experimental conditions that differed from clinical use (low power level, special system balance). Periodic control measurements with further developed LED or lamp phantoms under clinical conditions (i.e., at higher power levels) revealed deviations from the projected distributions in different regards (see Fig. 11.6 as an illustration) (WUST et al. 1990, 1995c):

1. Clear decentering effects typical of the system occur in the synchronized state (i.e., feeding all channels with the same phase and amplitude). For example in system A in a German university clinic there is a downward focus deviation (Fig. 11.6, top), whereas system B exhibits a pronounced upward deviation of the focus (Fig. 11.6, bottom).
2. Further minor changes can accumulate in the case of measurements of the same system at different times, yet the basic behavior of the system (for example a tendency for the focus to deviate downward) remains constant. Repeated checks can also reveal "unfavorable" system states in which phase balancing will hardly improve centering. Such changes could indicate technical shortcomings such as tube defects.

As expected, no one method (VSIE, FDTD, or FIT) can correctly describe the SAR distributions measured (E field sensor scans) in Fig. 11.7 over the entire frequency range. This is understandable since numerical simulations

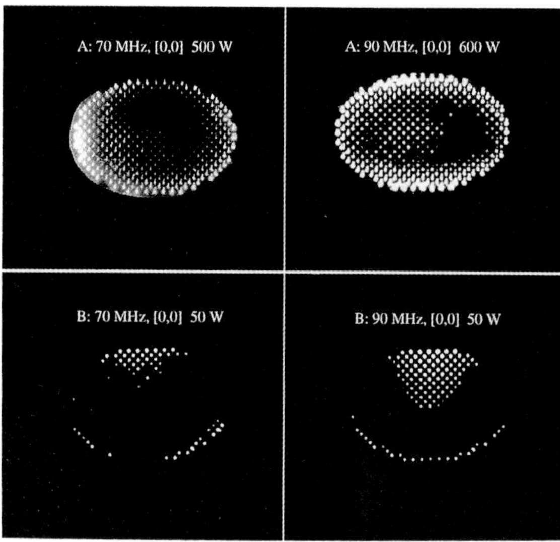

Fig. 11.6. Visualized SAR distributions from a lamp phantom for two synchronous configurations (70 and 90 MHz). Completely different behavior is found for systems A and B at two hospitals in Germany. System A has a deviation to the bottom and left. Conversely, system B has a severe offset to the top, which might be caused by coupling to the surroundings (WUST et al. 1994d)

consider only an idealized applicator model, while in an experimental setting different systems will behave differently despite having the same applicator.

The synchronous system states and their theoretical descriptions represent an extremely difficult test case. As Fig. 11.7 shows, there are marked qualitative deviations between visualized distributions and theoretical predictions even disregarding the decentering of the focus. This applies particularly to frequencies outside the resonance frequency, for example 70 MHz. Thus various numerical procedures predict either excessive lateral or vertical values that do not at all describe the actual situation. In the case of 70 MHz in particular, the predicted focusing ability is better than that actually observed in the E field sensor scan (Fig. 11.7, 70 MHz). This could have to do with the cross-talk effects mentioned above. Note that the SAR scans in Fig. 11.7 concur well with the visual distributions (Fig. 11.6A). In the VSIE method two different antenna models were used (NADOBNY 1993). Either identical cosinoidal current distributions over the antennas were assumed (VSIE, J), or calculations were based on identical E fields at the antenna feeding points (VSIE, U). In two-dimensional model calculations these assumptions will lead to totally different power deposition patterns. However, in three-dimensional model calculations the differences will not be as large (Fig. 11.7).

The marked difference between two systems at different locations was surprising, and cannot be explained by system errors. The most probable cause would seem to be more or less significant differences in the antenna network (Fig. 11.2), including malfunction of high-frequency components and coupling phenomena, as well as environmental influences that obviously can form an additional coupling with the antennas. Further informations are found in WUST et al. (1995c). At times the steering capability of a system is greatly impaired. Thus for system B in Fig. 11.8 (bottom) it is seen that despite forced downward steering (by phase shifting) hardly any change in the power deposition pattern could be achieved in comparison to the initial state.

Despite a downward drift the steering capability of the system is much less restricted in system A. Standard configurations can be set as in Fig. 11.8 (top) (for a dorsal rectal carcinoma). In many measurements it became apparent that describing the system by means of model calculations is easier in the case of eccentric SAR distributions. Obviously, introducing phase offsets reduces the coupling between the antennas. This facilitates a description using simulation calculations. Generally, eccentric power deposition patterns in phantoms can be satisfactorily described even by two-dimensional models (WUST et al. 1993b).

In system A the steering capability increases further when damping is introduced. This can be achieved with a bolus of water with minimal conductivity (tap water). In this case almost ideal

Fig. 11.7. E field sensor scans along the major and minor axis for the same setup of system A, i.e., 70 and 90 MHz (Fig. 11.6). Good agreement is obtained between E field scans and visualized patterns of Fig. 11.6. Three-dimensional calculations are shown for the same phantom (with the specifications: major axis 2a = 38 cm, minor axis 2b = 27 cm, plus 1 cm fat-equivalent ring axial length 60 cm; σ = 0.55 S/m, ε_r = 78 inside; σ = 0.04 S/m, ε_r = 10 in the layer; antenna length 46 cm): VSIE method with two diferent antenna models (NADOBNY 1993) and FDTD method (SULLIVAN 1990, 1991). No numerical method is able to describe all the measurements correctly. This is attributed to unpredictable coupling effects which effect modifications of the control parameters themselves in the feeding points of the antennas

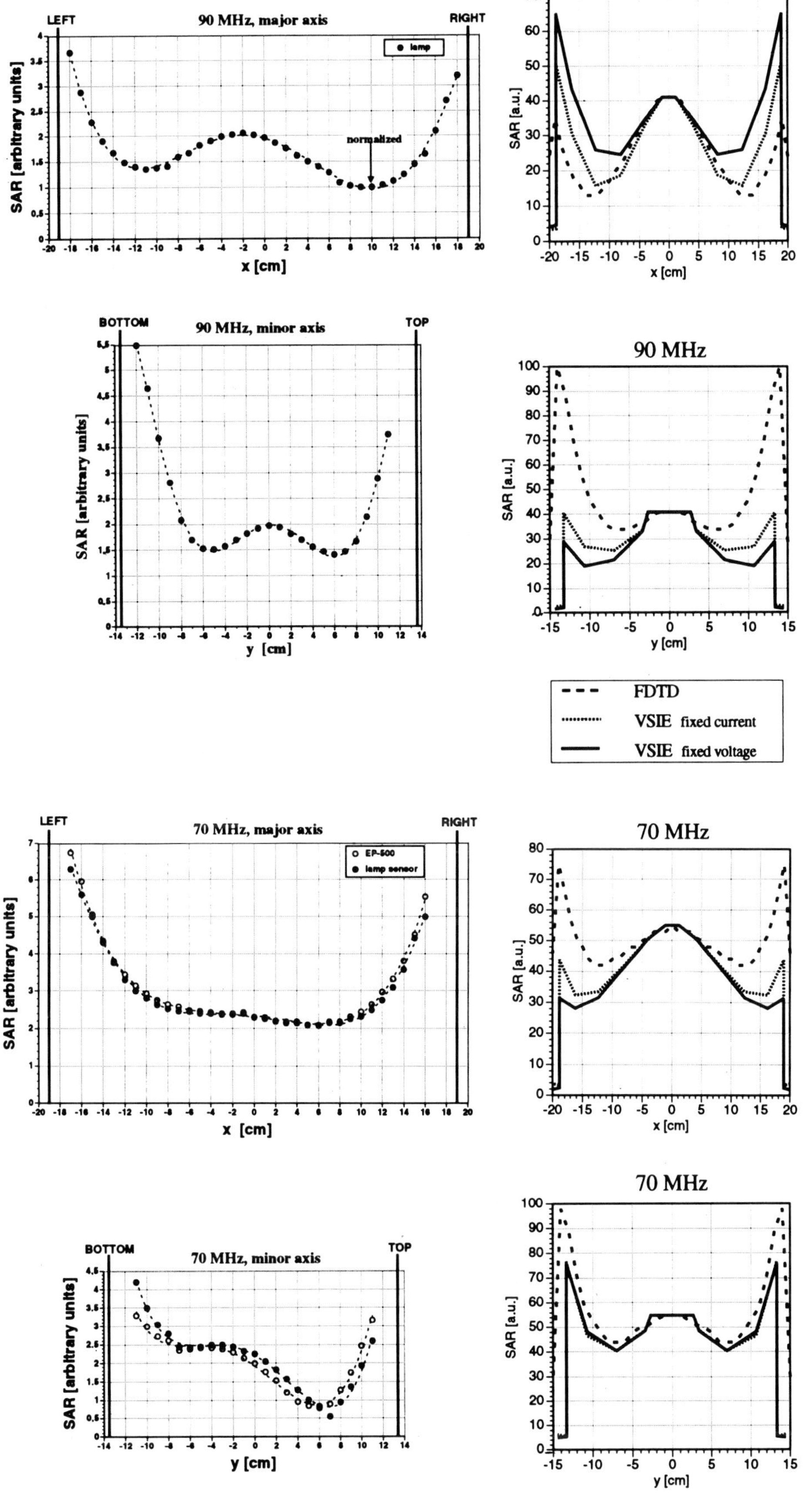

LEFT
90 MHz, major axis
RIGHT
lamp
normalized
SAR [arbitrary units]
x [cm]
90 MHz
SAR [a.u.]
x [cm]
BOTTOM
90 MHz, minor axis
TOP
SAR [arbitrary units]
y [cm]
90 MHz
SAR [a.u.]
y [cm]
FDTD
VSIE fixed current
VSIE fixed voltage
LEFT
70 MHz, major axis
RIGHT
EP-500
lamp sensor
SAR [arbitrary units]
x [cm]
70 MHz
SAR [a.u.]
x [cm]
BOTTOM
70 MHz, minor axis
TOP
SAR [arbitrary units]
y [cm]
70 MHz
SAR [a.u.]
y [cm]

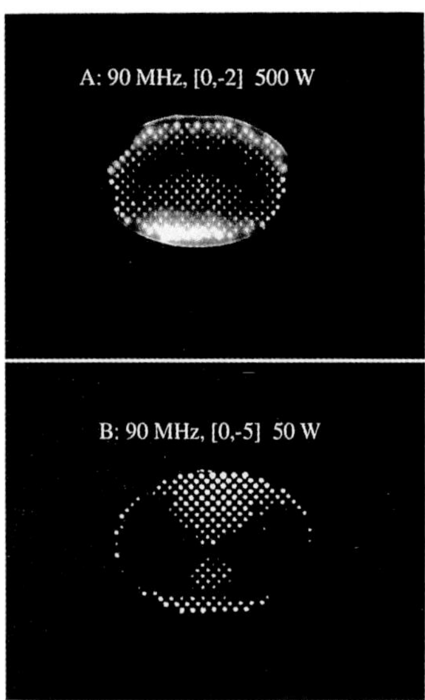

Fig. 11.8. Standard adjustment of system A (see Fig. 11.6) for a posteriorly located target volume. A target point of [0, −2] is selected resulting in the phases on the figure above. The visualized SAR pattern is fairly described by two-dimensional modeling calculations and SAR control appears satisfactory. Conversely, SAR control in system B is severely limited. Even a vigorous steering to the bottom by selecting a target point of [0, −5] does not change the pattern significantly in comparison to the "synchronous" pattern [0, 0] in Fig. 11.6 (see also text)

distributions can be achieved for the synchronous system states, but at higher power levels.

Our comparative phantom measurements illustrate two SIGMA systems with fundamentally different characteristics. The steering capability of system A is only slightly influenced by environmental factors, primarily outside the resonance frequency of 90 MHz. This system proved to be variable and unstable over time. On the other hand, the power deposition pattern can be controlled within limits by controlling the phases appropriately, and these eccentric deposition patterns can even be described theoretically by two-dimensional model calculations. The steering capability of system B is severely impaired by a (reversible) malfunction (probably poor connector contact). The power deposition patterns are not described merely by the applicator model alone. Only by taking the whole network as well as the environment into account can we arrive at a satisfactory description of the measurements. It should be noted that such system behavior does not necessarily have to be a disadvantage for clinical applications, since in the specific case of system B the focus was extremely stable. The only requirement is that the tumor can be localized in this focus.

Our intent has been to demonstrate how closely measuring, technical knowledge, and theoretical description depend on one another. Obviously it is almost impossible to make correct predictions with so complex an applicator as the SIGMA applicator solely on the basis of theoretical analysis. Even though all the methods employed (VSIE, FDTD, and FIT) allow for the antennas coupling with each other and with the heterogeneous medium (albeit in different ways), models make assumptions about control parameters (e.g., E fields) in the feeding points of the antennas which obviously differ from the true values. Figure 11.9 summarizes assumptions about the feeding point of an antenna. Only recording the E fields at the base points of all antennas (with known geometry) will provide complete information about the final E field pattern. Conversely, assuming current sources or voltage sources at the base points (i.e., assuming currents or voltages) will only provide incomplete information, since exact specification of the antenna impedances $\underline{Z}$ at the feeding points is virtually impossible. Whereas this value should correspond to the output impedance of the amplifier (i.e., 50 Ω), various influences can cause a mismatch between generator and antenna which affects assumed control parameters at the base point of the antenna. This leads to the relevant deviations between the theoretically predicted pattern and the one that is actually measured. Changes in the control parameters can lead to significant changes in the power deposition pat-

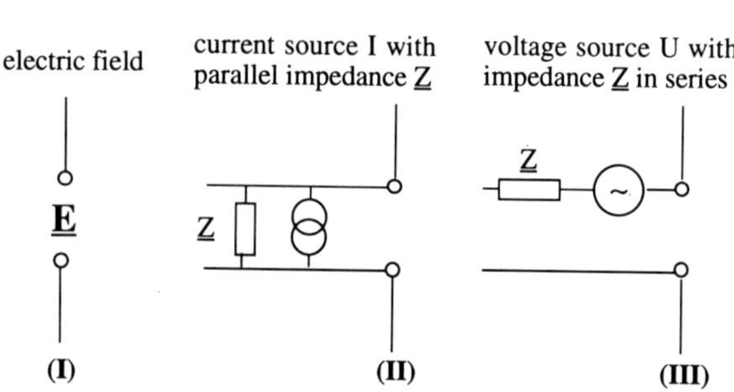

Fig. 11.9. The feeding point of a dipole antenna can be electrically characterized by a *current* or *voltage* source (II or III). The information is not complete if the impedance $\underline{Z}$ is unknown. Knowledge of the actual E field in the feeding point provides complete information about the radiation characteristic of an antenna

tern, particularly near synchronous system states. When there are eccentric shifts in the power deposition patterns, minor phase changes will no longer be able to influence the power deposition pattern significantly.

The realization that the sum of coupling effects can no longer be described theoretically led to an improved scheme of online quality control. The antenna characteristics can be completely ascertained by measuring E fields between the antenna and the medium (phantom or patient). The electro-optical sensor described above, which can measure the phase and amplitude of E fields, has already been developed for this purpose. The actual control parameters at the antenna base points can now (without any knowledge of the couplings) be determined in two ways: (a) If a suitable antenna model is available, the base point parameters in the antennas can be calculated from a finite number of E field measurements (the number of measurements must correspond to the number of antennas). (b) If the phase and amplitude of the E field have been measured on a closed curve (two-dimensional) or surface (three-dimensional) around the problem area, no antenna model will be needed at all. In this case the E field measurements can be used as a boundary condition to calculate the SAR distribution lying within the curve or surface by means of the FE method. This process is demonstrated in Fig. 11.10 using a homogeneous elliptical phantom. The phases and amplitudes of the E field were measured in angle increments of $\approx 10°$. The phase measurement is particularly characteristic, whereas the amplitude measurement does not contain much information. The FE calculation produces quite a good representation of the visualized SAR. This measuring method has since been extended. Further details can be found in WUST et al. (1995b).

11.3.5 Clinical Evaluation

Table 11.4 provides an overview of in vivo measurements in over 40 patients treated in 200 regional hyperthermia sessions with the SIGMA applicator (WUST et al. 1995a). The following in vivo quantities were extracted from the temperature–time curves by a computer-assisted graphical process (Fig. 11.5): SAR, effective perfusion, and relative SAR (SAR/total power). Determination of effective perfusion from temperature–time curves and its clinical relevance have been discussed in WATERMAN et al. (1987), WATERMAN (1987), LAGENDIJK et al. (1988), WONG et al. (1988), SAMULSKI et al. (1987b, 1989), ROEMER (1990b), FELDMANN et al. (1992), and WUST et al. (1995a). In regional hyperthemia a reasonable determination of perfusion from temperature–time curves is possible because of moderate thermal gradients. Reference methods are given in ACKER et al. (1990) and FELDMANN et al. (1992).

A comparison between the relative SAR at the beginning and at the end of regional hyperthermia gives us a sobering picture of the ability to control the SAR with the SIGMA applicator. In fact the relative SAR can be neither significantly increased in the tumor nor lowered in the normal tissue (rectum, vagina, and bladder). However, it becomes apparent that the initial setting already differentiates between tumor tissue and normal tissue within certain limits and an "optimum" has obviously already been attained. These are generally standard settings which have been determined in advance on the basis of phantom measurements (such as are shown in Figs. 11.6 and 11.8).

To further evaluate SAR steering capability the appropriate CT scans for the temperature measuring points were also analyzed. The following variables were determined graphically: the size of the CT cross-section (related to absorption), minimum absorption distance from the measuring point to the outer contour (this describes the eccentricity of the measuring point), the visual angle from the measuring point to the surrounding bony structures (related to shielding), and the thickness of the fat layer. In addition to this, clinical variables such as age, sex, Karnofsky index, histology, and previous treatments to date (especially previous radiation treatments) were recorded.

The most important in vivo measured quantities in Table 11.4 are the relative SAR (as a measure of the technical accessibility of a tumor for radiofrequency hyperthermia) and the temperature increase dT (as a measure of the therapeutic effectiveness attained). As dependent variables, both measured quantities were subjected to a variance analysis in which all in vivo measured quantities, CT data, and clinical parameters were taken into consideration. The hypothesis of whether the group means of a dependent variable (such as relative SAR or dT) depend equally on

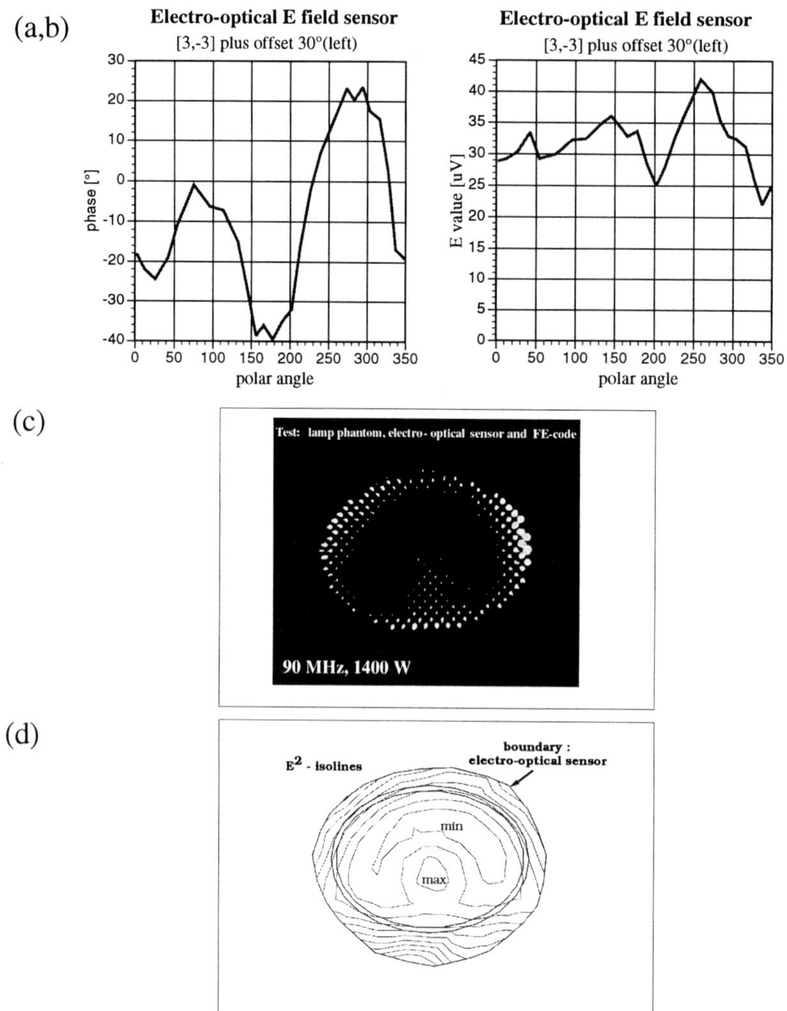

Fig. 11.10a–d. Use of an electro-optical E field sensor for noninvasive determination of SAR distribution in the interior of an elliptical phantom (Wust et al. 1994c). **a,b** Phases and amplitudes of E field are measured on a closed curve around the phantom in the midplane. The phase curve provides more information about the SAR distribution than the amplitude curve. **c** SAR distribution as visualized by a lamp phantom. **d** Using the measured curves as boundary condition in an FE algorithm results in a calculated SAR pattern in **a** which agrees reasonably with the actual visualized pattern

Table 11.4. Survey of in vivo measurements deduced from temperature/time curves (mean values and standard deviations from 200 hyperthermia treatments in 43 patients) (from Wust et al. 1993d)

	Tumor	Normal tissue
Rel. SAR (start) (mW/g/100 W)	8.0 ± 7.1	5.9 ± 3.3
Rel. SAR (end) (mW/g/100 W)	8.3 ± 7.0	5.6 ± 2.9
SAR (mW/g)	38 ± 22	35 ± 15
Perfusion (start) (ml/100 g/min)	10.3 ± 7.0	8.3 ± 7.7
Perfusion (end) (ml/100 g/min)	12.8 ± 9.7	14.7 ± 9.3
Temperature elevation (°C) (above basal temperature)	4.0 ± 1.4	3.7 ± 0.9

specified factors (extracted from the independent variables) was tested in a univariate analysis. Negating the null hypothesis with an appropriate level of significance shows the dependence on the respective factor (main effects) or a combination of two factors (two-way interactions).

The results of such a variance analysis for the relative SAR are summarized in Table 11.5. As was expected, it was revealed that the relative SAR was significantly dependent on factors that characterize the absorption. In particular, tumors situated in the center of large cross-sections are associated with low relative SARs. This effect

Table 11.5. Analysis of variances for intratumoral relative SAR (mW/g/100 W) achieved (289 measurements, from WUST et al. 1995a)

Factor		Attributed variance (%)	Group mean	*P* level
Cross-section *A*	≤575/>575 cm^2	7.8	10.7/5.3	0.000
Absorption d_{min}	≤6.7/>6.7 cm	5.2	10.5/5.3	0.000
Shielding *s*	≤13%/≤13%	1.8	9.3/6.8	0.006
Two-way interaction	$A \otimes d_{min}$	5.9	–	0.000
Preirradiation	−/+	1.5	10.6/5.2	0.001
Histology	Squamous/adeno/sarcoma	7.6	5.6/5.7/11.9	0.000
Sex	Female/male	5.0	9.6/5.9	0.000
Age	≤50/>50 years	2.4	10.7/5.9	0.000
Karnofsky score	<80%/≥80%	1.9	5.9/9.4	0.000

Table 11.6. Analysis of variances for intratumoral temperature elevation (°C) achieved (149 measurements, from WUST et al. 1995a)

Factor		Attributed variance (%)	Group mean	*P* level
Effective perfusion W_{eff}	≤10/>10 ml/100 g/min	25	4.6/3.3	0.000
Power deposition SAR	≤35/>35 mW/g	16	3.7/4.4	0.000
Thermoregulation *d*W	≤0/>0 ml/100 g/min	1.6	4.6/3.8	0.06
Two-way interaction	$SAR \otimes W_{eff}$	2.0	–	0.04
Preirradiation	−/+	3.2	3.9/4.1	0.02
Histology	Squamous/adeno/sarcoma	3.3	4.3/3.5/4.2	0.07

is already clear from a two-dimensional point of view (Sect. 11.1). Clarifying the entire three-dimensional problem is necessary for understanding how the relative SAR is dependent on the topographical proximity of bony structures (see below). It is interesting that the relative SAR is dependent on previous treatment of the tumor. Presumably previous radiation treatment causes progressive fibrosis in the tumor, decreasing its electrical conductivity and thus reducing the relative SAR. Indirect dependence on other factors (histology, age, sex, Karnofsky index) also exists via the main factors (absorption, tumor localization, previous radiation). It follows from this that the relative SAR is determined to a great extent by geometrical and anatomical factors, which partially explains the small degree of steering capability observed.

The variance analysis of the intratumoral temperature increase dT, which finally determines the effectiveness of the hyperthermia (Table 11.6), has important consequences. It becomes apparent that the perfusion and SAR are almost equally predictive for dT. In follows from this that sufficiently high SAR can compensate for higher perfusions in tumors. Since the relative SAR can hardly be influenced at present (see above), this is achieved by increasing the total power. An analysis of the factors limiting power will follow below. Interestingly, the thermal regulation in tumors (i.e., the increase in intratumoral perfusion under hyperthermia) is not a very important factor in the temperature increases that are finally attained. Since according to present knowledge the perfusion can hardly be influenced at all, it follows from the analysis summarized in Table 11.6 that future research must focus on increasing the SAR.

One way to do this could be by increasing the relative SAR. The limits can be seen in the results in Table 11.5, which demonstrates a strong dependency on anatomical conditions such as absorption and shielding. This is substantiated by a three-dimensional simulation study conducted with the VSIE method (Fig. 11.11). In the frontal section, the three-dimensional test case of a presacral tumor exhibits a very slight qualitative change in the SAR distribution at the transition from

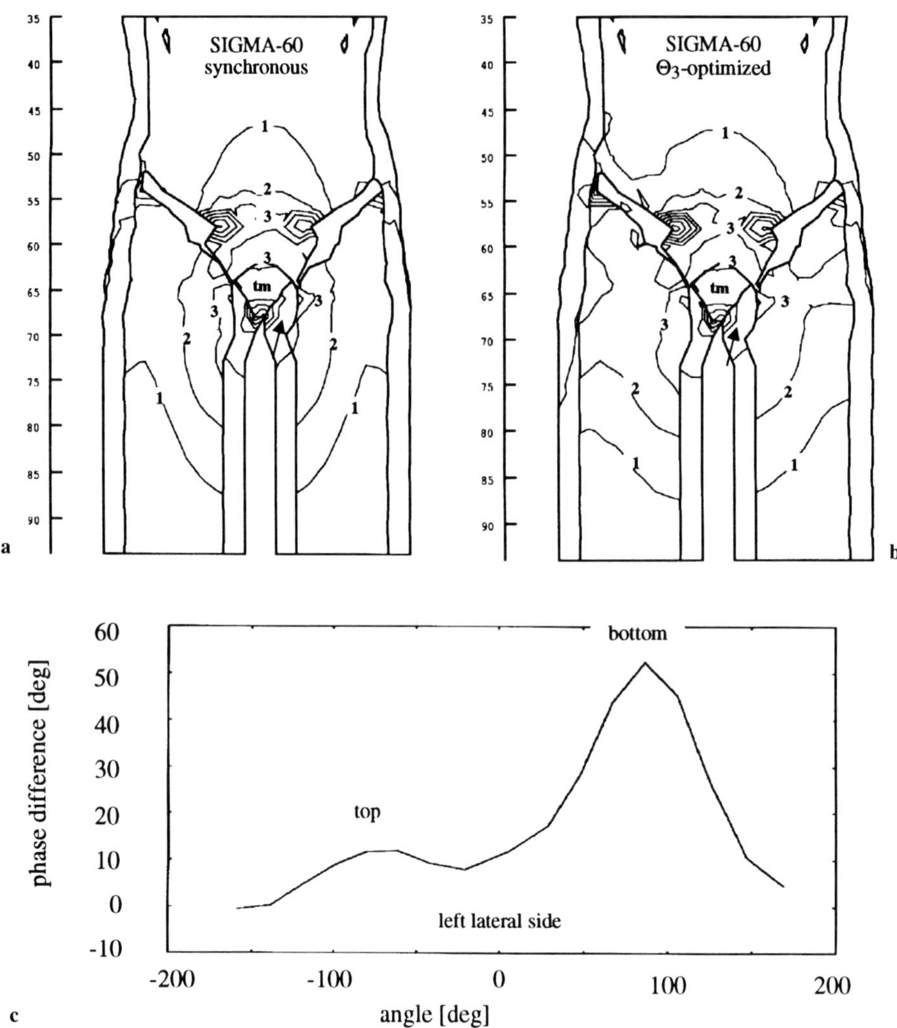

Fig. 11.11a–c. Simulation study performed according to the VSIE method, showing limited SAR contorl. In particular, SAR elevations at electrical boundaries (hot-spot phenomena) are documented Note that the VSIE method (Wust et al. 1993a; Nadobny 1993) works on a tetrahedron grid generated from a contour model. Thus E fields at electrical boundaries are very precisely calculated. **a** SAR isolines in a frontal cross-section across a presacrally located tumor for a standard setup of the SIGMA applicator (synchronous radiation at 90 MHz). The *arrow* indicates a critical point where at first the temperature threshold of 44°C in normal tissue is exceeded (perineal fat). This estimation is based on perfusion assumptions in every tissue (e.g., Wust et al. 1991a) and an FE calculation of temperature using the bioheat transfer equation. **b** Phases and amplitudes of all four channels of the SIGMA applicator are optimized with respect to Θ_3 (see Table 11.9). Only a minor difference from the synchronous patterns is seen. **c** Phase difference between both patterns (at body surface) indicates a strong phase delay to the bottom by about 50° (defined with a positive sign), corresponding to a standard adjustment such as shown for a phantom in Fig. 11.8. Obviously, phantom measurements suggest a higher steering capability than is found in VSIE modeling calculations

synchronous antenna control to antennas steered in a dorsal direction (Fig. 11.11a,b). Figure 11.11c documents the significant phase shift at the antennas. Careful inspection of Figs. 11.11a and 11.11b reveals that the SAR distribution is determined to a large extent by the electrical boundaries of the heterogeneous medium despite this external control. In particular, SAR peaks appear at certain anatomical structures (for example the inner pelvic girdle) virtually independent of external steering. These E field peaks have been termed "hot spot phenomena", they are caused by the axial polarization of the primary incident electrical field in conjunction with the electrical boundaries perpendicular to it (i.e., transitions between markedly different electrical media, particularly bone/muscle boundaries). The analysis of this test case will be continued in the next section. Hot spot phenomena are dealt with in FELDMANN et al. (1991) and BEN-YOSEF et al. (1992) and were previously analyzed experimentally in TURNER (1984).

That fact that the SAR distribution is model-dependent has already been mentioned in 11.3.2 (a regular grid in the FDTD method versus a tetrahedron grid with specified contours in the VSIE or FE methods). The great emphasis placed on the electrical boundaries in the VSIE method led to the prediction that the relative SAR's degree of steering capability would be slight. This appears to concur with clinical experience (see Table 11.4).

Test measurements during a heat treatment conducted in vivo within the invasive hyperthermia catheter using the EP-500 E field sensor (BSD Medical Corporation) also confirm the existence of boundary phenomena as predicted by the VSIE method. Figure 11.12 shows a strong shielding effect at the tip of the catheter ($R = 0$ cm) and a pronounced E field peak in the vicinity of the muscle/bone boundary ($R = 5$ cm). Both measuring points are represented in the appropriate CT cross-sections. Note that the catheter was implanted in oblique direction to the transverse plane and in consequence has a distinct axial component (i.e., in the main direction of polarization). These in vivo phenomena (shielding, E field peaks at boundaries) can be neither re-

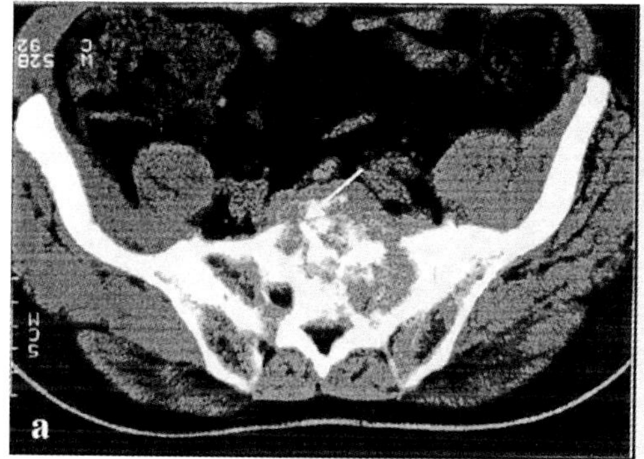

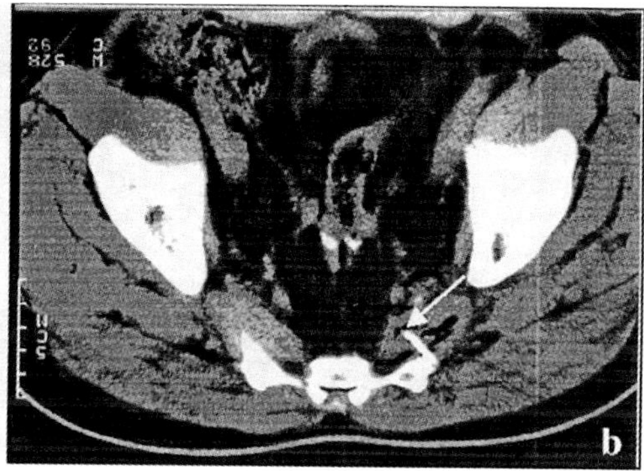

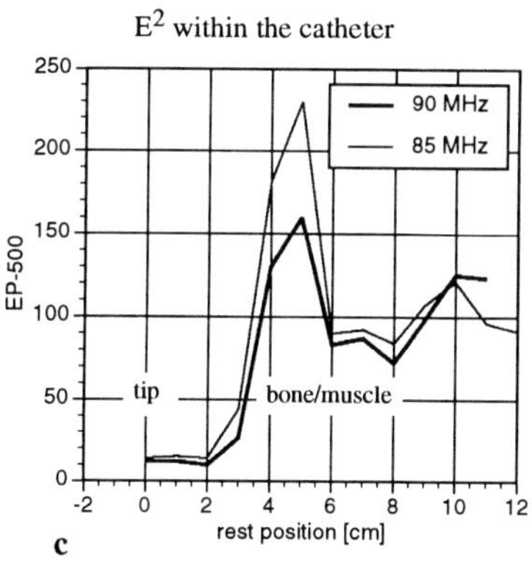

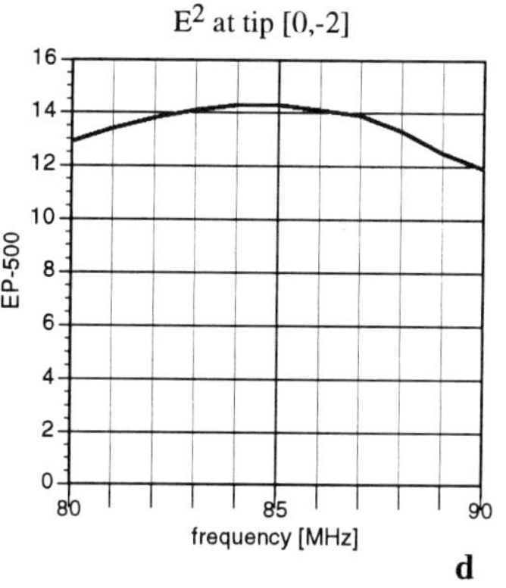

Fig. 11.12a–d. Use of a high-resistive E field sensor (EP-500, BSD Med. Corp.) for invasive E^2 scan within a hyperthermia catheter in a rectal recurrence which has destroyed the pelvic bone. The catheter has a strong component along the patient axis which is the dominant E field direction. **a** Transverse section across the catheter tip (see arrow). The measurement point is shielded by bone. **b** Transverse section 5 cm away from the tip. This measurement point is in close proximity to a bone–muscle interface (see arrow). **c** The E^2 field sensor scan within the catheter shows very low values at the up and a pronounced maximum at rest position 5 cm which corresponds to the electrical boundary. A target point selection of [0, −2] and frequency 90 MHz is chosen. **d** SAR at the tip (**a**) has only a slight dependency on frequency, with a maximum at 85 MHz. However, for 85 MHz a considerably higher E field is seen at the bone–muscle interface (see **c**)

produced by two-dimensional calculations nor represented by three-dimensional calculations on a voxel model (see Sect. 11.4). The search for the correct model in radiofrequency hyperthermia must continue.

Classification and analysis of the acute limiting factors in radiofrequency hyperthermia confirms the existence of hot spot phenomena associated with boundaries (WUST et al. 1993b, 1995a). Table 11.7 shows that in the case of the SIGMA applicator the power-dependent toxicity dominates, particularly in that clinical form presumably corresponding to hot spot phenomena. Patients typically perceive such phenomena not as an excessively high temperature or a heat sensation, but rather as a localized sensation of discomfort or pressure, burning, or even pain. It can sometimes be very difficult to distinguish this from mechanical pressure (for example from the bolus) in the course of differential diagnosis. With the SIGMA applicator these complaints are more often localized at the edge of the applicator (thigh, hip and trochanter major, inguinal region, suprapubic region, and perineum) or in anatomical regions with electrical boundaries (scar areas or the sacral region).

The *toxicity spectrum* differs significantly for the hyperthermia systems in clinical use and provides valuable information for a possible further development of RF hyperthermia. A significant difference between the various systems is the *size of the treatment volume*, which manifests itself in the axial SAR distribution in the homogeneous phantom. The axial applicator length (FWHM of the SAR) is about 17 cm for the operating frequency of 90 MHz on the SIGMA-60 applicator as well as for 70 MHz on the four-waveguide applicator (SCHNEIDER 1993, personal communication) and almost twice that, 30 cm (DELEEUW et al. 1990), for the operating frequency of 70 MHz on the TEM applicator. These significantly differing treatment volumes result in differences in clinical application, as listed in Table 11.8 (DELEEUW 1993, personal communication; VAN DIJK 1993, personal communication) for pelvic tumors. The local power-dependent toxicity is inversely proportional to the treatment volume. However, the systemic toxicity, and thus the required and tolerated total power, predictably increses with the treatment volume.

The ability of an applicator to create localized SAR distributions is not necessarily an advantage, since under certain circumstances the local side-effects increase (as documented with the SIGMA applicator). This was also indicated by a simulation study (albeit two-dimensional) by WUST et al. (1991a) where defined threshold conditions (violation of temperature limits, corresponding to power-limiting factors) were avoided by defocusing the SAR distributions. Obviously there is an optimum treatment volume that is a function of the specific tumor case. This is another degree of freedom which can prove important in the further development of regional hyperthermia (see Sect. 11.4).

The differing spectrum of side-effects with the TEM applicator on the one hand and the SIGMA or four-waveguide applicator on the other is also influenced by the applicator design. By completely filling the space between the patient and the antenna with water, the TEM applicator's improved coupling appears to reduce the applicator edge effects and thus the local toxicity. Besides this, fewer positioning problems that could also be limiting factors in clinical application occur with the TEM applicator.

Table 11.7. Classification of acute treatment-limiting factors for the SIGMA-60 applicator

		Specific cause	Handling
Power-related toxicity	80%		
Hot spot phenomena	40%	Electrical boundaries Applicator edge	Change of geometry Applicator design
Tumor-related pain	30%	Tumor swelling	Analgosedation Corticosteroids
Heat sensation	20%	Larger tissue volumes > 43°–44°C	SAR steering (phase, amplitude)
Systemic stress	10%	Circulatory stress by thermoregulation	Treatment volume Patient selection
Maintenance of position	30%	Water bolus pressure	Applicator design

Table 11.8. Comparison of TEM applicator (DeLeeuw 1993, personal communication), SIGMA-60 applicator, and four-waveguide applicator (MPA, van Dijk 1993) for heat treatments of pelvic tumors

	TEM	SIGMA-60	MPA
Operating frequency (MHz)	70	90	70
Axial length (cm)	30	17	17
Power-limiting factors			
Local toxicity	10%	80%	33%
Systemic stress	20%	<10%	17%
Technical reasons	35%	∅	∅
Below tolerance level	35%	10%	50%
Average power	1.5 kW	600 W	600–850 W
Positioning problems	∅	30%	∅
Intratumoral temperatures			
<42°C	54%	34%	52%
42°–43°C	30%	45%	29%
⩾43°C	16%	21%	19%
Tumor entities			
Rectal cancer	70%	30%	34%
Cervical cancer	4%	30%	20%
Sarcomas	∅	30%	5%
Prostatic cancer	15%	2%	1%
Other	11%	8%	40%

It remains to be mentioned that the SIGMA applicator's predecessor, the BSD-1000 APA system (typical operating frequency 70 MHz) lies between the TEM applicator and the SIGMA-60 applicator. The four-waveguide applicator, on the other hand, has a treatment volume comparable to that of the SIGMA-60 applicator (Table 11.8). This also influences the side-effect spectrum of the four-waveguide applicator in which the local toxicity dominates as well. We note again that the temperatures attained with a regional hyperthermia system (Table 11.8) are not necessarily decisive for the technical efficiency of the system, since a broad spectrum exists with respect to both the heterogeneity of the tumor treated and the clinical application.

Thus it can be seen from Table 11.7 that the tolerance threshold for local toxicity can be raised within limits by medical interventions such as analgosedation (Issels et al. 1990, 1991). This might explain the deviation in the temperatures attained in Table 11.2. Above all, note that appropriate selection of patients may make systems that theoretical analysis must clearly rate as inferior appear in a favorable light (see capacitive systems, Table 11.2).

11.4 Schemes for Further Development of Current Radiofrequency Technique

11.4.1 Introduction

Given the technical and clinical status of RF hyperthermia systems described in the last section, further development is desirable. Improving SAR steering capabilities is conceivable only by increasing the degrees of freedom. The resulting increase in the complexity of such a system implies adequate patient-specific planning and optimization and appropriate verification during therapy. Accordingly, a technical advance can only consist in an integrated overall scheme including components for hyperthermia planning, online control, and an improved applicator. All three components will be briefly discussed in the following section. Further information can be found in Chaps. 16–21 of this volume.

11.4.2 Patient-Specific Hyperthermia Planning

The first hyperthermia planning system was implemented by Sullivan in Stanford in 1991 (Sullivan 1991; Sullivan et al. 1993). The SAR distribution was calculated by the FDTD method on a regular grid produced by averaging over the voxels of a series of CT scans. Each voxel is assigned a low water content (fat and bone) or a high one (muscle, tumor, etc.) according to its Hounsfield units with the electrical parameters $\varepsilon_r = 10$, $\sigma = 0.02\,\mathrm{S/m}$ or $\varepsilon_r = 80$, $\sigma = 0.8\,\mathrm{S/m}$.

An alternative model of a patient is generated by interactively entering contours between the various tissue compartments (tumor, fat, bone, muscle, etc.). Both regular grids and tetrahedron grids can be created from such contour stacks (SEEBASS 1990). The VSIE and FE methods make use of tetrahedron grids. Figure 11.13 summarizes the options of a patient-specific hyperthermia planning system as it is structured in the clinic for radiology at the Rudolf Virchow University Hospital in Berlin (SEEBASS et al. 1993b). It includes the FDTD method on a voxel model according to SULLIVAN et al. (1993) as an option.

Figure 11.14 shows a very clear graphical form of representation for the SAR distribution achieved by coloring the CT scans (color wash method). What strikes the observer are the dramatic differences resulting from utilization of different models (voxel model, contour model). Apparently the more statistically oriented voxel model will produce significantly more optimistic distributions (averaging of voxels of high and low water content). In contrast, the contour model emphasizes more strongly the boundary effects that lead to hot spot phenomena at critical boundaries (when E fields have strong components perpendicular to bone/muscle or fat/muscle interfaces). The greater interaction at these boundaries simultaneously results in greater

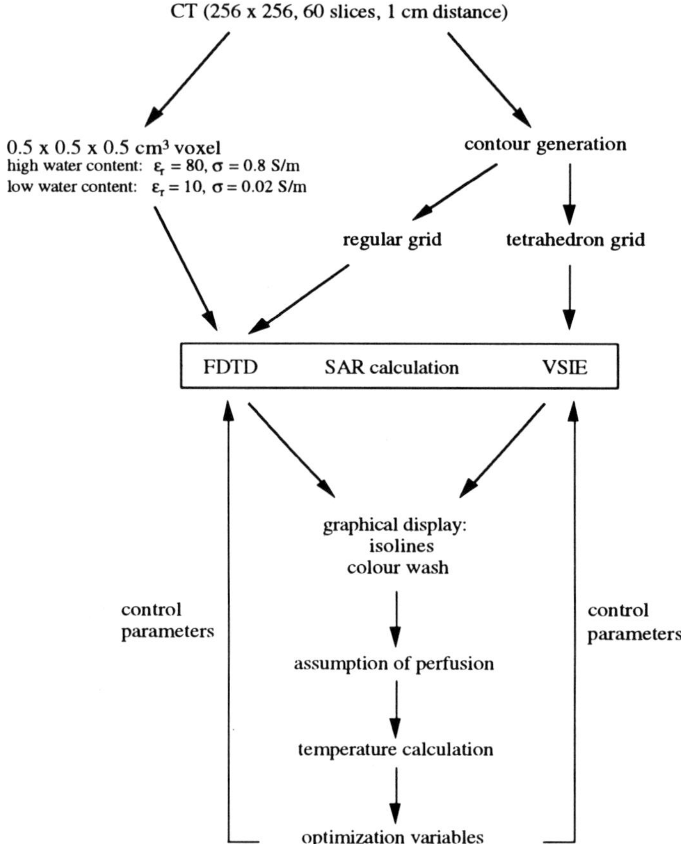

Fig. 11.13. Design of a patient-specific hyperthermia treatment planning system which has been developed at the Rudolf Virchow Clinic. One part of this system originates from the Stanford 3D Hyperthermia Treatment Planning system (SULLIVAN et al. 1993), which employs the FDTD method to calculate the SAR distribution on a regular grid. Further development especially concerning the graphic options has been referred to as the Berlin system (SEEBASS et al. 1993b). Other parts deal with optimization routines which are mainly based on estimations of temperature distributions (WUST et al. 1991a). The VSIE method, which makes use of a tetrahedron grid (NADOBNY et al. 1993), is also included into the treatment planning system. Thus, different patient models are employed for simulations such as a voxel model or a contour model

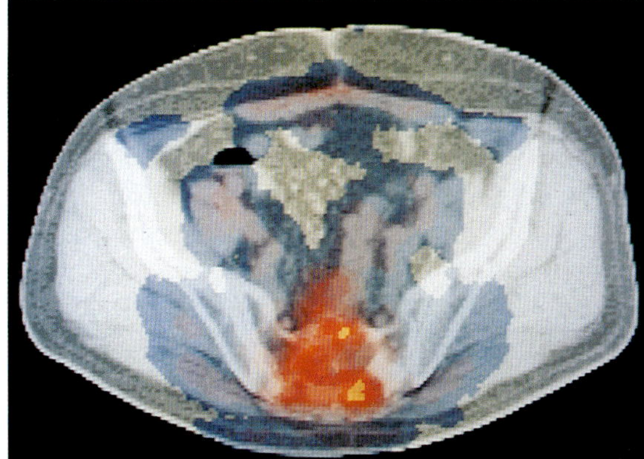

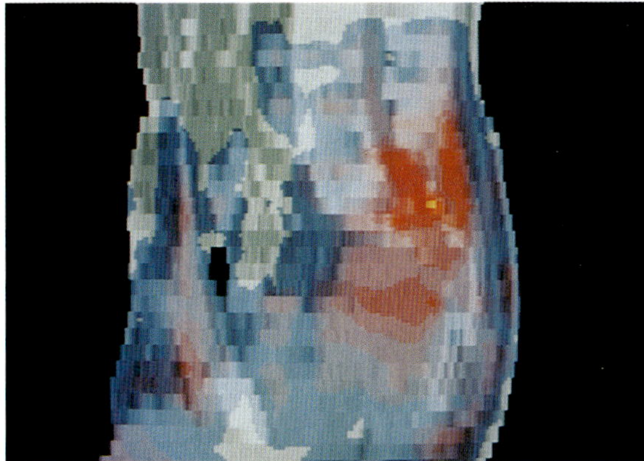

a

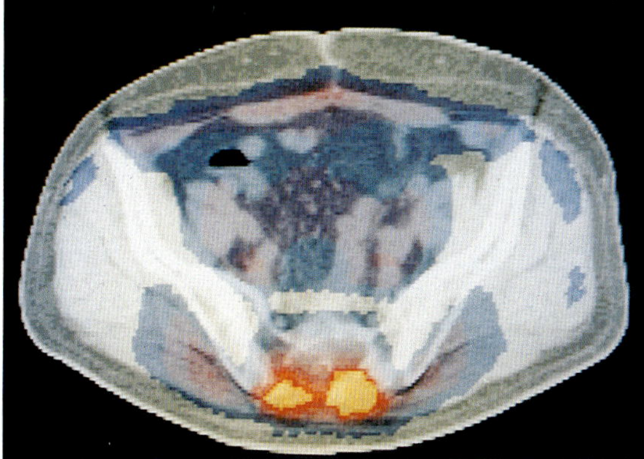

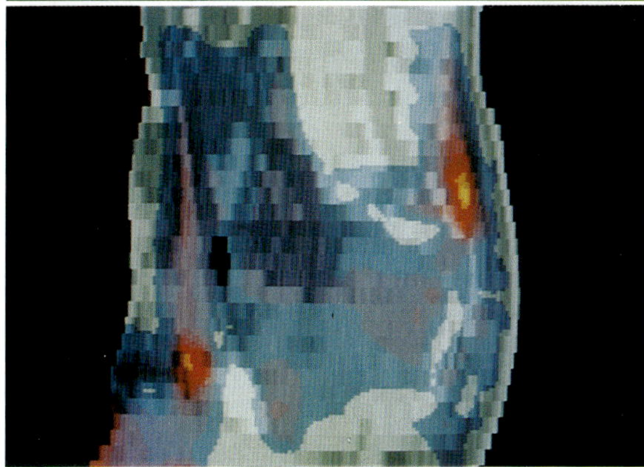

b

shielding/attenuation with respect to areas beyond the boundaries. This explains the relatively unsatisfactory SAR distribution in Fig. 11.14b.

Interestingly, the predictions of the FDTD method on a contour model qualitatively agree better with clinical experience. Thus it appears that the boundary effects in a voxel model tend to be underestimated. It is even possible that numerical methods best describe conditions when they make a particularly careful analysis at electrical boundaries, as does the VSIE method or the FE method. Such three-dimensional effects dominate the restrictions of SAR control which are induced by coupling (as outlined in Sect. 11.3). On the one hand for uncomplicated geometrical structures a satisfactory agreement has been found between SAR measurements and numerical simulations with FDTD method (SULLIVAN et al. 1992). However, comparison of the different numerical methods with respect to patient-specific hyperthermia planning is still incomplete. In particular, the best patient model has not yet been clearly specified.

According to Fig. 11.13, a temperature calculation can be made after calculating the SAR distribution based on perfusion in the tissues by solution of the bioheat transfer equation (SEEBASS 1990; BORNEMANN 1991, 1992), thus forming a basis for optimizing the SAR distribution. Table 11.9 shows several optimization variables (i.e., quan-

Fig. 11.14a,b. Patient-specific SAR calculations for a patient with recurrent rectal cancer (destroying the sacral bone) by use of the FDTD method (SULLIVAN et al. 1993). The calculations are performed for the SIGMA-60 applicator at 90 MHz with a reduced ventral amplitude (80%) and a target point selection of [0, −1] according to an appropriate standard pattern for a dorsal tumor. Two different patient models are assumed: **a** In a *voxel model* for every voxel electrical parameters are either $\sigma = 0.8$ S/m. $\varepsilon_r = 78$ (high water content tissue, for Hounsfield units $0 < \mathrm{HU} < 100$) or $\sigma = 0.02$ S/m, $\varepsilon_r = 10$ (low water content tissue, $\mathrm{HU} \leqslant 0$ or $\mathrm{HU} \geqslant 100$). The electrical parameters of the regular grid are determined by averaging over the constituent voxels. Results from this model are quite optimistic and do not show hot spots related to electrical boundaries. **b** In a *contour model* for the same patient organs and tissues are specified by contours interactively and every region is characterized by typical σ, ε_r. Therefore electrical boundaries are inherently accentuated and less optimistic results are obtained with hot spot phenomena and shielding effects. The difference between both models is documented for this case of recurrent rectal cancer destroying the sacral bone. Higher SAR in the tumor which is largely surrounded by bone is predicted by the FDTD method on a voxel model

Table 11.9. Optimization variables that are maximized by variation of phases and amplitudes of independent antennas[a]

Optimization variables for SAR distribution
$\pi_1 = \int \mathrm{SAR(tumor)} d^3r / \int \mathrm{SAR}$ (normal tissue)d^3r
$\pi_2 =$ SAR(tumor center)/ $\mathrm{SAR_{max}}$ (normal tissue)
$\pi_3 =$ SAR(tumor center)/ total power
Optimization variables for T distribution
$\Theta_1 = -\int \| 43 - T(\mathrm{tumor}, \leqslant 43°\mathrm{C}) \|^2 d^3r$
$\Theta_2 = \Theta_1 - \int \| 42 - T(\mathrm{normal\ tissue}, \geqslant 42°\mathrm{C}) \|^2 d^3r$
$\Theta_3 =$ %tumor $\geqslant$ 43°C

[a] Search for phases and amplitudes is performed by a standard gradient routine. Temperature distributions are calculated by the bioheat transfer equation assuming catalogized perfusion values in tumors and normal tissues (Wust et al. 1991a). As a restricting condition, total power is limited by specified threshold temperatures in normal tissues (44°C in muscle and fat; 42°C in intestine). An example of such an optimization procedure is given in Table 11.10

tities for maximization using appropriate search routines) that are derived from either SAR distributions or temperature distributions. Developing suitable optimization strategies is a difficult problem (Wust et al. 1991a). It becomes apparent that the use of SAR optimization variables (π_1, π_2, π_3), while at first glance suitable, does not lead to favorable results concerning the achieved temperature distributions. For this optimization strategy, local peaks often result (hot spot formation), particularly in the area around the tumor, limiting increase of total power. Conversely, the temperature distribution optimization variables (Θ_1, Θ_2, Θ_3) generally lead to a defocusing of the power deposition pattern. This avoids hot spots, permitting an increase in total power and thus improved overall temperature distribution. The development of suitable optimization strategies remains an unsolved problem of hyperthermia planning.

11.4.3 Online Control

As was described in the preceding section, the many factors and variables in RF hyperthermia and their complex interaction make verification of a setting essential during heat therapy even where sufficiently precise patient-specific planning has been developed. Previous methods such as with E field sensor arrays on the patient's skin (EP-400, BSD Medical Corp.) are not sensitive enough for this purpose. For this reason an electro-optical E field sensor that registers the phase and amplitude of the electrical field and is suitable for recording a closed curve/surface around the cross-section of the patient (boundary condition) has been developed (Meier et al. 1992, 1994). In the case of an elliptical homogeneous phantom, SAR distributions have already been determined with good precision from such boundary conditions using the FE method (Wust et al. 1995b; see also Fig. 11.10).

However, this procedure cannot be easily applied to a patient due to the fact that the calculated internal SAR distribution is model-dependent, as has been described above. Therefore the dielectric distribution of the heterogeneous medium must be sufficiently known. At present there is no definitive information available regarding the range of fluctuation or imprecision of the dielectric tissue parameters in vivo.

The numerical and measuring procedures developed can be used directly for reconstructing dielectric distributions or for testing patient models. Figure 11.15 (upper part) shows how the recording of a boundary curve can be used for testing and determining an assumed dielectric distribution in the interior of the heterogeneous medium if a suitable antenna model (with known incident field E_{inc}) is available. An estimated dielectric distribution can be modified iteratively in such a manner that it will finally accurately describe all measurements in the framework of a given model. The precision of the reconstruction process increases with the number of antennas (projections). Furthermore, Haacke et al. (1991) have outlined a method to extract electrical parameters from magnetic resonance imaging which might be suitable as starting dielectric distribution.

On the basis of a reconstructed dielectric distribution, the SAR distribution can be determined by means of an FE algorithm from a complete boundary condition that has been measured (Fig. 11.15, lower part). Here, there are close links between the patient-specific planning, patient model utilized, reconstruction method, and measuring procedure. Some aspects of this problem are discussed in Bolomey and Hawley (1990; there called "generalized imaging") and Wang and Takagi (1991).

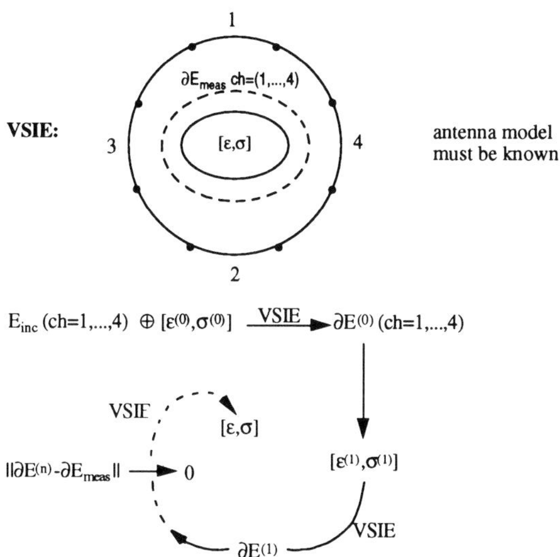

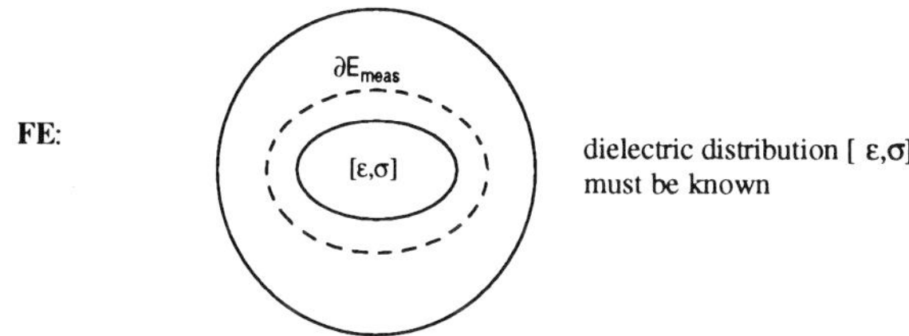

Fig. 11.15. A proposed concept for noninvasive control of hyperthermia using an electro-optical E field sensor (Fig. 11.10). Realization of this concept demands highly advanced numerical methods as well as measuring technology: Firstly, the dielectric distribution of the cross-section is only crudely known and must be better determined. If incident fields of antennas are known, for every single antenna and assumed dielectric distribution the E field on a closed curve can be calculated (using a numerical method with open boundaries such as the VSIE method) and compared with measured curves (using the electro-optical E field sensor). By an iterative numerical procedure the starting dielectric distribution is improved stepwise (Wang and Takagi 1991). Secondly, for every setup the SAR distribution can be achieved from a measured closed curve/surface if the interior dielectric distribution is known. The FE method or FDTD methods can be used for this task

11.4.4 Improving the Application in Radiofrequency Hyperthermia

The contour model in conjunction with the FDTD or VSIE method suggests that the SAR distribution and in consequence efficiency as well as tolerance can be significantly improved by suitably modifying the polarization directions of the radiators in relation to the electrical boundaries. Such an approach is illustrated in Fig. 11.16. The number of degrees of freedom has been expanded (polarization direction, number of antennas) in comparison to the fixed antenna configuration, e.g., of the SIGMA applicator (see Fig. 11.3). The further development of the optimization problem has two main goals with respect to such a complex antenna system: (a) circumventing shielding effects and the hot spots associated with them by adapting the radiation directions, and (b) minimizing clinically relevant local toxicity in the total therapy volume. The latter case can also consist in avoiding applicator edge effects. The goal of minimizing hot spots is to permit an increase in total power. At present total power is known to be almost the only control parameter for the SAR in the tumor (Sect. 11.3).

It has already been demonstrated in model calculations that increasing the number of degrees of freedom can improve effectiveness. Table

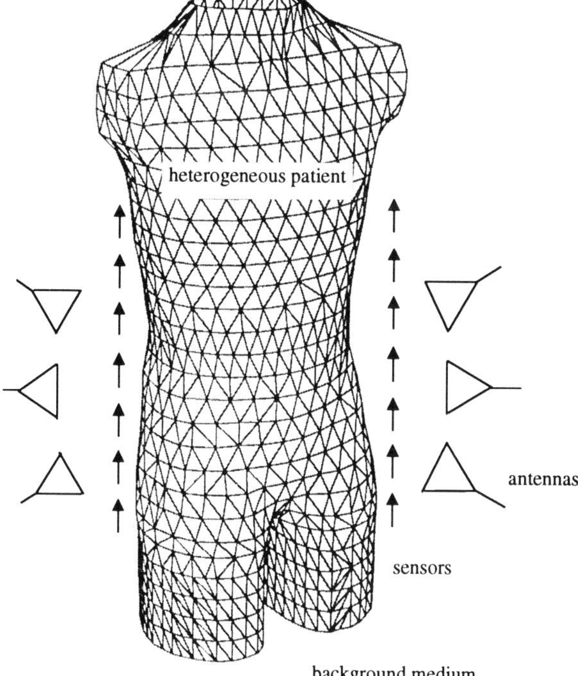

Fig. 11.16. Schematic description of an applicator with improved three-dimensional radiation scheme for regional hyperthermia: there is optimized orientation and position of single antennas, with sensors between antennas and patient for noninvasive control, such as that discussed in conjunction with Figs. 11.10 and 11.15

Table 11.10. Improvement of index temperatures (OLESON et al. 1989; ISSELS et al. 1990) by different optimization strategies (see Table 11.9). For the current system SIGMA-60 with eight antennas, SAR and temperature-oriented variables were used for optimization.

Optimization	8 antennas			24 antennas
	π_2	→Sync.	→ Θ_2	→Θ_2
T_{80} (°C)	40.1	40.2	40.5	41.4
T_{20} (°C)	41.9	42.0	42.3	43.0
Power (W)	300	350	415	450

Variables maximizing SAR in the tumor (π_2) are less favourable and restrict the total power (early violation of temperature limits in normal tissues near the tumor because of stronger focusing). Even a synchronous pattern is superior. However, only a slight improvement is achieved by maximizing temperature-oriented variables (Θ_2) with current technology. For a fictious ring applicator with a larger number of 24 antennas, i.e., a three-fold segmentation of every antenna of the SIGMA ring (Fig. 11.4), considerable improvement is obtained: T_{80} is increased nearly 1°C if Θ_2 is used as the optimization variable

11.10 illustrates such an example in which the number of antennas of the SIGMA applicator was increased from eight to 24. The SAR distributions for a three-dimensional VSIE patient model (contour model, tetrahedron grid) attained with the original SIGMA-60 applicator have already been shown in Fig. 11.11. In the continuation of this test case, Table 11.10 shows how a clear improvement in the temperature/volume histogram can be induced by introducing 24 independently controlled antennas. The index temperatures are significantly improved accordingly on the order of 1°C. The improvement is partially based on hot spot reduction that circumvents power-limiting conditions and permits further increase in total power. Allowing for all degrees of freedom in patient-specific simulation calculations is an extremely challenging task on which work is now progressing. Again, note that such optimization strategies depend on the "right" patient model.

The applicator design also influences other important characteristics such as *positioning of the patient* and *antenna coupling*. For instance in clinical use of the TEM applicator positioning of the patient in water was seen to reduce positioning problems significantly. Particularly with the TEM applicator no reductions in therapy time due to positioning problems were observed (see Table 11.8). In contrast, the bolus with the SIGMA applicator not only produces clinically relevant constriction of the patient, but also gives rise to specific side-effects at the applicator edge which may be eliminated by improved coupling conditions (such as changing the bolus form).

Finally, it was demonstrated in the previous section that the coupling between the antennas and the electrical environment can be diminished by a *reduction in the Q value* of the applicator. This can be achieved by introducing liquid with minimal conductivity (tap water) into the bolus or by employing absorbing walls. Manipulations of this sort will necessarily result in an increase in the power required.

Another important degree of freedom for optimizing radiofrequency hyperthermia is the *treatment volume*. Varying this parameter requires additional applicator options (applicator size, antenna size, and frequency). Local and systemic toxicity behave oppositely with respect to the size of the treatment volume (see Table 11.8). A systematic analysis will be required to determine the extent to which local effects and thermal gradients can be lessened by an increase in the treatment volume. Presumably an "optimum" treatment volume can be determined for a specific tumor case (i.e., cross-section size, localization, perfusion assumptions, and clinical prerequisites).

The underlying thermodynamic problem (Fig. 11.17) is further complicated by the interaction of the organism with the environment. The applied power and thermal interaction affect the *systemic temperature*, which significantly influences the attainable absolute intratumoral temperatures and thermal gradients. Precise influencing of the thermal interaction and thus an increase in systemic temperature can be achieved via thermal insulation and ambient temperature (particularly in the coupling medium). This dictates further requirements with respect to applicator development. It is possible that increasing the systemic temperature is the missing link required in increasing efficiency in regional hyperthermia. The physiological and regulatory mechanisms that come into action in such a state of "partial body hyperthermia" are still largely unexplained. The potential for improvement in regional radiofrequency hyperthermia can be seen as sufficiently great to warrant working towards further technological development of existing systems.

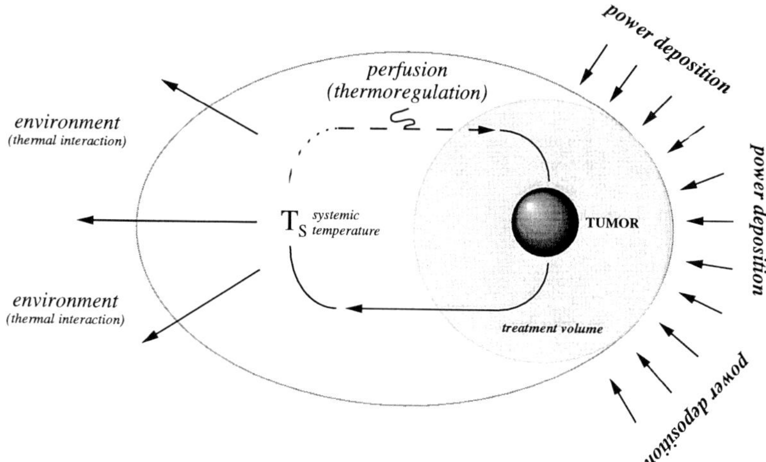

Fig. 11.17. Regional hyperthermia is part of a general thermodynamic problem. The intratumoral temperature distribution depends on many variables such as power deposition patterns, perfusion, regulation of perfusion, systemic temperature, and thermal regulation of the whole organism. Obviously, a trade-off exists between teatment volume and systemic load. The final systemic temperature T_s is a result of total power (depending on the treatment volume, see Table 11.8) and thermal interaction with the environment. By specific manipulations, e.g., thermal isolation, systemic temperature can be influenced. Systemic temperature might become an additional degree of freedom for regional hyperthermia

11.5 Summary

- Radiofrequency systems based on phased array applicators (frequency range 50–100 MHz) are most suitable for regional hyperthermia of pelvic and abdominal regions.
- Available systems today are poor at controlling relative SAR distributions; SAR is predominantly increased by increasing total power.
- In clinical practice, enhancement of total power often is limited by SAR maxima at electrical tissue boundaries such as muscle-bone or muscle-fat, so-called hot spots. Systemic stress and local discomfort in present systems are inversely correlated.
- The antenna network of phased array applicators is most effectively calibrated and controlled by visualizing phantoms (LEDs or lamps).
- Sophisticated treatment planning systems are required for further system evaluation and technological development including numerical tools for patient-specific calculation of SAR, temperature and optimization tools. Correct calculations are a prerequisite for realistic patient models.
- The VSIE (volume surface integral equation) method based on a contour model is currently the most accurate method for calculating power deposition patterns in three-dimensional heterogenous media.
- Thermal optimization variables are required for reasonable optimization routines.
- Phase control in the direction of the patient axis by increasing the antenna and channel number permits better SAR control and reduction of hot spots.
- Treatment volume and systemic body temperature are important variables to be considered in advanced hyperthermia systems.
- Improved applicators are required that take more variables into account (antennas, channels, treatment volume, systemic temperature) and provide better positioning options for the patient.
- Development and exploitation of phase-sensitive E-field measurement techniques together with advanced planning tools might be used in the future to control and optimize power deposition patterns in patients.

Acknowledgements. The authors are very grateful for valuable financial support for this research from the Deutsche Krebshilfe (M38/85/Fe1, M6/90/Fe6, M100/91/Fe7) and the Deutsche Forschungsgemeinschaft (SFB 273). We appreciate the important technical assistance of Mr. H. Fähling, and the help of Mrs. H. Ganter in preparing the manuscript and various figures.

References

Acker JC, Dewhirst MW, Honoré GM, Samulski TV, Tucker JA, Oleson JR (1990) Blood perfusion measurements in human tumors: evaluation of laser Doppler methods. Int J Hyperthermia 6: 287–304

Allen S, Kantor G, Bassen H, Ruggera P (1988) CDRH RF phantom for hyperthermia systems evaluations. Int J Hyperthermia 4: 17–23

Bach Andersen JB (1985) Theoretical limitations on radiation into muscle tissue. Int J Hyperthermia 1: 45–55

Bassen HI, Smith GS (1983) Electric field probes – a review. IEEE Trans Ant Prop 31: 710–718

Ben-Yosef R, Sullivan DM, Kapp DS (1992) Peripheral neuropathy and myonecrosis following hyperthermia and radiation therapy for recurrent prostatic cancer: correlation of damage with predicted SAR pattern. Int J Hyperthermia 8: 175–185

Bolomey JC, Hawley MS (1990) Noninvasive control of hyperthermia. In: Gautherie M (ed) Methods of hyperthermia control. Springer, Berlin Heidelberg New York, pp 35–111

Bornemann F (1991) An adaptive multilevel approach to parabolic equations. Part II. variable-order time discretization based on a multiplicative error correction. IMPACT Comput Sci Eng 3: 93–122

Bornemann F (1992) An adaptive multilevel approach to parabolic equations. Part III. 2D-error estimation and multilevel preconditioning. IMPACT Comput Sci Eng 4: 1–45

Brezovich IA, Young JH, Atkinson WJ, Wang M (1982) Hyperthermia considerations for a conducting cylinder heated by an oscillating electric field applied parallel to the cylinder axis. Med Phys 9: 746–748

Brezovich IA, Atkinson WJ, Chakraborty DP (1984) Temperature distributions in tumor models heated by self-regulating nickel-copper alloy thermoseeds. Med Phys 11: 145–152

Corry PM, Barlogie B (1982) Clinical application of high frequency methods for local tumor hyperthermia. In: Nussbaum GH (ed) Physical aspects of hyperthermia. Medical Physics Monograph No. 8. Published for the American Association of Physicists in Medicine by the American Institute of Physics, pp 307–328

Corry PM, Jabboury K, Kong JS, Armour EP, McGraw FJ, LeDuc T (1988) Evaluation of equipment for hyperthermia treatment of cancer. Int J Hyperthermia 4: 53–74

Deuflhard P, Leinen P, Yserentant H (1989) Concepts of an adaptive hierarchical finite element code. IMPACT Comput Sci Eng 1: 3–35

De Leeuw AAC, Lagendijk JJW (1987) Design of a clinical deep-body hyperthermia system based on the 'coaxial TEM' applicator. Int J Hyperthermia 3:413–421

De Leeuw AAC, Lagendijk JJW, van den Berg PM (1990) SAR distribution of the "coaxial TEM" system with variable aperture width: measurements and model computations. Int J Hyperthermia 6: 445–451

De Leeuw AAC, Mooibroek J, Lagendijk JJW (1991) Specific absorption rate steering by patient positioning in the "coaxial TEM" system: phantom investigation. Int J Hyperthermia 7: 605–611

Dohlus M (1992) Ein Beitrag zur Berechnung elektromagnetischer Felder im Zeitbereich. Dissertation, Inst. f. HF-Technik, Fachgebiet Theorie elektromagnetischer Felder, Technische Hochschule Darmstadt

Feldmann HJ, Molls M, Adler S, Sack H (1991) Hyperthermia in eccentrically located pelvic tumors: excessive heating of the perineal fat and normal tissue temperatures. Int J Radiat Oncol Biol Phys 20: 1017–1022

Feldmann HJ, Molls M, Höderath A, Krümpelmann F, Sack H (1992) Blood flow and steady state temperatures in deep seated tumors and normal tissues. Int J Radiat Oncol Biol Phys 23: 1003–1008

Feldmann HJ, Molls M, Heinemann H-G, Romanowski R, Stuschke M, Sack H (1993) Thermo-radiotherapy in locally advanced deep seated tumors – thermal parameters and treatment results. Radiother Oncol 26: 38–44

Field SB, Franconi C (eds) (1987) Physics and technology of hyperthermia. Martinus Nijhoff, Dordrecht

Gibbs FA (1987) Regional hyperthermia in the treatment of cancer. In: Paliwal BR, Hetzel FW, Dewhirst MW (eds) Biological, physical and clinical aspects of hyperthermia. AAPM Medical Physics Monograph 16: 330–344

Gibbs FA, Sapozink MD, Gates KS, Stewart JR (1984) Regional hyperthermia with an annular phased array in the experimental treatment of cancer: report of work in progress with a technical emphasis. IEEE Trans Biomed Eng 31: 115–119

González González D, van Dijk JDP, Oldenburger F, Hulshof MCCM, Schneider C, Blank LECM (1992) Results of combined treatment with radiation and hyperthermia in 111 patients with large or deep seated tumors. Hyperthermic oncology 1992, vol 1, Summary papers, Berner EW (ed) Avizona Board of Regents, p 415b

Grant JP, Clarke RN, Symm GT, Spyrou NM (1989) A critical study of the open-ended coaxial line sensor technique for RF and microwave complex permittivity measurements. J Phys E Sci Instrum 22: 757–770

Haacke EM, Petropoulos LS, Nilges EW, Wu DH (1991) Extraction of conductivity and permittivity using magnetic resonance imaging. Phys Med Biol 36: 723–734

Hand JW (1990) Biophysics and technology of electromagnetic hyperthermia. In: Gautherie M (ed) Methods of External Hyperthermic Heating. Springer Berlin Heldelberg New York, pp 1–59

Hand JW, James JR (eds) (1986) Physical techniques in clinical hyperthermia. Research Studies Press, Letchworth, Herts., England

Hand JW, Vernon CC, Prior MV (1992) Early experience of a commercial scanned focussed ultrasound hyperthermia system. Int J Hyperthermia 8: 587–607

Harari PM, Hynynen KH, Roemer RB, Anhalt DP, Shimm DS, Stea B, Cassady JR (1991) Development of scanned focussed ultrasound hyperthermia: clinical response evaluation. Int J Radiat Oncol Biol Phys 21: 831–840

Hiraoka M, Jo S, Akuta K, Nishimura Y, Takahashi M, Abe M (1987) Radiofrequency capacitive hyperthermia for deep-seated tumors. Cancer 60: 121–127

Hornsleth SN (1993) The finite difference time domain method and its application to hyperthermia simulations, Hyperthermic oncology 1992, vol 2, Gerner EG, Cetas TC (eds) Arizona Board of Regents, pp 271–273

Howard GCW, Sathiaseelan V, King A, Dixon K, Anderson A, Bleehen NM (1986) Regional hyperthermia for extensive pelvic tumours using an annular phased array applicator: a feasibility study. Br J Radiol 59: 1195–1201

Issels RD, Prenninger SW, Nagele A et al. (1990) Ifosfamide plus etoposide combined with regional hyperthermia in patients with locally advanced sarcomas: a phase II study. J Clin Oncol 8: 1818–1829

Issels RD, Mittermüller J, Gerl A et al. (1991) Improvement of local control by regional hyperthermia combined with systemic chemotherapy (ifosfamide plus etoposide) in advanced sarcomas: updated report on 65 patients. J Cancer Res Clin Oncol 117 (Suppl IV): S141–S147

James BJ, Sullivan DM (1992a) Direct use of CT scans for hyperthermia treatment planning. IEEE Trans Biomed Eng 39: 845–851

James BJ, Sullivan DM (1992b) Creation of three-dimensional patient models for hyperthermia treatment planning. IEEE Trans Biomed Eng 39: 238–242

Jordan A, Wust P, Fähling H, John W, Hinz A, Felix R (1993) Inductive heating of ferromagnetic particles and magnetic fluids: physical evaluation of their potential for hyperthermia. Int J Hyperthermia 9: 51–68

Kapp DS, Fessenden P, Samulski TV et al. (1988) Stanford University Institutional Report. Phase I evaluation of equipment for hyperthermia treatment of cancer. Int J Hyperthermia 4: 75–115

Klodt H (1990) Nahfeldantennen für die Hyperthermiebehandlung von Hirntumoren. Diplomarbeit, Institut f. Hochfrequenztechnik, Technische Universität Berlin

Lagendijk JJW, Hofman P, Schipper J (1988) Perfusion analysis in advanced breast carcinoma during hyperthermia. Int J Hyperthermia 4: 479–495

Lynch DA, Paulsen KD, Strohbehn JW (1985) Finite element solution of Maxwell's equations for hyperthermia treatment planning. J Comput Phys 58: 246–269

Leybovich LB, Myerson RJ, Emami B, Straube WL (1991) Evaluation of the Sigma 60 applicator for regional hyperthermia in terms of scattering parameters. Int J Hyperthermia 7: 917–935

Marsland TP, Evans S (1987) Dielectric measurements with an open-ended coaxial probe. IEEE Proc 134: 341–349

Meier T, Kostrzewa C, Schüppert B, Petermann K (1992) Electro-optical E-field sensor with optimized electrode structure. Electronics Letters 28: 1327–1328

Meier T, Kostrzewa C, Petermann K, Schüppert B (1995) Integrated optical E-field probes with segmented modulator electrodes. J Lightwave Technology

Müller C (1969) Foundations of the mathematical theory of electromagnetic waves. Springer, Berlin Heidelberg New York

Myerson RL, Leybovich L, Emami B, Grigsby PW, Straube W, von Gerichten D (1991) Phantom studies and preliminary clinical experience with the BSD-2000. Int J Hyperthermia 7: 937–951

Nadobny J (1993) Berechnung und Optimierung elektromagnetischer Felder im Patienten bei regionalen Hyperthermie-Anwendungen. Dissertation, Fachbereich Elektrotechnik, Technische Universität Berlin

Nadobny J, Seebass M, Wust P, Felix R (1992) The essential importance of appropriate definition and 3D-modeling of E-M-sources for clinical 3D-hyperthermia planning. 6th International Congress on Hyperthermic Oncology. Hyperthermic oncology 1992, Gerner EW (ed) Arizona Board of Regents vol 1 (Summary Papers), p 226

Nishimura Y, Hiraoka M, Akuta K et al. (1992) Hyperthermia combined with radiation therapy for primarily unresectable and recurrent colorectal cancer. Int J Radial Oncol Biol Phys 23: 759–768

Nussbaum GH (ed) (1982) Physical aspects of hyperthermia. Medical Physics Monograph No. 8, Published for the American Association of Physicists in Medicine by the American Institute of Physics

Oleson JR, Heusenkveld RS, Manning MR (1983) Hyperthermia by magnetic induction: clinical experience with concentric electrodes. Int J Radiat Oncol Biol Phys 9: 549–556

Oleson JR, Sim DA, Conrad J, Fletcher AM, Gross EJ (1986) Results of a phase I regional hyperthermia device evaluation: microwave annular array versus radiofrequency induction coil. Int J Hyperthermia 2: 327–336

Oleson JR, Dewhirst MW, Harrelson JM, Leopold KA, Samulski TV, Tso CY (1989) Tumor temperature distributions predict hyperthermia effects. Int J Radiat Oncol Biol Phys 16: 559–570

Oleson JR, Samulski TV, Leopold KA, Clegg ST, Dewhirst MW, Dodge RK, George SL (1993) Sensitivity of hyperthermia trial outcomes to temperature and time: implications for thermal goals of treatment. Int J Radiat Oncol Biol Phys 25: 289–297

Paulsen KD (1990) Calculation of power deposition patterns in hyperthermia. In: Gautherie M (ed) Thermal dosimetry and treatment planning. Springer, Berlin Heidelberg New York, pp 57–118

Paulsen KD, Ross MP (1990) Comparison of numerical calculations with phantom experiments and clinical measurements. Int J Hyperthermia 6: 333–349

Paulsen KD, Lynch DR, Strohbehn JW (1988a) Three-dimensional finite boundary and hybrid element solutions of the Maxwell equations for lossy dielectric media. IEEE Trans Microwave Theor Tech 36: 682–693

Paulsen KD, Strohbehn JW, Lynch DR (1988b) Theoretical electric field distributions produced by three types of regional hyperthermia devices in a three-dimensional homogeneous model of man. IEEE Trans Biomed Eng 35: 36–45

Petrovich Z, Langholz B, Gibbs FA et al. (1989) Regional hyperthermia for advanced tumors: a clinical study of 353 patients. Int J Radiat Oncol Biol Phys 16: 601–607

Pilepich MV, Myerson RJ, Emami BN, Perez CA, Leybovich L, von Gerichten D (1987) Regional hyperthermia: a feasibility analysis. Int J Hyperthermia 3: 347–351

Raskmark P, Larsen T, Hornsleth SN (1994) Multi-applicator hyperthermia system description using scattering parameters. Int J Hyperthermia 10: 143–151

Roemer RB (1990a) Thermal dosimetry. In: Gautherie M (ed) Thermal dosimetry and treatment planning. Springer Berlin Heidelberg New York, pp 119–214

Roemer RB (1990b) The local tissue cooling coefficient: a unified approach to thermal washout and steady-state "perfusion" calculations. Int J Hyperthermia 6: 421–430

Roemer RB, Fletcher AM, Cetas TC (1985) Obtaining local SAR and blood perfusion data from temperature measurements: steady state and transient techniques compared. Int J Radiat Oncol Biol Phys 11: 1539–1550

Samulski TV, Kapp DS, Fessenden P, Lohrbach A (1987a) Heating deep seated eccentrically located tumors with an annular phased array system: a comparative clinical study using two annular array operating configurations. Int J Radiat Oncol Biol Phys 13: 83–94

Samulski TV, Fessenden P, Valdagni R, Kapp DS (1987b) Correlations of thermal washout rate, steady state temperatures, and tissue type in deep seated recurrent or metastatic tumors. Int J Radiat Oncol Biol Phys 13: 907–916

Samulski TV, Cox RS, Lyons BE, Fessenden P (1989) Heat loss and blood flow during hyperthermia in normal canine brain. II. Mathematical model. Int J Hyperthermia 5: 249–263

Sapozink MD, Gibbs FA, Egger MJ, Stewart JR (1986) Regional hyperthermia for clinically advanced deep-seated pelvic malignancy. Am J Clin Oncol 9: 162–169

Sapozink MD, Gibbs FA, Gibbs P, Stewart JR (1988) Phase I evaluation of hyperthermia equipment: University of Utah Institutional Report. Int J Hyperthermia 4: 117–132

Sapozink MD, Joszef G, Astrahan MA, Gibbs FA, Petrovich Z, Stewart JR (1990) Adjuvant pelvic hyperthermia in advanced cervical carcinoma. I. Feasibility, thermometry and device comparison. Int J Hyperthermia 6: 985–996

Schneider CJ, van Dijk JDP (1991) Visualization by a matrix of light-emitting diodes of interference effects from a radiative four-applicator hyperthermia system. Int J Hyperthermia 7: 355–366

Schneider CJ, De Leeuw AAC, van Dijk JDP (1992) Quantitative determination of SAR profiles from photographs of the light-emitting diode matrix. Int J Hyperthermia 8: 609–619

Schneider CJ, van Dijk JDP, De Leeuw AAC, Wust P, Baumhoer W (1994) Quality assurance in various radiative hyperthermia systems applying a phantom with LED-matrix. Int J Hyperthermia 10: 143–151

Seebass M (1990) 3D-Computersimulation der interstitiellen Mikrowellen-Hyperthermie von Hirntumoren, Bericht Nr.CVR 1/90, Institut für Radiologie und Pathophysiologie, Deutsches Krebsforschungszentrum, Heidelberg

Seebass M, Nadobny J, Wust P, Felix R (1992) 2D and 3D finite elements mesh generation for hyperthermia generation, 6th International Congress on Hyperthermic Oncology (ICHO), Hyperthermic Oncology 1992, vol 1 (Summary Papers). Gerner EW (ed) Avizona Board of Regents, p 229

Seebass M, Schlegel W, Wust P, Nadobny J (1993a) Thermal modeling for brain tumors. In: Seegenschmiedt HM, Sauer R (eds) Interstitial and intracavitary hyperthermia in oncology. Springer, Berlin Heidelberg New York, pp 143–146

Seebass M, Sullivan D, Wust P, Deuflhard P, Felix R (1993b) The Berlin Extension of the Stanford hyperthermia treatment planning program, Konrad-Zuse-Zentrum, Preprint SC93-35

Shimm DS, Cetas TC, Oleson JR, Gross ER, Buechler DN, Fletcher AM, Dean SE (1988) Regional hyperthermia for deep-seated malignancies using the BSD annular array. Int J Hyperthermia 4: 159–170

Storm FK, Harrison WH, Elliott RS, Kaiser LR, Silberman AW, Morton DL (1981) Clinical radiofrequency hyperthermia by magnetic-loop induction. J Microw Power Electromagn Energy 16: 179–184

Strohbehn JW, Paulsen KD, Lynch DR (1986) Use of the finite element Method in computerized thermal dosimetry. In: Hand JW, James JR (eds) Physical techniques in clinical hyperthermia. Research Studies Press, Letchworth Herts England, pp 383–451

Strohbehn JW, Curtis EH, Paulsen KD, Lynch DR (1989) Optimization of the absorbed power distribution for an annular phased array hyperthermia system. Int J Radiat Oncol Biol Phys 16: 589–599

Sullivan DM (1990) Three-dimensional computer simulation in deep regional hyperthermia using the FDTD method. IEEE Trans Microwave Theor Tech 38: 204–211

Sullivan DM (1991) Mathematical methods for treatment planning in deep regional hyperthermia. IEEE Trans Microwave Theor Tech 39: 864–872

Sullivan DM, Borup DT, Gandhi OP (1987) Use of the finite-difference time-domain method in calculating EM absorption in human tissues. IEEE Biomed Eng 34: 148–157

Sullivan DM, Buechler D, Gibbs FA (1992) Comparison of measured and simulated data in an annular phased array using an inhomogeneous phantom. IEEE Trans Microwave Theor Tech 40: 600–604

Sullivan DM, Ben-Yosef R, Kapp DS (1993) The Stanford 3-D hyperthermia treatment planning-technical review and clinical summary. Int J Hyperthermia 9: 627–643

Turner PF (1984a) Hyperthermia and inhomogeneous tissue effects using an annular phased array. IEEE Trans Microwave Theor Tech 32: 874–882

Turner PF (1984b) Regional hyperthermia with an annular phased array. IEEE Trans Biomed Eng 31: 106–114

Turner PF, Schaefermeyer T (1989) BSD-2000 approach for deep local and regional hyperthermia: clinical utility. Strahlenther Onkol 165: 700–704

van der Ploeg SK, Broekmeyer-Reurink MP, Rietveld PJM, van Rhoon GC, Verloop-van't Hof EM, van der Zee J (1993) Temperature distribution during deep hyperthermia. 13th ESHO Conference, June 16–19, Brussels, Book of Abstracts, p 56

van Dijk JDP, González-González D, Blank LECM (1989) Deep local hyperthermia with a four aperture array system of large waveguide radiators. Results of simulation and clinical applicatoin. In: Sugahara T, Saito M (eds) Hyperthermic oncology 1988, vol I: Summary papers. Taylor & Francis, London, pp 573–575

van Rhoon GC, Visser AG, van den Berg PM, Reinhold HS (1988) Evaluation of ring capacitor plates for regional deep heating. Int J Hyperthermia 4: 133–142

van Rhoon GC, Raskmark P, Hornsleth SN, van den Berg PM (1994) Radiofrequency ring applicator: energy distributions measured in the CDRH phantom. Med Biol Eng Comput

Wang J, Takagi T (1991) Iterative determination of complex permittivity and SAR distribution of two-dimensional biologiclal body. Electronics Letters 27: 112–113

Waterman FM (1987) Measurement of perfusion in human tumors. In: Paliwal BR, Hetzel FW, Dewhirst MW (eds) Biological, physical and clinical aspects of hyperthermia. AAPM, Medical Physics Monograph 16: pp 182–207

Waterman FM, Nerlinger RE, Moylan DJ, Leeper DB (1987) Response of human tumor blood flow to local hyperthermia. Int J Radiat Oncol Biol Phys 13: 75–82

Weiland T (1984) On the numerical solution of Maxwell's equations and applications in the field of accelerator physics. Particle Accelerators 15: 245–292

Weiland T (1986) Die Diskretisierung der Maxwell-Gleichungen. Phys Bl 42: 191–201

Wong TZ, Mechling JA, Jones EL, Strohbehn JW (1988) Transient finite element analysis of thermal methods used to estimate SAR and blood flow in homogeneously and nonhomogeneously perfused tumor models. Int J Hyperthermia 4: 571–592

Wust P, Nadobny J, Fähling H, Riess H, Koch K, John W, Felix R (1990) Einflußfaktoren und Störeffekte bei der Steuerung von Leistungsverteilungen mit dem Hyperthermie-Ringsystem BSD-2000. I. Klinische Observablen und Phantommessungen. Strahlenther Onkol 166: 822–830

Wust P, Nadobny J, Felix R, Deuflhard P, Louis A, John W (1991a) Strategies for optimized application of annular-phased-array systems in clinical hyperthermia. Int J Hyperthermia 7: 157–173

Wust P, Nadobny J, Fähling H, Riess H, Koch K, John W, Felix R (1991b) Einflußfaktoren und Störeffekte bei der Steuerung von Leistungsverteilungen mit dem Hyperthermie-Ringsystem BSD-2000. II. Meßtechnische Analyse. Strahlenther Onkol 167: 172–180

Wust P, Nadobny J, Seebass M, Dohlus M, John W, Felix R (1993a) 3D-computation of E-fields by the Volume-surface integral equation (VSIE) method in comparison to the Finite-integration theory (FIT) method. IEEE Trans Biomed Eng 40: 745–759

Wust P, Nadobny J, Seebass M, Fähling H, Felix R (1993b) Potentials of radiofrequency hyperthermia: planning, optimization, technological development. In: Gerner EW (ed) Hyperthermic oncology 1992, vol 2. University of Arizona

Wust P, Fähling H, Jordan A, Nadobny J, Seebass M, Felix R (1994a) Development and testing of SAR-visualizing phantoms for quality control in RF hyperthermia. Int J Hyperthermia 10: 127–142

Wust P, Stahl H, Löffel J, Seebass M, Riess H, Felix R (1995a) Clinical, physiological and anatomical determinants for radiofrequency hyperthermia. Int J Hyperthermia 11: 151–167

Wust P, Meier T, Seebass M, Fähling H, Petermann K, Felix R (1995b) Noninvasive prediction of SAR distributions with an electro-optical E field sensor. Int J Hyperthermia 11: 295–310

Wust P, Fähling H, Felix R, Rahman S, Issels RD, Feldmann H, van Rhoon G, van der Zee (1995c) Quality control of the SIGMA applicator using a lamp phantom: a four-center comparison. Int J Hyperthermia 11: in press

Zwamborn APM, van den Berg PM (1991) A weak form of the Conjugate Gradient FFT method for 2-D TE scattering problems. IEEE Trans Microwave Theor Tech 39: 953–960

Zwamborn APM, van den Berg PM (1992) The three-dimensional weak form of the Conjugate Gradient FFT method for solving scattering problems. IEEE Trans Microwave Theor Tech 40: 1757–1766

12 Ultrasound Heating Technology

K. Hynynen

CONTENTS

12.1 Introduction

Ultrasound has several characteristics which make it well suited for the induction of thermal therapy. These include the feasibility of constructing applicators of virtually any shape and size, and the good penetration of ultrasound at frequencies where the wavelengths are on the order of millimeters. The small wavelengths allow the beams to be focused and controlled. The major disadvantages of ultrasound are high absorption in bone and reflection from gas interfaces, which make treatments difficult to execute. These competing features require that ultrasound therapy systems be fairly complex in order to execute a treatment optimally. Only a few clinical systems have attempted to utilize the flexibility of ultrasound and thus, it has not yet been widely tested. Moreover, there are no clinical systems which are fully optimized for treatment of a given tumor.

12.2 Basic Physics of Ultrasound

Ultrasound is a form of vibrational energy (more than 18000 cycles/s) that is propagated as a mechanical wave by the motion of particles within the medium. The wave causes compressions and rarefactions of the medium, thus propagating a pressure wave along with the mechanical movement of the particles. The characteristics of the wave are a function of both the original disturbance generating the motion and the acoustic properties of the medium through which it travels. The propagating wave can be either longitudinal or transverse (shear wave), depending on whether the particles vibrate along or across the direction of the propagation. During an ultrasound hyperthermia treatment the waves are primarily longitudinal, with shear waves being generated only under special circumstance such as soft tissue-bone interfaces. Only the basic principles of longitudinal waves will be reviewed here; further theoretical details may be found elsewhere (see, for example, Hueter and Bolt 1995; Wells 1969, 1977).

12.2.1 Particle Motion

In order to understand ultrasound propagation, consider a particle in a simple harmonic motion oscillating around its rest position (Fig. 12.1). For

K. Hynynen, PhD, Department of Radiology, Brigham and Women's Hospital, Harvard Medical School, 75 Francis Street, Boston, MA 02115, USA

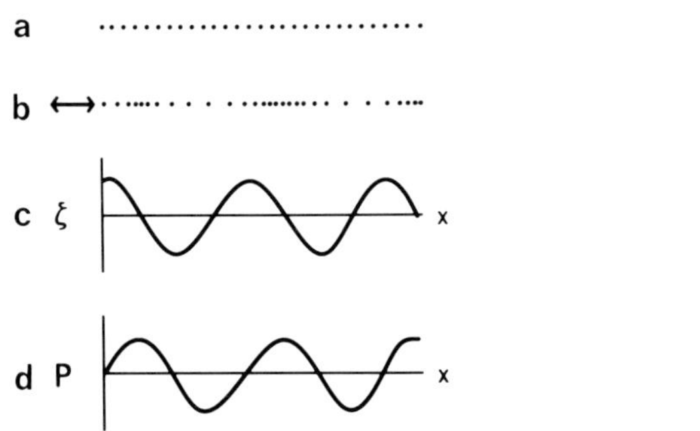

Fig. 12.1a–d. Ultrasound propagation in a medium. **a** Particles in their rest positions. **b–d** The particle positions (**b**), displacements (**c**), and pressure (**d**) at one time point during wave propagation

such a motion, the particle displacement (ζ) relative to the origin of the coordinate system is given as a function of time by the relation:

$$\zeta = \zeta_a \sin(\omega t + \phi), \tag{12.1}$$

where ω is the angular frequency, the quantity of $\omega t + \phi$ is called the phase, and thus ϕ is the initial phase at $t = 0$. The displacement varies between $+\zeta_a$ and $-\zeta_a$. The maximum displacement, ζ_a, is called the amplitude of the harmonic motion. The particle displacement repeats itself with certain time intervals as characterized by the sine function. This time interval is called the period of motion (τ). The frequency of the oscillations (f) is equal to the number of complete cycles per unit time:

$$f = 1/\tau. \tag{12.2}$$

Each particle in the medium will oscillate around its rest position with the frequency of the propagating wave. The wavelength (λ) is defined as the minimum distance between particles that are in the same phase of motion. The wavelength can be calculated from the propagation speed of the wave (c) in the medium and either the period (τ) or the frequency (f) of the wave:

$$\lambda = c\tau = c/f. \tag{12.3}$$

The speed of ultrasound is not frequency dependent and has an average magnitude of 1550 m s^{-1} in most soft tissues. The speed in fatty tissues is less than in other soft tissues, being about 1480 m s^{-1}, while in the lungs, the air spaces reduce the speed to about 600 m s^{-1}. The highest values have been measured in bone, between 1800 and 3700 m s^{-1}. Thus, the wavelength in soft tissues is about 1.5 mm at the frequency of 1 MHz, and about 0.5 mm at 3 MHz.

12.2.2 Acoustic Impedance

An important consideration during sonication of tissues is the reflection of ultrasound beams from the interface of two media with different acoustic impedances. The acoustic impedance of the medium (Z) is defined as the ratio of the sound pressure $p = \rho c v$ to the particle velocity v at any point in the field. Thus, $Z = \rho c$, where ρ is the density.

When an ultrasound beam meets the interface of two media it may be partly reflected and partly transmitted (Fig. 12.2). The incident angle (θ_i) and the angle of reflection (θ_r) are always equal. The transmission angle (θ_t) can be determined from Snell's law as follows:

$$\sin\theta_t/\sin\theta_i = c_2/c_1, \tag{12.4}$$

where c_1 and c_2 are the speed of sound in medium 1 and 2, respectively. The ratio between the reflected (p_r) and the incident acoustic pressure (p_i) of the wave depend on the incidence angle and the acoustic impedance of each medium. For plane waves it is defined as:

$$p_r/p_i = (Z_2\cos\theta_i - Z_1\cos\theta_t)/ \\ Z_2\cos\theta_i + Z_1\cos\theta_t). \tag{12.5}$$

This relation applies when the wavelength of the plane wave is smaller than the dimensions of the reflecting object. When the wavelength is comparable to or greater than the dimensions of the object, the wave is scattered in all directions. The

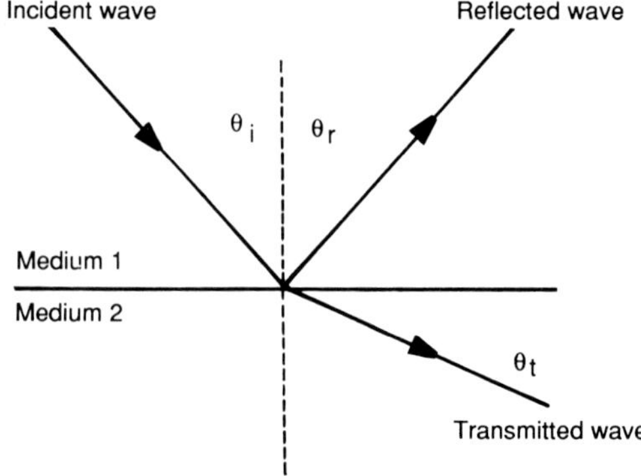

Fig. 12.2. Ultrasound reflection at a flat interface of two media

total scattered acoustic power depends on the size, shape, and acoustic properties of the object.

Generally, most of the soft tissues have an impedance roughly equal to that of water, having a density around $1000\,kg\,m^{-3}$ and an acoustic impedance of $1.6 \times 10^6\,kg\,m^{-2}s^{-1}$. Fat has a slightly lower impedance value of $1.35 \times 10^6\,kg\,m^{-2}\,s^{-1}$ due to its lower density and lower speed of sound. This means that the ultrasound beam does not suffer large reflection losses while penetrating from one soft tissue to another (FAN and HYNYNEN 1992). Bone and lung tissues have impedances that are significantly higher and lower, respectively. About 33%–39% of the energy is reflected at soft tissue – bone interfaces at an incident angle of 0°. At a tissue – gas interface, all the energy is reflected back into the tissue.

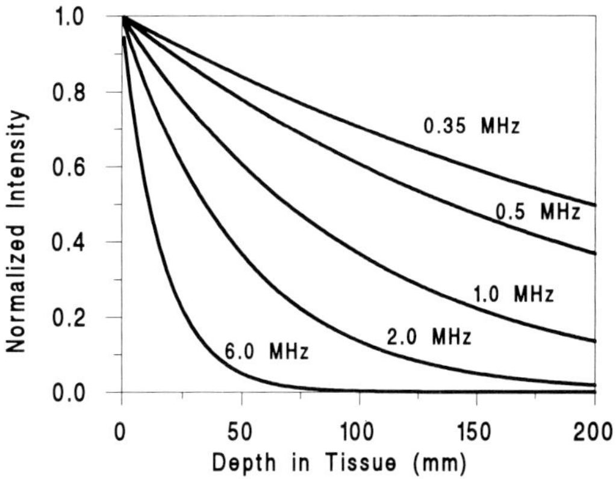

Fig. 12.3. The simulated ultrasound intensity from a planewave source as a function of depth and frequency in soft tissues. The attenuation value used in the calculations was $5\,Np\,m^{-1}\,MHz^{-1}$

12.2.3 Wave Propagation in Tissue

In tissue, ultrasound energy is attenuated according to an exponential law. The rate of energy flow through a unit area normal to the direction of the wave propagation is called the acoustic intensity (I). For a plane wave, assuming that there is no wave distortion, the intensity $I(x)$ at the depth x is described by:

$$I(x) = I(0)e^{-2\mu x}, \tag{12.6}$$

where $I(0)$ is the intensity at the surface and μ is the amplitude attenuation coefficient per unit path length ($Np\,m^{-1}$ or m^{-1}) (Fig. 12.3). Ultrasonic attenuation in tissues is the sum of the losses due to absorption and scattering. In the scattering process, the elastic discontinuities within the tissue absorb the energy and then re-emit it away from its original direction of propagation.

In an idealistic, purely elastic medium, the energy in an ultrasonic field is in either kinetic or potential form, and the pressure wave is in phase with the particle velocity. In a real medium there are also viscous forces between the moving particles which cause a lag between the particle pressure and velocity (or change in density). Therefore, an energy loss during each cycle will result. The absorption in a viscoelastic medium should depend on the square of the frequency (f^2). This is true in many liquids but not in tissues, where the absorption has been shown to increase almost linearly as a function of frequency:

$$\alpha = \alpha_o(f)^m, \tag{12.7}$$

where α_o is the absorption coefficient at 1 MHz and f is the frequency in MHz. α_o and m are dependent on the tissue type and m has been found experimentally to be between 1 and 1.2 for soft tissue(Goss et al. 1979). The absorption and attenuation values measured for different tissues are summarized in Table 12.1. The measured absorption coefficient values are significantly larger ($3–10\,m^{-1}$ at 1 MHz) than those estimated based on the classic absorption theory (around $0.1\,m^{-1}$ at 1 MHz). Thus, there must also be other absorption mechanisms in tissues in addition to the viscous one. During the compressive part of the cycle, energy is stored in the medium in a number of forms, such as lattice vibrational energy, molecular vibrational energy, and translational energy. During the expansion part of the cycle, this stored energy is returned to the wave and the medium temperature returns to the original level. However, in tissue the increased kinetic energy of the molecules is not in balance with the environment, and the system tries to redistribute the energy. The transfer of energy takes time and thus, during the decompression cycle, energy will return out of phase to the wave and absorption results. In addition, a portion of the stored energy remains in various forms within the medium. This mechanism of energy absorption is called relaxation. The ultrasonic absorption mechanism in tissues has been reviewed in detail by DUNN (1976) and WELLS (1977).

Table 12.1. Acoustic properties of mammalian tissues at a temperature of 37°C and frequency of 1 MHz (data from Goss et al. 1978, 1979, 1980; Chivers and Parry 1978; Lyons and Parker 1988; Wells 1977)

Tissue	Absorption ($Np\,m^{-1}$)	Attenuation ($Np\,m^{-1}$)	Density ($kg\,m^{-3}$)	Speed ($m\,s^{-1}$)
Bone	–	150–350	1380–1810	1500–3700
Brain	1.2–6.4	4–29	1030	1516–1575
Fat	–	5–9	921	1400–1490
Kidney	3.3	3–10	1040	1564–1640
Liver	2.3–3.2	3.2–18	1060	1540–1640
Lung	7	430–480	400	470–658
Muscle	2–11	4.4–15	1070–1270	1508–1630
Tendon	14	30–70	1200	1750

In experimental studies, the attenuation coefficient has been found to follow the frequency in a similar manner to that of the absorption. However, the attenuation values have been found to be larger than those of absorption. Scatter accounts for part of this difference, but some of it has been explained as due to attenuation measurement errors (Carstensen et al. 1981; Lyons and Parker 1988).

12.2.4 Tissue Temperature Elevation Induced by Ultrasound

For any continuous, single-frequency ultrasound field, when the effects of interfaces and shear viscosity are small, the temporal average absorbed power density $\langle q \rangle$ depends on the square of the acoustic pressure amplitude p_a as follows:

$$\langle q \rangle = \alpha p_a^2 / \rho_o c, \tag{12.8}$$

where ρ_o is the density of the medium without the sound field (Nyborg 1981). In a plane wave situation, this can be expressed as:

$$\langle q \rangle = 2\alpha I. \tag{12.9}$$

where α is the amplitude absorption coefficient. Thus, the amount of absorbed energy is determined by the pressure amplitude (or intensity) of the incident ultrasound beam, the ultrasound absorption coefficient of the tissue, and the heat transfer mechanisms of the tissue.

The situation is quite different at soft tissue – bone interfaces, where about 33%–39% of the incident energy is reflected back at normal incidence. In addition, the amplitude attenuation coefficient of ultrasound is about 10–20 times higher in bone than in soft tissues. This causes the transmitted beam to be absorbed rapidly, creating a significant temperature increase. There are several studies showing preferential heating of the bone surface during sonication with a nonfocused physiotherapy transducer operating at 1 MHz (Nelson et al. 1950; Lehmann et al. 1966, 1967). Similar hot spots also appear during scanned focused ultrasound hyperthermia when weakly focused, low-frequency beams are used to heat tissues in front of bones (Hynynen and DeYoung 1988) (Fig. 12.4). This can be avoided, or at least reduced to an acceptable level, if the intensities at the bone surface are only between 10% and 50% of the value at the back of the target volume. (This depends on the tumor perfusion rate, the intesity at the bone surface should be lower in well-perfused tumors.) Reduced intensity at the bone surfaces can be achieved in many cases with multiple focused beams, high frequencies, or more sharply focused transducers. Since the hot spot is mainly caused by absorption in the bone, it can also be decreased by reducing the amount of energy transmitted into the bone through the interface. This can be done effectively by increasing the incident angle (Davis and Lele 1987).

Soft tissue–gas interfaces create a similar problem by reflecting all of the incident energy. This means that the absorbed power will be doubled close to the interface, and, therefore, the average power density of the beam has to be smaller than one-half of the value at the treatment volume (again, this depends on the perfusion of the tumor and the tissues close to the interface) (Hynynen 1990). At lower frequencies the beams can propagate long distances in tissues; therefore, gas interfaces can reflect the beams into unexpected locations, which sometimes results in patient discomfort.

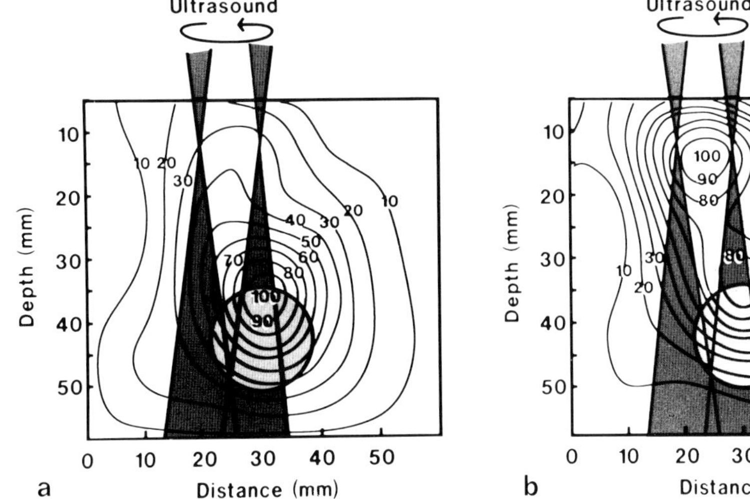

Fig. 12.4. The normalized temperature distribution along the axial plane of a 10-mm-diameter scan during 1 MHz (**a**) and 3.6 MHz (**b**) ultrasound in dog's thigh muscle and bone in vivo. The strong ultrasound absorption in the bone caused a hot spot at the muscle–bone interface when the 1 MHz frequency was used. (From HYNYNEN and DEYOUNG 1988)

12.3 The Ultrasonic Field

An ideal point source of ultrasonic energy emits radiation equally in all directions, resulting in a spherical wave front. The ultrasonic field from a real source can be analyzed with Huygen's principle by modeling it as a large number of point sources situated very close together, and then analyzing the resultant wave front (ZEMANEK 1971). The finite size of transducers causes various boundary phenomena (reflection, refraction, and diffraction), which, when combined with the inhomogeneities of the transducer material, cause a deviation of a real acoustic field from a theoretical one.

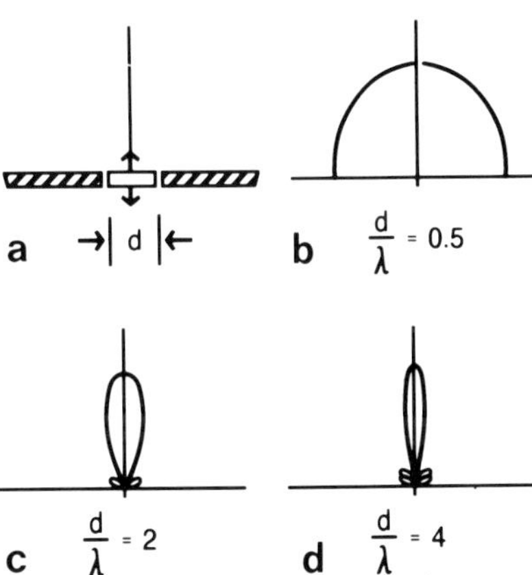

Fig. 12.5a–d. The ultrasound field emitted by a circular piston vibrating at different frequencies **a** Diagram of the piston; **b–d** the field patterns

12.3.1 Unfocused Ultrasonic Fields

The ultrasound field emitted by a circular piston transducer (diameter d, radius a) depends on the ratio between the diameter of the piston and the wavelength. The beam becomes more and more directed when the diameter increases with respect to the wavelength (Fig. 12.5). Transducers that have $d >> \lambda$ have two zones in the ultrasound fields that they emit. In general the region between the transducer and the last axial maximum (the near field or Fresnel zone) has pressure maxima and minima rings symmetric around the central axis, causing the distribution of acoustic energy to be nonuniform. The number of maxima and minima across the beam depends upon the values of x, the distance from the transducer surface, and a/λ. Generally, the frequency of the peaks increases with decreasing x and increasing values of a/λ. As one can see from Fig. 12.6, the number of pressure maxima across the beam increases from one at the last axial maximum, to two at the last axial minimum and three at the second to last axial maximum, etc. The beam also narrows towards the last axial maximum,

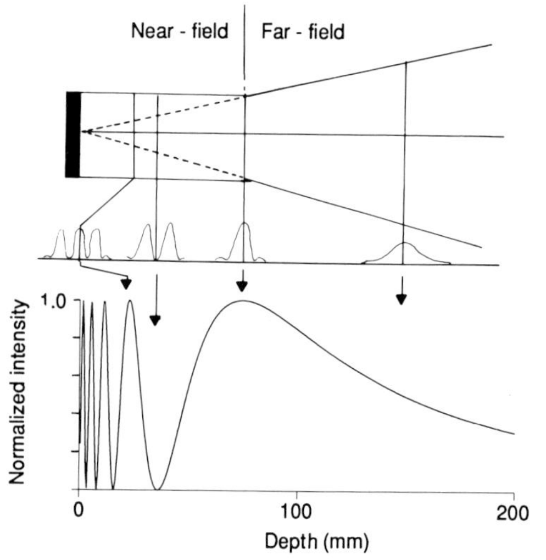

Fig. 12.6. The ultrasound field distribution from a flat circular transducer with **d** >> λ. *Top*: the beam outline; *middle*: the cross-sectional (pressure amplitude)^2 distributions; *bottom*: the axial (pressure amplitude)^2 distribution

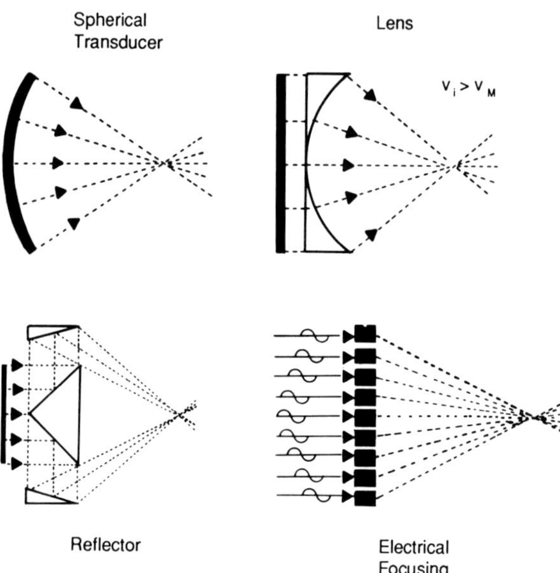

Fig. 12.7. Ultrasonic focusing systems

being about one-quarter of the diameter of the transducer (−3 dB beam diameter) at the last axial maximum. The last axial maximum occurs at the distance defined by:

$$x_{max} = (4a^2 - \lambda^2)/4\lambda$$
$$= a^2/\lambda \text{ (when } a >> \lambda).$$

The ultrasonic field beyond the last axial maximum (the far field or Fraunhofer zone) is diverging, and the intensity follows the inverse square law, $I(x) \sim 1/x^2$, at large distances. The intensity distribution across the beam in the far field can be approximated by a Gaussian distribution with roughly 84% of the energy in the main lobe. The rest of the energy is distributed through side lobes. Most of the plane wave ultrasound hyperthermia aplicators are between 3 and 10 cm in diameter and operate between 0.5 and 5 MHz. Thus, the heated region is in the near field. At these frequencies, especially above 1 MHz, the pressure maxima and minima are so close to each other that the thermal conduction smooths the temperature distribution. If the ultrasonic disc is properly mounted and functioning correctly, the average energy distribution should be fairly uniform and cover almost the whole surface area of the applicator. It is also well known that the energy deposition pattern can be smoothed by slightly varying the driving frequency around the resonant frequency (Munro et al. 1982).

12.3.2 Focused Ultrasonic Fields

The shape of an ultrasound beam emitted by a transducer can be modified by focusing. In a fashion similar to those used in optics, the ultrasonic beams can be focused by using self-focusing radiators, lenses or reflectors. Focusing can also be achieved by using transducer arrays that are driven with signals having the proper phase difference to obtain a common focal point (electrical focusing) (Fig. 12.7). The wavelength imposes the limitation on the size of the focal region and the sharpness of the focus is determined by the ratio between the aperture of the array to the wavelength.

12.3.2.1 Spherically Curved Transducers

The theory of spherically curved transducers vibrating with uniform normal surface velocity was developed by O'Neil (1949). The theory shows that it is only possible to focus energy in the near field of an equivalent plane transducer, due to the finite size of the wavelength. The focused acoustic field is very complex between the acoustic focus and the transducer, resembling the near field of a plane wave transducer (Figs. 12.8, 12.9). Beyond the focus, the field behaves in a similar fashion to that of the far field of a plane transducer,

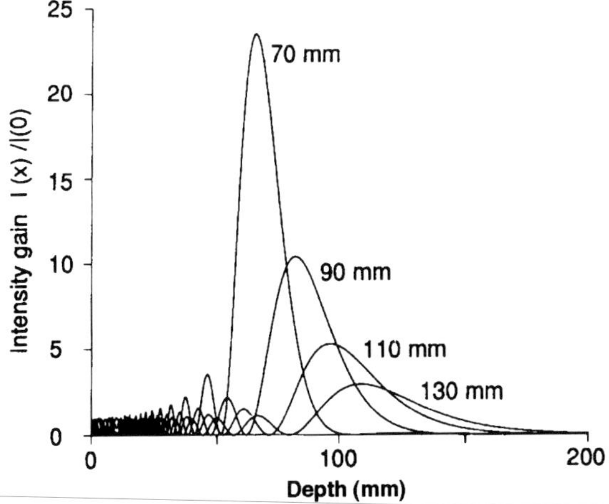

Fig. 12.8. The simulated axial intensity distribution in tissue from a focused transducer (diameter = 60 mm, frequency 1 MHz) for various values of radius of curvature

except that the divergence of the beam beyond the focus is dominated by the geometrical divergence angle of the transducer. The shape of the focus is long and narrow. These dimensions are dependent on the focusing properties of the transducer, i.e., its diameter, radius of curvature, and frequency. For spherically curved radiator an approximate half-intensity beam width (d_t) at the focus is obtained from:

$$d_t = 1.417\left(\frac{R}{2a}\right)$$

where R in the radius of curvature and $2a$ is the diameter of transducer. The axial length of the focus (d_x) is

$$d_x = 7.17\left(\frac{R}{2a}\right)^2$$

(Hunt 1987). By increasing the radius of curvature, the maximum intensity can be pushed deeper into the tissue, but the focal region becomes longer and the peak intensity smaller. This is due to the reduced focusing effect of the transducer and the attenuation within the tissue, respectively. It is possible to induce an intensity maximum at any practical depth in soft tissues with a suitable

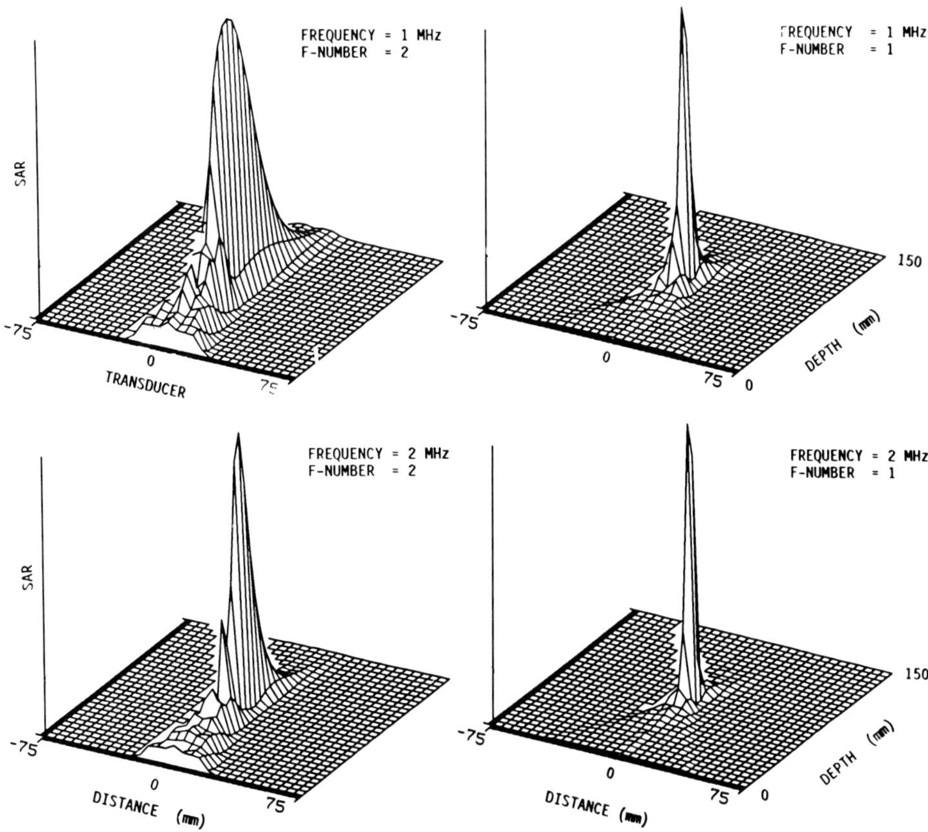

Fig. 12.9. The simulated ultrasound field distribution in tissue in the axial plane of different focused transducers. The frequency and the F-number (= diameter/radius of curvature) are given in the graph

choice of the transducer parameters, as long as the beam entry is not restricted by gas or bone.

12.3.2.2 Ultrasonic Lenses

Similar to those used in optics, acoustic lenses are made of materials in which the speed of sound (c_L) is different from that in the coupling medium (c_m), causing the ultrasound beam to focus. Lenses made of solids, e.g., plastics, metals, or liquids, where the speed of sound is higher (solids) or lower (liquid) than in water, have been used. The ideal shape of a lens is planoconcave (Fig. 12.7), with $c_L > c_m$, where the generating curve of the concave surface is elliptic. The advantage of lenses over spherically curved transducers is that a desired ultrasonic field can be produced from a single transducer by choosing the appropriate lens.

It is also possible to form a line focus or multiple foci by using special lenses (LALONDE et al. 1990).

12.3.2.3 Reflectors

The absorption losses in lenses can be avoided by using acoustic reflectors made of material with either a much higher or much lower acoustic impedance than the propagating medium. Reflectors have rarely been used for hyperthermia purposes. However, they may offer some advantages such as minimal attenuation of x-rays for applicators used with simultaneous radiation therapy (MONTES and HYNYNEN 1992).

12.3.2.4 Electrical Focusing

Ultrasonic beams can be focused by using one- or two-dimensional arrays of transducers, with each element driven by a signal of specified phase so that the hemispherical waves emitted by each element (small enough compared with wavelength in order to act as a point source) are in phase at the desired focal point. This principle is illustrated in Fig. 12.10, where a one-dimensional array is shown.

The phased array construction is limited by the center-to-center spacing of the elements. This sets limits on the maximum size of the elements. Similar to the microwave phased arrays, the maximal spacing between the centers of neighboring elements is one-half of a wavelength in order to avoid grating lobes (STEINBERG 1976) (Fig. 12.11). If focusing only along the central axis is desired, then element spacing up to one wavelength can be used. However, there are ways to make the element size larger (up to two wavelengths) by utilizing curved arrays (EBBINI and CAIN 1991a,b; EBBINI et al. 1988). This means that element sizes around 1.5–6 mm are required for an operating frequency of 0.5 MHz.

Perhaps the biggest advantage of phased arrays over any other transducer is that the ultrasound field distribution can be controlled as desired. One can move the focal spot to a desired spot or scan it around. Multiple simultaneous foci can be created or one focus can be made larger. The field can also be reduced in desired locations by setting up destructive interference patterns. Therefore, one has a lot of freedom to generate desirable ultrasound fields with a two-dimensional array. In practice, the desired field distribution can be described in selected locations (control points) in the field and the optimal phase and amplitude distribution of the driving signal can be calculated by using pseudoinverse techniques as proposed by EBBINI and CAIN (1989).

12.4 Ultrasound Transducers

12.4.1 Structure of an Ultrasound Hyperthermia Transducer

Figure 12.12 shows the general structure of a high-power ultrasound transducer. The thickness of the plate of piezoelectric material determines the operating frequency. Both surfaces of the transducer are covered by thin metal electrodes. The transducer plate is mounted on the holder in such a way that it has maximum freedom to move. On the front surface there can be a one-quarter wavelength matching layer that reduces the acoustic mismatch between the transducer and the coupling media. However, it is optional and adequate power outputs can be obtained without it. An air space behind the plate provides a low impedance backing. This space can also house the electrical matching circuit. Maximum electrical efficiency of the transducer can be obtained when the transducer is matched to the electrical impedance of the driving amplifier and the ele-

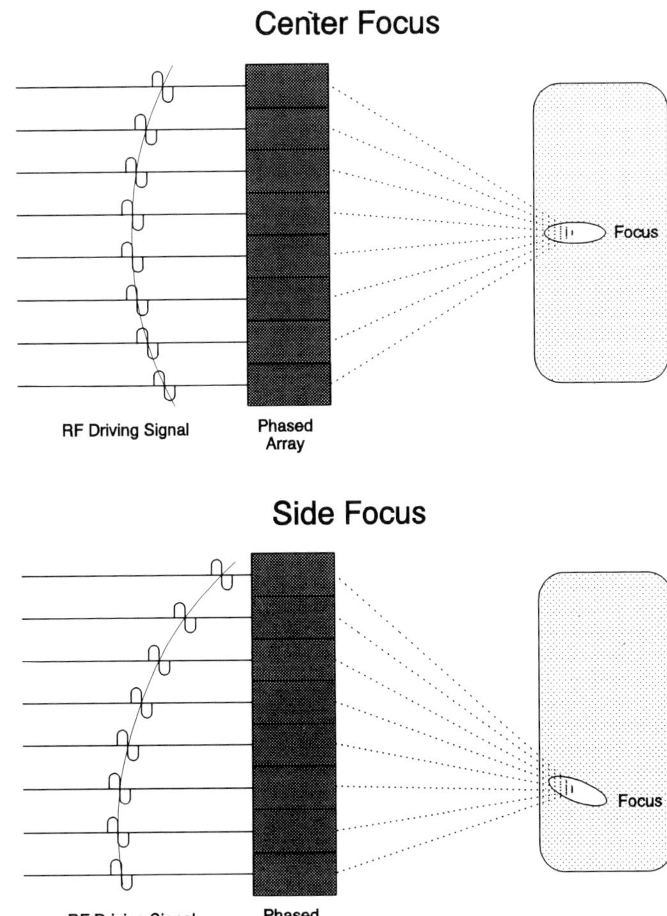

Fig. 12.10. A diagram of a one-dimensional phased array

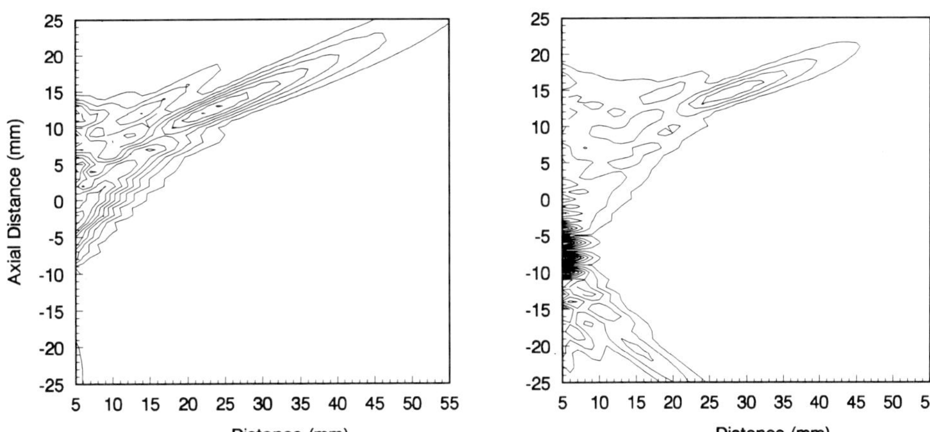

Fig. 12.11. The measured ultrasound field distribution from a one-dimensional, 16-element phased array at the frequency of 0.5 MHz, with the beam focused 15 mm off the central axis. The center-to-center spacing of the elements was 2.5 mm (*right*) and 1.8 mm (*left*). (From BUCHANAN and HYNYNEN 1994)

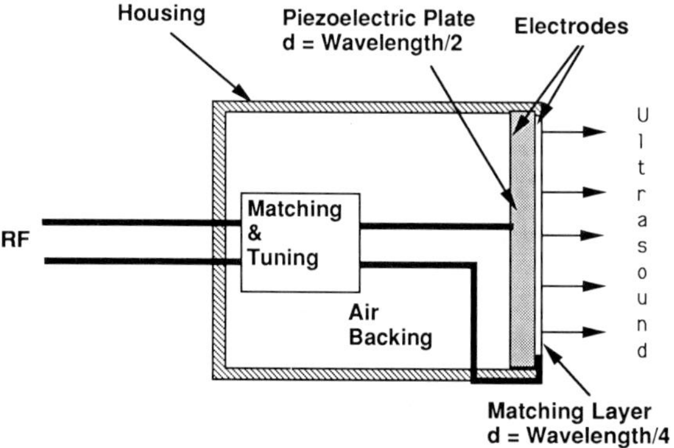

Fig. 12.12. Diagram of an ultrasound therapy transducer

ctrical and mechanical resonances of the transducer are tuned together.

12.4.2 Piezoelectric Materials

Certain materials which lack a center of symmetry in their lattice structure, have the property that the application of pressure causes an electrical voltage to appear across the crystal. The voltage is proportional to the applied pressure within the elastic limits of the material. This phenomenon is called the piezoelectric effect. Similarly, the application of an electrical voltage across the crystal causes a mechanical deformation (inverse of the piezoelectric effect). When an electrical voltage is applied across the crystal the positively charged particles, or positive end of the dipole, tend to move towards the negative voltage and the negative particles towards the positive side. The crystal deforms until the elastic forces between the particles counter balance the electrical forces. Reversing the voltage induces an opposite effect. Thus, by applying a changing voltage across a piezoelectric crystal, electrical energy can be converted to mechanical thickness changes of the crystal.

For hyperthermia, transducers capable of producing high-power, single-frequency, continuous waves for extensive periods are needed. Lead zirconate titanate (or PZT) has been the most widely used. In addition to the piezoelectric material, the mechanical structure of the transducer is very important for meeting these requirements. The maximum stress wave is obtained when the thickness of the plate $d = \lambda/2$ or an odd multiple of $\lambda/2$. The frequency which corresponds to the half wavelength thickness is called the fundamental resonant frequency of the transducer. If the transducer is driven at a frequency which is three times its fundamental frequency, it is operating at its third harmonic, and so on.

12.5 Ultrasound Systems for Induction of Hyperthermia

The following section is a summary of the hyperthermia devices that utilize ultrasound as the method of heating. Only the systems' characteristics that are important for the understanding of their function will be given. The generation of the RF signals to be converted into mechanical motion is in principle similar in all systems; therefore, a typical system diagram is presented in Fig. 12.13. The RF signal is generated by a signal generator or an oscillator and is amplified by an RF amplifier. The forward and reflected electrical power are measured after amplification in order to obtain the total acoustic power output. The signal enters the transducer through a matching and tuning network that couples the electrical impedance of the transducer to the output im-

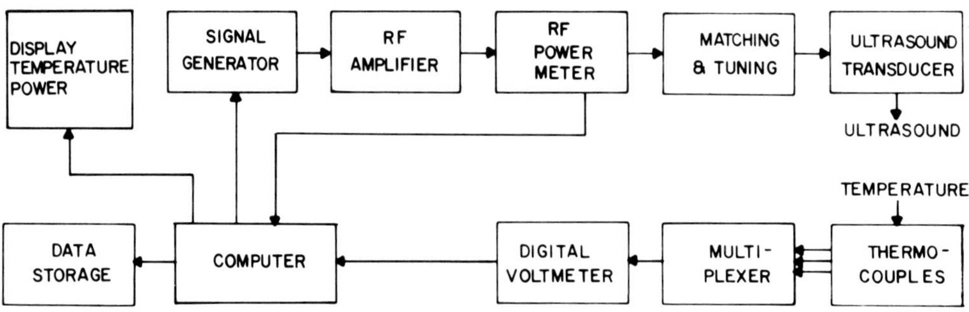

Fig. 12.13. Block diagram of an ultrasound hyperthermia system

pedance of the power amplifier. The power output is controlled by the amplitude and duty cycle of the RF voltage.

12.5.1 Superficial Heating Systems

12.5.1.1 Planar Transducer Systems

The first clinical ultrasound systems utilized single circular and planar transducers, which were sonicating through a temperature-controlled water column to the patient (MARMOR et al. 1979; CORRY et al. 1982). A diagram of such a device is presented in Fig. 12.14. The main advantages of these applicators are: First, they are simple to construct and operate. Second, the energy penetration is good and applicators with different frequencies allow some control over the depth of the heated region (frequencies of 1 – 3 MHz are commonly used). Finally, the energy deposition pattern is well collimated and relatively uniform power output can be obtained over the whole transducer surface (provided that the applicator construction has been done properly) (MUNRO et al. 1981). The main disadvantage is that there is no control over the energy deposition as a function of lateral location and thus hot spots (such as are generated on bone surfaces or on scar tissue) often limit power output, resulting in subtherapeutic temperatures. More control over the power deposition patterns was obtained when the applicator was divided into concentric rings. Controlling the power to each ring individually has been demonstrated to result in a small improvement in the temperature distributions (RYAN et al. 1991).

In order to heat larger tumors and gain better control over the energy deposition, multielement applicators with independent power input to each transducer element can be used. This allows a variable power output over the heated area to compensate somewhat for variations in the cooling by blood flow and thermal conduction, and to adapt to the geometry of the tumor. A 16-square element (4 × 4) array described by UNDERWOOD et al. (1987) has been tested clinically and is now commercially available. The individual element size is 36 mm × 36 mm and they operate at either 1 or 3 MHz. Since the tumor is always within the near field of the transducer, the beam is well collimated and propagates to the volume in front of each element. This allows good control over the power deposition pattern. However, the disappointing clinical temperature distributions (SAMULSKI et al. 1990) indicate that more control over the power field is needed. This can be achieved by using smaller elements, and allowing variable frequency control for each element.

12.5.1.2 Mechanically Scanned Fields

A mechanically scanned system can also be used for the treatment of superficial tumors with several theoretical advantages. First, the ultrasound power can be controlled as a function of the scan location with good spatial resolution. Second, since the energy deposition is scanned, the patient can identify locations which cause pain, allowing the system to reduce power in these locations. Third, the penetration depth as a function of location can be controlled by using multiple frequencies. Finally, the heated region can be tailored to cover the tumor and even large volumes can be treated. The major disadvantage is that such systems are expensive to build and that there are no systems that are commercially available. The initial clinical trials utilizing a scanned

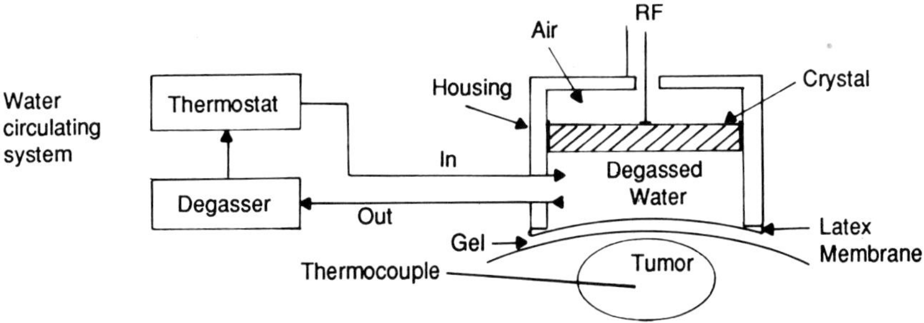

Fig. 12.14. A planar ultrasound hyperthermia transducer system

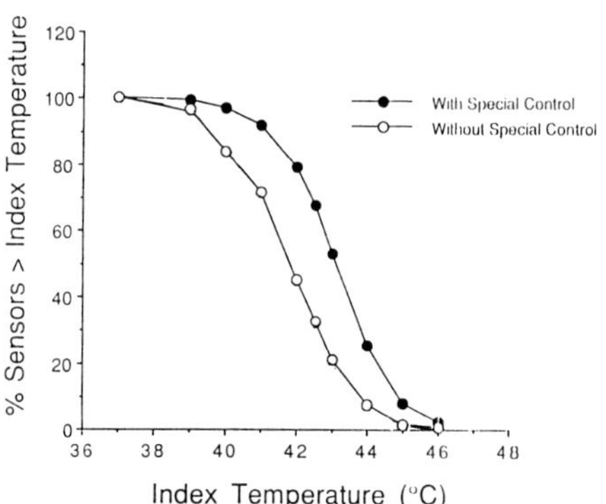

Fig. 12.15. A summary of the temperatures measured during scanned ultrasound treatments of chest wall tumors. (From ANHALT et al. 1993)

transducer system (Fig. 12.15) are encouraging (ANHALT et al. 1993).

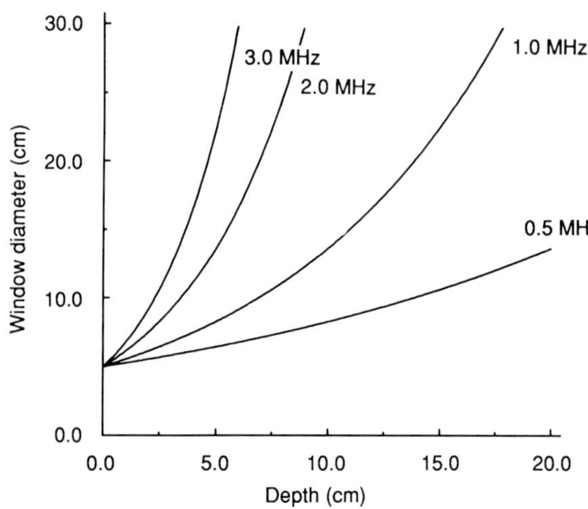

Fig. 12.16. The diameter of the ultrasonic window required for compensating the attenuation losses in soft tissues as a function of depth for various frequencies. The diameter of the target volume was 5 cm

12.5.2 Deep Heating Systems

There are several common requirements for all systems which are used for heating deep tumors. First, the effective beam diameter has to decrease to compensate for the attenuation losses in the tissue. In order to obtain a higher temperature in the tumor than in the the overlying tissues, more convergence and intensity gain is required. Second, the energy deposition pattern has to be controllable in order to reduce hot or cold spots. Finally, the patient–system interface has to be such that accurate localization of the tumor can be achieved.

The theoretical geometrical gain to overcome the attenuation losses can be calculated easily, if the attenuation coefficient(s) is known. The surface window diameter required as a function of depth for various frequencies and target volume diameters is presented in Figs. 12.16 and 12.17, assuming representative attenuation values from Table 12.1. These graphs indicate the minimum surface window diameter required to obtain equal absorbed power density at the surface and at depth. It is clear that the required geometrical gain depends strongly on the operating frequency and also on the target volume diameter. The window size sets practical limitations on the size of tumors that can be heated at depth. The optimal frequency for deep heating is between 0.5 and 1.5 MHz. In practice the highest possible frequency should be selected to minimize the hot spots at bone surfaces behind the tumor.

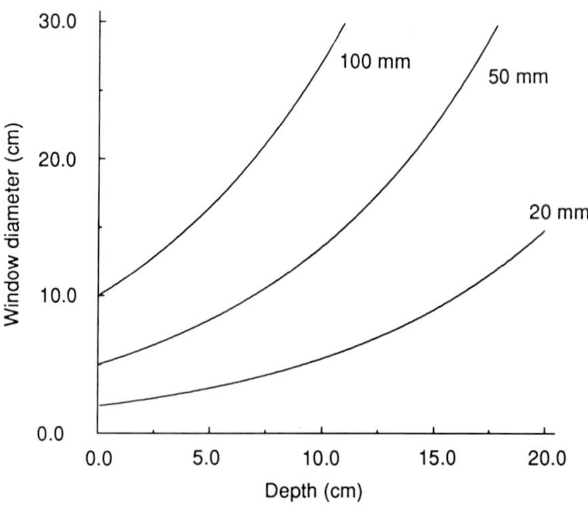

Fig. 12.17. The diameter of the ultrasonic window required for compensating the attenuation losses in soft tissues as a function of depth for various target volume diameters. The frequency was 1 MHz

12.5.2.1 Mechanical Focusing

A mechanically focused ultrasound system can be used to overcome the effect of attenuation and to deliver more energy into deep tumors. This can be done by using multiple beams overlapping at depth, using spherically curved transducers or lenses. The first clinical system evaluated was constructed from six 350 kHz circular plane transducers (diameter 70 mm). Because the beams could be aimed independently they could be adjusted to all overlap at one location or form a larger, more dispersed focus (FESSENDEN et al. 1984). However, this system is not presently used in the clinic, due to the large number of treatments limited by pain (30% pain limited). The low frequency used (350 kHz) penetrates deep into the tissues and propagates beyond the focal region. This can induce hot spots at bone or air interfaces beyond the target volume. Similar experimental systems, but with more mechanical control, have subsequently been designed to operate in the frequency range of 0.5–1.0 MHz. These utilize either focused (HYNYNEN et al. 1983; SEPPI et al. 1985) or planar multiple stationary beams (Labthermics Technologies, Urbana, Ill., USA; SVENSSON et al. 1992). None of these systems have been fully tested in a clinical setting to evaluate their effectiveness.

Another approach used to increase the size of the heated volume is to scan a focused transducer in such a manner that the focus travels throughout the whole tumor. This allows good control over the power deposition pattern, since the power can be controlled as a function of the location. Thus, the power output can be tailored for each tumor to give the desired temperature distribution, provided that temperatures are measured in an adequate number of locations. A significant advantage of this method over many of the current hyperthermia techniques is that because the scanning is usually executed under computer control, the shape and size of the treated volume can be accurately controlled. Only three mechanical scanning devices have been tested in clinical trials (Figs. 12.18, and 12.19) (LELE 1983; HYNYNEN et al. 1987, 1990; HARARI et al. 1991; GUTHKELCH et al. 1991; HAND et al. 1992), and there are no commercially available devices. These systems heated some tumors well and almost always at least part of the tumor reached

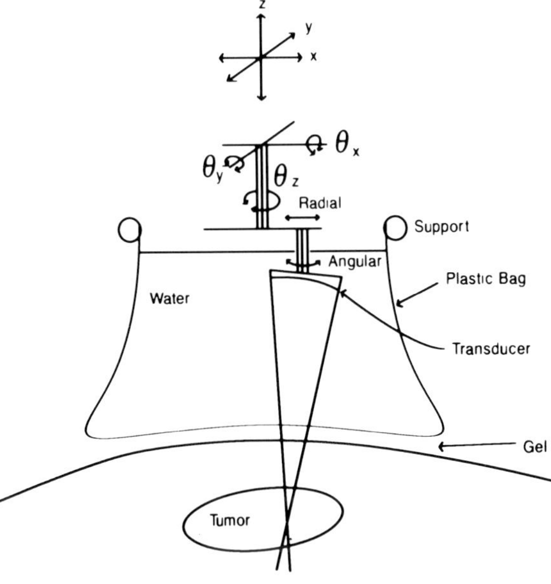

Fig. 12.18. A diagram of the first scanned and focused ultrasound hyperthermia system. (From LELE 1983)

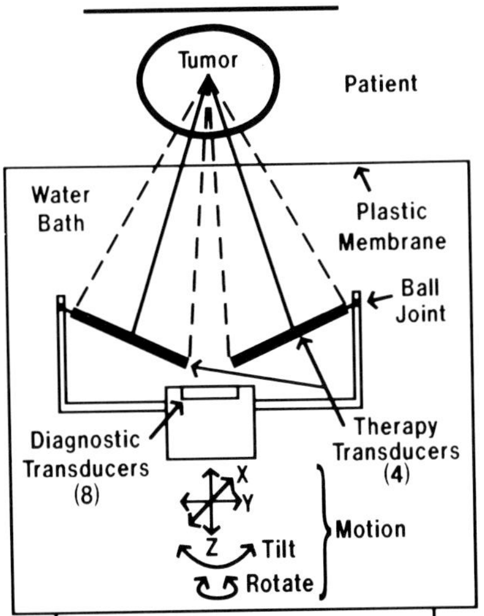

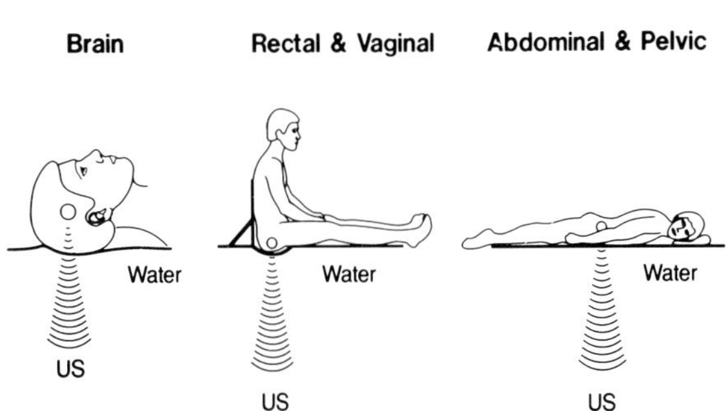

Fig. 12.19. A clinical scanned focused ultrasound system combined with ultrasound imaging: **a** diagram of the sonication head; **b** diagram of different treatment positions. (From HYNYNEN et al. 1987)

therapeutic temperatures. However, they were not optimized and do not utilize the full potential of mechanically scanned systems. Some of the issues related to the scanned focused systems have been investigated and there are guidelines for scanning speed (HYNYNEN et al. 1986; MOROS et al. 1988) and pattern (MOROS et al. 1990; LIN et al. 1992). The potential benefits of using multiple entrance sites has also been demonstrated in a simulation study for the treatment of neck tumors (TU et al. 1994).

12.5.2.2 Electrical Focusing

The required beam convergence can also be obtained by using phased array applicators. Some of these applicators have been extensively studied and hold significant promise. However, none have yet been clinically used.

The first attempts to utilize electrical focusing in ultrasound hyperthermia were made by DO-HUUN and HARTEMANN (1982). They constructed a concentric ring transducer, where each ring was driven with a different signal. This approach offered an acoustic focus at a desired distance on the central axis. The focus was scanned along the axis but not in any other directions. According to the simulation study of CAIN and UMEMURA (1986) such an array is capable of generating a ring focus, but it also creates a secondary focus both in front and behind the focal plane on the central axis of the beam. An interesting approach that avoids the secondary foci of the concentric ring device is to combine electrical focusing with a mechanically focused transducer (lens system or spherically curved transducer) (CAIN and UMEMURA 1986). The principle of this system is shown on the far right of Fig. 12.20. For this device, a circular transducer is divided into sectors, each of which has an individual driving circuitry with a lens placed in front of the transducer to focus the beam. Then, the phase differences between the driving signals of the various transducer elements can be set such that the pressure amplitude along the central axis is zero and the energy is focused into a ring at the focal plane.

The most flexible, although expensive way of utilizing electrical focusing is to use a two-dimensional array of small transducers, each of which has a separate amplitude and phase control. In order to reduce the amount of required electronics, several methods have been developed. OCHELTREE et al. (1984) reported a stacked array approach and BENKESER et al. (1987) used tapered arrays (Fig. 12.20). Both techniques drive only a part of the array at one time and then cover the complete array in a sequence. This reduces geometric gain since the focusing is achieved only along the length of the array. Another method of reducing the number of transducer elements is to utilize both mechanical and electrical focusing. Simulations and experiments have shown that a cylindrical or spherical section array of transducers could provide a flexible way of focusing and scanning the ultrasonic field electrically (EBBINI et al. 1988, 1991).

The full utilization of phased arrays requires several hundred transducer elements and driving lines. These hardware requirements can be met easily by using modern circuit board construction techniques and components. This makes electrical

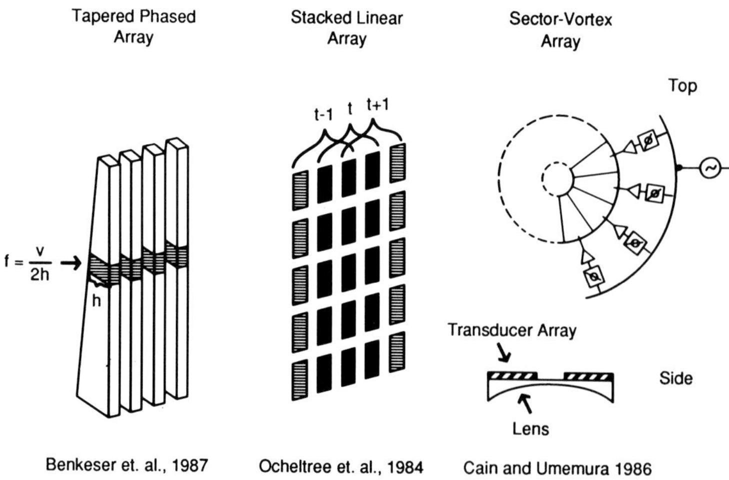

Fig. 12.20. Three different ways to reduce the number of driving channels with phased array ultrasound hyperthermia applicators

ultrasound field control an attractive alternative to the mechanically focused systems (EBBINI and CAIN 1991a,b).

12.5.3 Ultrasound Intracavitary Applicators

The technical feasibility of constructing transducers of almost any shape and size has made it possible to develop small intracavitary ultrasound applicators. The piezoelectric ceramic can be manufactured in the shape of a cylinder with electrodes on both inner and outer surfaces. When an RF voltage is applied on the electrodes, the cylinder wall thickness will expand and contract with the voltage. This generates a cylindrical ultrasound wave which propagates radially outward. The directivity of this wave will depend on the ratio between the cylinder length and the wavelength (Fig. 12.21). In order to obtain an ultrasound beam that is well collimated, the cylinder length has to be on the order of ten wavelengths. Multiple cylinders can be joined together to form arrays. Each element in such an array can be driven independently at desired power output levels. This will allow the power deposition pattern to be modified in order to obtain the desired temperature distribution. Applicators as small as 1 mm in diameter have been constructed (HYNYNEN and DAVIS 1993). The coupling between the applicator and the cavity wall can be provided by an inflatable water bolus encased by a flexible, ultrasound-transparent membrane. The temperature of the cavity wall can be controlled by circulating the coupling water through a heat exchanger. The operating frequency and the bolus temperature allow some control over the heating depth (Fig. 12.22). Applicators with sectors of cylinders can also be constructed for applications where the tumor is only on one side of the cavity (Figs. 12.23, 12.24). Segmenting the cylinders or sectors also in the

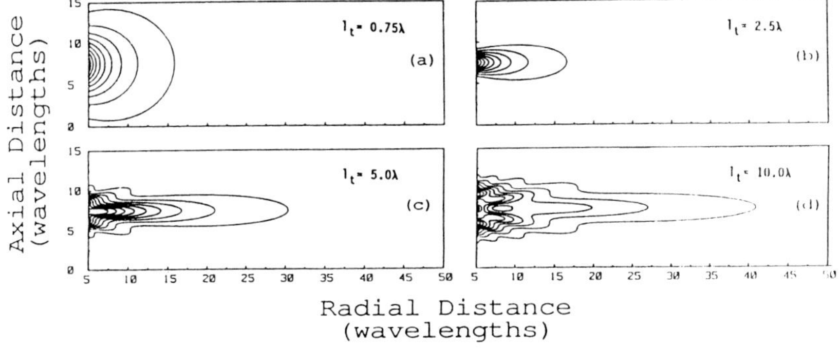

Fig. 12.21a–d. Simulated ultrasound field distributions along a single cylindrical element of various lengths. (From DIEDERICH and HYNYNEN 1990a)

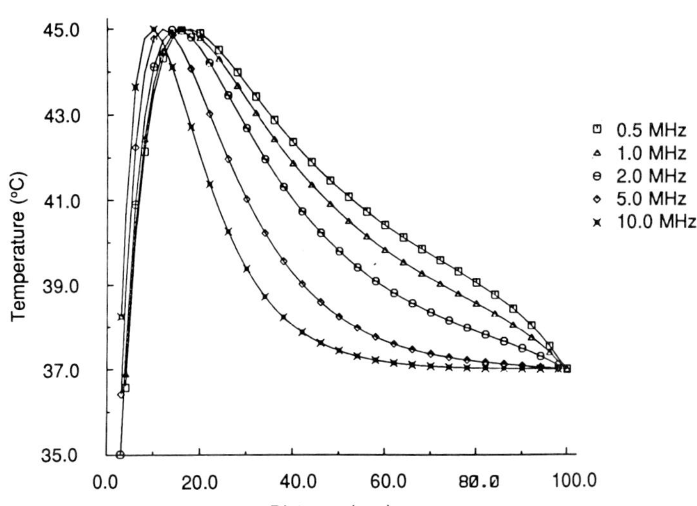

Fig. 12.22. Theoretical radial temperature distributions induced by a cylindrical intracavitary applicator as a function of the operating frequency. (From DIEDERICH and HYNYNEN 1987)

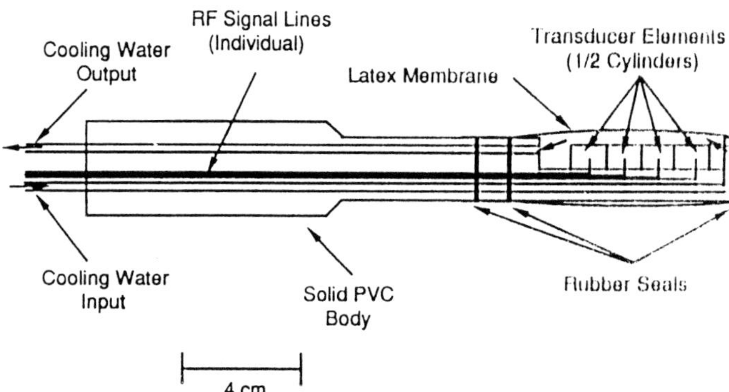

Fig. 12.23. A diagram of a four-element intracavitary applicator used in clinical prostate treatments. (From DIEDERICH and HYNYNEN 1990a)

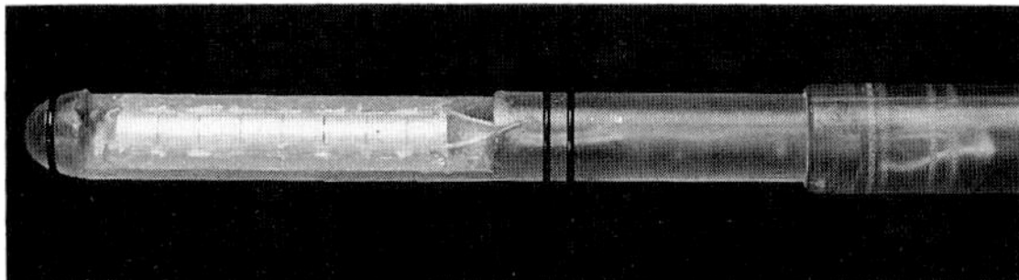

Fig. 12.24. A photograph of an eight-element intracavitary applicator used for prostate treatments

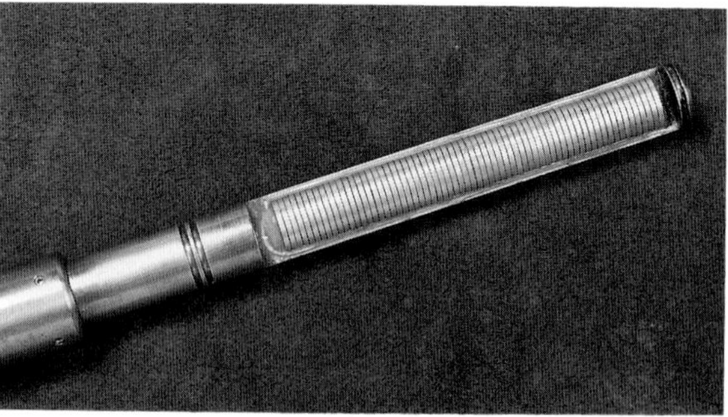

Fig. 12.25. A 500-kHz, 64-element intracavitary ultrasound hyperthermia array. (From BUCHANAN and HYNYNEN 1994)

angular direction offers more control over the heating pattern (DIEDERICH and HYNYNEN 1987, 1989, 1990a).

A complete intracavitary system has been constructed and is under clinical testing for the treatment of prostate (FOSMIRE et al. 1993), vaginal, and rectal tumors. These clinical applicators were later combined with a diagnostic ultrasound applicator to help in the aiming of the ultrasound fields. This was found useful in the treatment of the prostate tumors.

It is also possible to utilize electrically focused ultrasound arrays in a cavity. The theoretical feasibility and the physical properties of such an array were investigated by DIEDERICH and HYNYNEN (1991). A 64-element array and driving hardware and software was constructed and tested in vitro and in vivo (BUCHANAN and HYNYNEN 1994) (Fig. 12.25). The results demonstrated that practical intracavitary phased arrays are feasible (Fig. 12.26) and that they may significantly improve the depth of heating.

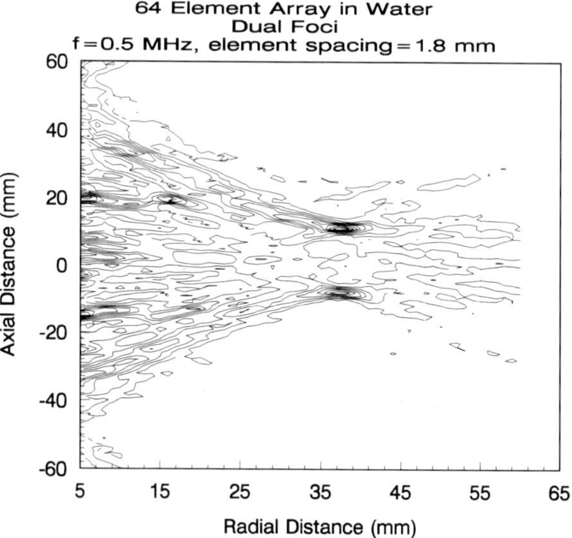

Fig. 12.26. A measured ultrasound field with two focal points from the array in Fig. 12.25

12.5.4 *Interstitial Ultrasound Hyperthermia*

A more precise way of delivering energy into a tumor is to implant small energy sources directly into the target volume. The placement can be done during surgery, or percutaneously. It has been proposed that interstitial ultrasound hyperthermia could be induced either by delivering the energy from an external source into the tumor via an interstitial wave guide (JAROSZ 1990) or by using small cylindrical ultrasound sources interstitially (Fig. 12.27) (Hynynen 1992; Hynynen and Davis 1993; Diederich and Hynynen 1993).

In the first approach an ultrasound wave guide is utilized to transmit the energy from a planar ultrasound transducer outside of the tissue into the catheter. The formation of standing waves will generate a radially propagating wave at the bare tip section of the wave guide.

In the second approach, small (outside diameter = 1 mm) cylindrical ultrasound sources were developed in a similar manner as the intracavitary applicators described earlier (Fig. 12.28). These applicators can be inserted directly into standard brachytherapy catheters which are filled with water. The water can be circulated and cooled to obtain better depth of penetration. Arrays of multiple elements can offer power control as a function of the length of the applicator. The temperature measurements obtained from in vitro perfused kidneys showed that therapeutic temperature elevations could be induced in perfused tissues. The radial extent of the therapeutic zone could be increased by circulating water around the applicators, thus avoiding high temperatures on the applicator surface. It was also shown that some control over the temperature distribution along the length of the applicator could be achieved by using a two-element applicator. An array of four applicators implanted in a square pattern with the spacing of 25 mm between the catheters was able to heat the tissue volume

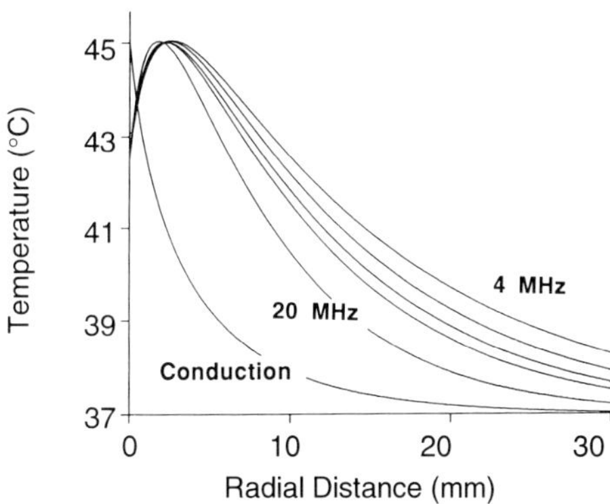

Fig. 12.28. The radial temperature distribution from a cylindrical interstitial ultrasound source at operating frequencies of 4, 6, 8, 10, and 20 MHz and for a hot source (conduction). (Hynynen 1992)

inside of the implant (Fig. 12.29) (Hynynen and Davis 1993). Similar and even larger spacing appears feasible based on theoretical calculations (Diederich and Hynynen 1993).

Additional discussion of interstitial ultrasound technology appears elsewhere in this volume (Chap. 13, Sect. 13.5).

12.5.5 Intraoperative Systems

The first ultrasound applicators used intraoperatively were similar to the single-element superficial applicators described earlier (Collacchio et al. 1990). This system was later upgraded to use

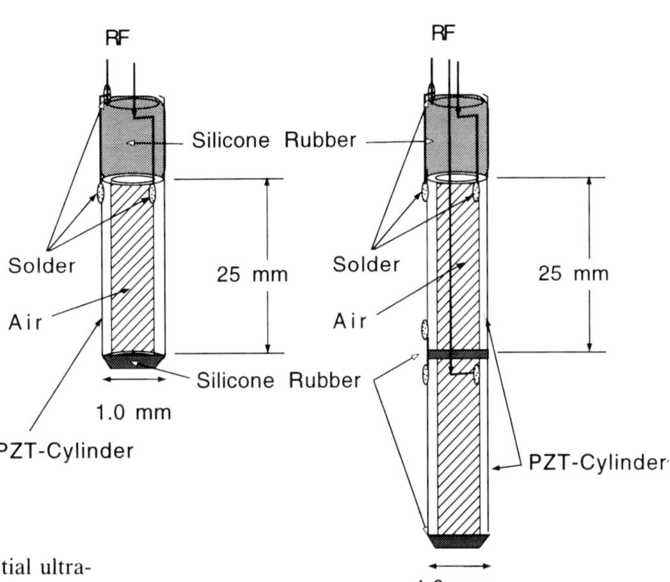

Fig. 12.27. A diagram of the cylindrical interstitial ultrasound sources

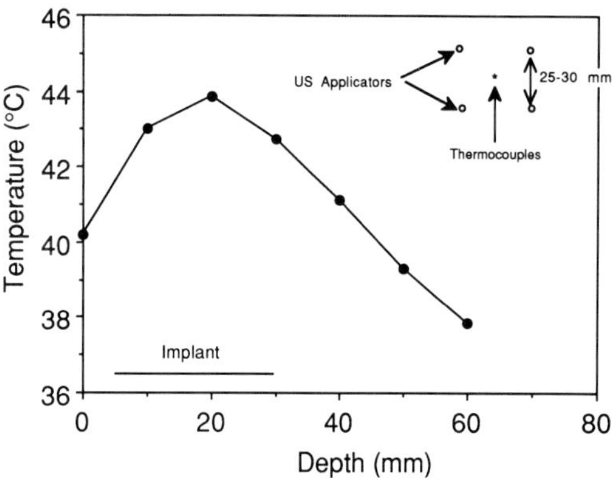

Fig. 12.29. A temperature distribution measured in vivo along the central axis of the implant in a spontaneous dog tumor

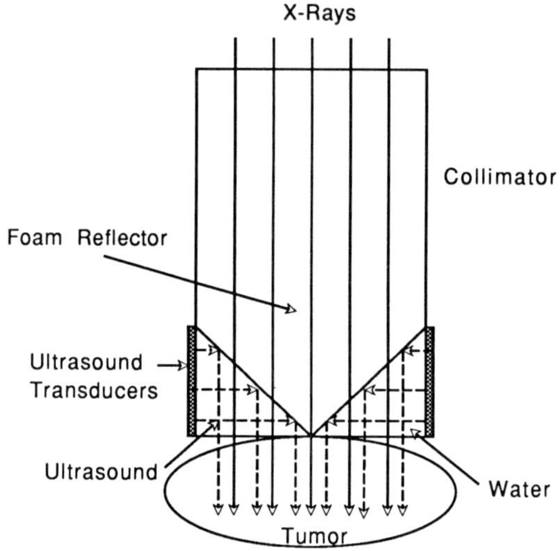

Fig. 12.30. A diagram of an intraoperative ultrasound hyperthermia system that allows simultaneous radiation therapy treatment. (From Montes and Hynynen 1992)

multiple elements and computer feedback (Ryan et al. 1991; Hartov et al. 1993). Another intraoperative ultrasound hyperthermia system which could be used simultaneously with orthovoltage x-ray radiation was also developed (Montes and Hynynen 1992). In this system the ultrasound transducers are mounted in the walls of a cylinder that is used to collimate the radiation beam. The transducers sonicate towards the center of the cylinder where a foam reflector is located. This reflector (transparent to the x-ray radiation) converts the ultrasound to propagate parallel with the radiation beam (Fig. 12.30). This system is now in the final experimental stages and should be tested clinically in the near future.

12.5.6 High Temperature Hyperthermia

A method of reducing the thermal exposure variations due to perfusion is to perform the treatment in such a short period that the perfusion

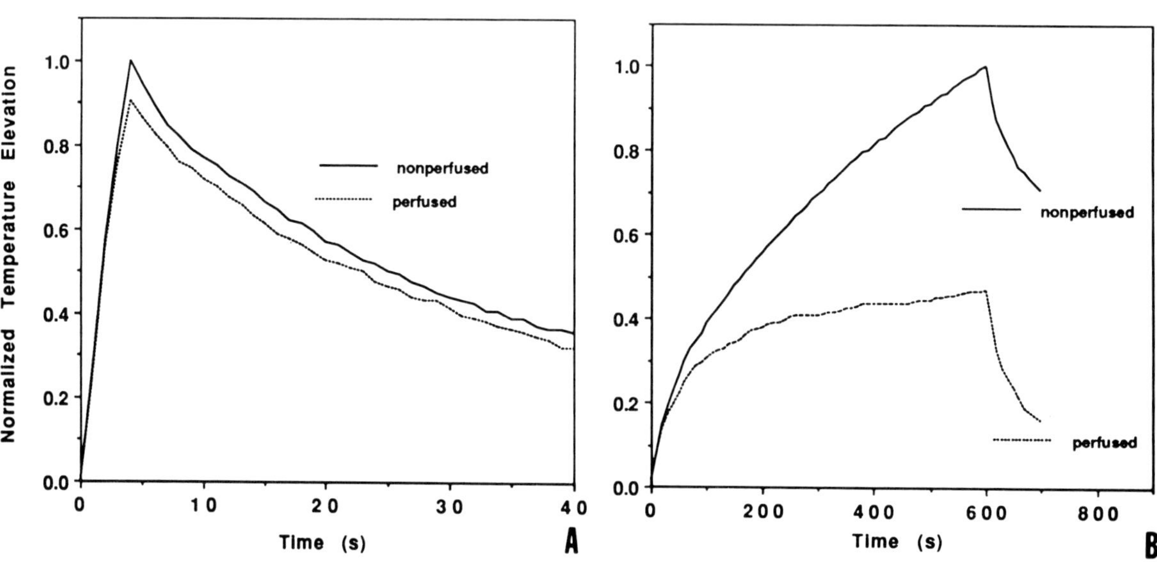

Fig. 12.31A,B. The measured temperature elevation in in vivo dog thigh muscle with perfusion and immediately after the animal was sacrificed. **A** A 4-s sonication and **B** a 10-min sonication in the same location. (From Billard et al. 1990)

and large blood vessel effects can be neglected. The physical principle of this technique is that the mass of blood which is heated and removed from tissue (carries energy away) is small compared with the mass of the tissue if the energy input is short (a few seconds). The effect of perfusion becomes large during longer exposures associated with regular hyperthermia treatments (typically 30–60 min) because the mass of blood heated by the energy input increases whereas the mass of the solid tissue stays constant as time increases (Figs. 12.31, 12.32). For example in kidney, which has a high perfusion rate (1–3 ml/g/min), the mass of blood would be only 1.7%–5% of the total mass of the tissue during a 1-s exposure. This approach seems particularly reasonable because the tissue density, specific heat, and thermal conduction (the factors determining the temperature elevation during energy input in addition to blood flow) are fairly well known for tissues and do not vary to the same extent as the blood perfusion rate. Similarly, good dose uniformity can be obtained close to large blood vessels, which is not possible with longer hyperthermia treatments (DORR and HYNYNEN 1992) (Fig. 12.33).

Relatively high temperatures and intensities (Fig. 12.34) are required during a few-second exposure to deliver a thermal dose equivalent to that given during the hyperthermia treatments at a lower temperature. The sensitivity of the temperature elevation to the perfusion increases with increasing focal spot size such that only

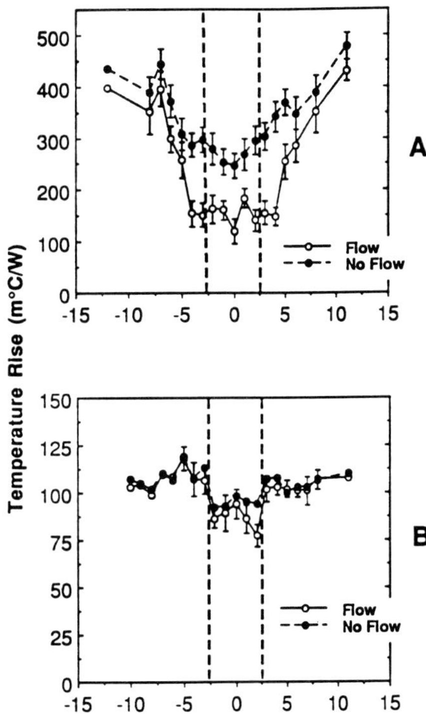

Fig. 12.33A,B. The temperature elevation/acoustic power for a line of sonications across a femoral artery of a dog. Both the full flow case and the case when the artery was closed are shown for 180 s (**A**) and 5 s (**B**) sonications. (From DORR and HYNYNEN 1993)

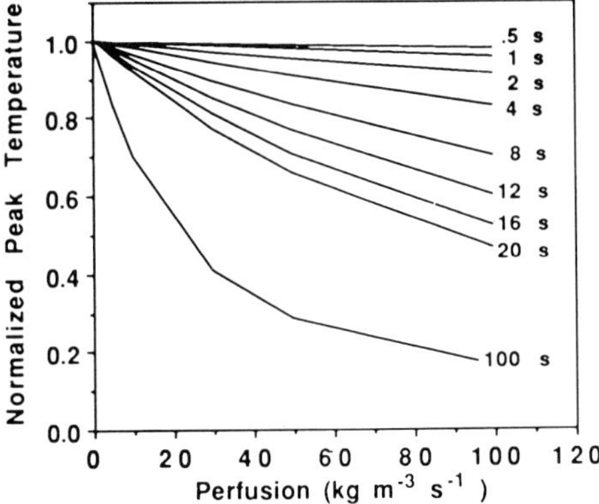

Fig. 12.32. The simulated normalized peak temperature (normalized to the nonperfused case) as a function of perfusion for pulse lengths ranging from 0.5 s to 100 s. The half-power beam width was 7.65 mm. (From BILLARD et al. 1990)

relatively small beam diameters (a few millimeters) can be used (BILLARD et al. 1990). Thus, multiple exposures have to be used to cover the whole target volume. If multiple sonications are repeated within a short time interval, undesirable temperature elevations could result between the skin and the focal depth. To avoid tissue damage in the near field, the sonications should be separated by at least 30-s intervals (DAMIANOU and HYNYNEN 1993).

High temperature hyperthermia originated from the use of ultrasound for lesion production (e.g., FRY et al. 1955) and was subsequently proposed for hyperthermia treatments of brain tumors by BRITT et al. (1984). The theoretical analysis, experimental in vitro verification with perfused organs, and also in vivo studies were done by BILLARD et al. (1990). Theoretical evaluation of some aspects of the therapy have also been performed by DAVIS and LELE (1989) and HUNT et al. (1991). The studies were expanded to investigate the effect of large blood vessels (DORR and HYNYNEN 1992).

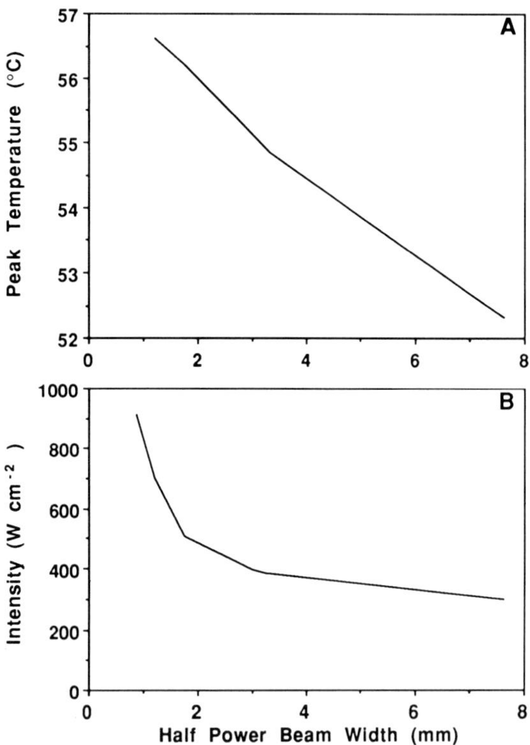

Fig. 12.34. A Required peak temperatures to achieve an equivalent thermal dose of 60 min at 43°C during a 2-s exposure as a function of the half-power beam width. **B** The required intensities to achieve the temperatures presented in **A**. (From BILLARD et al. 1990)

12.5.7 Thermal Surgery Systems

Focused high-power ultrasound beams are well suited for noninvasive local coagulation of deep target volumes. First, the energy can be focused precisely so that the boundaries of the necrotic volume are sharply demarcated without damage to the overlying or surrounding tissues. Second, the tissue necrosis is almost instantaneous without late effects. Finally, the focus can be made very small (diameter less than 1 mm) and multiple sonications can be used to tailor the tissue necrosis to cover the desired target volume.

Since the early experiments of LYNN et al. (1942), ultrasound has been extensively tested for trackless surgery of the brain in both animals (FRY et al. 1955; BASAURI and LELE 1962) and humans (FRY 1965; HEIMBURGER 1985). In spite of the promising results, it has never been widely adopted for clinical use. During the past few years new experimental studies (FRIZZELL 1988; CHAPELON et al. 1992; SANGHVI et al. 1992; YANG et al. 1992; TER HAAR et al. 1991) and clinical trials using ultrasound for noninvasive surgery of tumors (FOSTER et al. 1993; VALLENCIEN et al. 1992) have shown promise. A transrectal surgery applicator for prostate treatment and the external surgery applicator have been developed and commercial prototype devices are now undergoing clinical trials. Both of these systems utilize diagnostic ultrasound to guide the therapy. In addition, the coupling to the patient is roughly similar to the hyperthermia systems described earlier. A third ultrasound device utilizes MRI to guide and monitor the surgery. The main advantage of MRI is that it is also capable of monitoring the temperature elevation during the treatment. This allows targeting at low power levels and monitoring of the temperature elevation outside of the focal zone. The MRI contrast of many soft tissue tumors is excellent and allows precise aiming of the beam. Finally, it may even be possible to see the coagulation necrosis in the images after the sonication (Fig. 12.35) (HYNYNEN et al. 1992, 1993; DARKAZANLI et al. 1993; CLINE et al. 1993).

12.6 Feedback Control

It is generally known that the blood perfusion rate varies from tumor to tumor and also within a tumor (JAIN and WARD-HARDLEY 1984). This can cause variations in the induced temperature

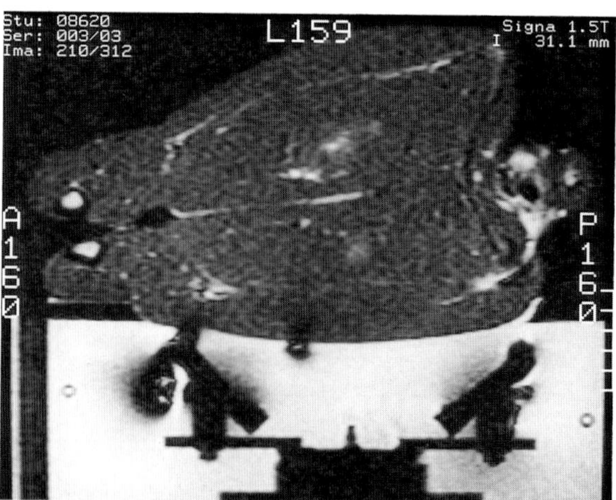

Fig. 12.35. A T2-weighted magnetic resonance image after sonication of a dog thigh muscle in vivo showing the necrosed tissue volume. (From HYNYNEN et al. 1993)

distribution even with a uniform power deposition pattern. Thus, exposing the tumor with constant power does not necessarily induce uniform temperatures. For example, subtherapeutic temperatures have been measured in most of the large, deep, tumors heated with scanned focused ultrasound without computerized feedback (HYNYNEN et al. 1990). The first obvious way to improve the temperature distributions achieved by hyperthermia treatments is to use the measured temperatures to control the power output as a function of location. Thus, tumor volumes where the measured temperatures are lower than the target temperature would receive more power while locations where the temperatures are too high would be allowed to cool by reducing the power level (DAS and LELE 1984; JOHNSON et al. 1990; LIN et al. 1992; HARTOV et al. 1983) (Fig. 12.36).

During clinical treatments the number of temperature sensors is limited and thus power control is often inadequate. Therefore many treatments are limited by patient tolerance in tissue volumes where temperatures are not measured. It has been proposed that patent pain can also be used to control (reduce) the local power to a level which can be tolerated. This kind of spatial power control using both the temperatures and patient pain has been implemented in the treatment of chest wall tumors (see ANHALT et al. 1993), with good initial results.

Another aspect of the spatial control is to be able to control the operating frequency as a function of location due to the variations of tumor thickness. This is especially important in the chest wall, where bone is located behind the tumor. It is fairly difficult to construct ultrasound transducers that have a wide-frequency bandwidth. A simple way to achieve some control over the operating depth is to use separate transducers operating at different frequencies. Similar result can be achieved by switching the driving frequency of a given transducer between its fundamental and odd harmonic frequencies (HYNYNEN et al. 1990a; HYNYNEN 1992). By controlling the amplitude of each of the frequencies, the penetration depth and, thus, the temperature distribution as a function of depth, can be controlled on-line during the scanning (Fig. 12.37). This frequency control can be combined with the temperature and pain feedback control algorithms to optimize the power delivery during the treatment.

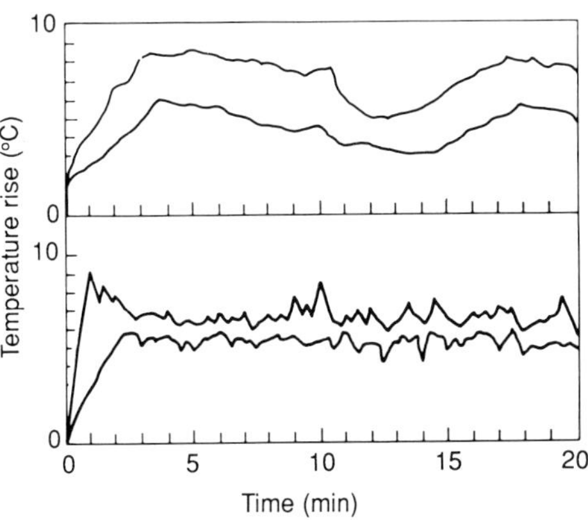

Fig. 12.36. The maximum and minimum temperature elevations in the target volume during an ultrasound hyperthermia experiment in dog's thigh muscle in vivo. *Top*: manual control of the total power; *bottom*: automatic multiregional feedback controller. (From JOHNSON et al. 1990)

12.7 Aiming the Therapy

Targeting of the therapy beam is mostly an unsolved problem in all of the clinical devices. On-line ultrasound imaging has been used to help to aim the therapy in some devices (Fig. 12.38). Ultrasound imaging has been found to be adequate in about 50% of the tumors treated (HYNYNEN et al. 1989). Imaging with CT in the treatment position prior to the therapy can be used to reduce uncertainties in the treatment geometry (HYNYNEN and LULU 1990). The effectiveness of the treatment is strongly dependent on the accuracy of the therapy delivery. Thus, accurate aiming of the beams should be an integral part of every clinical hyperthermia device. Unfortunately this is not yet the case.

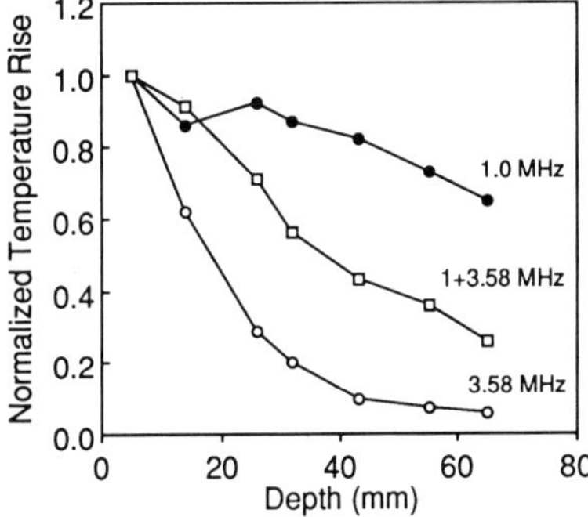

Fig. 12.37. The normalized temperature distributions in dog thigh muscle in vivo obtained using a two-frequency system. (From HYNYNEN 1992)

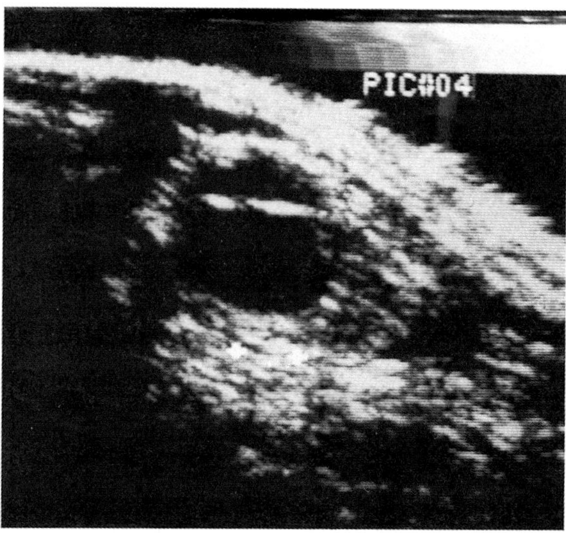

Fig. 12.38. An ultrasound image of a superficial human tumor. Note the thermocouple probe passing through the tumor. The image was obtained with the system described by Hynynen et al. (1987)

12.8 Future Developments in Ultrasound Hyperthermia

So far, only some of the potential of ultrasound as a method to induce elevated temperatures in tissue has been utilized, and the systems developed have not been optimal. However, the possibilities have been demonstrated with laboratory systems. Clinical trials have been encouraging, showing that ultrasound beams can penetrate deep and that the power deposition pattern can be controlled. Good temperatures have been measured in many superficial and deep tumors. Now commercial devices suitable for routine clinical therapy need to be manufactured.

12.9 Summary

Based on the current theoretical, experimental and clinical experience the following conclusions can be made:

- Ultrasound can be used to induce hyperthermia safely and effectively.
- The ultrasound field propagation in soft tissues is predictable and controllable. The ultrasound field can be tailored to cover a desired tumor volume accurately.
- The ultrasound beams can be focused to deep target volumes. This allows selective heating of deep tumors and control over the heating fields.
- Ultrasound applicators can be made in practically any shape and size. Thus, special applicators for different sites can be made. The feasibility of manufacturing external, intracavitary, intraoperative and interstitial ultrasound sources has been demonstrated.
- The accurate control over the heating field allows complex control methods to be used to optimize the energy deposition during the treatment.
- Ultrasound applicators can be combined with diagnostic ultrasound transducers or MRI scanners. This allows accurate energy delivery and potential for noninvasive temperature monitoring and control.
- At the present time there are no commercial devices that fully utilize the potential of ultrasound in the induction of hyperthermia. Therefore, it is not possible to explore the clinical effectiveness of ultrasound induced hyperthermia.

References

Anhalt DP, Hynynen K, Roemer RB, Nathanson S, Stea B, Cassady JR (1993) Scanned ultrasound hyperthermia for treating superficial disease. Hyperthermic oncology 1992, Arizona Board of Regents, Tuscon, AZ, vol 2, pp 191–192

Basauri L, Lele PP (1962) A simple method for production of trackless focal lesions with focused ultrasound: statistical evaluation of the effects of irradiation on the central nervous system of the cat. J Physiol 160: 513–534

Benkeser PJ, Frizzell LA, Ocheltree KB, Cain CA (1987) A tapered phased array ultrasound transducer for hyperthermia treatment. IEEE Trans Ultrasonics, Ferroelectrics and Frequency Control 34: 446–453

Billard BE, Hynynen K, Roemer RB (1990) Effects of physical parameters on high temperature ultrasound hyperthermia. Ultrasound Med Biol 16: 409–420

Bowman FH (1982) Heat transfer mechanisms and thermal dosimetry. Natl Cancer Inst Monogr 61: 437–445

Britt RH, Pounds DW, Lyons BE (1984) Feasibility of treating malignant brain tumors with focused ultrasound. Prog Exp Tumor Res 28: 232–245

Buchanan MT, Hynynen K (1994) The design and evaluation of an intracavitary ultrasound phased array for hyperthermia. IEEE Trans Biomed Eng 41: 1178–1187

Cain CA, Umemura S-A (1986) Concentric-ring and sector vortex phased array applicators for ultrasound hyperthermia therapy. IEEE Trans Microwave Theory Tech 34: 542–551

Carstensen EL, Becroft SA, Law WK, Barber DB (1981) Finite amplitude effects on thresholds for lesion production in tissues by unfocussed ultrasound. J Acoust Soc Am 70: 302–309

Chapelon JY, Margonari J, Vernier F, Gorry F, Ecochard R, Gelet A (1992) In vivo effects of high-intensity ultrasound on prostatic adenocarcinoma dunning R3327. Cancer Res 52: 6353–6357
Chivers RC, Parry RJ (1978) Ultrasonic velocity and attenuation in mammalian tissues. J Acoust Soc Am 63: 940–953
Cline HE, Schenck JF, Watkins RD, Hynynen K, Jolesz FA (1993) Magnetic resonance guided thermal surgery. Magn Res in Medicine 30: 98–106
Colacchio TA, Coughlin C, Taylor J, Douple E, Ryan T, Crichlow RW (1990) Intraoperative radiation therapy and hyperthermia. Morbidity and mortality from this combined treatment modality for unresectable intra-abdominal carcinomas. Arch Surg 125: 370–375
Corry PM, Barlogie B, Tilchen EJ (1982) Armour EP, Ultrasound induced hyperthermia for the treatment of human superficial tumors. Int J Radiat Oncol Biol Phys 8: 1225–1229
Damianou C, Hynynen K (1993) Near-field heating during pulsed high temperature ultrasound hyperthermia treatment. Ultrasound Med Biol 19: 777–787
Darkazanli A, Hynynen K, Unger E, Schenck JF (1993) On-line monitoring of ultrasound surgery with MRI. Magn Reson Imaging 3: 509–514
Das H, Lele PP (1984) Design of a power modulator for control of tumor temperature. In: Overgaard J (ed) Hyperthermic oncology 1984, vol 1, pp 707–714
Davis BJ, Lele PP (1987) Bone-pain during hyperthermia by ultrasound. Proc. 35th Ann. Meeting Radiation Research Soc Atlanta Georgia, p 11
Davis BJ, Lele PP (1989) A theoretical study of rapid hyperthermia by scanned focussed ultrasound. Winter Annual Meeting of ASME, San Francisco, CA, December 10–15 1989
Diederich C, Hynynen K (1987) Induction of hyperthermia using an intracavitary ultrasonic applicator. Proc IEEE Ultrasonic Symp, pp 871–874
Diederich C, Hynynen K (1989) Induction of hyperthermia using an intracavitary multielement ultrasonic applicator. IEEE Trans Biomed Eng 36: 432–438
Diederich C, Hynynen K (1990a) The development of intracavitary ultrasonic applicators for hyperthermia: a theoretical and experimental study. Med Phys 17: 626–634
Diederich CJ, Hynynen K (1990b) The feasibility of interstitial ultrasound hyperthermia. Proceedings of the 38th Ann. Meeting of the Radiation Research Society and 10th Ann. Meeting of the North American Hyperthermia Group, New Orleans, Louisiana, April 7–12, p 92
Diederich C, Hynynen K (1991) The feasibility of using electrically focussed ultrasound arrays to induce deep hyperthermia via body cavities. IEEE Trans Ultrasonics Ferroelectrics and Frequency Control 38: 207–219
Diederich CJ, Hynynen K (1993) Ultrasound technology for interstitial hyperthermia. In: Seegenschmiedt MH (ed) Interstitial and intracavitary hyperthermia in oncology. Springer, Berlin Heidelberg New York, pp 55–61
Do-Huun JP, Hartemann P (1982) Deep and local heating induced by an ultrasound phased array transducer. Proc IEEE Ultrasonic Symp, pp 735–738
Dorr LN, Hynynen K (1992) The effect of tissue heterogeneities and large blood vessels on the thermal exposure induced by short high power ultrasound pulses. Int J Hyperthermia 8: 45–59
Dunn, F (1976) Ultrasonic attenuation, absorption, and velocity in tissues and organs. In: Linzer M (ed) Ultrasonic tissue characterization. NBS Spec Publ, 453, Washington, pp 21–28
Ebbini ES, Cain CA (1989) Multiple-focus ultrasound phased-array pattern synthesis: optimal driving-signal distributions for hyperthermia. IEEE Trans Ultrasonics Ferroelectrics Frequency Control 36: 540–548
Ebbini ES, Cain CA (1991a) Experimental evaluation of a prototype cylindrical section ultrasound hyperthermia phased-array applicator. IEEE Trans Ultrasonics Ferroelectrics Frequency Control 38: 510–520
Ebbini ES, Cain CA (1991b) A spherical-section ultrasound phased array applicator for deep localized hyperthermia. IEEE Trans Biomed Eng 38: 634–643
Ebbini ES, Umemura S-I, Ibbini M, Cain C (1988) A cylindrical-section ultrasound phased array applicator for hyperthermia cancer therapy. IEEE Trans Ultrasonic, Ferroelectrics Frequency Control 35: 561–572
Ebbini E, Wang H, O'Donnell M, Cain C (1991) Acoustic feedback for hyperthermia phased-array applicators: aberration correction, motion compensation and multiple focusing in the presence of tissue inhomogeneities. Proc IEEE Ultrasonics Symp, pp 1343–1346
Ebbini ES, Seip R, Iasemidis L, O'Donnell M, Cain CA (1992) Cancer treatment with high intensity focused ultrasound: a combined therapy/imaging system for precision noninvasive lesion formation. Proc 14th Ann Internat Conf IEEE/EMBS, Oct 29–Nov 1, 1992, Paris, France, IEEE Catalog Number 92CH3207-8, pp 352–353
Fan X, Hynynen K (1992) The effects of wave reflection and refraction at soft tissue interfaces during ultrasound hyperthermia treatments. J Acoust Soc Am 91: 1727–1736
Fessenden P, Lee ER, Anderson TL, Strohbehn JW, Meyer JL, Samulski TV, Marmor JR (1984) Experience with a multitransducer ultrasound system for localized hyperthermia of deep tissues. IEEE Trans Biomed Eng 31: 126–135
Fosmire H, Hynynen K, Drach GW, Stea B, Swift P, Cassady JR (1993) Feasibility and toxicity of transrectal ultrasound hyperthermia in the treatment of locally-advanced adenocarcinoma of the prostate. Int J Radiat Oncol Biol Phys 26: 253–259
Foster RS, Bihrle R, Sanghvi NT, Fry FJ, Donohue JP (1993) High-intensity focused ultrasound in the treatment of prostatic disease. Eur Urol 23 (Suppl 1): 29–33
Frizzell LA (1988) Threshold dosages for damage to mammalian liver by high intensity focussed ultrasound. IEEE Trans Ultrasonics Ferroelectrics Frequency Control 35: 578–581
Fry FJ (1965) Recent developments in ultrasound at biophysical research laboratory and their application to basic problems in biology and medicine. In: Kelly E (ed) Ultrasound energy. University of Illinois Press, Urbana, pp 202–228
Fry FJ (1978) Intense focused ultrasound: its production, effects and utilization. In: Fry FJ (ed) Ultrasound: its applications in medicine and biology, part II. Elsevier, New York, pp 689–736
Fry WJ, Wulff VJ, Tucker D, Fry FJ (1950) Physical factors involved in ultrasound induced changes in living systems: I. Identification of non-temperature effects. J Acoust Soc Am 22: 867–871
Fry WJ, Barnard JW, Fry FJ, Krumins RF, Brennan JF (1955) Ultrasonic lesions in the mammalian central nervous system. Science 122: 517–518

Goss SA, Frizzell LA, Dunn F (1979) Ultrasonic absorption and attenuation of high frequency sound in mammalian tissues. Ultrasound Med Biol 5: 181–186
Goss SA, Johnson RL, Dunn F (1978) Comprehensive compilation of empirical ultrasonic properties of mammalian tissues. J Acoust Soc Am 64: 423–457
Goss SA, Johnson RL, Dunn F (1980) Compilation of empirical ultrasonic properties of mammalian tissues. II. J Acoust Soc Am 68: 93–108
Guthkelch AN, Carter LP, Cassady JR et al. (1991) Treatment of malignant brain tumors with focussed ultrasound hyperthermia and radiation: results of a phase I trial. J Neurooncol 10: 271–284
ter Haar G, Rivens I, Chen L, Riddler S (1991) High intensity focused ultrasound for the treatment of rat tumors. Phys Med Biol 36: 1495–1501
Hand JW, Vernon CC, Prior MV (1992) Early experience of a commercial scanned focused ultrasound hyperthermia system. Int J Hyperthermia 8: 587–607
Harari PM, Hynynen K, Roemer RB, Anhalt DP, Shimm DS, Stea B, Cassady JR (1991) Scanned focussed ultrasound hyperthermia: clinical response evaluation. Int J Radiat Oncol Biol Phys 21: 831–840
Hartov A, Colacchio TA, Strohbehn JW, Ryan TP, Hoopes PJ (1993) Performance of an adaptive MIMO controller for multiple-element ultrasound hyperthermia system. Int J Hyperthermia 9: 563–579
Heimburger RF (1985) Ultrasound augmentation of central nervous system tumor therapy. Indiana Med 78: 469–476
Hueter TF, Bolt RH (1955) Sonics; techniques for the use of sound and ultrasound in engineering and science. John Wiley, New York
Hunt JW (1987) Principles of ultrasound used for hyperthermia. In: Field SB, Franconi C (eds) Physics and technology of hyperthermia. NATO ASI Series E: – No. 127, Martinus Nijhoff Publishers, Boston, pp 354–389
Hunt JW (1990) Principles of ultrasound used for generating localized hyperthermia. In: Field SB, Hand JW (eds) An introduction to the practical aspects of clinical hyperthermia. Taylor and Francis, London, pp 371–422
Hunt JW, Lalonde R, Ginsberg H, Urchuk S, Worthington A (1991) Rapid heating: critical theoretical assessment of thermal gradients found in hyperthermia treatments. Int J Hyperthermia 7: 703–718
Hynynen K (1990) Hot spots created at skin-air interfaces during ultrasound hyperthermia. Int J Hyperthermia 6: 1005–1012
Hynynen K (1991) The threshold for thermally significant cavitation in dog's thigh muscle in vivo. Ultrasound Med Biol 17: 157–169
Hynynen K (1992) The feasibility of interstitial ultrasound hyperthermia. Med Phys 19: 979–987
Hynynen K, Davis KL (1993) Small cylindrical ultrasound sources for induction of hyperthermia via body cavities or interstitial implants. Int J Hyperthermia 9: 263–274
Hynynen K, DeYoung D (1988) Temperature elevation at muscle-bone interface during scanned, focused ultrasound hyperthermia. Int J Hyperthermia 4: 267–279
Hynynen K, Lulu BA (1990) State of the art in medicine: hyperthermia in cancer treatment. Invest Radiol 25: 824–834
Hynynen K, Watmough DJ, Shammari M et al. (1983) A clinical hyperthermia unit utilizing an array of seven focussed ultrasonic transducers. Proc IEEE Ultrasonic Symp, pp 816–821
Hynynen K, Roemer R, Moros E, Johnson C, Anhalt D (1986) The effect of scanning speed on temperature and equivalent thermal exposure distributions during ultrasound hyperthermia in vivo. IEEE Trans Microwave Theory Techniques 34: 552–559
Hynynen K, Roemer R, Anhalt D, Johnson C, Xu ZX, Swindell W, Cetas TC (1987) A scanned, focussed, multiple transducer ultrasonic system for localized hyperthermia treatments. Int J Hyperthermia 3: 21–35
Hynynen K, Roemer RB, Anhalt D et al. (1990a) Practical techniques to improve temperature distributions during scanned focussed ultrasound hyperthermia treatments. Abstracts of the 38th Ann. Meeting of the Radiation Res. Soc. and 10th Ann. Meeting of the North American Hyperthermia Group, New Orleans, Louisiana, 7–12 April, p 15
Hynynen K, Shimm D, Anhalt D, Stea B, Sykes H, Cassady JR, Roemer RB (1990b) Temperature distributions during clinical scanned, focussed ultrasound hyperthermia treatments. Int J Hyperthermia 6: 891–908
Hynynen K, Damianou C, Darkazanli A, Unger E, Levy M, Schenck JF (1992) On-line MRI monitored noninvasive ultrasound surgery. Proc. 14th Ann. Inter. Conf. IEEE engineering in Medicine and Biology Society, Paris, Fance, 29 Oct–1 Nov 1992, pp 350–351
Hynynen K, Darkazanli A, Unger E, Schenck JF (1993) MRI-guided noninvasive ultrasound surgery. Med Phys 20: 107–115
Jain RK (1984) Ward-Hartley K, Tumor blood flow-characterization, modifications, and role in hyperthermia. IEEE Trans. Sonics and Ultrasonics, SU-31: 504–526
Jarosz BJ (1990) Rate of heating in tissue in vitro by interstitial ultrasound. Proc. 12th Ann. Int. Conf. IEEE Engineering in Medicine and Biology Soc, IEEE 90CH2936-3: 274–275
Johnson C, Kress R, Roemer RB, Hynynen K (1990) Multipoint feedback control system for scanned, focussed ultrasound hyperthermia. Phys Med Biol 35: 24–834
Lalonde R, Worthington A, Hunt JW (1990) Hyperthermia: field conjugate acoustic lenses for deep heating. Proc. 1990 IEEE/EMBS Conference, Philadelphia, Pennsylvania, pp 235–236
Lehmann JF, deLateur BJ, Silverman DR (1966) Selective heating effects of ultrasound in human beings. Arch Phys Med Rehabil 47: 331–339
Lehmann JF, deLateur BJ, Warren CG, Stonebridge JS (1967) Heating produced by ultrasound in bone and soft tissue. Arch Phys Med Rehabil 48: 397–401
Lele PP (1983) Physical aspects and clinical studies with ultrasound hyperthermia. In: Storm FK (ed) Hyperthermia in cancer therapy. Hall Medical, Boston, pp 333–367
Lele PP (1987) Effects of ultrasound on solid mammalian tissues and tumors in vivo. In: Repacholi MH, Grandolfo M, Rindi A (eds) Ultrasound: medical applications, biological effects and hazard potential. Plenum Press, New York, pp 275–306
Lele PP, Parker KJ (1982) Temperature distributions in tissues during local hyperthermia by stationary or steered beams of unfocussed or focussed ultrasound. Br J Cancer 45 (Suppl V): 108–121
Lin WL, Roemer RB, Hynynen K (1990) Theoretical and experimental evaluation of a temperature controller for scanned focussed ultrasound hyperthermia. Med Phys 17: 615–625
Lin WL, Roemer RB, Moros EG, Hynynen K (1992) Optimization of temperature distributions in scanned

focussed ultrasound hyperthermia. Int J Hyperthermia 8: 61–72

Lynn JG, Zwemer RL, Chick AJ, Miller AE (1942) A new method for the generation and use of focused ultrasound in experimental biology. J Gen Physiol 26: 179–193

Lyons ME, Parker KJ (1988) Absorption and attenuation in soft tissues II – experimental results. IEEE Trans Ultrasonics, Ferroelectrics Frequency Control 35: 511–521

Marmor JB, Pounds D, Postic TB, Hahn GM (1979) Treatment of superficial human neoplasms by local hyperthermia induced by ultrasound. Cancer 43: 188–197

Montes HZ, Hynynen K (1992) A system for the simultaneous delivery of intraoperative radiation and ultrasound hyperthermia. In: Gerner EW (ed) Hyperthermic oncology 1992, vol 1, p 279

Moros EG, Roemer RB, Hynynen K (1988) Simulations of scanned focussed ultrasound hyperthermia: the effect of scanning speed and pattern. IEEE Trans Ultrasonics, Ferroelectrics Frequency Control 35: 552–560

Moros EG, Roemer RB, Hynynen K (1990) Pre-focal plane high temperature regions induced by scanning focussed ultrasound beams. Int J Hyperthermia 6: 351–366

Munro P, Hill RP, Hunt JW (1982) The development of improved ultrasound heaters suitable for superficial tissue heating. Med Phys 9: 888–897

Nelson PA, Herrick JF, Krusen FH (1950) Temperatures produced in bone marrow, bone and adjacent tissues by ultrasound diathrmy. Arch Phys Med 31: 687–695

Nyborg WL (1981) Heat generation by ultrasound in a relaxing medium. J Acoust Soc Am 70: 310–312

Ocheltree KB, Benkeser JP, Frizzell LA, Cain CA (1984) An ultrasound phased array applicator for hyperthermia. IEEE Trans Sonics Ultrasonics 31: 526–531

O'Neil HT (1949) Theory of focussing radiators. J Acoust Soc Am 21: 516–526

Ryan TP, Hartov A, Colacchio TA, Coughlin CT, Stafford JH, Hoopes PJ (1991) Analysis and testing of a concentric ring applicator for ultrasound hyperthermia with clinical results. Int J Hyperthermia 7: 587–603

Samulski TV, Grant WJ, Oleson JR, Leopold KA, Dewhirst MW, Vallario P, Blivin J (1990) Clinical experience with a multi element ultrasonic hyperthermia system: analysis of treatment temperatures. Int J Hyperthermia 6: 909–922

Sanghvi NT, Foster RS, Fry FJ, Bihrle R, Hennige C, Hennige LV (1992) Ultrasound intracavitary system for imaging, therapy planning and treatment of focal disease. Proceedings IEEE Ultrasonics Symp., IEEE 92CH3118-7, pp 1249–1253

Seppi E, Shapiro E, Zitelli L, Henderson S, Wehlau A, Wu G, Dittmer C (1985) A large aperture ultrasonic array system for hyperthermia treatment of deep-seated tumors. Proc IEEE Ultrasonics Symp, pp 942–949

Steinberg BD (1976) Principles of aperture and array system design. John Wiley, New York

Svensson GK, Hansen JL, Delli Carpini D, Bornstein B, Herman T, Bowman F, Newman W (1992) SAR and temperature distributions for a spherical focused, segmented ultrasound machine (FSUM). Hyperthermic oncology 1992. Proceedings of the Sixth International Hyperthermia Conference, Tucson, Arizona, 26 April–1 May 1992, vol 1, p 335

Tu S, Hynynen K, Roemer RB (1994) The simulation of bidirectional ultrasound hyperthermia treatments of neck tumors. Int J Hyperthermia 10: 707–722

Underwood HR, Burdette EC, Ocheltree KB, Magin RL (1987) A multi-element ultrasonic hyperthermia applicator with independent element control. Int J Hyperthermia 3: 257–267

Vallancien G, Harouni M, Veillon B, Mombet A, Prapotnich D, Bisset JM, Bougaran J (1992) Focused extracorporeal pyrotherapy: feasibility study in man. J Endourol 6: 173–180

Wells PNT (1969) Physical principles of ultrasonic diagnosis. Academic Press, London

Wells PNT (1977) Biomedical ultrasonics. Academic Press, London

Yang R, Reilly CR, Rescorla FJ, Sanghvi NT, Fry FJ, Franklin TD, Grosfeld JL (1992) Effects of high-intensity focused ultrasound in the treatment of experimental neuroblastoma. J Pediatr Surg 27: 246–251

Zemanek J (1971) Beam behavior within the nearfield fo a vibrating piston. J Acoust Soc Am 49: 181–191

13 Interstitial Heating Technologies

P.R. Stauffer, C.J. Diederich, and M.H. Seegenschmiedt

CONTENTS

13.1 Introduction

Invasive interstitial heating techniques offer a number of advantages over external heating approaches for localizing heat into small tumors at depth. Over the past two decades, nine distinctly different interstitial heating modalities have emerged in response to changes in surgical implant techniques, clinical treatment protocols, and brachytherapy hardware. They consist of: (1) implantable microwave (MW) antennas operating between 0.4 and 2.5 GHz, (2) resistively coupled RF electrodes driven at 0.3–3 MHz for local current field (LCF) heating, (3) capacitively coupled RF electrodes (CC-RF) driven at 8–27 MHz, (4) internal LCF-type electrodes coupled inductively to external 6- to 13-MHz power sources via receiving loop antennas implanted under the skin (IC-RF), (5) 5- to 12-MHz tubular ultrasound (US) radiators, (6) laser illuminated, fiberoptic coupled crystal diffusers (Laser), and three "Hot Source" techniques: (7) hot water tubes (HW), (8) DC voltage driven resistance wires (RW), and (9) inductively coupled, thermoregulating ferromagnetic implants (Ferroseeds).

In most cases, the development and optimization of these technologies specifically for hyperthermia treatment of cancer have been extremely rapid. The average time separating the first report of clinical results from the initial publication of laboratory device development is just under 3 years, as seen in Table 13.1. Along with the rapid development of physical devices, there has been a parallel evolution of clinical treatment protocols which has stimulated continuing modification of the techniques. Numerous technical challenges remain to implement and take full advantage of the theoretically predicted gains in heating uniformity from recent advances and to optimize the clinical combination of interstitial heat and brachytherapy.

This chapter reviews the underlying principles of operation for each technique only briefly to complement the in depth coverage of interstitial heating modalities given in previous reviews (Strohbehn and Mechling 1986; Strohbelhn 1987; Stauffer 1990, 1991, 1992; Hand et al. 1991; Trembly et al. 1991; Handl-Zeller 1992; Seegenschmiedt and Sauer 1993) and in the associated primary literature. A description of the design evolution of interstitial heating devices is presented as an aid to understanding the current

P.R. Stauffer, MD, Department of Radiation Oncology, University of California, P.O. Box 0226, San Francisco, CA 94143, USA

C.J. Diederich, PhD, Department of Radiation Oncology, University of California, P.O. Box 0226, San Francisco, CA 94143, USA

M.H. Seegenschmiedt, MD, Department of Radiation Oncology, University of Erlangen-Nürnberg, Universitätsstraße 27, 91054 Erlangen, FRG

Table 13.1. Interstitial heating modalities: year of first publication

Effort	RF-LCF electrodes	Microwave antennas	Ferroseeds	Laser	Hot water, tubes	Resistance wires	CC-RF electrodes	Ultrasound transducer
Preclinical	1976	1977	1982	1983	–	1990	1989	1990
Clinical	1980	1981	1988	1986	1987	1989	1989	–

state of the art as well as the future potential of these technologies, with a focus on interstitial hyperthermia. Intracavitary and thermal ablation procedures are presented elsewhere in this volume (see Chaps. 12 and 14). Issues of appropriate thermometry and quality assurance procedures for the interstitial technologies are also covered elsewhere (IBBOTT et al. 1989; SHRIVASTAVA et al. 1989; CETAS 1990; STAUFFER 1990; EMAMI et al. 1991; PRIONAS and KAPP 1992; ESHO 1993; HAND 1993). The current effort updates the status of device development and summarizes heating performance characteristics for each of the nine interstitial techniques. Major developments in each field are highlighted and representative references from key investigators are given for more in depth study. The chapter ends with general recommendations for the appropriate clinical applications of each modality, as derived from the current physical capabilities and limitations of each technique.

13.2 Implantable Microwave Antennas

At frequencies above approximately 300 MHz, tissue acts as a lossy dielectric and the predominant mode of propagation for electromagnetic waves is radiative rather than conductive. In order to localize MW radiation to a tumor-sized volume, several miniature antenna designs have evolved based on ≤1.5-mm-diameter coaxial cable feedlines implanted in tissue inside insulating plastic catheters, with the preferred return path for the current incorporated as part of the design. Minor modifications to the tip portion of the implanted cables cause significant variations in the radiation patterns of single antennas as well as in the interaction of antenna arrays. These are discussed below.

13.2.1 Dipole Antennas

The simplest antenna structure useful for interstitial implantation is a length of semirigid coaxial cable with a section of outer conductor removed to expose a length of inner conductor at the distal end (Fig. 13.1). This open-ended coaxial cable radiates most efficiently if implanted a distance of about $\lambda/4$ for use as a monopole above a skin surface ground plane (TAYLOR 1978), or if implanted to a depth of approximately twice the exposed conductor length. In this case, the structure operates as a half-wave dipole with current minimums at the tip and skin entrance points, and a maximum near mid-depth at the "junction" of the inner and outer conductor sections. This produces a symmetric gaussian prolate spheroid (football) shaped heating pattern in tissue around the dipole (Fig. 13.2). At the most commonly used microwave frequencies (f) of 433, 915, and 2450 MHz, the wavelength of radiation in tissue (λ_T) is shortened from that occurring in free space ($\lambda_o = c/f$) to about $\lambda_T = \lambda_o/(\varepsilon_r)^{.5} \cong 10$, 4.5, and 1.7 cm respectively. Since the antennas are normally placed inside implant catheters ($\varepsilon_r \approx$ 2–4) surrounded by a variable amount of air ($\varepsilon_r \approx$ 1), the effective wavelength of radiation into the catheter–air–tissue load is lengthened over that of a bare antenna in tissue (ε_r for muscle tissue is about 50). In typical use, the resonant $\lambda/2$ length of an insulated dipole antenna in human soft tissue is about 6–8 cm at 915 MHz. Effects of catheter thickness, diameter, and material on the radiation pattern, input impedance, and efficiency of dipole antennas have been studied extensively (STROHBEHN et al. 1979; DE SIEYES et al. 1981; CASEY and BANSAL 1986; JONES et al. 1988; ZHANG et al. 1988; ISKANDER and TUMEH 1989; WONG and TREMBLY 1994). Because the clinical application of this technique requires that heating lengths be adjusted to fit variable tumor sizes, many have also studied the effects of varying dipole antenna insertion depths. Reports indicate that the dipole antenna radiation pattern is significantly affected by differences in insertion depth both for single antennas and for antenna arrays (DENMAN et al. 1988; CHAN et al. 1989; JAMES et al. 1989; RYAN et al 1990; ZHANG et al. 1991b). MECHLING et al. (1992) have simulated the effects of these power

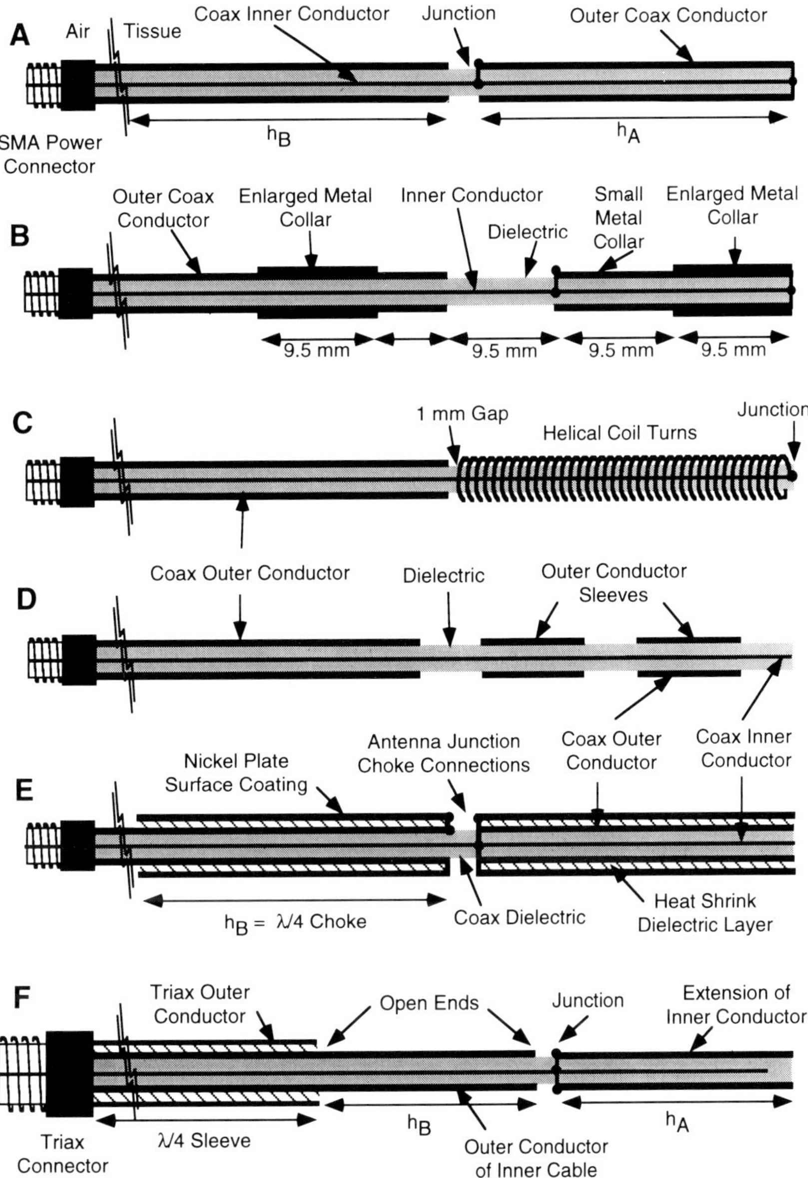

Fig. 13.1A–F. Schematic drawings of coaxial cable mounted interstitial microwave antennas intended for insertion inside insulating catheters into lossy tissue. **A** Dipole antenna showing extension of the coax inner conductor (h_A) and implanted length of outer conductor (h_B), separated at the "junction" (King et al. 1983). **B** Dipole with enlarged diameter collars for increased capacitive coupling through the catheter wall, which helps extend the heating pattern axially away from the junction (Turner 1986). **C** Helical coil antenna with fine wire coil approximately 1 turn per mm axial length. The coil attaches to the inner conductor at the tip and has a 1-mm separation gap to the outer conductor (Satoh and Stauffer 1988). **D** Multinode antenna with short sections of outer conductor removed to expose inner conductor "nodes" (Lee et al. 1986) for extending the heating pattern axially. **E** Dipole antenna with quarter-wavelength chokes made from metallic coating on the outer dielectric surface over both the h_A and h_B antenna sections (Ryan et al. 1990). **F** Sleeve dipole antenna with quarter-wavelength sleeve and transformed open end (Hurter et al. 1991)

deposition pattern changes on the ability to heat realistic tumor volumes.

The power deposition rate in tissue around the antennas is determined from $P_D = \sigma\ |\mathbf{E}_T|^2/2\rho$ where σ and ρ are the tissue electrical conductivity and density, and $\mathbf{E}_T = \Sigma \mathbf{E}_i$ is the total electric field vector summed from all antenna sources. For a single insulated dipole in a dissipative medium,

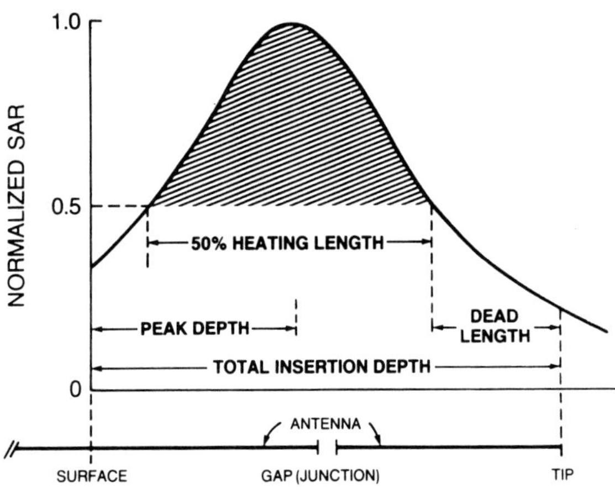

Fig. 13.2. Characteristics of a typical SAR profile around a single microwave antenna as measured in a catheter parallel and approximately 5 mm distant from the antenna. The 50% heating length quantifies the total length along the antenna axis that is heated effectively (at least 50% of the maximum SAR). The dead length refers to that portion of the profile adjacent to the antenna tip which is heated less than 50% of the maximum SAR. Reprinted from SATOH, STAUFFER, FIKE (1988) with kind permission from Elsevier Science Ltd. The Boulevard, Langford Lane, Kidlington 0 × 5 1 GB, UK

$\mathbf{E}_T$ has a significant radial field component (E_{Tr}) along much of the antenna length, which together with the dominant axial component (E_{Tz}) forms an elliptically polarized field close to the antenna (KING and IIZUKA 1963; KING et al. 1983). This complex field varies along the antenna length in both magnitude and direction and approaches linear polarization only in the far field at large distance from the antenna. Thus for interstitial heating applications, there is an unavoidable variation of $\mathbf{E}_T$ along the dipole length, which causes a rapid falloff of power deposition axially as well as radially from the peak near the inner/outer conductor junction. The point receiving 50% of the maximum SAR occurs within 2–3 mm of the antenna junction (KING et al. 1983; BABIJ et al. 1991). Methods for increasing the effective radial penetration of heating using air (EPPERT et al. 1991; TREMBLY et al. 1991; YEH et al. 1994) or water (MORIYAMA et al. 1988; GENTILI et al. 1991) cooling of the antenna–tissue interface are under investigation. Control of surface temperature should improve the uniformity of heating around each antenna by homogenizing surface temperature along the entire antenna length as well as moving the point of maximum temperature rise away from the antenna surface to broaden the effectively heated region.

To heat typically sized tumor volumes, antennas may be placed in an array around the target volume and driven either noncoherently to avoid interference effects, or with phase-adjusted (coherent) signals to obtain higher field strengths at distance from the antennas where the individual field components (E_i's) add constructively. Because power deposition increases as the square of the total field ($\mathbf{E}_T$), SAR can be significantly enhanced near mid-depth in the array center where the electric fields are all directed predominantly parallel to the axes of the coherently driven antennas. Progressively less enhancement of SAR is obtained with increasing distance in either direction from the junction plane due to the increasing proportion of E_r field components that do not add constructively. The theoretical SAR patterns possible with these coherently phased arrays of dipole antennas have been studied by numerous investigators (STROHBEHN et al. 1982; TREMBLY 1985; TURNER 1986; WONG et al. 1986; ZHANG et al. 1988; JONES et al. 1989; MECHLING et al. 1992). Figure 13.3 from JAMES et al. (1989) demonstrates the theoretical power deposition characteristics of a four antenna array implanted in homogeneous tissue and driven in-phase at 915 MHz. Note the dramatic focusing of power deposition centrally between antennas for $\lambda/2$ insertion depth (Fig. 13.3a) and the shift of heating further from the antenna tips when the antennas are placed deeper in tissue (Fig. 13.3b). The accompanying requirement for precise control of antenna phase relationship accentuates uncertainties in the power deposition pattern which result from unavoidable imperfect clinical conditions, such as nonparallel implant orientation, unmatched antenna impedances, efficiencies or insertion depths, and tissue heterogeneities. For example, CLIBBON et al. (1993) reported significant perturbations of array heating patterns when one antenna of a four-antenna array was shifted axially a distance of 1–2 cm from perfect alignment. Additionally, WILKINSON et al. (1990) reported on the results of site visits by the Hyperthermia Physics Center (HPC), indicating that microwave antenna efficiency of commercially supplied dipole antennas varied by as much as 35% within single-institution sets of "identical" antennas. This emphasizes that equal power application to "in-phase" antenna arrays will not necessarily produce the theoretically expected central hot spot and

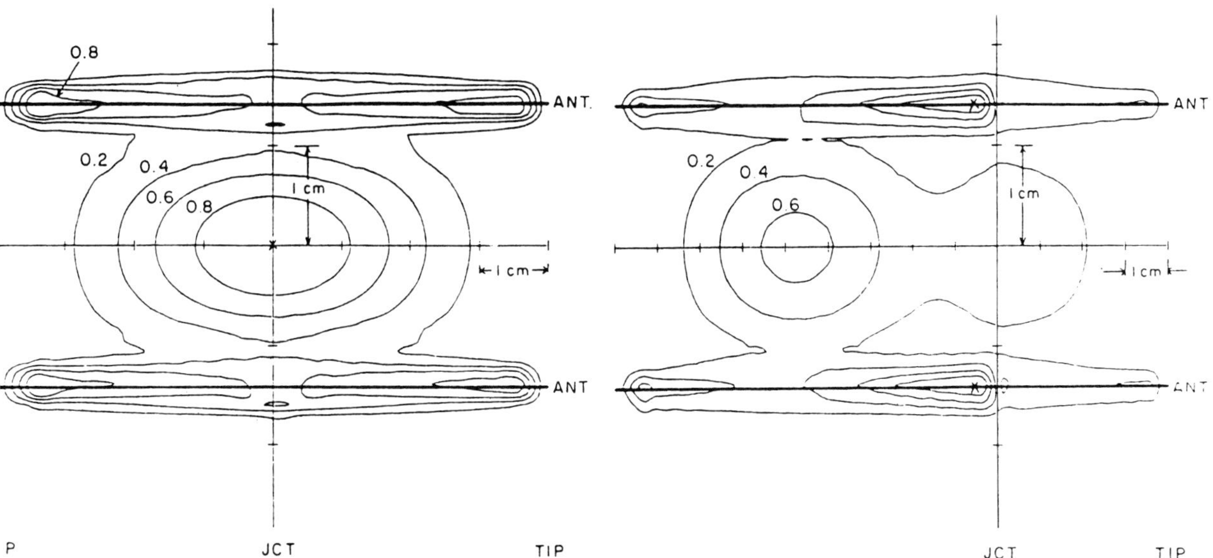

Fig. 13.3. Cross-section of the longitudinal SAR pattern in the diagonal plane of four in-phase 915-MHz dipole antennas at the corners of a 2-cm-square array: **a** 7.5 cm insertion depth (resonant $\lambda/2$ ID for the $h_A = h_B$ 3.9-cm antennas in 2.2-mm-OD catheters); **b** 12.7 cm ID. Reproduced with permission, all rights reserved (from JAMES et al. 1989)

suggests tht independent power and phase control of antennas is required.

As a means of reducing the uncertainties of imperfect antenna and tissue conditions while at the same time improving the uniformity of SAR within the implant volume, investigators have suggested the use of phase modulation to sequentially rotate in-phase "hot spots" around within the array (TREMBLY et al. 1986, 1988, 1994; ZHANG et al. 1990, 1991). Figure 13.4 from ZHANG et al. (1990) demonstrates the ability to eliminate the phase focused peak in the center of the array by sequentially applying 180° phase differences between time varying in-phase pairs of antennas. For the phase modulation scheme simulated in Fig. 13.4, the 50% of maximum SAR contour includes the entire cross section of the implant array and even extends 7 mm outside the array boundary. This is significantly better uniformity of power deposistion than can be obtained with four in-phase or noncoherent phase antennas for the same 2 cm array spacing. In fact, CAMART et al. (1992) reported that the volume heated above 41.5°C can theoretically be increased 300% over that obtained with a fixed in-phase array by using appropriately calculated phase shifts and phase rotation sequences. Practical problems which have slowed the introduction of phase rotation schemes into the clinic are the added hardware requirements for independent phase and amplitude control of microwave sources in the clinic, and the associated increase in thermometry required for monitoring and controlling the more complex treatment configuration. Even so, one very innovative system has been employed recently in a phase II clinical trial using computer-planned, time-modulated phase delays to four-antenna arrays which incorporate automatic temperature control by multifrequency radiometry (CAMART et al. 1993; FABRE et al. 1993; PREVOST et al. 1993). Additionally, since varying the insertion depth of one antenna in an array was found to produce an effect equivalent to introducing a phase shift to that antenna, an alternative method of producing controllable phase modulation by appropriate sequencing of insertion depth changes of the dipoles has been proposed (CLIBBON et al. 1993). Such cyclic scanning of antennas might be expected to provide improved homogenization of heating within the array due to controllable variation of power deposition along each catheter as well as phase modulation of the antenna array focal hot spot.

In an effort to improve control over the power deposition pattern along the antenna length, several alternatives to the basic dipole antenna structure have been investigated. Modifications include the use of multiple active sections to extend the heating pattern (LEE et al. 1986), partial wavelength chokes to restrict radiation

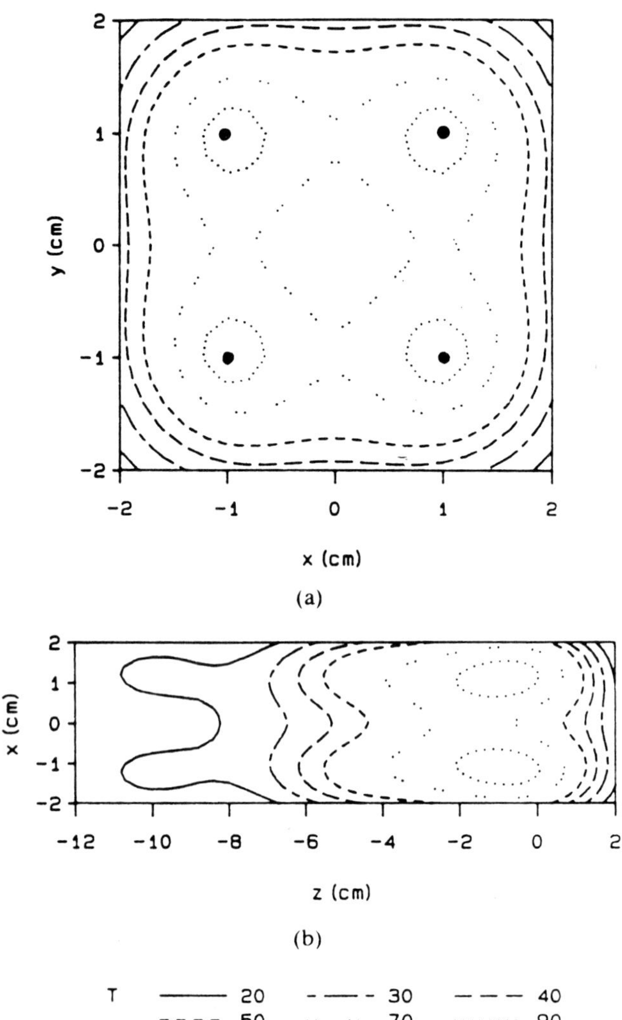

Fig. 13.4. Cross-section of SAR calculated for the mid-depth "junction" plane of four phase-modulated antennas driven at 915 MHz. Note the shift of SAR away from the array center compared to four in-phase antennas, due to the sequential rotation of phase differences between antennas. (From ZHANG et al. 1990)

back along the feedline (LIN and WANG 1987; HURTER et al. 1991; WONG and TREMBLY 1994), and enlarged diameter sleeves for preferential (capacitive) coupling of current through selected portions of the catheter insulation (TURNER 1986; ROOS and HUGANDER 1988; CERRI et al. 1993). Although efforts have produced improvements in tip heating and restriction of feedline heating, most test results of dipole-based antenna arrays demonstrate a residual dependence of heating pattern on insertion depth in tissue, and little ability to change the effective heating length (50% HL) controllably outside the range of 3–5 cm for antennas driven at 915 MHz. Current dipole-type antennas should be appropriate for heating tumors approximately 3–5 cm in length where the situation can benefit from phase addition of fields centrally (or peripherally with dynamic phase rotation) and where the antenna can be inserted 1–1.5 cm past the deep tumor margin (MECHLING et al. 1991, 1992).

13.2.2 Helical Coil Antennas

An alternative design consisting of a helical coil of wire wound tightly over the distal portion of the inner conductor and connected to the coaxial cable feedline at the tip (STAUFFER et al. 1987b; SATOH and STAUFFER 1988; SATOH et al. 1988) or at both ends of the coil (WU et al. 1987; ASTRAHAN et al. 1991) has also been investigated (Fig. 13.1). Analytical formulations of the fields surrounding noninsulated electrically small helical antennas radiating in lossy tissue have been developed (CASEY and BANSAL 1988; MIROTZNIK et al. 1993) and the results compared with experimental SAR measurements. Depending on the appropriate combination of coil length, diameter, and winding pitch for a given operating frequency, efficient coil radiators that restrict heating to a cylindrical region immediately surrounding each coil may be constructed for most practical size tumours. Numerous experimental studies of helical coil antennas have demonstrated both independence of heating pattern on insertion depth in tissue and an improved extension of heating out to the antenna tip as compared to dipole-type radiators (STAUFFER et al. 1987b); SATOH and STAUFFER 1988; SATOH et al. 1988; RYAN 1991; RYAN et al. 1991a; SATHIASEELAN et al. 1991). Figure 13.5 shows the linear SAR profiles along the antenna length at a radial distance of $r = 5$ mm in tissue-equivalent phantom. Note the close correspondence of SAR to the length and position of the coils (ranging from 1.1 to 3.0 cm long) which results from improved heating at the antenna tip and lack of overheating near the tissue surface even for antennas implanted just 5 mm beneath the surface. Despite the advantages of improved heat localization around variable length coils, helical coil antennas are not optimum for all applications. Since the antennas are normally driven with noncoherent microwave sources to limit interaction of the complex circularly polarized fields, the peak SAR occurs adjacent to each coil rather than in the tissue midway between antennas. Several independent studies have reported comparative evaluations of heating patterns from the above antennas (SATOH et al. 1988; TUMEH and ISKANDER 1989; RYAN 1991; RYAN et al. 1991, 1992; SATHIASEELAN et al. 1991). In general, the data support the following recommendations: helical coil antennas may be preferable for heating smaller tumors (1–4 cm diameter) in critical tissues where factors such as heating out to the antenna tip and steep gradients proximal to the coil section are more important than maximizing the separation of antennas. Dipole antennas may be preferable for situations benefitting from phase focusing of heat in tissue between antennas when the antenna tips can be extended into normal tissue beyond the tumor.

13.2.3 Microwave Power Distribution

Initially, single-channel microwave sources were used with combinations of two-way and four-way power splitters to divide the generator output into separate "in-phase" signals for each antenna. Problems with this configuration derive from the inability to adjust relative power and phase of each antenna and the potential for obtaining

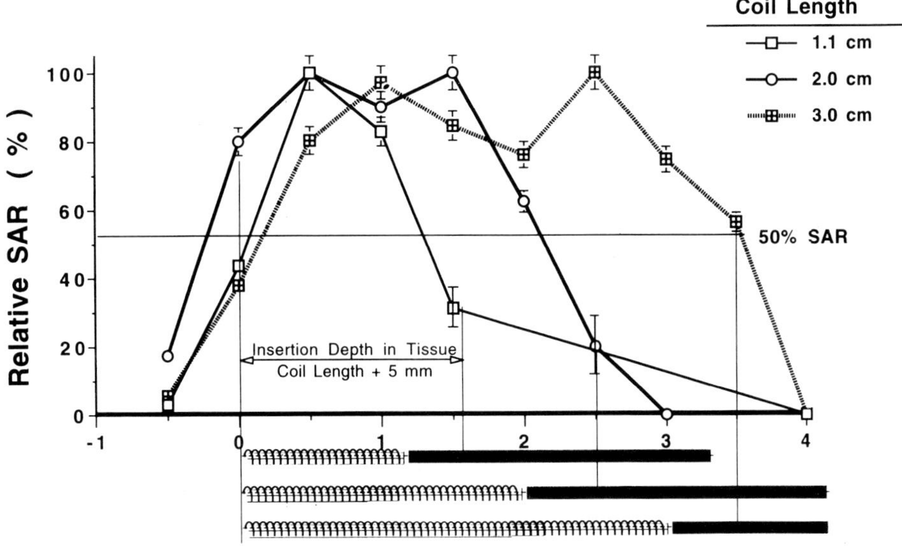

Fig. 13.5. Measured relative SAR profiles at r = 5 mm distance from three different length helical coil antennas in 915-MHz muscle equivalent phantom. Insertion depth for each antenna was the helical coil length plus 5 mm. Standard deviations are for three independent trials. Similar curves were obtained for helical coil antennas with 1.3-, 1.5-, 2.5-, and 3.5-cm-long coils (data not shown for clarity) and for antennas inserted deeper in the tissue

fixed out-of-phase drive signals due to minor temperature- and power-dependent phase shifts in the power splitters and/or cable connections. These problems can be accentuated by the variability of input impedances and efficiencies of commercial antennas (Wilkinson et al. 1990), and the effects of tissue heterogeneity. Ryan and Wright (1989) describe an improved system using computer-controlled high-speed PIN diode switches to control average power to each antenna by varying duty cycle. This type of system provides significantly improved phase and amplitude balance between antennas of an array, though care must still be taken to accommodate extra fixed phase shifts between channels resulting from variable tissue, antenna, or connection cable characteristics. Commercial systems providing even more control flexibility through computer-controllable phase and amplitude adjustments of multiple independent microwave generators are just becoming available (Camart et al. 1992; Diederich and Stauffer 1993; Fenn et al. 1993). Regardless of the power system used, thermometry requirements of feedback control of the treatment increase dramatically to take advantage of the independent power and phase adjustments. Thus, systems incorporating thermometry inside the catheter with each independently controlled antenna (Astrahan et al. 1988; Fabre et al. 1993) or sensors that are regularly spaced within the target tissue (Engler et al. 1987; Ryan et al. 1911) are highly desirable to supplement the normally sparse tissue measurements possible with fixed position fiberoptic probes.

13.2.4 Key Developments

1. 915-MHz (Strohbehn et al. 1979), 2450-MHz (Samaras 1984), and 433-MHz (Trembly 1985) interstitial microwave heating systems.
2. Clinically practical implantable antenna designs, including dipole (Taylor 1978; de Sieyes et al. 1981), multinode (Lee et al. 1986), $\lambda/4$ choke (Lin and Wang 1987; Hurter et al. 1991; Wong and Trembly 1994), variable diameter (Turner 1986; Roos and Hugander 1988), and helical coil (Li et al. 1984; Wu et al. 1987; Satoh and Stauffer 1988; Astrahan et al. 1991; Mirotznik et al. 1993) styles.
3. Antenna surface cooling via circulating air (Trembly et al. 1991) or water (Moriyama et al. 1988; Gentili et al. 1991) for increased axial homogeneity and radial penetration of therapeutic heating.
4. Improved uniformity of SAR within an implant array volume by cyclic modulation of phase differences between adjacent antennas (Trembly et al. 1988; Zhang et al. 1991a; Camart et al. 1993).
5. Tissue temperature monitoring and feedback control by multifrequency radiometry from within the interstitial antenna sources (Mizushina et al. 1992; Fabre et al. 1993).

13.3 Radiofrequency Electrodes

Radiofrequency current heating is normally accomplished at frequencies between 0.3 and 30 MHz where the mechanism of power absorption in tissue is resistive losses from conduction currents between electrodes. Frequencies at the lower end of the range are generally used for inducing current between pairs of metallic electrodes in direct galvanic contact with the tissue, while the upper end of the range is useful for capacitive coupling of current from electrode sections located inside insulating catheters. A hybrid technique, hereafter labeled inductively coupled RF (IC-RF), is also described.

13.3.1 Resistively Coupled Electrodes (RF-LCF)

Analytical solutions for the case of ohmic heating of tissue with RF currents between needle implants have been presented previously (Brezovich and Young 1981; Hand et al. 1991; Visser et al. 1993) along with numerical calculations of the power deposition patterns for several idealized (parallel, equal depth, regularly spaced) electrode configurations (Strohbehn 1983; Zhu and Gandhi 1988; Prior 1991). Practical considerations for heating with clinically realizable LCF electrode arrangements are given below.

Previous theoretical work has clearly shown that for two parallel equal-length needles in homogeneous tissue, an applied RF potential difference produces a uniform electric field at a given radial distance from the needle surface (neglecting end effects). Although the magnitude of the electric field falls off in tissue roughly as the inverse distance from each needle, the field and hence the distribution of electric current is uniform along the needle length in homogeneous tissue.

For practical configurations with nonparallel needles in heterogeneous tissue, current will preferentially flow along the paths of least resistance which result from regions of low-resistivity tissue or decreased separation between needles. Conversely, current will tend to avoid low water content tissues with high resistivity such as fat and bone. These basic principles are shown diagrammatically in Fig. 13.6. Power is deposited directly in tissue according to the simple relation $P_D = \rho |J|^2/2$ where $\rho = 1/\sigma$ is the tissue resistivity and J is the current density which is highest at the point of smallest cross-sectional area through which the RF current must flow (i.e., needle–tissue interface). Thus, power absorption is concentrated near the electrode–tissue interface and falls off rapidly with distance, roughly as $1/r^2$ depending on specific array geometry. Typical electrical impedances for the circuit consisting of two 1.5-mm-diameter metal electrodes implanted either 5 or 14 cm deep in tissue and spaced up to 4 cm apart are given in Table 13.2. At both 0.5-MHz and 5-MHz frequencies, the electrical impedance of the interstitial electrode circuit is determined primarily by the two needle–tissue interfaces and the intervening tissue resistance is small, though significant, being on the order of 2–3 Ω for each added centimeter of separation. Numerical calculations show that the power deposited between electrode pairs separated by only 1 cm drops to less than 10% of the maximum power deposition rate within a radial distance of 1.5 or 3 mm from 1- or 2-mm-diameter electrodes respectively (STROHBEHN 1983). While this leads to highly nonuniform power deposition patterns, the resulting tissue temperature distribution is considerably more uniform due to thermal conduction and convective redistribution of thermal energy within the array volume. In fact, for electrical conductivity, thermal conductivity, and blood perfusion values typical of human soft tissue, fairly uniform temperature distributions (with minimum tem-

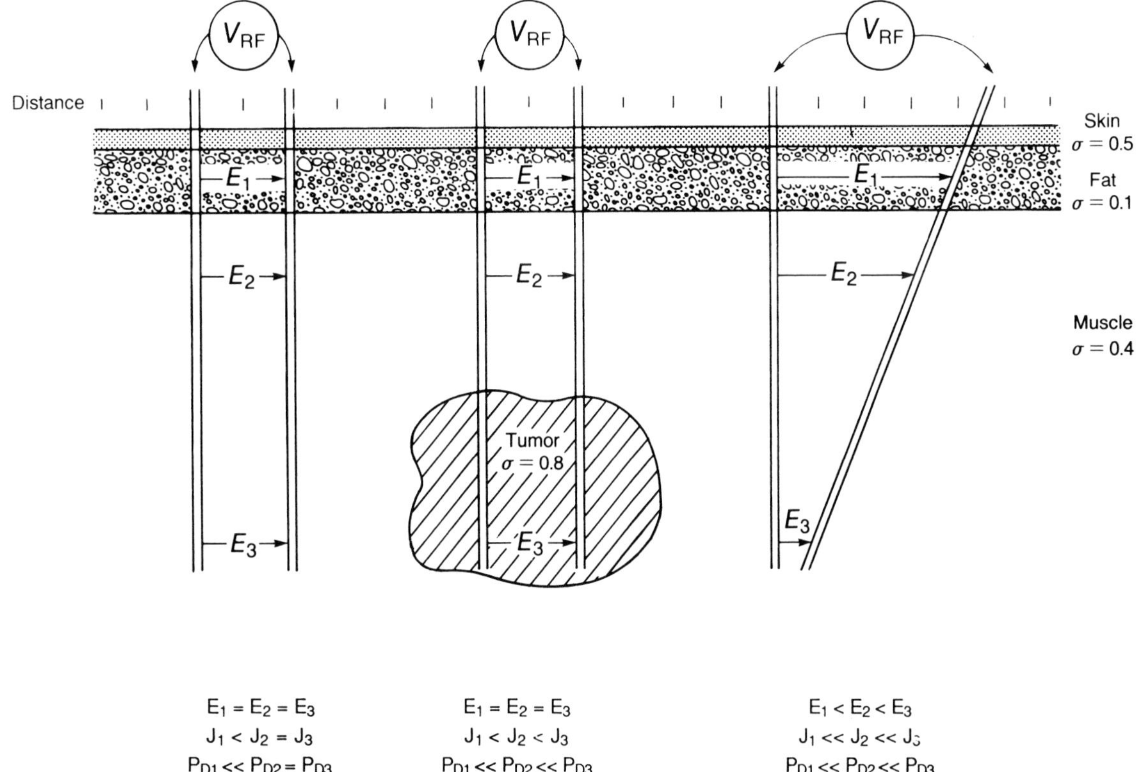

Fig. 13.6. Basic principles of ohmic heating with RF currents between metal needle electrodes. Note that electric field distributions at the individual points (E_1, E_2, E_3) vary according to the separation between electrodes while the current density $J = \sigma E$ and hense power deposition, also depends on variability of tissue electrical conductivity σ. Power deposition preferentially avoids high-resistivity fat tissue relative to regions of higher electrical conductivity or close electrode spacing

Table 13.2. Input impedance of LCF needle pair circuit in two different in vivo tissues

Electrode spacing	Canine muscle (5 cm ID)		Human tumor (14 cm ID)	
	500 kHz	10 MHz	500 kHz	5 MHz
1 cm	–	–	12.3 Ω ∠−6°	10 Ω ∠+5.5°
2 cm	20.5 Ω ∠−19°	16.1 Ω ∠+4.9°	14.5 Ω ∠−6°	13 Ω ∠+7.5°
3 cm	21.8 Ω ∠−19°	17.5 Ω ∠+8.9°	16.5 Ω ∠−5°	15 Ω ∠+7°
4 cm	–	–	20.2 Ω ∠−5.5°	18.5 Ω ∠+7°

perature rises between needles at least 50% of the maximum temperature rise) may be obtained in homogeneous tissues with this nonuniform power deposition pattern for electrode spacings up to 1.5 cm, as demonstrated with both numerical simulations (Strohbehn 1983) and in vivo measured data (Fig. 13.7).

13.3.1.1 LCF Electrode Design

A number of electrode styles have been used to date as shown schematically in Fig. 13.8. The simplest and most common implant has been an array of rigid 1.5- to 2-mm-diameter stainless steel needles originally manufactured for ^{192}Ir or ^{125}I brachytherapy implants. When inserted approximately normal to the high-resistance fat layer as shown in Fig. 13.6, little current flows in the fat layer and heating may be concentrated in deeper tissues which have lower resistance and/or where needles are closer together from convergence of the implant. While power is deposited in the thin layer of lower resistance skin, this superficial tissue tends to cool sufficiently due to intact blood perfusion and convective losses into air. For planar implants where the electrodes are entirely in or near superficial tissue, however, the twisting and pulling of skin at the angled needle entrance sites can cause significant overheating of the skin due to restriction of essential blood perfusion cooling. In either case, a snug-fitting catheter (Corry et al. 1989) or thin dielectric coating (Kapp and Prionas 1992; Prionas et al. 1994) may be installed over portions of the needles to minimize power deposition in well-innervated skin and to localize heat in the tumor at depth. Cosset et al. (1984) developed an alternative electrode insulation technique consisting of a tumor-length metal tube with sections of plastic tubing glued to either end. Electrical contact to the central "active" section was made with a metal stylet inserted through one of the plastic leaders. A flexible version of the insulated sleeve electrode was constructed for applications allowing through-implants by attaching a fine wire braid over the outside of a plastic catheter leader, and then covering the metal braid with dielectric (Kapp et al. 1988; Goffinet et al. 1990). After removal of a tumor-length section of outer insulation, the electrode was drawn into the target tissue behind an implant needle and heating obtained between exposed sections of wire braid. Further improvement in control of SAR within the implant array should be possible using segmented electrodes (Prionas et al. 1989, 1993) to adjust heating along the third dimension. These short segments should provide a means of varying power deposition along the implant length, with the potential to better accommodate heterogeneous tissue properties and variable separation of nonparallel implant needles (Kapp and Prionas 1992). One example of the control possible with segmented electrodes is shown in Fig. 13.9 (Prionas et al. 1993) as the measured SAR distributions between two parallel four-segment electrodes of 2.4 mm diameter and 1.0 cm center-to-center separation. In this case, power deposition was effectively localized to the regions between the outer two powered segments of each electrode and less than 5% of the maximum SAR was obtained between the two central segments with zero power.

13.3.1.2 LCF Power Distribution

Over the past decade there has been an evolution of systems used to distribute power to interstitially implanted electrodes. The simplest approach used was to connect all needles together into two to four rows, or concentric rings, and apply power to adjacent rows from a single RF amplifier (Doss and McCabe 1976; Cetas et al. 1980; Milligan

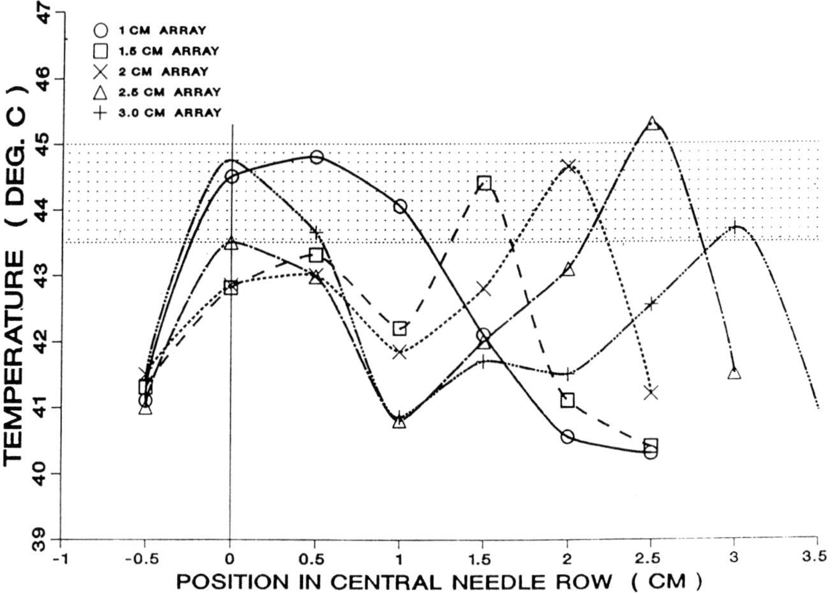

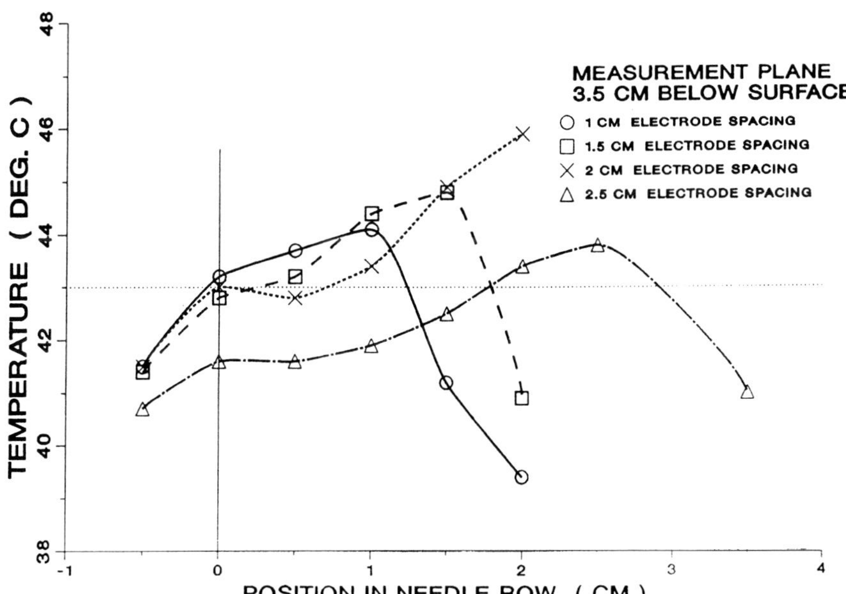

Fig. 13.7a,b. Study of temperature drop between RF electrodes for several separations in two different perfusion pig tissues in vivo. Note the acceptable uniformity of heating between electrodes for 1.0 and 1.5 cm spacing, with increasing droop in the tissue and difference between the two needle temperatures for larger spacings. **a** Steady state temperatures were measured mid-depth in the central row of three parallel rows of 17-gauge needles inserted 3.5 cm in pig liver. "Effective cooling rates" (Milligan et al. 1983; Stauffer et al. 1987a) as determined from thermal washout data measured at a reference point in tissue 5 mm from a heating needle remained essentially constant at 77 ± 8 ml/100 g per min throughout all heat trials which were repeated for each different needle spacing, implying very high surrounding tissue perfusion. **b** Steady state temperatures measured mid-depth in the central row of three parallel rows of 17-gauge needles inserted 7 cm deep into pig thigh muscle. Effective cooling rates measured 5 mm from a central row heating needle were 20.9 ± 2.3 ml/100 per min, throughout the heat trials, implying moderately low perfusion. Note the significantly higher temperatures obtained between implants as compared to the higher perfusion tissue in **a** , though temperature differences between needles of each pair are still large for electrode spacings > 1.0–1.5 cm

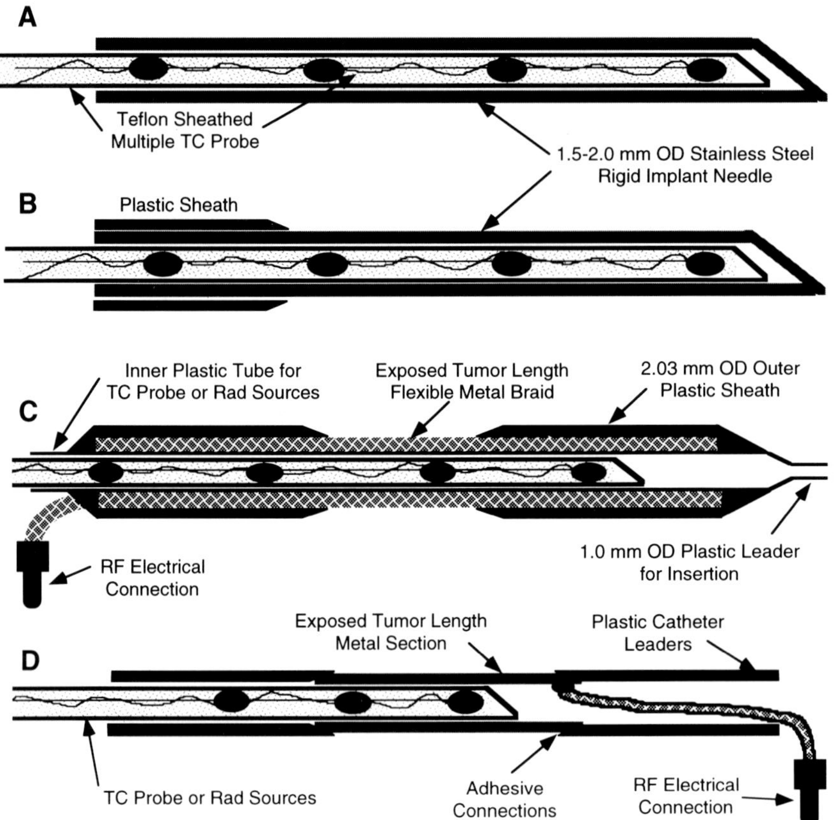

Fig. 13.8A–D. Schematic drawing of RF-LCF electrode designs with central lumen for multisensor temperature probes during heat treatment (as drawn) or subsequently for radioactive seeds during brachytherapy. **A** 1.5- to 2.0-mm-diameter (17- to 15-gauge) stainless steel needles with plastic coated multijunction thermocouples inside for treatment monitoring and control. **B** Plastic-coated or catheter-covered proximal portion of simple metal needle electrode for restricting heating of overlying normal tissue. **C** Stanford/Oximetrix flexible metal braid electrode with inner plastic tube for thermometry or radiation sources and outer plastic insulating layer for restricting heating to the tissue between bare metal sections in contact with tissue (Kapp et al. 1988). **D** Tumor length metal electrode with plastic tubing leaders glued to either end. Wire connections to the deep electrode section are made through one plastic leader and thermometry or radiation seed access through the other (Cosset et al. 1984)

and Dobelbower 1984; Stauffer 1984). An alternative configuration of electrodes utilized a single external ground plate, belt, or intracavitary obturator for the return currents from an interstitial array of needles which were all connected together to the power source (Cetas et al. 1980; Brezovich and Young 1981). Since resulting tissue temperatures tended to be nonuniform (in relation to the heterogeneity of tissue properties), control over the induced temperature distribution was extremely poor, especially if a large number of electrodes were connected together (Manning et al. 1982; Manning and Gerner 1983).

A second power distribution scheme provided significantly improved control of SAR by connecting a single power source to a number of computer-controlled relays which were hard-wire connected to preplanned needle pairs (Astrahan and George 1980; Astrahan and Norman 1982). During treatment, the computer operated each relay sequentially to apply power to each electrode pair for a short time (0–0.5 s), adjusted automatically in response to temperature feedback. Since power was applied to each needle pair for only a brief time and then interrupted for a much longer time (sufficient to cycle through all other pairs), this system had an inherent temporal variation of temperature which could cause more patient pain at an equivalent average tissue temperature than the more recent power distribution schemes with more constant output. Additionally, because of the hard-wire connections, there was no mechanism to correct for temperature differences between needles of each pair that resulted

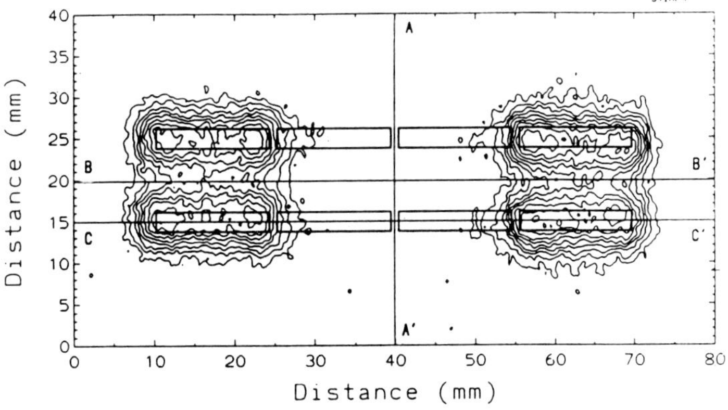

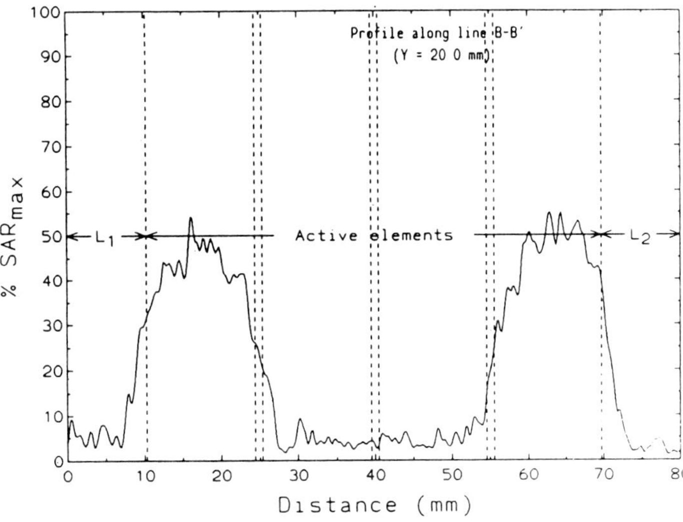

Fig. 13.9A,B. Measured relative SAR pattern around a pair of four segment radiofrequency electrodes spaced 1.0 cm apart in 500-kHz tissue eqùivalent phantom. Electrode diameter 2.4 mm; segment length 1.4 cm; 60 W to segment pairs 1 and 4 and 0 W to central pairs 2 and 3. **A** Contour plot of SAR; **B** SAR profile along central cut *B-B'* showing effective localization between the activated elements. (From PRIONAS et al. 1994)

from different tissue properties around each needle. The effects of even small differences in tissue properties are demonstrated in Fig. 13.7, which indicates that quite different tissue temperatures were obtained even in well-controlled parallel needle arrays in essentially homogeneous tissue – if needle spacings greater than 1–1.5 cm were used. Even so, time-multiplexed hard-wire pair RF systems have been commercialized and used successfully in the clinic (VORA et al. 1982) with a temporal ripple of typically 2°C or less at the needle surface for ≤1.5 cm electrode spacing in moderately perfused tissue, and a spatial variation within the array quite similar to other interstitial heating modalities (STAUFFER et al. 1989). In fact, for a small number of implants, temporal ripple was almost nil as seen in the time–temperature plots for a two-pair needle array in normal muscle tissue (STAUFFER et al. 1987a). Eventually, however, a third approach was introduced which provided separate well-isolated power amplifiers for hard-wire connection to each preplanned electrode pair. This approach offered significant advantages in that all pairs could be heated simultaneously to minimize temporal ripple and multiple temperature feedback signals could be used to control the power of each amplifier separately, but still required preplanned hard-wire pairing of electrodes. This configuration has been implemented successfully into clinical systems which provide independent control of up to 16 fixed-connection needle pairs, or which power needles individually by using a common external return electrode (Cosset et al. 1985).

Subsequently, a fourth drive scheme was introduced which utilizes a single power source and multiplexed current paths to sequentially connect variable combinations of electrodes together under computer control (Kapp et al. 1988; Corry et al. 1989; Prionas et al. 1994). During treatment, power deposition around each electrode is controlled by changes to the duty cycle for current paths involving that electrode. Since this computer-controlled multiplexer technique allows very simple expansion of channels (determined by the number of low-cost switching relays in the multiplexer), this system appears well suited for driving segmented electrode arrays which require a large number of independently controllable channels. Due to the single power source configuration, however, all electrodes are in one of three states at any particular moment – either disconnected or at the high or low RF potential. Thus, multiple current paths from each electrode are unavoidable (unless all electrodes except a single pair are disconnected) and may include undesirable currents between segments that were not intended to be paired together. Future systems may provide even more control of SAR with a fifth hybrid power generation scheme utilizing separate well-isolated power amplifiers for nearby electrode segments along with computer-controlled multiplexing of dynamically variable electrode pairing.

Depending on the electrode style chosen, there are a number of restrictions on implantation and applied power schemes which must be observed for low-frequency RF heating. Since LCF electrodes are normally connected to the generator in pairs (either by hardware or time-sequenced multiplexing), the conducting portion of each electrode should be nearly the same length to avoid overheating of tissue near the electrode with less contact area. Additionally, the electrode sections should be positioned both parallel and at about the same depth below the tissue surface in order to avoid concentration of current between the closest edges of adjacent electrode sections. This requires extra caution when planning allowable power connections for segmented RF electrode arrays. Regardless of electrode style used, further improvement in both patient tolerance and tumor heating uniformity is predicted for electrodes which include circulating temperature-regulated water to cool the electrode surface (Prior 1991). The ability to control electrode temperature should allow use of higher current densities and thus increased power deposition at distance from the electrodes for an equivalent maximum implant temperature, as well as equilibrate tissue interface temperatures along the implant length in heterogeneous tissue.

13.3.1.3 Key Developments

1. Metal needle implants with single-channel RF generators (Doss and McCabe 1976; Cetas et al. 1980; Milligan and Panjehpour 1983).
2. Time-sequenced computer-controlled multichannel power sources (Astrahan and George 1980; Astrahan and Norman 1982; Vora et al. 1982).
3. Insulated flexible electrodes (Cosset et al. 1984; Goffinet et al. 1990).
4. Computer-controlled multiplexing of single power source allowing simultaneous independent power control of electrodes (Kapp et al. 1988; Corry et al. 1989; Kapp and Prionas 1992).
5. Segmented rigid and flexible electrodes (Kapp and Prionas 1992; Prionas and Kapp 1992; Prionas et al. 1993).
6. Theoretical simulations of heating with water-cooled RF electrodes (Prior 1991).
7. Template-mounted circuit board with one to two (multiwire) quick connects for making electrode power connections with reduced treatment setup complexity (Corry et al. 1989).

13.3.2 Capacitively Coupled Electrodes (CC-RF)

By moving to higher RF frequencies, electrical current may be coupled capacitively from a metal electrode through plastic catheter insulating layers into the surrounding tissue. In contrast to the direct galvanic contact of LCF electrodes, the high capacitive impedance of the 27-MHz electrode–catheter–tissue interface produces a surface of nearly uniform current density which exhibits little sensitivity to variations in the much lower resistance of intervening tissue. In addition, the high impedance catheter layer helps diffuse otherwise high current densities occurring at the ends of implanted electrodes. Thus, the SAR pattern of capacitively coupled electrodes is substantially independent of separation distance and relative orientation of adjacent electrodes. In fact, relatively uniform SAR patterns have been demonstrated for a number of implant geometries that would be unusable for lower frequency LCF systems, such as angled, curved, co-linear, and even intersecting electrodes (VISSER et al. 1989; DEURLOO et al. 1991). As in RF heating with LCF electrodes, the radial falloff of power deposition is extremely sharp, with SAR reduced to <10% of its maximum within 2 mm of the implant surface (MARCHAL et al. 1989).

13.3.2.1 Electrode Design

At least five electrode styles have been used during the evolution of this technique (Fig. 13.10). Initially, heating was accomplished using a single wire electrode inserted inside a snug-fitting plastic catheter (MARCHAL et al. 1989). A well-coupled external ground plate was used for the return current from this single-ended electrode to restrict radiation to the desired region and to avoid unintentional current paths through inadvertent patient contact with nearby grounded objects (including operating personnel). Two improvements to this basic wire implant were described by VISSER et al. (1989). The first involved the use of flexible coaxial cable with the inner conductor removed and replaced with a fiberoptic temperature sensor. With the outer coax cable dielectric entirely removed, the exposed wire braid was inserted into the implant catheter and current paths established using an external ground plate. While this enabled monitoring of temperature inside each implant catheter, heating resulted along the entire implanted length with no sparing of overlying normal tissue. An alternative design left the central conductor and surrounding dielectric of the coax intact for connection to the outer braid at the electrode tip. In order to restrict heating to this distal section, the outer wire braid was removed from the implanted length proximal to the target tissue and current effectively localized to the distal section where the implant catheter fit tightly over the wire braid. A practical improvement over this design, consisting of a plastic catheter coated with conducting paint over the distal section, was described by DEURLOO et al. (1991). Activation of the tip electrode was accomplished with a thin wire extending through the lumen of the catheter alongside a probe for monitoring temperature. LAGENDIJK (1990) and LAGENDIJK et al. (1994) describe a "dual-electrode" configuration having two active sections in the same catheter driven 180° out of phase. As in the previous design, the active metal sections were driven by thin wires running alongside a multipoint thermometry probe in the central lumen of the applicator, as shown in Fig. 13.10. With this electrode, longitudinal control of the SAR distribution became possible using separate generators for the two segments. Theoretically, this design should readily accommodate more than two segments per catheter for increased spatial resolution of longitudinal control.

13.3.2.2 Power Distribution

Initially, 27.12-MHz interstitial heating systems used a separate power source with transformer-isolated connections to one interstitial electrode and one external ground electrode. In order to obtain sufficient isolation of power sources and minimize cross-talk between implanted electrodes, the external ground plate was segmented and each return connection isolated from the others. Electrical matching of electrode circuits was accomplished via individual tuning coils. In practice, the external plate position is not critical due to the long wavelength at 27 MHz. To minimize undesirable heating of superficial tissues under the edges of the external electrodes, the surface area of each plate should be at least 10 times greater than the surface area of the interstitial electrode and should be coupled to the skin with a saline-filled bolus bag to provide a more uniform capacitively loaded impedance for diffusing current near the edges. An alternative drive scheme was introduced which avoided the complexities of external plates by allowing two internal applicators to be paired together and driven from a single generator. This configuration was shown to be more sensitive to relative length and orientation of the paired electrodes, however (DEURLOO et al. 1991). An improved "hybrid" drive scheme evolved using an additional external return plate for each internal electrode pair to define the ground reference potential and provide a return path for any unbalanced current between interstitial electrodes (LAGENDIJK 1990; LAGENDIJK

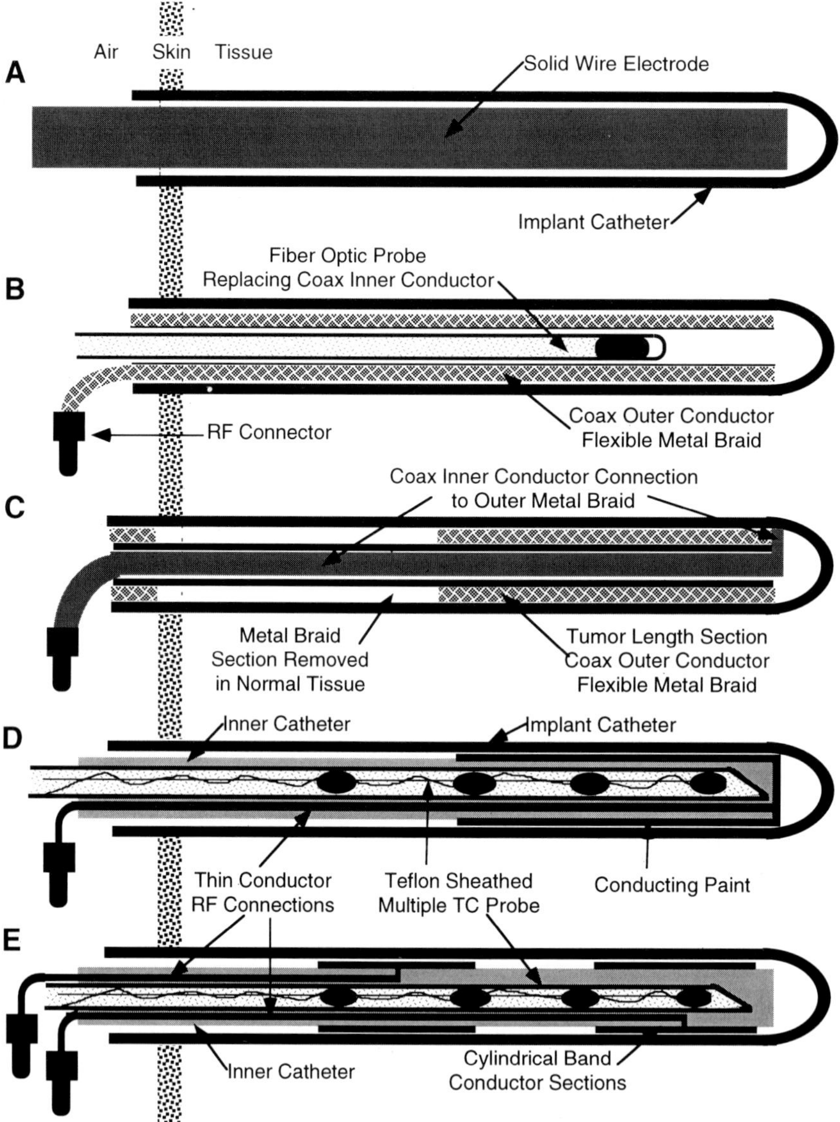

Fig. 13.10A–E. Schematic drawing of the evolution of CC-RF electrode designs. All applicators are inserted inside an insulating plastic catheter and driven at 13.56–27.12 MHz. **A** Metal wire style with no provision for depth localization (MARCHAL et al. 1989). **B** Flexible coaxial cable applicator with temperature probe in place of inner conductor; no provision for depth localization (VISSER et al. 1989). **C** Coaxial cable with outer conductor stripped away except for active tip section (VISSER et al. 1989). **D** Active heating section consists of conductive coating on catheter surface with temperature sensors (or radiation sources) in central lumen (DEURLOO et al. 1991). **E** Dual-electrode design with multiple conducting cylinders on outside of catheter with temperature sensors or radiation sources inside (LAGENDIJK 1990)

et al. 1995). This allowed the use of separate generators for each internal electrode for improved lateral and/or longitudinal control of SAR. The external plate also helped confine heating to the region near the implanted electrodes rather than allow unstable current paths through ill-defined and undesirable external patient ground points. Schematic illustrations of these power distribution schemes have been given previously (VISSER et al. 1993).

13.3.2.3 Key Developments

1. 27-MHz unrestricted length, flexible, single-ended electrodes with individual external

ground plates and individual power control (MARCHAL et al. 1989; VISSER et al. 1989).
2. "Dual-electrode" applicator design with two independently driven segments per catheter and external ground plate (LAGENDIJK 1990; LAGENDIJK et al. 1995).
3. Balun-balanced interstitial electrode pairs with no external plate (DEURLOO et al. 1991).

13.3.3 Inductively Coupled Electrodes (IC-RF)

A third interstitial RF modality was introduced to facilitate repeated heatings of permanently implanted, connectorless electrodes. In this approach, current is inductively coupled from an external loop antenna into a surgically implanted loop just under the skin, which is connected by coaxial cable to an electrode pair within the tumor (DOSS and MCCABE 1986, 1988). Due to practical limitations in body surface area available for implantation of subdermal receiving antennas, this technique is intended for only a small number of implanted circuits, preferably one. Thus the technique must use either parallel rows of electrodes connected together, or implanted plates surrounding the target volume. Heating of tissue around the metal electrodes is accomplished via resistively coupled currents between electrodes, just as in the lower frequency LCF technique. Concerns nearly identical to those presented in Sect. 13.3.1 apply regarding the need for parallel, equal length electrodes. While GREENBLATT (1987) and PISCH (1994) have defined appropriate methods for surgical implantation of biocompatible implants fixed into parallel rows in the tumor bed using absorbable layers of vicryl mesh, uniformity of heating is still adversely affected by the number of electrodes connected together to a single power source (CETAS et al. 1980; MANNING and GERNER 1983). Thus, this technique appears appropriate for treatment of small volumes which can benefit from the ability to be reheated periodically from a small number of electrodes without externalized connections.

Initial "passive hyperthermia implant" (PHI) systems have used external power source frequencies of 6.78 MHz and 13.56 MHz (DOSS and MCCABE 1986, 1988). For small tissue volumes ($<25\,cm^3$), sufficient power transfer was achieved using transmitting and receiving loop antennas of 14 cm diameter separated by 1.5 mm. For somewhat larger tumor volumes, DOSS and MCCABE (1988) proposed connecting concentric parasitic loops in parallel with the primary receiving loop to increase the gain of the receiving circuit. Because of the transformer coupling of internal and external loop antennas, induced current in the receiving loop(s) helped cancel eddy currents which would otherwise contribute to superficial tissue heating under the transmitting antenna. Depending on the target volume, the ratio of power deposition around the implanted electrodes to that obtained from eddy current heating of superficial tissue around the receiving antenna varied in the range of 5:1 to 10:1, allowing power transfer to the internal electrode circuit in excess of 50 W per multiple loop antenna.

An integral feature of the PHI system was the ability to remotely estimate volume-averaged tissue temperature between electrodes by the change in phase of electrode input impedance as seen at the external coupled antenna terminals (DOSS and MCCABE 1986). In addition, DOSS and MCCABE (1988) described an independent implantable circuit for accurately determining a single point temperature within the tumor. This "passive temperature implant" (PTI) consisted of a thermistor connected to a second subdermally implanted loop which was coupled inductively to an external antenna and 10-MHz low-power source for interrogating the thermistor sensor. This remote single-point temperature monitoring capability may find future application in combination with other interstitial or external heating techniques as well.

13.3.3.1 Key Developments

1. 6- to 13-MHz "PHI" system for connectorless LCF heating of a surgically implanted array of electrodes via energy coupled inductively through the skin, and for connectorless monitoring of average tissue temperature around the electrodes (DOSS and MCCABE 1986).
2. 10-MHz "PTI" system for adding remote single-point temperature measurement capability to the above PHI system (DOSS and MCCABE 1988).

13.4 Thermal Conduction "Hot Source" Techniques

Hot source techniques constitute the most basic form of interstitial heating in that no power is deposited directly in tissue and the resulting temperature distributions are dependent only on tissue thermal parameters rather than heterogeneous electrical or acoustical tissue properties. For these techniques, maximum tissue temperature is readily determined as the surface temperature of the implanted sources, and minimum tissue temperature is dictated by the implant geometry and thermal properties which vary both spatially and temporally during heat treatment. In principle, Hot Source implants may be considered either "constant temperature" or "constant power." Tissue temperatures adjacent to constant power sources vary directly with surrounding perfusion changes since the constant power generation along the source provides no accommodation for variable thermal loading. Constant temperature implants may provide somewhat more uniform heating of tissues with heterogeneous thermal properties due to their ability to provide more or less thermal energy output in response to changes in thermal loading (perfusion). Important geometry considerations include relative spacing and orientation of sources, and source length. As with all interstitial heat sources, heat is lost axially off the ends due to thermal conduction, producing a tapering off of temperature between sources near the ends compared to that near the middle, even for constant temperature sources. As source separation increases or source length decreases, the axial direction temperature profiles become increasingly peaked centrally and show less heating near the ends (Fig. 13.11). Since Hot Source techniques have no mechanism for increasing power deposition directly in tissue, at least one of the following approaches must be used to minimize low temperature regions at either end of an implanted target: (a) the sources may be placed closer together; (b) the sources may be extended beyond the target volume in both directions so that the target is located within the centrally uniform region; or (c) the sources may be broken into multiple sections and the ends maintained at higher temperature to counter the extra heat losses. These approaches have been studied theoretically by numerous investigators and shown to produce significantly improved temperature uniformity within the target for denser implant spacing (Matloubieh et al. 1984; Hand et al. 1991; Prior 1991), when the implants extend at least 1–1.5 cm beyond the target (Matloubieh et al. 1984; Chin and Stauffer 1991), or when higher temperature elements are placed at either end of the implant (Patel et al. 1991). While segmented sources can provide the most adjustable, and potentially uniform, elevation of tissue temperature along the implant length, not all Hot Source techniques are capable of varying temperature along the implant surface. The following sections describe three techniques which rely similarly upon basic thermal redistribution of heat within an array of implants, but which differ in methodologies used to heat the implants as well as in the controllability of temperature along each source.

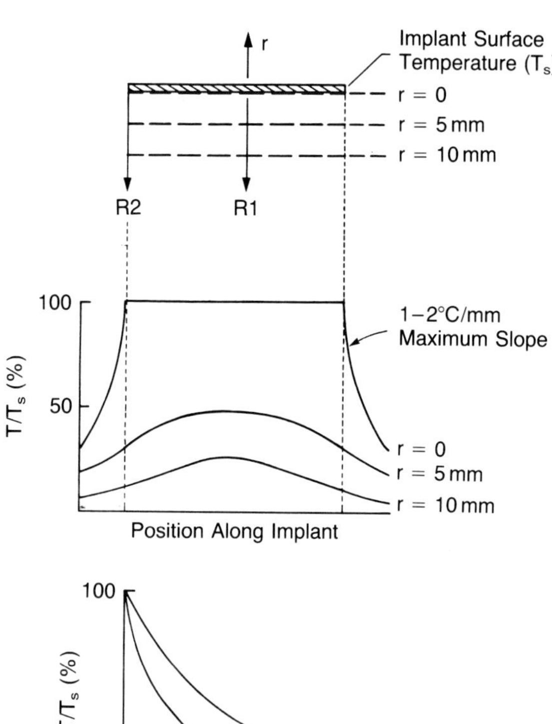

Fig. 13.11. Temperature distribution in tissue adjacent to a finite length "equal-temperature" heat source. Note rapid shortening of effectively heated length at increasing radial distance. (From Stauffer 1990) Reproduced with permission. All rights reserved

13.4.1 Hot Water Tubes

One of the most straightforward approaches to interstitial conductive heating is to circulate water at a fixed hyperthermic temperature through an array of needles or catheters. Due to the mechanics of nonturbulent water flow through a tube, there is a velocity profile across the lumen such that flow is fastest in the center and slowest near the tubing wall. For the case of hot water losing energy to cooler tissue, there is a corresponding temperature profile across the tube as well as along its implanted length. To minimize temperature gradients around the tube, water flow should be sufficiently rapid that turbulent flow is obtained to thoroughly mix the fluid for maximum energy transfer across the tube wall and minimum transit time and temperature drop along the length. For a tube with an internal diameter of 1.5 mm implanted 10 cm deep in moderately perfused tissue, this requires a water flow rate of roughly 2.5 ml/s to limit the temperature drop to approximately 0.3°–0.5°C (HAND et al. 1991).

13.4.1.1 Applicator and Water Distribution System Design

Initially, hot water was circulated through hollow metal or plastic tubes to create surfaces of nearly uniform temperature (BREZOVICH et al. 1988). HANDL-ZELLER et al. (1988) introduced an improved applicator having three separate channels: one for introducing hot water to the catheter tip section around a fixed position radioactive source, a second for injecting cold water at a point just proximal to the radiation source for cooling overlying normal tissue, and a third to serve as return path for the mixture of hot and cold water. This design was further modified as shown in Fig. 13.12 to allow separate channels for radiation sources. (From HANDL-ZELLER and HANDL 1992) (© 1992 Springer-Verlag)

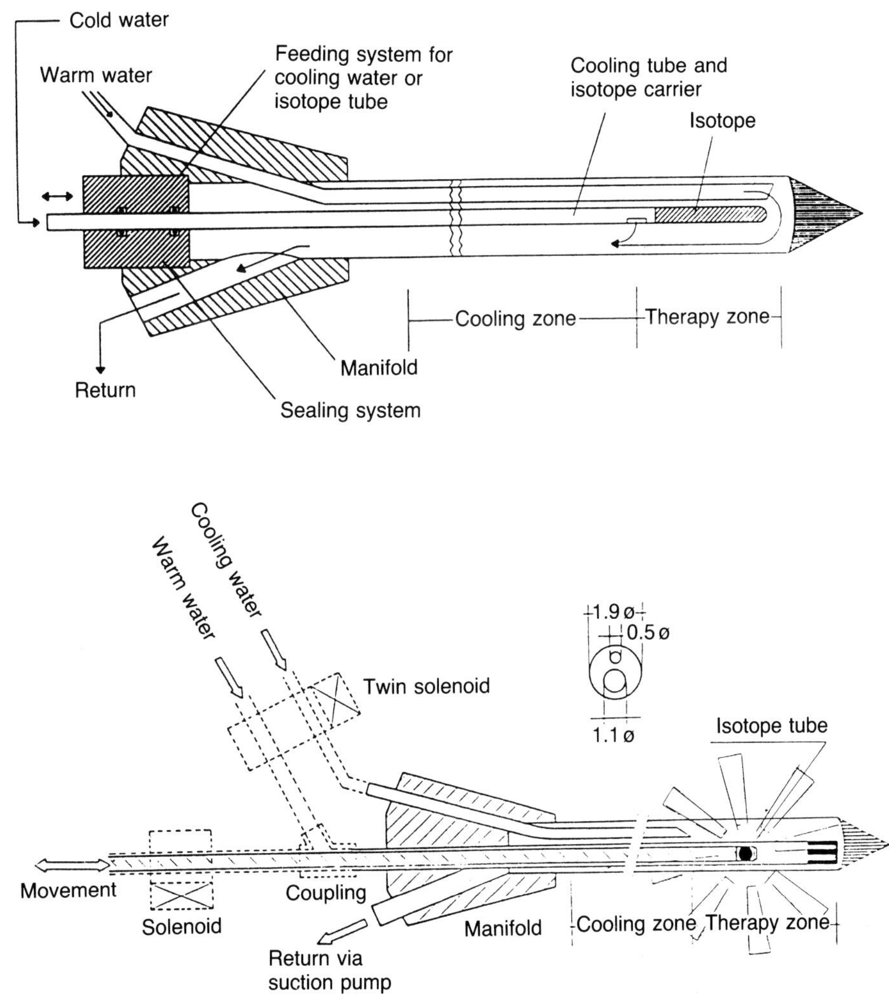

Fig. 13.12. Schematic drawing of dual-chamber hot water applicators with provisions for cooling of overlying normal tissue and simultaneous treatment with LDR or HDR

circulating the hot and cold water in addition to an isolated central channel for afterloading low dose rate (LDR), pulsed dose rate (PDR), or high dose rate (HDR) sources during treatment (Handl-Zeller and Handl 1991, 1992; Handl-Zeller 1993).

Initial clinical water distribution systems used a single temperature-regulated reservoir and pump to circulate water into a distribution manifold having equal size output ports for generating approximately equivalent flow rates through a parallel array of identical length and diameter tubes (Brezovich et al. 1988; Schreier et al. 1990). This type of system was subsequently upgraded to include a second similar distribution manifold for circulating water at a cooler temperature to the proximal portions of the implant tubes which traverse normal tissue (Handl-Zeller and Handl 1991).

13.4.1.2 Key Developments

1. Theory of required water flow rates and heat transfer characteristics (Hand et al. 1991).
2. Clinically viable manifold system for distributing water to multiple constant temperature implant tubes (Brezovich et al. 1988; Schreier et al. 1990).
3. Implant catheters with channels for separate hot and cold water sources as well as a port for afterloading a radiation source for simultaneous LDR, PDR, or HDR therapy (Handl-Zeller and Handl 1991; Handl-Zeller 1993).

13.4.2 Resistance Wire Heaters

The basic mechanism of source heating is ohmic losses from an electrical current flowing through a length of high-resistance material which is normally in coiled wire form to increase the total length and resistance of axially short elements. The power available for heat generation in each resistance wire section is $P = I^2R$ where I is the series current flowing through the wire of total resistance R from end to end. This interstitial technique is distinguished from other electrical wire implants by the use of simple DC voltage sources to drive direct current through the resistance elements, which avoids the complexity of electromagnetic power deposition in tissue.

13.4.2.1 Applicator Design

Initially, clinical applicators consisted of tightly wound coils of high resistance wire coated with a plastic catheter sheathing for electrical insulation from the tissue (Baumann and Zumwalt 1989; Marchosky et al. 1990a,b). A thermistor sensor was attached to the inner surface of the heating coil, and small diameter electrical connections from the heating coil and thermistor extended through the inner lumen of the applicator to the system electronics. This design evolved into dual-purpose applicators with a wire coil wrapped around a central catheter large enough to accommodate radioactive sources for simultaneous thermoradiotherapy (Fearnot et al. 1990). For a given resistance wire material formed into a tightly wound coil, resistance is distributed uniformly along the element length and for any given current there is a corresponding uniform power loss per unit length of the implant. While existing commercial resistance wire applicators have no provision for varying power dissipation along the length, this could be implemented in one of three ways: (a) vary the spacing of heating coil turns along the axial length with lower turns density near the center or wherever less heating power is desired; (b) fuse together multiple sections of different resistivity material and connect them in series to the power source to yield higher temperatures around the sections with higher resistivity wire (e.g., at the ends); or (c) use multiple coil elements in each catheter with separate drive electronics for each. Patel et al. (1991) described the theoretical advantages of segmented two- and three-section heater coils connected in series to a single power source for increasing source temperature at either end of the implant (Fig. 13.13).

Resistance wire heat sources offer some unique capabilities over other Hot Source techniques. Due to the ability to accurately monitor both implanted catheter temperature and applied power, there is sufficient information to calculate approximately the effective thermal conductivity of surrounding tissues, which can then be related to volume averaged blood perfusion. Software has been written to predict minimum tumor temperature between implants from knowledge of implant spacing and real time measurements of implant power dissipation and surface temperatures (Babbs et al. 1990), and furthermore to use these calculations for real time control of

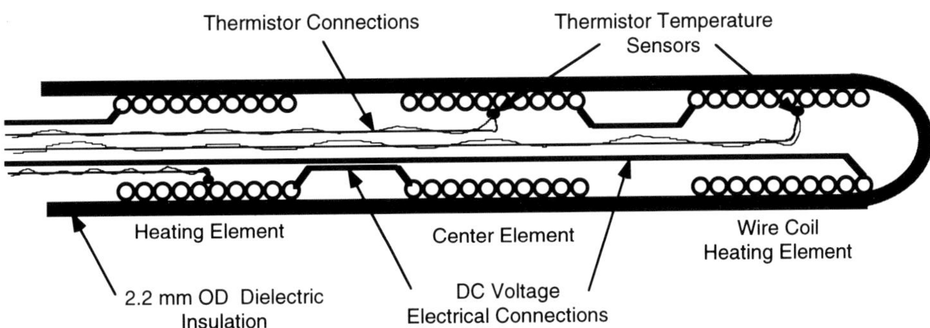

Fig. 13.13. Schematic drawing of three-section resistance wire heater. The heating elements are connected in series to a DC power supply with the outer two elements having higher resistivity to produce higher temperatures at either end of the applicator. (Adapted from PATEL et al. 1991)

power to each implant (DEFORD et al. 1991a,b). Although temperature can vary along the length of the "constant power" source in relation to variations in perfusion, fairly accurate knowledge of maximum tissue temperature is available from thermistor measurements of heating coil temperature which can be made at several points along the length. Substantially more temperature information is estimated from the bioheat transfer equation-based algorithm used to predict the "droop," or variation of temperature between implants. DEFORD et al. (1992) have indicated that in general, variations of about 10% in the thermal properties or implant geometry cause errors in the estimates of minimum tissue temperature of less than 1°C. In an evaluation of 22 patient treatments, DEFORD et al. (1991a) reported an average estimation error of the minimum tumor temperature between implants of just 0.4°C.

13.4.2.2 Key Developments

1. Hardware for controlling DC voltage distribution to multiple implanted resistance wire implants with sufficient control and stability for use in long-duration heat protocols (BAUMANN and ZUMWALT 1989; MARCHOSKY et al. 1990a).
2. Algorithm for feedback control of power to each implant, derived from computer-predicted minimum tissue temperatures based on measured implanted catheter temperatures and associated power levels (BABBS et al. 1990; DEFORD et al. 1990).
3. Applicator design for simultaneous heat and radiation (FEARNOT et al. 1990) with multiple heating elements (PATEL et al. 1991).

13.4.3 Ferromagnetic Seed Implants

In principle, magnetic fields may be generated quite easily with an RF current in a wire coil. These fields can be used to couple energy inductively into any lossy conductor in the field with no direct contact. Over the past three decades, a number of medical applications have emerged for magnetic induction heating systems in the range of 20 kHz to 27 MHz. Initial investigations reported on the use of magnetic fields at frequencies between 37 and 600 kHz to inductively couple energy and heat small 1- to 2-mm-diameter ferromagnetic "seed" implants. These connectorless implants were heated to temperatures of 100°C or more for thermal ablation treatment of small focal neurological disorders (BURTON et al. 1966; WALKER and BURTON 1966; BURTON et al. 1971; MOIDEL et al. 1976). Subsequently, higher power systems were developed for heating large internal organs or tumor masses that had been injected with iron powder-impregnated "ferrosilicone" solutions to localize the power absorption (RAND et al. 1977, 1981). Due to the small size of particles that could be injected intra-arterially upstream of the tumor mass, RF frequencies were lowered to the range of 20–56 kHz to minimize eddy current heating of surrounding normal tissues while generating sufficient heat loss in the particles. Subsequent investigations have continued this research on injectable heating solutions and produced materials with significantly higher power absorption efficiency, such as ferromagnetic colloidal particles (CHAN et al. 1993) and subdomain ferrite particle suspensions (JORDAN et al. 1993). These materials are currently under investigation for producing local hyperthermia of deep-seated regions (entire organs or large tumor masses) without the trauma of interstitial needles, and potentially with the microscopic particles concentrated in tumor via tumor-specific antibodies or liposome encapsulations. Recently, a large development effort of one group has focused on delivering hyperthermia via a small ferromagnetic seed implant that has been remotely maneuvered along the path of minimum neurological trauma from a small burr hole in the skull to the desired target in surgically inaccessible deep brain (Malloy et al. 1990, 1991; Quate et al. 1991; Ritter et al. 1992). This project has required the integration of several related technologies including: (a) noncontact DC magnetic field manipulation of the position of a small implanted ferromagnetic seed, (b) real time visualization of seed position using stereo fluoroscopic imaging superimposed over preoperative MRI scans, and (c) RF magnetic field induced eddy current heating of the ferromagnetic seed. A number of applications in interstitial heat-activated therapy have been suggested (Grady et al. 1990a,b; Ritter et al. 1992). Alternatively, several investigators have studied the use of inductively coupled fields at frequencies above about 10 MHz to produce intentional eddy current heating of tissues in the absence of implanted material (Guy et al. 1974; Elliott et al. 1982; Oleson 1982; Ruggera and Kantor 1984; Tiberio et al. 1988; Kato et al. 1990). The following discussion will focus on the production of interstitial hyperthermia using induction heating systems which couple energy into percutaneously implanted, finite size "ferroseed" implants that are compatible with needle or catheter implant techniques.

13.4.3.1 Coupling Energy to the Load

For ferromagnetic cylinders oriented parallel to a magnetic field, seed heating results due to ohmic losses from circumferential eddy currents induced on the implant surface (Brezovich et al. 1984; Stauffer et al. 1984a; Haider et al. 1991). Power absorption per unit length is dependent on seed characteristics (radius a, length L, magnetic permeability μ, electrical conductivity σ) and the frequency (ω) and strength (H_o) of the magnetic field. For cylindrical seeds implanted in a regular array with 1-cm spacing, each 1-cm length must heat 1 cm^3 of tissue along the central portion of the implant volume. For these conditions, the average power absorbed into a 1-cm^3 tissue volume surrounding a cylindrical metal seed has been derived previously (Smythe 1950; Stauffer et al. 1984a):

$$P_I = \pi a(\omega\mu/2\sigma)^{1/2} H_o^{\,2} \times 10^{-2}\,\mathrm{W/m^3}. \qquad (13.1)$$

Similarly, it has been shown (Davies and Simpson 1979; Oleson 1982) that the power deposited directly into a 1-cm^3 volume of tissue at distance r from the center of a dielectric tissue mass of generally uniform electrical conductivity σ_T and permeability μ_T is:

$$P_T = \omega^2 \mu_T^{\,2} r^2 \sigma_T H_o^{\,2} \times 10^{-6}\,\mathrm{W/m^3}. \qquad (13.2)$$

This normalization to 1 cm^3 of tissue in each case allows direct comparison of power absorbed by a metal implant and conducted out into the surrounding tissue with the power that would be deposited directly in the same tissue volume without the presence of the seed. The predominant difference is seen to be their functional dependencies on frequency and radius of eddy current loops. The power absorbed in tissue by these two mechanisms is compared graphically in Fig. 13.14, which gives separate curves for a range of typical ferroseed radii and magnetic permeabilities along with curves for direct tissue absorption in three different size tissue loads. It is readily seen that frequencies below 500 kHz should be used for localized heating of small implanted ferromagnetic materials, and frequencies above about 10 MHz for efficient heating of tissue directly from the magnetic field. Stauffer et al. (1984b) proposed the use of intermediate frequencies (1–10 MHz) for applications that might benefit from simultaneous regional eddy current tissue warming with local heat boost to the tumor implant. Atkinson et al. (1984) have discussed additional considerations for the appropriate frequencies to be used in induction heating applications.

Design of induction heating equipment for generating magnetic fields around the tumor implant is relatively straightforward and is covered in general electrical engineering reference books. Stauffer et al. (1994) have reviewed the induction heating coil configurations that can provide optimum coupling into ferroseed arrays located at any depth or orientation in the body, and have described appropriate electrostatic shielding techniques for safe operation of magnetic induction heating coils in the patient clinic.

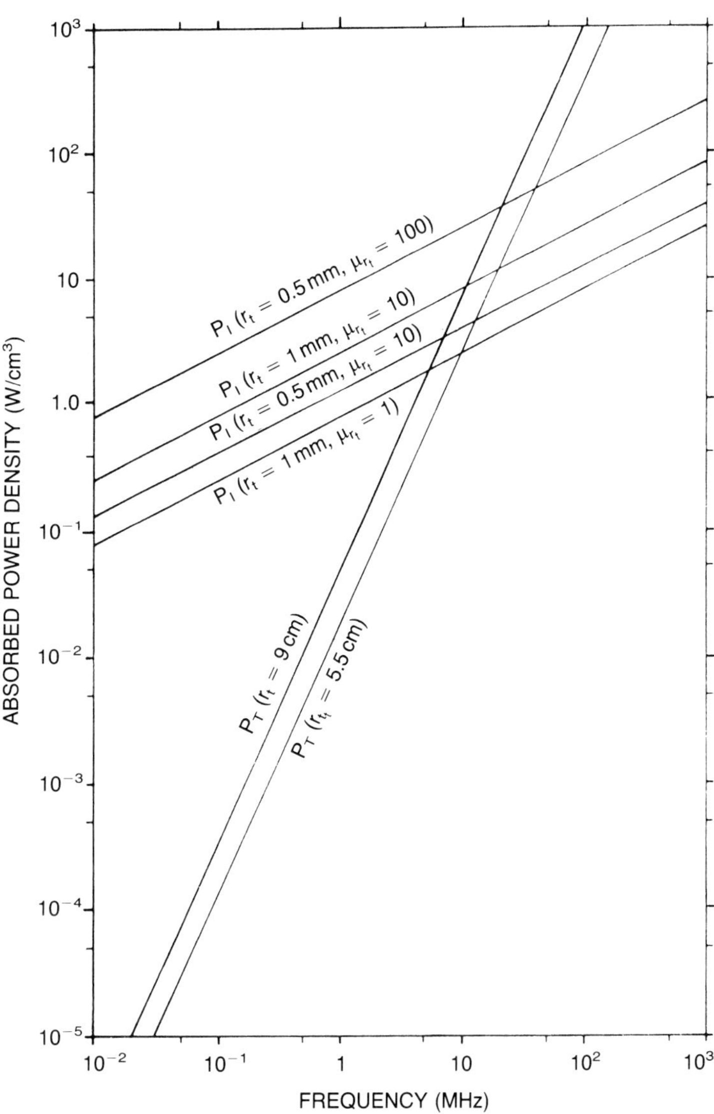

Fig. 13.14. Frequency dependence of absorbed power density in 1 cm^3 of tissue from magnetic field-induced eddy currents directly in tissue at distance r_t from the center of the tissue mass, or from inductively coupled eddy current heating of a 1-cm-long cylindrical ferroseed implant of permeability μ_t, radius r_t. (From STAUFFER et al. 1984) (© 1984 IEEE)

13.4.3.2 Thermoseed Design

While most of the parameters in Eq. 13.1 are not easily varied during treatment, different seed power absorption rates can be preplanned by changes in seed permeability and/or electrical conductivity. One such change occurs naturally as a consequence of heating the seed. The permeability of any ferromagnetic material drops rapidly as it is heated up to its "Curie point." As this temperature is reached, heating efficiency drops, allowing the material to cool below its Curie point and regain lost permeability. By alloying together a highly permeable material (iron, nickel, or cobalt) with another metal having a lower Curie point, the resulting Curie point can be lowered to a temperature suitable for therapeutic hyperthermia. This produces, in effect, inherent proportional temperature control with a gradient dependent on constituent materials and alloying techniques (CHEN et al. 1988).

A number of investigators have contributed to the evolution of ferroseed materials for medical applications requiring interstitial heating. BURTON et al. (1966), WALKER and BURTON (1966), MERRY et al. (1973), and MOIDEL et al. (1976) all described studies of high permeability materials such as #430 stainless steel, hysterloy, and carbon steel which could be implanted in tissue and heated via magnetic fields for thermal ablation of neurological disorders. BURTON et al. (1971) continued the development of brain implant materials by introducing the first thermoregulating seeds made from an alloy of palladium-nickel (Pd-Ni) which exhibited a sharp transition from magnetic to nonmagnetic properties between 95° and 110°C. BREZOVICH et al. (1984) introduced thermoregulating nickel-copper (Ni-Cu) seeds with steep transitions around 46°C which were intended for interstitial hyperthermia rather than thermal ablation. Others worked on optimizing the alloying techniques for improving the sharpness of transition and reproducibility of fabrication for a family of different temperature nickel-silicon (Ni-Si) thermoseeds in the range of 46°–65°C (DESHMUKH et al. 1984; DEMER et al. 1986; CHEN et al. 1988). These Ni-Si alloys demonstrated moderately steep transitions with power absorption falling from about 90% to 10% of its maximum value over a 7°–10°C range of temperature just below their Curie point (or a maximum slope of −7% to −12%/°C). KOBAYASHI et al. (1986) returned to the study of Pd-Ni alloys and reported successful compositions having Curie points in the range of 40°–60°C, with power absorption transitions on the order of −20%/°C. Evolving clinical protocols suggested the need for ferroseeds that could be used inside needles rather than catheters, so MATSUKI and KURAKAMI (1985) reported the development of high permeability ferrite materials loaded inside high electrical conductivity outer sheaths with power absorption transitions over temperature ranges as small as 3°C (−33%/°C). Recent work with Ni-Pd alloys (VAN DIJK 1993; MEIJER et al. 1995) has produced further improvement in the transition slope, with current seeds demonstrating slopes on the order of −30%/°C as shown in Fig. 13.15. While alloys with steeper transitions should improve results, even seeds with moderately steep transitions provide considerable homogenization of temperatures on the seed surface and in the immediate surroundings and can accommodate relatively large variations in applied magnetic field strength or thermal loading from tissue perfusion. The experimental data of Fig. 13.16

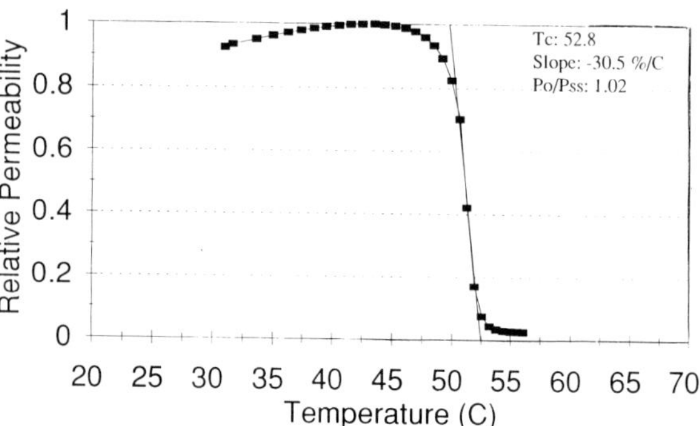

Fig. 13.15. Relative permeability (proportional to power absorption) of nickel palladium alloy (17% Ni, 83% Pd) as a function of temperature. Note the sharp reduction of power absorption (−30.5%/°C) as the Curie point temperature is reached. Data supplied by T.C. Cetas (personal communication)

demonstrate the benefits of thermoregulation obtained using Ni-Si seeds with a maximum power absorption transition of −7%/°C. Theoretical analysis by HAIDER et al. (1993) has also demonstrated that tissue temperature between implants absorbing power with a transition slope of −10%/°C drops only 2°–3°C below that obtained for the optimum case of perfectly thermoregulating (constant temperature) sources for blood perfusion rates encountered clinically. Theoretical advantages of constant temperature sources as opposed to implants which absorb a constant power per unit length have been discussed previously (BREZOVICH et al. 1984; MATLOUBIEH et al. 1984; HAIDER et al. 1993).

In parallel with efforts to improve thermoregulation capabilities, there has been an evolution of seed design to keep pace with changing clinical protocols. The first improvement over basic high permeability stainless steel implant needles was the fabrication of strings of 1-cm-long thermoregulating segments held end to end in plastic heat shrink catheters. This configuration provided flexible implants of arbitrary length with the capability of interspersing different temperature seeds, or even radioactive seeds, along the length before afterloading into the implant catheters (STAUFFER et al. 1984b). Evolution of ferroseed design continued with the introduction of multistranded wires having higher power absorption per unit length due to the increased surface area available for eddy current losses (HAIDER et al. 1991). For clinical use, the thermoregulating wire strands were twisted together into a single

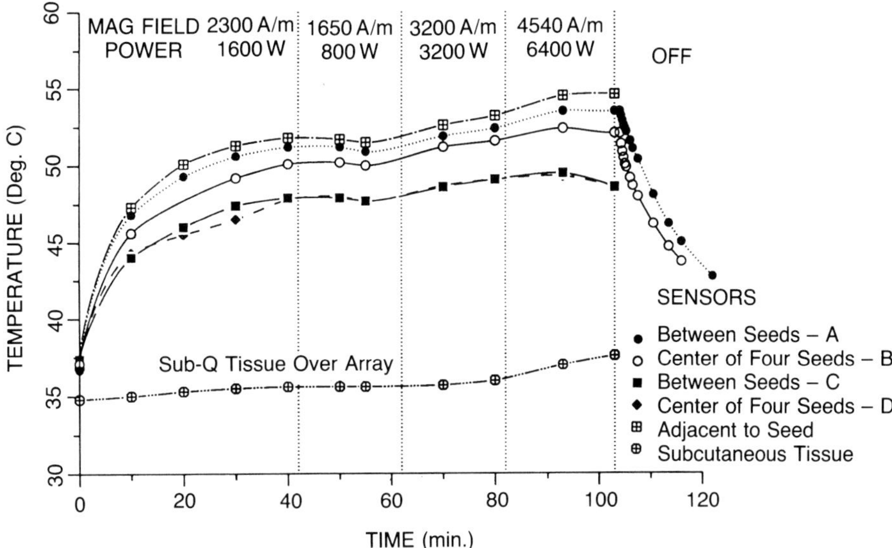

Fig. 13.16. Thermoregulating characteristics of a 1-cm-spaced array of Ni-Si thermoseeds in normal pig muscle in vivo. Points *A* and *C* are midway between two seeds and points *B* and *D* record "minimum tissue temperature" centered among four seeds. All sensors are mid-depth in the 5-cm-long array with 2 cm separation from the subcutaneous tissue probe. Note the 47°C minimum tissue temperature for 52°–53°C thermoseeds, and the minimal 2°C change in seed temperature for a factor of 8 increase in applied power

1.4-mm-diameter tumor length source, and glued to the end of a 1.4-mm-diameter plastic catheter for afterloading into the #14- or 15-gauge (1.95- to 2.15-mm-OD) implant catheters (Stea et al. 1990). Matsuki and Kurakami (1985) described an alternative seed configuration consisting of a thermoregulating ferrite rod inserted inside an outer nonmagnetic copper cylinder. This "soft heating" approach has great potential for applications requiring rigid needle implants since tumor length sections of ferrite may be afterloaded (perhaps with interspersed radioactive seeds) into nonmagnetic implant needles for localized treatment of deep sites.

The ferromagnetic seed heating technique exhibits several unique capabilities:

1. Ferroseed sources of any length may be implanted at any depth without the need for externalized connections.
2. Ferroseeds may be broken into short segments, each with a different thermoregulating temperature, for custom tailoring the axial temperature profile.
3. Due to inherent temperature regulation near their Curie point, ferroseeds act more like constant temperature sources than constant power sources.
4. Connectorless self-regulating seeds may allow heat treatments without external temperature monitoring.

While previous clinical applications have failed to take advantage of some of these capabilities, desirable protocols involving repeated reheating of permanently implanted sources left in tumor bed following surgery for combination with fractionated radiotherapy or activation of multiple drug cycles may require accelerated development of these capabilities. For permanent implants, issues of seed migration and biological toxicity of ferromagnetic metals must be resolved first. Brezovich et al. (1990) reported no clinical ill-effects after long-term implantation (14 months) of in vivo rat liver tissues with gold-plated Ni-Cu thermoseeds, though increased levels of Ni and Cu were found in tissue near the implants. Additional biocompatibility studies are required to optimize methods for permanent ferroseed implants, including investigation of heating with ferrite materials completely encased in inert stainless steel tubes (Matsuki et al. 1987; Satoh et al. 1989). Problems of migration of loose seeds from the original implant site have also been reported (Brezovich et al. 1990), so that methods of fixing the implants in place, such as those suggested by GREENBLATT (1987) and PISCH (1994) must also be investigated.

13.4.3.3 Key Developments

1. High-temperature ferromagnetic seed materials for thermal ablation (BURTON et al. 1966; WALKER and BURTON 1966; MERRY et al. 1973; MOIDEL et al. 1976).
2. Practical induction coil designs for interstitial hyperthermia applications in a variety of tissue sites (KAMINISHI and NAWATA 1981; STAUFFER et al. 1984b, 1994).
3. Thermoregulating ferromagnetic seed materials in the hyperthermic temperature range (BREZOVICH et al. 1984; DESHMUKH et al. 1984; KOBAYASHI et al. 1986; CHEN et al. 1988).
4. Theory of heat source spacing, temperature preplanning (MATLOUBIEH et al. 1984; HAIDER et al. 1987, 1993; PALIWAL et al. 1989; CHIN and STAUFFER 1991; CHEN et al. 1992).
5. Theory of induction heating principles as applied to clinical hyperthermia, frequency, and power deposition considerations (OLESON 1982; OLESON et al. 1983; ATKINSON et al. 1984).
6. "Soft heating" method of inserting high permeability thermoregulating core inside nonferrous tubing for implants requiring rigid metal needles (MATSUKI and KURAKAMI 1985; SATOH et al. 1989).
7. Magnetic colloidal solutions for regionally localized heating (RAND et al. 1981; CHAN et al. 1993; JORDAN et al. 1993).
8. Interstitial heating following magnetic field stereotaxic positioning of ferromagnetic implants in deep tissue sites (GRADY et al. 1989; HOWARD et al. 1989; MALLOY et al. 1991).

13.5 Implantable Ultrasound Radiators

Several types of interstitial ultrasound applicators are currently under investigation which can be classified into one of two basic design schemes: devices which consist of tubular piezoceramic transducers, or acoustic waveguide antennas. The general characteristics of three implementations of these designs are shown schematically in Fig. 13.17 and described in the following sections. Additional discussion of interstitial ultrasound technology appears elsewhere in this volume (Chap. 12, Sect. 12.5.4).

13.5.1 Tubular Transducer Arrays

Within the first classification are design schemes which utilize single-element or multielement arrays of tubular piezoceramic transducers which are placed either within a brachytherapy implant catheter and surrounded by a coupling fluid (HYNYNEN 1992; DIEDERICH and HYNYNEN 1993), or directly in the tissue (DIEDERICH et al. 1993, in press). The transducers are thin-walled piezoceramic tubes which resonate across the wall thickness, emitting energy in the radial direction which is well-collimated to the boundaries of the transducer length. For interstitial heating applications, transducers ranging from 1 to 2.5 mm in diameter and operated at frequencies between 5 and 12 MHz have been investigated. Power deposition from these devices falls off proportionally as $\exp\{-2\alpha fr\}/r$, where r is the radial distance from the catheter, f is the frequency in MHz, and α ($\mathrm{Np\,m^{-1}\,MHz^{-1}}$) is the attenuation coefficient of the surrounding tissue (DIEDERICH and HYNYNEN 1989). For most soft tissues and tumors, α ranges between 4 and 15 $\mathrm{Np\,m^{-1}\,MHz^{-1}}$ (GOSS et al. 1978). The radial falloff is due primarily to geometrical losses, with the 50% SAR_{max} for a 2.2-mm-diameter 7-MHz applicator occurring at approximately 1 mm distance in soft tissue. This compares favorably to the 27% SAR_{max} value obtained 1 mm from comparable RF-LCF electrodes. The power level can be controlled separately for each cylindrical transducer segment and can be varied during treatment. The length and number of transducers within an applicator can be selected depending on the desired overall length of heating and longitudinal resolution of control. The major constraints arise from the maximum number of RF lead wires that can be passed through the central lumen of the tubular transducers, and the requirement that each tube be at least 10λ (10λ = 3 mm @ 5 MHz; 10λ = 1.5 mm @ 10 MHz) in length to ensure effective collimation of the beam profile (DIEDERICH and HYNYNEN 1990).

13.5.1.1 Catheter-Coupled Devices

Initial design schemes consisted of applicators with one or two transducers (PZT material, 1 mm OD, 9.5 MHz) attached end-to-end, sealed tightly to ensure air backing, and with RF lead wires placed within the inner lumen (HYNYNEN

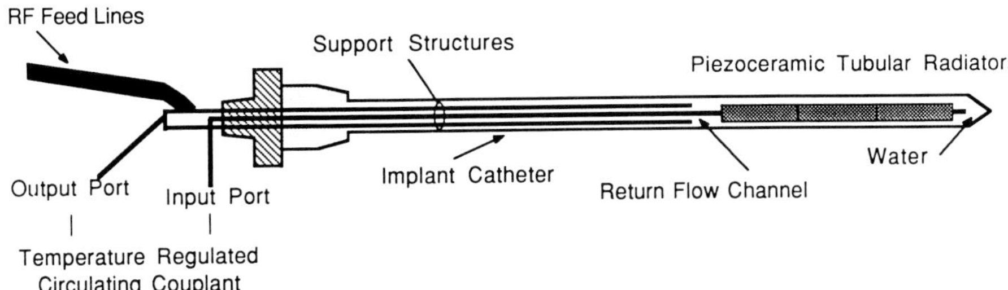

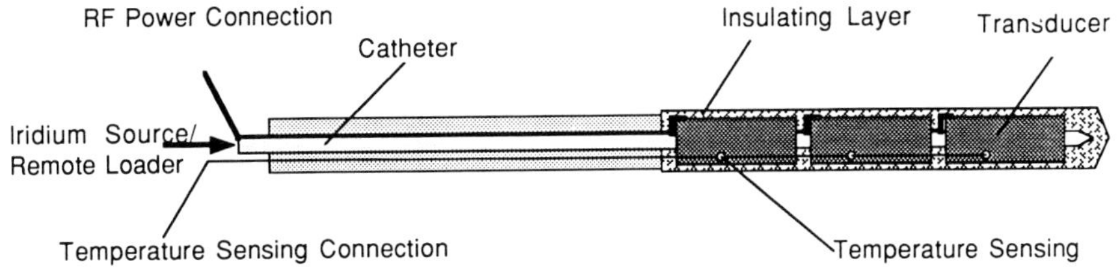

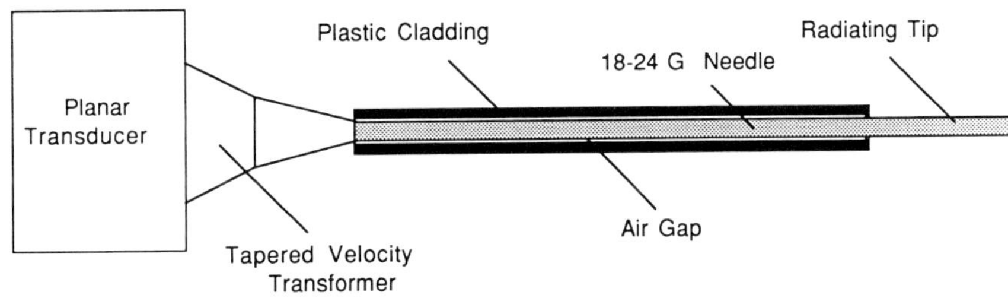

Fig. 13.17. Schematic diagrams of three types of interstitial ultrasound applicators: catheter-coupled transducers with circulating water cooling; direct-coupled transducers for smaller diameter applicators allowing simultaneous brachytherapy; and acoustic waveguide antenna with plastic/air gap insulation of overlying normal tissue region

1992; Diederich and Hynynen 1993; Hynynen and Davis 1993). These applicators could be placed either within open-end catheters having temperature-controlled water circulated through the catheter, or within a closed-end catheter filled with static water. Devices with temperature-controlled circulating fluid to couple the ultrasound energy and control temperature of the catheter–tissue interface demonstrated improved heating distributions. A modified design consisting of 1.5-mm-diameter PZT tubular radiators (8–11 MHz) mounted in semiflexible segmented arrays was described (Diederich et al. 1993; Diederich in press), as shown schematically in Fig. 13.17. Separate channels for the circulating water coolant and electrical connections to the transducers and thermocouples were integrated within the support structure to enable insertion of the entire assembly into a thin-walled 14-gauge closed-end implant catheter.

Theoretical simulations of tissue temperature distributions from these multielement ultrasound applicators have clearly demonstrated that catheters may be spaced further apart than other interstitial techniques to cover a given implant volume due to increased radial penetration of energy from each source (Diederich and Hynynen 1993; Diederich et al. 1993; Diederich in press). The simulations indicate that for typical 2-cm applicator spacing in a 2×2 implant array, T_{90} temperatures $\geqslant 42°C$ can be obtained within the array for a $T_{max} \leqslant 45°C$ using 5- to 9-MHz ultrasound applicators in high perfusion tissue ($10\,kg\,m^{-1}\,s^{-1}$). The simulations also demonstrate the potential improvement in volume heating uniformity that is possible from individual control of power to each segment of the multielement applicators, as illustrated in Fig. 13.18. Simulated heating characteristics were verified with measurements of acoustic parameters and temperature distributions in water, in in vitro perfused tissue phantoms, and in spontaneous canine tumors (HYNYNEN 1992; DIEDERICH et al. 1993; HYNYNEN and DAVIS 1993; DIEDERICH in press). Measurements of relative pressure squared distributions in degassed water have demonstrated the effective collimation of beam patterns and the ability to control longitudinal power distributions of tubular transducer linear array applicators (Fig. 13.19A). The pressure-squared measurements are proportional to SAR and are useful for determining the shape of the energy deposition in tissue. The diffraction peaks prominent in pressure-squared distributions will be thermally smeared in perfused tissue so as to produce significantly more uniform temperature distributions, as shown in Fig. 13.19B. Additional in vitro perfused phantom studies by this group have demonstrated that therapeutic temperature distributions are still possible using larger implant array spacings up to 2.5–3.0 cm. Although transducer power requirements increase dramatically for larger array spacing, current 1.5-mm-diameter tubes can provide almost 5 W per cm length, which should be sufficient to produce therapeutic temperatures in tissues of moderate to high perfusion (5–8 $kg\,m^{-3}s^{-1}$) (DIEDERICH et al. 1993; DIEDERICH in press).

While feasibility has clearly been demonstrated, several technical challenges remain before widespread clinical use is practical. First, a very tight tolerance on the variation of tube wall thickness is

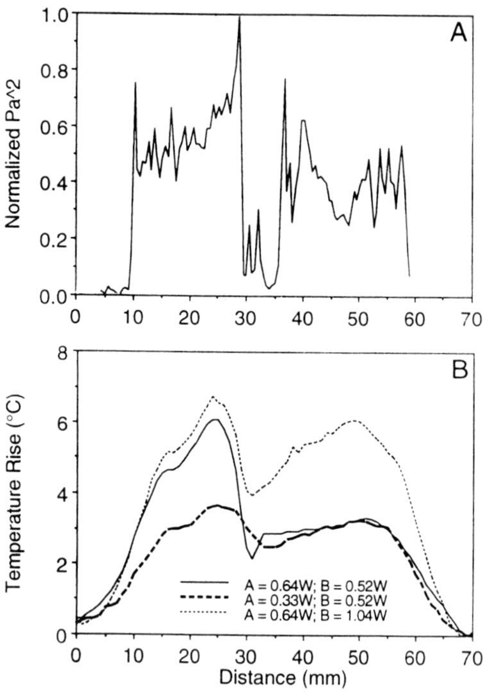

Fig. 13.19. A Relative pressure squared distributions in water along a multiple-element linear array ultrasound applicator with two 1.0-mm-OD × 2.5 cm-long PZT-5 transducers. **B** Temperature distribution along the same applicator measured in a perfused in vitro tissue phantom 5 mm from the applicator. Note significant thermal smearing of intensity peaks from thermal conduction, and minor differences in transducer efficiency which required different power levels (*A*, left element; *B* right element) for equal power deposition Reproduced with permission, All rights reserved (from HYNYNEN and DAVIS 1993)

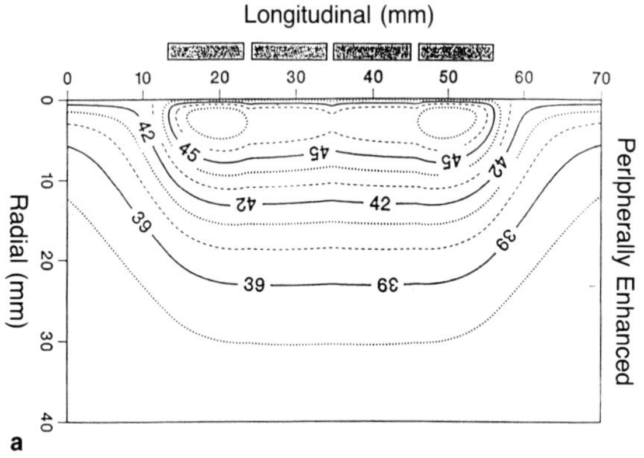

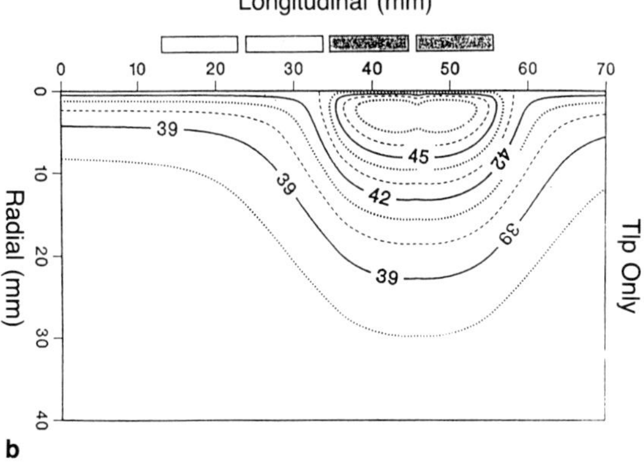

Fig. 13.18. Simulated temperature distributions along the length of a four-element catheter-coupled ultrasound applicator (1.5 mm OD × 1.0-cm-long tubular transducer @7.0 MHz, 2.2-mm-OD catheter, perfusion 2.0 $kg\,m^{-3}s^{-1}$). Applied power levels to the four elements were: **(a)** peripherally enhanced distribution (100%, 70%, 70%, 100%) and **(b)** tip heating only distribution (0%, 0%, 100%, 100%)

required during fabrication to ensure high efficiency and uniformity of beam distribution around the tube circumference as well as along the length. Tubes with sufficient uniformity have been tested but are not easily obtained from manufacturers due to production difficulties and low yields. Before ultrasound array applicators can be used clinically, RF systems with a large number of 10- to 15-W power amplifiers and independently adjustable frequency sources will be required to provide power for arrays of multielement applicators.

13.5.1.2 Direct-Coupled Devices

Diederich et al. (1993, in press) have described an alternative "direct-coupled" applicator design for applying heat simultaneously with standard Ir-192 brachytherapy (Fig. 13.17, middle). In this design, the transducer elements themselves form the outer wall of the applicator (with biologically and acoustically compatible thin insulation coating), for direct contact with the tumor. A catheter compatible with standard brachytherapy sources and remote afterloading devices forms the inner lumen of the tubular elements. Miniature thermocouple sensors are located on the surface of each transducer to monitor tissue interface temperatures. Due to the location of sensors on the applicator wall, effective thermal conductivity and blood perfusion estimates may be obtained in a manner similar to that described by BABBS et al. (1990) and DEFORD et al. (1991a) for resistance wire heaters. Simulations by DIEDERICH (in press) have demonstrated that these ultrasound devices can produce therapeutic temperature elevations up to 8 mm from the applicator surface. Preliminary experiments have verified that higher quality tubes capable of circumferentially uniform beam distributions are more easily obtained at this larger diameter. Heating performance of noncooled direct-coupled devices is highly sensitive to acoustic efficiency, however, since transducer self-heating reduces the effective radial penetration for a given T_{max} at the transducer surface. Current fabrication techniques provide acoustic efficiencies of 50%–70%.

13.5.2 Acoustic Waveguide Antenna

JAROSZ (1990, 1991) described a novel acoustic waveguide antenna design consisting of a 19-gauge needle coupled via a "tapered velocity transformer" to a 1-MHz, 1.3-cm-diameter planar disk piezoceramic transducer located outside the tissue (Fig. 13.17, bottom). The hypodermic needle was clad in plastic shrouding to prevent acoustic emissions except at the distal portion, which was left exposed. The length of the radiating tip could be altered by repositioning the plastic sleeve. Power distributions were shown to be well-collimated within the bounds of the exposed radiating section (JAROSZ 1991). Peak heating rates of 1.1°C/min and temperature elevations of 6°–8°C have been measured in vitro (JAROSZ 1990). Although the longitudinal power deposition is not readily varied along the length, advantages of this design stem from the minimal invasiveness of using small stainless steel needles for precise localization of heat in smaller target regions.

13.5.3 Key Developments

1. Design and evaluation of catheter-coupled tubular transducer devices (HYNYNEN 1992; DIEDERICH et al. 1993; HYNYNEN and DAVIS 1993; DIEDERICH in press).
2. Design and feasibility tests of direct-coupled tubular transducer applicators suitable for simultaneous thermoradiotherapy (DIEDERICH et al. in press).
3. Design and evaluation of acoustic waveguide antenna devices (JAROSZ 1990, 1991).

13.6 Fiberoptic Coupled Laser Illumination

The first use of lasers for invasive "interstitial heating" applications was reported by BOWN (1983a,b). For this application, laser light was transmitted via small-diameter (<1 mm) quartz fiberoptic cables into the tissue volume. Initial studies have used primarily neodymium yttrium garnet (Nd-YAG) lasers with a wavelength of 1064 nm, though there is increasing interest in other sources such as laser diodes (850 μm wavelength) and erbium-YAG lasers with 2094 μm wavelength (DICKINSON et al. 1991). Because the $1/e^2$ optical penetration depth of 1064 nm laser light ranges from only 3 to 8 mm for different tissues, photon energy incident on tissue is rapidly converted into heat and the principal interaction of laser light with tissue is thermal in nature

(Svaasand et al. 1985; McKenzie 1990). Matthewson et al. (1986) showed that biological effects are similar for continuous wave and pulsed laser output. For interstitial heating applications, critical components of the technology are the methods used to produce multiple implanted laser sources, and for diffusing laser light uniformly into the target volume surrounding each fiber.

The most controllable method of distributing laser energy to multiple fibers is by using multiple independent lasers. Although this method could provide the most uniform heating, system cost makes this impractical for large tumors. Alternatively, beam splitters may be used to illuminate several fibers from a single source. While this technique can produce a stable, fixed percentage of the total light output down each tube, the ratio cannot be altered during treatment. Work continues on the design of beam splitters (or star couplers) with higher power handling capability and more even splitting ratios. Current models can provide approximately ±20% output variability over the range of powers used when splitting the source into four or seven beams (Steger 1993). A potentially superior light distribution scheme is under investigation which could produce dynamic control over the laser splitting ratio by mechanically translating the group of optical fibers across the output of the laser source so that each fiber sequentially receives a variable proportion of the total output. For any of these distribution schemes, laser light is coupled to tissue at the end of the optical fiber as it emerges from the armor clad waveguide "light pipe." The light may be spread over a larger surface area by removing some of the protective cladding around the fiber tip section to let light escape back along the exposed fiber surface as well as from the open end. In order to diffuse the laser light more uniformly at the tip, several groups have investigated the use of diffusing crystals such as frosted quartz (Hashimoto et al. 1988; Nolsoe et al. 1992) and artificial sapphire (Daikuzono et al. 1987; Kanemaki et al. 1988; Panjehpour et al. 1990).

Due to the rapid falloff of SAR in tissue, thermal gradients are extremely steep around each fiber, especially for high-power short-duration laser applications which allow less time for thermal diffusion. Matthewson et al. (1987) reported temperatures as high as 100°C at the fiber surface to produce 43°–45°C at a radial distance of 8 mm from a single fiber. Steger (1993) estimated that fiber tip temperatures as high as 350°C are likely from the higher power laser sources. Thus, experimental work with "interstitial laser hyperthermia" (ILH) has focused primarily on the production of in situ necrosis (thermal ablation), rather than traditional interstitial hyperthermia within an array of sources <45°–55°C. Results of thermal ablation studies using interstitial, intracavitary, or intraoperative exposure have been reviewed recently (Steger 1993). Panjehpour et al. (1990) have reported the only work to date on controlled interstitial laser hyperthermia, in their investigation of heating dog muscle in vivo with an optical fiber-mounted 1.3-cm-long frosted synthetic sapphire diffusing tip. Using 3–5 W for 20–30 min, they reported satisfactory hyperthermia of cylindrical tissue volumes up to 3.5 cm^3 but concluded that larger diffuser crystals and multilaser sources were necessary for heating more realistically sized tumors. To date, only the thermal ablation work has continued into the human clinic (Masters et al. 1992).

13.6.1 Key Developments

1. Application of lasers to interstitial heating via fiberoptic cables (Bown 1983a,b) with control feedback for limiting temperature to hyperthermic range (Panjehpour et al. 1990).
2. Crystal diffuser tips for dispersing laser energy more uniformly from the fiber tip (Daikuzono et al. 1987; Kanemaki et al. 1988; Panjehpour et al. 1990).

13.7 Modality Selection Criteria

Interstitial hyperthermia treatment protocols vary widely between institutions as well as for different implant sites in the body. Some clinical situations demand stiff metal needles for accurate geometric implantation of deep tissue sites while others require flexible plastic catheters for improved patient comfort. The largest variables in determining optimum treatment configurations are tumor location and tissue properties, which vary from small <2 cm^3 lesions (Sneed et al. 1992) to large masses >200 cm^3 located either superficially or deep within the body (Vora et al. 1982; Stea et al. 1992). Temperature distributions vary not only from nonuniform power deposition in heterogeneous tissues but also from dynamic changes in blood perfusion during treatment. While providing overlapping capabilities, the present armamentarium of interstitial heating systems provides extremely useful flexibility of technical approach for the wide range of clinical treatment conditions. Although other combinations may exist, Table 13.3 presents a general guideline for matching current treatment protocols with most appropriate interstitial heating equipment in terms of the compatibility of devices with clinical procedures.

Considering heating performance capabilities, there are a number of differences in operational characteristics which further delineate the selection of best heating modality for each site. Figure 13.20 shows a direct comparison of radial temperature profiles obtained from 2.2-mm-OD interstitial sources using RF, microwave, ultrasound, and thermal conduction technologies, with the addition of surface cooling where possible. These one-dimensional thermal simulations were obtained using the bioheat transfer equation and theoretical expressions for SAR from RF-LCF electrode (MECHLING and STROHBEHN 1986), MW dipole–junction plane (B.S. Trembly, personal communication), and US transducer (DIEDERICH and HYNYNEN 1993) sources. While the radial penetration of effective heating from a single source is expanded significantly for water-cooled RF, MW, and US sources, there are a number of advantages to be gained from the use of hot source technologies which make arrays of thermal conduction sources a reasonable choice for many applications. Clinical applications for each of the technologies will be summarized below, as derived from physical device capabilities.

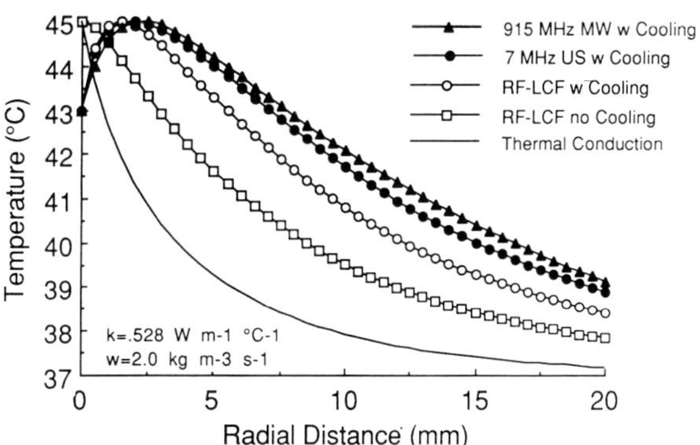

Fig. 13.20. Simulations of radial temperature gradients from single 2.2-mm-OD interstitial sources, comparing a catheter-coupled ultrasound transducer, 500-kHz LCF electrode, 915-MHz microwave dipole antenna (junction plane), and thermal conduction hot source. The curves were obtained using a one dimensional bioheat transfer equation model with perfusion = $2.0\,\mathrm{kg\,m^{-3}\,s^{-1}}$ and SAR distributions for the RF, MW, and US sources obtained from the literature (see text). A maximum tissue temperature of 45°C was enforced in each case

Because of power deposition directly in tissue at distance from the source, interstitial MW antennas appear best suited for small to moderate size tumors located near critical normal tissues where there is a need to minimize the number of implants and provide individual control of each source. They have worked well in treatments of deep tissue sites such as brain and prostate, and in sites requiring a small number of flexible and perhaps nonparallel catheter implants. Applications for implantable ultrasound radiators should be quite similar. Once the difficulties in obtaining small-diameter US transducers with angular symmetry of power deposition are resolved, these sources may assume some of

Table 13.3. Modality application guidelines: clinical protocols

	Sequential RT 30–60 min HT	Long term 2–3 day HT	Rapid heat 5–15 min HT	Simultaneous HT and RT	Heat source scanning	Permanent implants
Microwave	++		+		+	
RF-LCF	++	++	+	++		
CC-RF	++		+	+	+	
IC-RF	+			+		+
Ultrasound	+		+	+	+	
Res. Wire	++	++	+	++		
Ferroseeds	++		+	+	+	++
Hot Water	++	+	+	+		
Laser	+		+			

++, Currently in clinical use; +, clinical use feasible and practical with minor refinement of current systems

the applications treated previously with MW antennas due to the ability to measure source temperature and vary SAR along the implant length. In addition, hollow tubular ultrasound sources should enable use in applications requiring simultaneous heat and brachytherapy, or wherever precise control of the longitudinal SAR distribution is critical. While radiofrequency electrode systems do not produce heating as far radially from each source as the microwave and ultrasound techniques (Fig. 13.20), use of RF-LCF systems with reliable software-controlled electrode multiplexers in likely to continue for protocols involving simultaneous brachytherapy and long-duration, low-level heating of moderate to large tumors because of simplicity and reliability of equipment and minimal additional effort over existing brachytherapy procedures. Applications in the gynecological region are most common, with possibilities for large breast, neck, and extremity locations, as well as intraoperative abdominal or pelvic masses where uniformly spaced parallel arrays of electrodes can be implanted temporarily. Commercial availability of segmented flexible multielement electrodes should improve heating uniformity further without significant changes in site applicability, though at the expense of increased setup complexity. Raising the RF frequency to 27.12 MHz produces a number of advantages including independent source control and improved localization for applications requiring flexible, nonparallel, plastic catheter implants. DEURLOO et al. (1991) have demonstrated improved uniformity of heating between angled electrodes when driven in a transformer balanced configuration, suggesting applications in loop implants of the base of tongue or other head and neck sites.

For larger implant volumes, thermal conduction Hot Source techniques may be preferable to avoid the rapidly increasing complexity and costs of additional power generators and controlling thermometry for long multielement RF, MW, or US sources. Feedback control routines based on estimations of minimum tissue temperature derived from real time electrode power and temperature measurements have been implemented for the DC resistance wire technique suggesting potential tissue temperature control advantages over the other Hot Source techniques. Additionally, the commercial implementation of resistance wire technology has been demonstrated to provide reliable control for long-duration heat treatments applied simulaneously with radiation from sources within the coiled wire applicators. Applications for this "constant power" source technology include any size tumor of low to moderate perfusion that can be implanted with a densely spaced array of sources extending just beyond the outer tumor margin. Initial success in treating brain tumors suggests use in any implant site allowing densely spaced arrays. Ferromagnetic sources are now available in a variety of configurations including catheter-encased segmented ferroseed strings, stranded wires, and ferrite core activated metal needles, all of which provide accurate localization of heating to any size tumor at any depth in the body without the need for external connections other than minimal thermometry verification of minimum tissue temperatures. Some applications may benefit from the self-thermoregulation capabilities of Curie point ferroseeds which help homogenize temperature along the implant length even in nonparallel implants of heterogeneous tissue. While recent work has produced materials with steeper transitions of power absorption up to 30%/°C, the implants have not yet been proven sufficiently reliable to completely eliminate temperature monitoring. Combination with a noninvasive monitoring capability such as microwave radiometry or inductively coupled passive temperature implants may facilitate use in unique applications such as permanent implantation of radioactive ferroseed sources that can be heated repeatedly following surgery. Applications should continue in large-volume implants such as GYN, intact breast, and extremity, and eventually in permanent implants of difficult-to-reach sites such as brain, base of skull, and prostate. While there are no obvious unique applications for the hot water technique, clinical use of this technology should continue to expand due to simplicity of operation, availability of commercial equipment, and advantages of true constant temperature sources. Applications should be similar to those treated with ferroseed and resistance wire techniques. Because of developments supported by other medical applications such as interstitial and intracavitary thermal ablation, laser hyperthermia systems should continue to evolve, particularly for applications involving simultaneous heat and photodynamic therapy of small regions (WALDOW et al. 1985; MANG 1990; PANJEHPOUR et al. 1990) since both treatments employ the same equipment. These general characteristics of site applicability are summarized in Table 13.4, which lists general characteristics at the top and additional characteristics specific to each sub-heading toward the bottom.

Table 13.5 presents a comparative evaluation of the relative strengths and weaknesses of the above-named interstitial heating techniques for a list of 15 important characteristics of heating performance. In this chart, ratings are given separately for phase-modulated dipole and helical coil antenna arrays, and RF electrodes are split into separate categories for rigid needle and segmented water-cooled LCF electrodes, and capacitively coupled RF electrodes. These subjective ratings are intended to serve as a concise reference of relative heating performance for the different modalities and to facilitate identification of the most appropriate technique for each desired characteristic or group of characteristics.

13.8 Conclusions

The last decade has produced rapid progress in almost all the interstitial technology fields. Important technical advances are summarized in Table 13.6. Since companies have been slow to commercialize new developments, there are a number of significant improvements that must still be advanced from laboratory to clinical practice. Commercial implementation of these recent developments should facilitate increased use of treatment approaches that have great potential for increased local tumor toxicity, including simultaneous, long-duration interstitial heat and brachytherapy, permanent thermobrachytherapy implants of tumor bed following incomplete surgery, and heat with chemotherapy delivered either systemically, interstitially, or via liposomes for enhancement of local drug concentration. While engineering development is likely to continue in several of the fields due to ongoing in-house investigations, existing clinical systems involving resistively and capacitively coupled RF electrodes, microwave antenna, ferroseed, hot water, and resistance wire technologies are already capable of producing relatively uniform, well-localized hyperthermia of most deep tissue sites and are available for distribution to additional hyperthermia treatment facilities in current form. Ultrasound transducer linear array applicators should be available soon. Due to recently added capabilities, these interstitial heating technologies are primed and ready to begin new protocols aimed at maximizing the therapeutic potential of combined heat, radiation, and chemotherapy in the treatment of well-localized nonsuperficial disease.

13.9 Summary

- There are nine interstitial heating technologies with functional equipment systems in at least one institution. Some are still under development and require dedicated research personnel for safe operation while others are in routine clinical use.
- Past technical innovations in each field are summarized in Table 13.6 and guidelines for appropriate clinical use of the modalities in Tables 13.3 and 13.4. An evaluation of relative performance for a number of test criteria is given in Table 13.5.

Table 13.4. Modality selection criteria: site applicability

MW and US	RF electrodes	Hot Sources	
Small volume, any depth	Moderate volume, any depth	Any volume or depth	
Wider spacing allowed	Variable axial SAR	Variable axial SAR (except hot water)	
Nonparallel implants	Simultaneous HT/rads	Nonparallel implants allowed	
High perfusion tissues	Moderate perfusion tissues	Low–moderate perfusion tissues	
Implant inside margin	Implant to margin	Must implant outside margin	
Independent control possible		Knowledge/control of maximum tissue temperature	
US transducers	*LCF*	*Ferroseeds*	*Hot water*
Simultaneous HT/rads	Template and needles	Permanent implants	Localization more difficult
Variable axial SAR	Parallel equal length pairs		
Variable angular SAR	*CC-RF*	*DC wires*	*Laser*
	Nonparallel implants	Simultaneous HT/rads	Small volumes
	Independent control possible	Predicted T_{min} feedback	Simultaneous HT/PDT

Table 13.5. Comparative evaluation of heating performance characteristics

Performance characteristic	MW Dipole Phase-Mod	MW Helical Coil	RF LCF	Segmented LCF Water Cooled	CC-RF	Hot Water Tubes	Ferroseeds	Resistance Wires	Laser Crystals	Segmented US Water Cooled
Implant density requirements	++	+	−	−	+	−−	−−	−−	−−	++
Need for parallel implant alignment	+	++	−−	+	+	+	+	−	−	++
Insertion depth independence	−−	+	−	++	+	−	++	++	++	++
Knowledge of tissue T_{max}	−−	−−	−	−−	−	++	+	++	+	−−
Knowledge of tissue T_{min}	−−	−−	−	−−	−	+	+	+	+	−−
Current accuracy of 3D treatment planning	+	−−	−	+	+	++	++	++	−−	+
Potential accuracy of 3D treatment planning	+	+	+	+	+	++	++	++	+	++
Flexibility of possible heating lengths	−−	+	−	++	+	−	++	++	−−	++
Tip heating, axial uniformity	−−	+	−	++	+	−	+	−	−	++
Heating outside implant boundaries	++	+	−−	+	+	−−	−−	−−	−−	++
Expense, complexity of system	−−	−	+	−−	−	++	−	++	+	−−
Setup/planning/connections	−−	−	+	−−	+	+	++	++	++	−−
Thermometry requirements	−	−	+	−	−	+	++	++	+	−
Adjustability of lateral SAR (T) uniformity	++	+	+	+	+	−−	−	+	−	+
Adjustability of axial SAR (T) uniformity	−−	+[a]	−[a]	++	+[a]	−−	+[a]	+[a]	−−	++
Ease of real time control of array heating uniformity	−−	−[a]	−[a]	++	−[a]	−−	−[a]	−[a]	−−	++

++, Strong advantage of technique; +, advantage of technique; −, disadvantage of technique; −−, strong disadvantage of technique

[a] By replacing with a source of different temperature or heating length during treatment

Table 13.6. Abbreviated summary of technical innovations

MW antennas	*RF electrodes*	*Ferroseeds*	*Resistance Wires*
7-cm-long dipole antennas	Solid needle arrays, 1 source	Solid ferromagnetic needles	Embedded thermometry
Dipoles with chokes	Multiplexed power distribution	Thermoregulating materials	Hollow coiled wire implants
Large dia. sleeves/tip heating	Multipoint temperature control	Segmented multitemp. seeds	Predictive T_{min} control program
Multinode-extended length	Partially insulated electrodes	High output stranded wires	*Hot water tubes*
Helical coil-variable length	Multiplexed electrode pairing	Well-localized H fields	Single temp. water source
Rotating phase shift arrays	Water surface cooling	Injectable colloidal solutions	2nd source to cool surface
Air/water surface cooling	Prewired templates	*US transducers*	Dual-chamber catheters
Radiometry control	CC-RF needle to plate	Tubular linear arrays	*Laser*
	CC-RF needle to needle	Catheter coupled, water cooled	Variable length diffusers
	Inductively coupled RF implants	Hollow direct-coupled arrays	Multifiber splitters

- Recent technological developments have facilitated the introduction of new clinical approaches intended to increase the effectiveness of adjuvant heat, such as concurrent interstitial heat with radiation and/or drugs for either short (pulsed) or long-duration simultaneous therapy.
- Numerous implantable MW antennas are available now for routine clinical use, and commercial implementation of developments such as air or water cooling, phase modulation, and concurrent multifrequency radiometry should be available soon to further enhance volume heating effectiveness. Negative aspects for some applications stem from high system cost per channel, poor real time control of the longitudinal heating distribution, and incompatibility with simultaneous radiation sources.
- Several computer-controlled resistively- or capacitively-coupled RF systems (0.5–27 MHz) with up to 64 independent generators and segmented electrodes for higher resolution control of longitudinal power deposition are ready for commercial repackaging and distribution. Improvements to the clinical interface (e.g., template mounted multiwire quick connect for electrode connections, computer networked remote control) and enhancements such as water cooling should also be available soon.
- Several Hot Source techniques have reached maturity and are ready for new applications in current form. All are appropriate only for tissues with low to moderate perfusion that can be implanted with closely spaced arrays of implants out into the margin around the tumor. While handicapped by the inability to deposit power directly in tissue, the HS techniques have the potential to allow more accurate treatment planning based on knowledge of maximum array temperature.
  a) The dual temperature hot water tube system provides the least adjustable temperature control of any of the interstitial techniques, but offers advantages of hardware simplicity and true "constant temperature" sources.
  b) The DC voltage-driven resistance wire system is commercially available with relatively simple to use, variable heating length applicators and appears ready for new applications of interstitial heat delivered simultaneously with interstitial radiation and/or chemotherapy. New capabilities of real time power control from predictions of minimum tissue temperature between implants and independently-controlled segmented heater implants should be implemented soon.
  c) Ferromagnetic seed materials continue to evolve with improving thermoregulation and compatibility with evolving brachytherapy implant procedures. Current materials are approaching the performance of "constant temperature" sources and should be useful for applications requiring a high degree of localization with few externalized connections. Clinical induction heating equipment for producing external magnetic fields around the body have been built at a number of research institutions and appear to be available for distribution. Treatment

protocols which justify the more complex equipment by utilizing the unique potential of ferroseeds (permanent, connectorless implants with self-regulating temperature) have not yet been initiated.

- While medical grade laser equipment is widely available, appropriate interstitial applications for this technology have not been identified, except perhaps for interstitial hyperthermia combined with photodynamic therapy (Waldow et al. 1985; Mang 1990; Panjehpour et al. 1990). The optical fiber-coupled laser sources appear more suitable for intracavitary and intraoperative thermal ablation procedures than for lower temperature adjuvant hyperthermia.
- The feasibility of interstitial ultrasound transducer arrays has clearly been demonstrated with both direct-coupled and water-cooled applicator types. Commercial developers are still required for mass-producing the miniature catheter-mounted applicators and developing the associated power and control systems for driving multiple multi-transducer applicators with independently controlled frequency and amplitude. These sources should provide radial heating characteristics similar to those obtained with microwave antennas along with the advantages of very adjustable heating along the length, compatibility with simultaneous brachytherapy, and treatment control via source temperature feedback and real time estimation of tissue thermal parameters.

Acknowledgements. The authors would like to thank the numerous authors and collaborators who contributed significant research effort over the past 20 years toward the work summarized in this chapter. Apologies and special thanks also to the many additional researchers whose quality work helped further progress in the field but who did not receive adequate mention in the available space.

References

Astrahan MA, George FW (1980) A temperature regulating circuit for experimental localized current field hyperthermia systems. Med Phys 7: 362–364

Astrahan MA, Norman A (1982) A localized current field hyperthermia system for use with 192-iridium interstitial implants. Med Phys 9: 419–424

Astrahan MA, Luxton G, Sapoznik MD, Petrovich Z (1988) The accuracy of temperature measurement from within an interstitial microwave antenna. Int J Hyperthermia 4: 593–608

Astrahan MA, Imanaka K, Josef G et al. (1991) Heating characteristics of a helical coil microwave applicator for transurethral hyperthermia of benign prostatic hyperplasia. Int J Hyperthermia 7: 141–155

Atkinson WJ, Brezovich IA, Chakraborty DP (1984) Usable frequencies in hyperthermia with thermal seeds. IEEE Trans Biomed Eng 31: 70–75

Babbs CF, Fearnot NE, Marchosky JA, Moran CJ, Jones JT, Plantenga TD (1990) Theoretical basis for controlling minimal tumor temperature during interstitial conductive heat therapy. IEEE Trans Biomed Eng 37: 662–672

Babij TM, Hagmann JJ, Gottlieb CF et al. (1991) Evaluation of heating patterns of microwave interstitial applicators using miniature electric field and fluoroptic temperature probes. Int J Hyperthermia 7: 485–492

Baumann CK, Zumwalt CB (1989) Volumetric interstitial hyperthermia. Assoc Op Rm Nurses J 50: 258–274

Bown SG (1983a) Phototherapy of tumors. World J Surg 7: 700–709

Bown SG (1983b) Tumour therapy with the Nd: YAG laser. In: Joffe S, Muckerheide M, Goldman L (eds) Neodymium-YAG lasers in medicine and surgery. Elsevier, New York, pp 51–59

Brezovich IA, Young JH (1981) Hyperthermia with implanted electrodes. Med Phys 8: 79–84

Brezovich IA, Atkinson WJ, Chakraborty DP (1984) Temperature distributions in tumor models heated by self-regulating nickel-copper alloy thermoseeds. Med Phys 11: 145–152

Brezovich IA, Meredith RF, Henderson RA, Brawner W, Weppelmann B, Salter M (1988) Hyperthermia with water-perfused catheters. In: Sugahara T, Saito M (eds) Proceedings of 5th Intl. Symposium on Hyperthermic Oncology, 1988. Kyoto, vol 1, Taylor and Francis, London, pp 809–810

Brezovich IA, Lilly MB, Meredith RF et al. (1990) Hyperthermia of pet animal tumours with self – regulating feromagnetic thermoseeds. Int J Hyperthermia 6: 117–130

Burton CV, Mozley JM, Walker AE, Braitman HE (1966) Induction thermocoagulation of the brain: a new neurosurgical tool. IEEE Trans Biomed Eng 13: 114–120

Burton CV, Hill M, Walker AE (1971) The RF thermoseed–a thermally self-regulating implant for the production of brain lesions. IEEE Trans Biomed Eng 18: 104–109

Camart JC, Fabre JJ, Prevost FB, Pribetich J, Chive M (1992) Coaxial antenna array for 915 MHz interstitial hyperthermia: design and modelization – power deposition and heating pattern – phased array. IEEE Trans Microwave Theory Tech 40: 2243–2249

Camart JC, Dubois L, Fabre JJ, Vanloot D, Chive M (1993) 915 MHz microwave interstitial hyperthermia. II. Array of phase-monitored antennas. Int J Hyperthermia 9:445–454

Casey JP, Bansal R (1986) The near field of an insulated dipole in a dissipative dielectric medium. IEEE Trans Microwave Theory Tech 34: 459–463

Casey JP, Bansal R (1988) Finite length helical sheath antenna in a general homogeneous medium. Radio Sci 23: 1141–1151

Cerri G, DeLeo R, Primiani VM (1993) Thermic End-Fire interstitial applicator for microwave hyperthermia. IEEE Trans Microwave Theory Tech 41: 1135

Cetas TC, Connor WG, Manning MR (1980) Monitoring of tissue temperature during hyperthermia. Ann NY Acad Sci 335: 281–297

Cetas TC (1990) Thermometry. In: Field SB, Hand JW (eds) An introduction to the practical aspects of clinical hyperthermia. Taylor & Francis, London, pp 423–477

Chan KW, Chou CK, McDougall JA, Luk KH, Vora NL, Forell BW (1989) Changes in heating pattern of interstitial microwave antenna arrays at different insertion depths. Int J Hyperthermia 5: 499–507

Chan DCF, Kirpotin DB, Bunn PA (1993) Synthesis and evaluation of colloidal magnetic iron oxides for the site-specific radiofrequency-induced hyperthermia of cancer. J Magnetism Magnetic Materials 122: 374–378

Chen JS, Poirier DR, Damento MA, Demer LJ, Biencaniello F, Cetas TC (1988) Development of Ni-4 Wt. Prct. Si thermoseeds for hyperthermia cancer treatment. J Biomat Res 22: 303–319

Chen ZP, Roemer RB, Cetas TC (1992) Three-dimensional simulations of ferromagnetic implant hyperthermia. Med Phys 19: 989–997

Chin RB, Stauffer PR (1991) Treatment planning for ferromagnetic seed heating. Int J Radiat Oncol Biol Phys 21: 431–439

Clibbon KL, McCowen A, Hand JW (1993) SAR distributions in interstitial microwave antenna arrays with a single dipole displacement. IEEE Trans Biomed Eng 40: 925–932

Corry PM, Martinez A, Armour EP, Edmundson G (1989) Simultaneous hyperthermia and brachytherapy with remote afterloading. In: Martinez AA, Orton CG, Mould RF (eds) Brachytherapy HDR and LDR. Nucletron, Dearborn, MI, pp 193–204

Cosset JM, Dutreix J, Dufour J et al. (1984) Combined interstitial hyperthermia and brachytherapy: Intitut Gustave Roussy technique and preliminary results. Int J Radiat Oncol Biol Phys 10: 307–312

Cosset JM, Dutreix J, Haie C, Gerbaulet A, Janoray P, Dewar JA (1985) Interstitial thermoradiotherapy: a technical and clinical study of 29 implantations performed at the Institute Gustave-Roussy. Int J Hyperthermia 1: 3–13

Daikuzono N, Joffe SN, Tajiri H, Suzuki S, Tsunekawa H, Ohyama M (1987) Laserthermia: a computer-controlled contact Nd:YAG system for interstitial local hyperthermia. Med Instrum 21: 275–277

Davies J, Simpson P (1979) Induction heating handbook. McGraw-Hill, London, pp 307–340

de Sieyes DC, Douple EB, Strohbehn JW, Trembly BS (1981) Some aspects of optimization of an invasive microwave antenna for local hyperthermia treatment of cancer. Med Phys 8: 174–183

DeFord JA, Babbs CF, Patel UH, Fearnot NE, Marchosky JA, Moran CJ (1990) Accuracy and precision of computer-simulated tissue temperatures in individual human intracranial tumors treated with interstitial hyperthermia. Int J Hyperthermia 6: 755–770

Deford JA, Babbs CF, Patel UH, Bleyer MW, Marchosky JA, Moran CJ (1991a) Effective estimation and computer control of minimum tumor temperature during conductive interstitial hyperthermia. Int J Hyperthermia 7: 411–453

DeFord JA, Babbs CF, Patel UH, Fearnot NE, Marchosky JA, Moran CJ (1991b) Design and evaluation of closed-loop feedback control of minimum temperatures in human intracranial tumors treated with interstitial hyperthermia. Med Biol Eng Comput 29: 197–206

DeFord JA, Babbs CF, Patel UH (1992) Droop: a rapidly computable descriptor of local minimum tissue temperature during conductive interstitial hyperthermia. Med Biol Eng Comput 30: 333–342

Demer LJ, Chen JS, Buechler DN, Damento MA, Poirier DR, Cetas TC (1986) Ferromagnetic thermoseed materials for tumor hyperthermia. In: Robinson CJ, Kondraske GV (eds) Proceedings of IEEE Eng Med Biol Society Meeting. Fort Worth, TX, vol 2. IEEE Press, Piscataway, NJ, pp 1148–1153

Denman DL, Foster AE, Lewis GC et al. (1988) The distribution of power and heat produced by interstitial microwave antenna arrays. II. The role of antenna spacing and insertion depth. Int J Radiat Oncol Biol Phys 14: 537–545

Deshmukh R, Damento M, Demer L et al. (1984) Ferromagnetic alloys with curie temperatures near 50°C for use in hyperthermic therapy. In: Overgaard J (ed) Proceedings of 4th Int Symposium on Hyperthermic Oncology 1984, Arrhus, Denmark Taylor and Francis, London, pp 599–602

Deurloo IKK, Visser AG, Morawska M, van Geel CAJF, van Rhoon GC, Levendag PC (1991) Application of a capacitive-coupling interstitial hyperthermia system at 27 MHz: study of different applicator configurations. Phys Med Biol 36: 119–132

Dickinson MR, Charlton A, King TA, Freemont AJ, Bramley R (1991) Studies of er-YAG interactions with soft tissue. Lasers Med Sci 6: 125–132

Diederich CJ, Hynynen KH (1989) Induction of hyperthermia using an intracavitary multi-element ultrasonic applicator. IEEE Trans Biomed Eng 36: 432–438

Diederich CJ, Hynynen KH (1990) The development of intracavitary ultrasonic applicators for interstitial hyperthermia. Med Phys 17: 626–634

Diederich CJ, Hynynen KH (1993) Ultrasound technology for interstitial hyperthemia. In: Seegenschmiedt MH, Sauer R (eds) Interstitial and intracavitary thermoradiotherapy. Springer, Berlin Heidelberg New York, pp 55–61

Diederich CJ, Stauffer PR (1993) Pre-clinical evaluation of a microwave planar array applicator for superficial hyperthermia. Int J Hyperthermia 9: 227–246

Diederich CJ, Stauffer PR, Sneed PK, Phillips TL (1993) The design of ultrasound applicators for interstitial hyperthermia. 1993 IEEE Ultrasonics Symposium Proceedings, IEEE Press, Piscataway NJ, pp 1215–1219

Diederich CJ, Khalil IS, Stauffer PR, Sneed PK, Phillips TL (1995) Interstitial ultrasound applicators for simultaneous thermo-radiotherapy. Int J Hyperthermia, in press

Diederich CJ (1995) Ultrasound applicators for interstitial hyperthermia. Int J Hyperthermia, in press

Doss JD, McCabe CW (1976) A technique for localized heating in tissue: an adjunct to tumor therapy. Med Instrum 10: 16–21

Doss JD, McCabe CW (1986) Completely implantable hyperthermia applicator with externalized temperature monitoring: tests in conductive gel. Med Phys 13: 876–881

Doss JD, McCabe CW (1988) Total implants for hyperthermia application and thermometry. Int J Hyperthermia 4: 617–625

Elliott R, Harrison W, Storm F (1982) Hyperthermia: electromagnetic heating of deep-seated tumors. IEEE Trans Biomed Eng 29: 61–64

Emami B, Stauffer PR, Dewhirst MW et al. (1991) RTOG quality assurance guidelines for interstitial hyperthermia. Int J Radiat Oncol Biol Phys 20: 1117–1124

Engler MS, Dewhirst MW, Winget J, Oleson JR (1987) Automated temperature scanning for hyperthermia treatment planning. Int J Radiat Oncol Biol Phys 13: 1377–1382

Eppert V, Trembly BS, Richter HJ (1991) Air cooling for an interstitial microwave hyperthermia antenna: theory and experiment. IEEE Trans Biomed Eng 38: 450–460

ESHO (1993) Interstitial and intracavitary hyperthermia: a task group report of the European Society for Hyperthermia Oncology. In: Franconi C (ed) Tor Vergata Medical Physics Monograph Series, University of Rome, Rome

Fabre JJ, Chive M, Dubois L et al. (1993) 915 MHz microwave interstitial hyperthermia. I. Theoretical and experimental aspects with temperature control by multifrequency radiometry. Int J Hyperthermia 9: 433–444

Fearnot N, Marchosky J, Moran C, DeFord J, Babbs C, Sisken R (1990) A catheter for coincident interstitial hyperthermia and interstitial radiation. In: Proceedings of Tenth Annual Meeting of North American Hyperthermia Group. New Orleans, p 44

Fenn AJ, Diederich CJ, Stauffer PR (1993) An adaptive-focusing algorithm for a microwave planar phased-array hyperthermia system. Lincoln Lab J 6: 269–288

Gentili GB, Gori F, Lachi L, Leoncini M (1991) A water-cooled EM applicator radiating in a phantom equivalent tissue-experiments and numerical analysis. IEEE Trans Biomed Eng 38: 924–928

Goffinet DR, Prionas SD, Kapp DS et al. (1990) Interstitial 192-Ir flexible catheter radiofrequency hyperthermia treatment of head and neck and recurrent pelvic carcinomas. Int J Radiat Oncol Biol Phys 18: 199–210

Goss SA, Johnston RL, Dunn F (1978) Comprehensive compilation of empirical ultrasonic properties of mammalian tissues. J Acoust Soc Am 64: 423–457

Grady MS, Howard MA III, Malloy JA, Ritter RC, Quate EG, Gillies GT (1989) Preliminary experimental investigations of in vivo magnetic manipulation: results and potential application in hyperthermia. Med Phys 16: 263–272

Grady MS, Howard MA III, Broaddus WC et al. (1990a) Magnetic stereotaxis: a technique to deliver sterotactic hyperthermia. Neurosurgery 27: 1010–1015

Grady MS, Howard MA III, Malloy JA, Ritter RC, Quate EG, Gillies GT (1990b) Nonlinear magnetic stereotaxis: three-dimensional, in vivo remote magnetic manipulation of a small object in canine brain. Med Phys 17: 405–415

Greenblatt DR, Nori D, Tankenbaum A, Brenner H, Anderson LL, Hilaris BS (1987) New brachytherapy techniques using I-125 seeds for tumor bed implants. Endocurie/Hyp Oncol 3: 73–80

Guy AW, Lehmann JF, Stonebridge JB (1974) Therapeutic applications of electromagnetic power. Proc IEEE 62: 55–75

Haider SA, Chen ZP, Cetas TC, Roemer RB (1987) Interstitial ferromagnetic implant heating: practical guidelines for use. In: Leinberger J (ed) Proceedings of 9th Annual Conference of the Eng in Med and Biology Society, Boston, MA, vol 3. IEEE Press, Piscataway NJ, pp 1626–1628

Haider SA, Cetas TC, Wait JR, Chen JS (1991) Power absorption in ferromagnetic implants from radiofrequency magnetic fields and the problem of optimization. IEEE Trans Microwave Theory Tech 39: 1817–1827

Haider SA, Cetas TC, Roemer RB (1993) Temperature distribution in tissues from a regular array of hot source implants: an analytical approximation. IEEE Trans Biomed Eng 40: 408–417

Hand JW (1993) Invasive thermometry practice for interstitial hyperthermia. In: Seegenschmiedt MH, Sauer R (eds) Interstitial and intracavitary thermoradiotherapy. Springer, Berlin Heidelberg New York, pp 832–87

Hand JW, Trembly BS, Prior MV (1991) Physics of interstitial hyperthermia: radiofrequency and hot water tube techniques. In: Urano M, Douple E (eds) Hyperthermia and oncology. VSP, Zeist, pp 99–134

Handl-Zeller L (ed) (1992) Interstitial hyperthermia. Springer, Berlin Heidelberg New York

Handl-Zeller L (1993) Clinical experience of interstitial thermo-radiotherapy using hot-water-perfusion techniques. In: Gerner EW, Cetas TC (eds) Proceedings of 6th Intl. Congress on Hyperthermic Oncology, vol 2. Arizona Board of Regents, Tucson, AZ, pp 311–314

Handl-Zeller L, Handl O (1991) Combination of interstitial high and low dose rate irradiation with simultaneous hyperthermia. Endocurie/Hyp Oncol 7: 67–70

Handl-Zeller L, Handl O (1992) Simultaneous application of combined interstitial high- or low-dose rate irradiation with hot water hyperthermia. In: Handl-Zeller L (ed) Interstitial hyperthermia. Springer, Berlin Heidelberg New York, pp 165–170

Handl-Zeller L, Schreier K, Darcher K, Budihna M, Lesnicar H (1988) First clinical experience with the Viennese interstitial two zone hyperthermia system. In: Sugahara T, Saito M (eds) Proceedings of 5th Intl. Symposium on Hyperthermic Oncology, 1988, Kyoto, vol 1. Taylor and Francis, London, pp 814–816

Hashimoto D, Yabe K, Uedera Y (1988) Ultrasonic guided laser therapy for liver cancers – experimental temperature measurements and clinical application. In: Waidelich W, Waidelich R (eds) Proceedings of 7th International Society for Laser Surgery and Medicine 1987. Springer Berlin Heidelberg New York, pp 168–171

Howard III MA, Grady MS, Ritter RC, Gillies GT, Quate EG, Malloy JA (1989) Magnetic movement of a brain thermoceptor. Neurosurgery 24: 444–448

Hurter W, Reinbold F, Lorenz WJ (1991) A dipole antenna for interstitial microwave hyperthermia. IEEE Trans Microwave Theory Tech 39: 1048–1054

Hynynen K (1992) The feasibility of interstitial ultrasound hyperthermia. Med Phys 19: 979–987

Hynynen K, Davis KL (1993) Small cylindrical ultrasound sources for induction of hyperthermia via body cavities. Int J Hyperthermia 9: 263–274

Ibbott GS, Brezovich IA, Fessenden P et al. (1989) Performance evaluation of hyperthermia equipment, #26 AR. American Institute of Physics, New York

Iskander MF, Tumeh AM (1989) Design optimization of interstitial antennas. IEEE Trans Biomed Eng 36: 238–246

James BJ, Strohbehn JW, Mechling JA, Trembly BS (1989) The effect of insertion depth on the theoretical SAR patterns of 915 MHz dipole antenna arrays for hyperthermia. Int J Hyperthermia 5: 733–747

Jarosz BJ (1990) Rate of heating in tissue in vitro by interstitial ultrasound. In: Pedersen PC, Onaral B (eds) Proceedings of IEEE Engineering in Medicine and Biology Society Meeting. IEEE Press, Piscataway, NJ, pp 274–275

Jarosz BJ (1991) Temperature distribution in interstitial ultrasound hyperthermia. In: Nagel JH, Smith W (eds) Proceedings of IEEE Engineering in Medicine and

Biology Society Meeting. IEEE Press, Piscataway, NJ, pp 179–180
Jones KM, Mechling JA, Trembly BS, Strohbehn JW (1988) SAR distributions for 915 MHz interstitial microwave antennas used in hyperthermia for cancer therapy. IEEE Trans Biomed Eng 35: 851–857
Jones KM, Mechling JA, Trembly BS, Strohbehn JW (1989) Theoretical and experimental SAR distributions for interstitial dipole antenna arrays used in hyperthermia. IEEE Trans Microwave Theory Tech 37: 1200–1209
Jordan A, Wust P, Fahling H, John W, Hinz A, Felix R (1993) Inductive heating of ferrimagnetic particles and magnetic fluids: physical evaluation of their potential for hyperthermia. Int J Hyperthermia 9: 51–68
Kaminishi K, Nawata S (1981) Practical method of improving the uniformity of magnetic fields generated by single and double Helmholtz coils. Rev Sci Instr 52: 447–453
Kanemaki N, Tsunekawa H, Brunger C et al. (1988) Endoscopic Nd-YAG laserthermia: experimental study on carcinoma bearing BDF1 mice. In: Waidelich W, Waidelich R (eds) Proceedings of 7th Congress International Society of Laser Surgery and Medicine 1987. Springer, Berlin Heidelberg New York, pp 200–203
Kapp DS, Prionas SD (1992) Experience with radiofrequency-local current field interstitial hyperthermia: biological rationale, equipment development, and clinical results. In: Handl-Zeller L (ed) Interstitial hyperthermia. Springer, Berlin Heidelberg New York, pp 95–119
Kapp DS, Fessenden P, Samulski TV et al. (1988) Stanford University institutional report. Phase I evaluation of equipment for hyperthermia treatment of cancer. Int J Hyperthermia 4: 75–115
Kato H, Furukawa M, Uchida N et al. (1990) Development of inductive heating equipment using an inductive aperture-type applicator. Int J Hyperthermia 6: 155–168
King RWP, Iizuka K (1963) Field of a half-wave dipole in a dissipative medium. IEEE Trans Antennas Propagat 11: 275–285
King RWP, Trembly BS, Strohbehn JW (1983) The electromagnetic field of an insulated antenna in a conducting or dielectric medium. IEEE Trans Microwave Theory Tech 31: 574–583
Kobayashi T, Kida Y, Tanaka T, Kageyama N, Kobayashi H, Amemiya Y (1986) Magnetic induction hyperthermia for brain tumor using ferromagnetic implant with low Curie temperature. J Neurooncol 4: 175–181
Lagendijk JW (1990) A microwave-like LCF interstitial hyperthemia system. Strahlenther Onkol 166: 521
Lagendijk JW, Visser AG, Kaatee RSJP et al. (1995) The 27 MHz current source multielectrode interstitial hyperthermia method. Activity, Special Report 6, pp 83–90
Lee D, O'Neill MJ, Lam K, Rostock R, Lam W (1986) A new design of microwave interstitial applicator for hyperthermia with improved treatment volume. Int J Radiat Oncol Biol Phys 12: 2003–2008
Li KJ, Luk KH, Jiang HB, Chou CK, Hwang GZ (1984) Design and thermometry of an intracavitary microwave applicator suitable for treatment of some vaginal and rectal cancers. Int J Radiat Oncol Biol Phys 10: 2155–2162
Lin JC, Wang YJ (1987) Interstitial microwave antennas for thermal therapy. Int J Hyperthermia 3: 37–47
Malloy JA, Ritter RC, Grady MS, Howard III MA, Quate EG, Gilles GT (1990) Experimental determination of the force required for insertion of a thermoseed into deep brain tissues. Ann Biomed Eng 18: 299–313
Malloy JA, Ritter RC, Broaddus WC et al. (1991) Thermodynamics of movable inductively heated seeds for the treatment of brain tumors. Med Phys 18: 794–803
Mang T (1990) Combination studies of hyperthermia induced by the Neodymium: Yttrium-Aluminum-Garnet (Nd:YAG) laser as an adjuvant to photodynamic therapy. Lasers Surg Med 10: 173–178
Manning MR, Gerner EW (1983) Interstitial thermoradiotherapy. In: Storm FK (ed) Hyperthermia in cancer therapy. CK Hall, Boston, pp 467–477
Manning MR, Cetas TC, Miller RC, Oleson JR, Connor WG, Gerner EW (1982) Results of a phase I trial employing hyperthermia alone or in combination with external beam or interstitial radiotherapy. Cancer 49: 205–216
Marchal C, Nadi M, Hoffstetter S, Bey P, Pernot M, Prieur G (1989) Practical interstitial method of heating operating at 27.12 MHz. Int J Hyperthermia 5: 451–466
Marchosky JA, Babbs CF, Moran CJ, Fearnot NE, DeFord JA, Welsh DM (1990a) Conductive, interstitial hyperthermia: a new modality for treatment of intracranial tumors. In: Bicher HI et al. (eds) Consensus on hyperthermia for the 1990's. Plenum Press, New York, pp 129–143
Marchosky JA, Welsh DM, Moran CJ (1990b) Hyperthermia treatment of brain tumors. Missouri Med January: 29–33
Masters A, Steger AC, Lees WR, Walmsley KM, Bown SG (1992) Interstitial laser hyperthermia: a new approach for treating liver metastases. Br J Cancer 66: 518–522
Matloubieh AY, Roemer RB, Cetas TC (1984) Numerical simulation of magnetic induction heating of tumors with ferromagnetic seed implants. IEEE Trans Biomed Eng 31: 227–235
Matsuki H, Kurakami K (1985) High quality soft heating method utilizing temperature dependence of permeability and core loss of low curie temperature ferrite. IEEE Trans Magnetics 21: 1927–1929
Matsuki H, Murakami K, Satoh T, Hoshino T (1987) An optimum design of a soft heating system of local hyperthermia. IEEE Trans Magnetics 23: 2440–2442
Matthewson K, Coleridge-Smith P, Northfield TC, Bown SG (1986) Comparison of continuous wave and pulsed excitation for interstitial Nd:YAG induced hyperthermia. Lasers Med Sci 1: 197–201
Matthewson K, Coleridge-Smith P, O'Sullivan JD, Northfield TC, Bown SG (1987) Biological effects of intrahepatic Nd-YAG laser photocoagulation in rats. Gastroenterology 93: 550–557
McKenzie A (1990) Physics of thermal processes in laser-tissue interaction. Phys Med Biol 35: 1175–1209
Mechling JA, Strohbehn JW (1986) A theoretical comparison of the temperature distributions produced by three interstitial hyperthermia systems. Int J Radiat Oncol Biol Phys 12: 2137–2149
Mechling JA, Strohbehn JW, France LJ (1991) A theoretical evaluation of the performance of the Dartmouth IMAAH system to heat cylindrical and ellipsoidal tumour models. Int J Hyperthermia 7: 465–483

Mechling JA, Strohbehn JW, Ryan TP (1992) Three-dimensional theoretical temperature distributions produced by 915 MHz dipole antenna arrays with varying insertion depths in muscle tissue. Int J Radiat Oncol Biol Phys 22: 131–138

Meijer JG, van Wieringen N, Koedooder C, Nieuwenhuys GJ, van Dijk JDP (1995) The development of Pd Ni thermoseeds for interstitial hyperthermia. Med Phys 22(1): 1–4

Merry GA, Zervas NT, Hale R (1973) Induction thermocoagulation – a power seed study. IEEE Trans Biomed Eng 20: 302–303

Milligan AJ, Panjehpour M (1983) The relationship of temperature profiles to frequency during interstitial hyperthermia. Med Instrum 17: 303–306

Milligan AJ, Dobelbower RR (1984) Interstitial hyperthermia. Med Instrum 18: 175–180

Milligan AJ, Conran PB, Ropar MA, McCulloch HA, Ahuja RK, Dobelbower RR Jr (1983) Predictions of blood flow from thermal clearance during regional hyperthermia. Int J Radiat Oncol Biol Phys 9: 1335–1343

Mirotznik MS, Engheta N, Foster KR (1993) Heating characteristics of thin helical antennas with conducting cores in a lossy medium. I. Noninsulated antennas. IEEE Trans Microwave Theory Tech 41: 1878–1886

Mizushina S, Shimizou T, Sugiura T (1992) Precision of non-invasive temperature profile measurement using a multi-frequency microwave radiometric technique. In: Gerner EW (ed) Proceedings of 6th Intl. Conference on Hyperthermic Oncology, vol 1. Arizona Board of Regents, Tucson, AZ, p 212

Moidel RA, Wolfson SK, Selker RG, Weiner SB (1976) Materials for selective tissue heating in a radiofrequency electromagnetic field for the combined chemothermal treatment of brain tumors. J Biomat Res 10: 327–334

Moriyama E, Matsumi N, Shiraishi T et al. (1988) Hyperthermia for brain tumors: improved delivery with a new cooling system. Neurosurgery 23: 189–195

Nolsoe C, Torp-Pederson S, Olldag E, Holm HH (1992) Bare fibre low power Nd:YAG laser interstitial hyperthermia. Comparison between diffuser tip and non-modified tip. Lasers Med Sci 7: 1–8

Oleson JR (1982) Hyperthermia by magnetic induction. I. Physical characteristics of the technique. Int J Radiat Oncol Biol Phys 8: 1747–1756

Oleson JR, Cetas TC, Corry PM (1983) Hyperthermia by magnetic induction: experimental and theoretical results for coaxial coil pairs. Radiat Res 95: 175–186

Paliwal BR, Wang GB, Wakai RT et al. (1989) A pre-treatment planning model for ferromagnetic hyperthermia. Endocurie/Hyp Oncol 5: 215–220

Panjehpour M, Overholt BF, Milligan AJ, Swaggerty MW, Wilinson E, Kiebanow ER (1990) Nd:YAG laser induced interstitial hyperthermia using a long frosted contact probe. Lasers Surg Med 10: 16–24

Patel UH, DeFord JA, Babbs CF (1991) Computer-aided design and evaluation of novel catheters for conductive interstitial hyperthermia. Med Biol Eng Comput 29: 25–33

Pisch J, Berson A, Harvey J, Mishra S, Beattie E (1994) Absorbable mesh in placement of temporary implants. Int J Radiat Oncol Biol Phys 28: 719–722

Prionas SD, Kapp DS (1992) Quality assurance for interstitial radiofrequency-induced hyperthermia. In: Handl-Zeller L (ed) Interstitial hyperthermia. Springer Berlin Heidelberg New York, pp 77–94

Prionas SD, Fessenden P, Kapp DS, Goffinet DR, Hahn GM (1989) Interstitial electrodes allowing longitudinal control of SAR distributions. In: Sugahara T, Saito M (eds) Hyperthermic oncology, 1988. Taylor and Francis, London, vol 2, pp 707–710

Prionas SD, Kapp DS, Goffinet DR et al. (1993) Interstitial radiofrequency-induced hyperthermia. In: Gerner EW, Cetas TC (eds) Proceedings of 6th International Congress on Hyperthemic Oncology, vol 2. Arizona Board of Regents, Tucson AZ, pp 249–253

Prionas SD, Kapp DS, Goffinet DR, Ben-Yosef R, Fessenden P, Bagshaw MA (1994) Thermometry of interstitial hyperthermia given as an adjuvant to brachytherapy for the treatment of carcinoma of the prostate. Int J Radiat Oncol Biol Phys 28: 151–162

Prior MV (1991) A comparative study of RF-LCF and hot source interstitial hyperthermia techniques. Int J Hyperthermia 7: 131–140

Quate EG, Wika KG, Lawson MA et al. (1991) Goniometric motion controller for the superconducting coil in a magnetic stereotaxis system. IEEE Trans Biomed Eng 38: 899–905

Rand RW, Snyder M, Elliott DG, Snow HD (1977) Selective radiofrequency heating of ferrosilicone occluded tissue: a preliminary report. Bull Los Angeles Neurol Soc 41: 154–159

Rand RW, Snow HD, Elliot DG, Snyder M (1981) Thermomagnetic surgery for cancer. Appl Biochem Biotech 6: 265–272

Ritter RC, Grady MS, Howard III MA, Gillies GT (1992) Magnetic stereotaxis: computer-assisted, image-guided remote movement of implants in the brain. Innov Tech Biol Med 13: 437–449

Roos D, Hugander A (1988) Microwave interstitial applicators with improved longitudinal heating patterns. Int J Hyperthermia 4: 609–615

Ruggera PS, Kantor G (1984) Development of a family of RF helical coil applicators which produce transversely uniform axially distributed heating in cylindrical fat-muscle phantoms. IEEE Trans Biomed Eng 31: 98–106

Ryan TP (1991) Comparison of six microwave antennas for hyperthermia treatment of cancer: SAR results for single antennas and arrays. Int J Radiat Oncol Biol Phys 21: 403–413

Ryan TP, Wright W (1989) Design and performance of a high-speed driver circuit for PIN diode switches used in microwave hyperthermia. J Biomed Eng 11: 130–132

Ryan TP, Mechling JA, Strohbehn JW (1990) Absorbed power deposition for various insertion depths for 915 MHz interstitial dipole antenna arrays: experimental vs theory. Int J Radiat Oncol Biol Phys 19: 377–387

Ryan TP, Hoopes PJ, Taylor JH et al. (1991a) Experimental brain hyperthermia: techniques for heat delivery and thermometry. Int J Radiat Oncol Biol Phys 20: 739–750

Ryan TP, Wikoff RP, Hoopes PJ (1991b) An automated temperature mapping system for use in ultrasound or microwave hyperthermia. J Biomed Eng 13: 348–354

Ryan TP, James MS, Taylor MD, Coughlin CT (1992) Interstitial microwave hyperthermia and brachytherapy for malignancies of the vulva and vagina. I. Design and testing of a modified intracavitary obturator. Int J Radiat Oncol Biol Phys 23: 189–199

Samaras GM (1984) Intracranial microwave hyperthermia: heat induction and temperature control. IEEE Trans Biomed Eng 31: 63–69

Sathiaseelan V, Leybovich L, Emami B, Stauffer P, Straube W (1991) Characteristics of improved microwave interstitial antennas for local hyperthermia. Int J Radiat Oncol Biol Phys 20: 531–539

Satoh T, Masuki H, Hoshiono T, Yamada H, Takahashi M, Kimura K (1989) Experimental study on interstitial hyperthermia by soft heating method. In: Sugahara T, Saito M (eds) Hyperthermic oncology, 1988. Taylor and Francis, London vol 1, pp 848–850

Satoh T, Stauffer PR (1988) Implantable helical coil microwave antenna for interstitial hyperthermia. Int J Hyperthermia 4(5): 497–512

Satoh T, Stauffer PR, Fike JR (1988) Thermal dosimetry studies of helical coil microwave antennas for interstitial hyperthermia. Int J Radiat Oncol Biol Phys 15: 1209–1218

Schreier K, Budihna M, Lesnicar H et al. (1990) Preliminary studies of interstitial hyperthermia using hot water. Int J Hyperthermia 6: 431–444

Seegenschmiedt MH, Sauer R (eds) (1993) Interstitial and intracavitary thermoradiotherapy. Springer, Berlin Heidelberg New York

Shrivastava P, Luk K, Oleson J et al. (1989) Hyperthermia quality assurance guidelines. Int J Radiat Oncol Biol Phys 16: 571–587

Smythe WR (1950) Static and dynamic electricity. McGraw-Hill, New York, pp 397–400

Sneed PK, Gutin PH, Stauffer PR et al. (1992) Thermoradiotherapy of recurrent malignant brain tumors. Int J Radiat Oncol Biol Phys 23: 853–861

Stauffer PR (1984) Simple RF matching circuit for conversion of electrosurgical units or laboratory amplifiers to hyperthermia treatment devices. Med Instrum 18: 326–328

Stauffer PR (1990) Techniques for interstitial hyperthermia. In: Field SB, Hand JW (eds) An introduction to the practical aspects of clinical hyperthermia. Taylor & Francis, London, pp 344–370

Stauffer PR (1991) Interstitial hyperthermia: evolving technologies. In: Chapman JD, Dewey WC, Whitmore GF (eds) Radiation research: a twentieth century perspective. Academic Press, San Diego, pp 906–911

Stauffer PR (1992) Interstitial technology development: have we responded to the clinical needs. In: Gerner EW, Cetas TC (eds) Hyperthermic oncology 1992. Taylor and Francis, London, vol 2, 237–240

Stauffer PR, Cetas TC, Jones RC (1984a) Magnetic induction heating of ferromagnetic implants for inducing localized hyperthermia in deep seated tumors. IEEE Trans Biomed Eng 31: 235–251

Stauffer PR, Fletcher AM, DeYoung DW, Dewhirst MW, Oleson JR, Cetas TC (1984b) Observations on the use of ferromagnetic implants for inducing hyperthermia. IEEE Trans Biomed Eng 31: 76–90

Stauffer PR, Suen SA, Satoh T, Fike JR, Sneed PK (1987a) Validity of an in vivo tissue model for hyperthermia dosimetry. In: Leinberger J (eds) Proceedings of Ninth Annual Conference of the IEEE Engineering in Medicine and Biology Society, Boston. IEEE Press, Piscataway, NJ, pp 997–999

Stauffer PR, Satoh T, Suen SA, Fike JR (1987b) Thermal dosimetry characterization of implantable helical coil microwave antennas. In: Leinberger J (eds) Proceedings of Ninth Annual Conference of the IEEE Engineering in Medicine and Biology Society, Boston. IEEE Press, Piscataway, NJ, pp 1633–1635

Stauffer PR, Sneed PK, Suen SA et al. (1989) Comparative thermal dosimetry of interstitial microwave and radiofrequency-LCF hyperthermia. Int J Hyperthermia 5: 307–318

Stauffer PR, Sneed PK, Hashemi H, Phillips TL (1994) Practical induction heating coil designs for clinical hyperthermia with ferromagnetic implants. IEEE Trans Biomed Eng 41(1): 17–28

Stea B, Cetas TC, Cassady JR et al. (1990) Interstitial thermoradiotherapy of brain tumors: preliminary results of a phase I clinical trial. Int J Radiat Oncol Biol Phys 19: 1463–1471

Stea B, Shimm D, Kittelson J, Cetas TC (1992) Interstitial hyperthermia with ferromagnetic seed implants: preliminary results of a phase I clinical trial. In: Handl-Zeller L (ed) Interstitial hyperthermia. Springer, Berlin Heidelberg New York, pp 183–193

Steger AC (1993) Laser technology for interstitial hyperthermia. In: Seegenschmiedt MH, Sauer R (eds) Interstitial and intracavitary thermoradiotherapy. Springer, Berlin Heidelberg New York, pp 63–74

Strohbehn JW (1983) Temperature distributions from interstitial RF electrode hyperthermia systems: theoretical predictions. Int J Radiat Oncol Phys 9: 1655–1667

Strohbehn JW (1987) Interstitial techniques for hyperthermia. In: Field SB, Franconi C (eds) Physics and technology of hyperthermia. Martinus Nijhoff, Amsterdam, pp 211–240

Strohbehn JW, Mechling JA (1986) Interstitial techniques for clinical hyperthermia. In: Hand JW, James J (eds) Physical techniques in clinical hyperthermia. Research Studies Press, Letchworth, Herts, England, pp 210–287

Strohbehn JW, Bowers EW, Walsh JE, Douple EB (1979) An invasive antenna for locally induced hyperthermia for cancer therapy. J Microwave Power 14: 339–350

Strohbehn JW, Trembly BS, Douple EB (1982) Blood flow effects on the temperature distributions from an invasive microwave antenna array used in cancer therapy. IEEE Trans Biomed Eng 29: 649–666

Svaasand LO, Boerslid T, Oeveraasen M (1985) Thermal and optical properties of living tissue: application to laser induced hyperthermia. Lasers Surg Med 5: 589–602

Taylor L (1978) Electromagnetic syringe. IEEE Trans Biomed Eng 25: 303–304

Tiberio CA, Raganella L, Banci G, Franconi C (1988) The RF toroidal transformer as a heat delivery system for regional and focused hyperthermia. IEEE Trans Biomed Eng 35: 1077–1085

Trembly BS (1985) The effects of driving frequency and antenna length on power deposition within a microwave antenna array used for hyperthermia. IEEE Trans Microwave Theory Tech 32: 152–157

Trembly BS, Wilson AH, Sullivan MJ, Stein AD, Wang TZ, Strohbehn JW (1986) Control of SAR pattern with an interstitial microwave antenna array through variation of antenna driving phase. IEEE Trans Microwave Theory Tech 34: 568–571

Trembly BS, Wilson AH, Harvard JM, Sabatakakis K, Strohbehn JW (1988) Comparison of power deposition by in phase 433 and phase-modulated 915 MHz interstitial antenna array hyperthermia systems. IEEE Trans Microwave Theory Tech 36: 908–916

Trembly BS, Douple EB, Hoopes PJ (1991) The effect of air cooling on the radial temperature distribution of a single microwave hyperthermia antenna in vivo. Int J Hyperthermia 7: 343–354

Trembly BS, Ryan TP, Strohbehn JW (1992) Physics of microwave hyperthermia – microwave. In: Urano M, Douple E (eds) Hyperthermia and oncology, vol 3, Interstitial hyperthermia. VSP BV, Utrecht

Trembly BS, Douple EB, Ryan TD, Hoopes PH (1994) The effect of phase modulation on the temperature distribution of a microwave hyperthermia antenna array in vivo. Int J Hyperthermia 10(5): 691–705

Tumeh A, Iskander MF (1989) Perfomance comparison of available interstitial antennas for microwave hyperthermia. IEEE Trans Microwave Theory Tech 37: 1126–1133

Turner PF (1986) Interstitial equal-phased arrays for EM hyperthermia. IEEE Trans Microwave Theory Tech 34: 572–577

van Dijk J (1993) Magnetic induction heating of ferromagnetic seeds. In: Franconi C (ed) Interstitial and intracavitary hyperthermia. ESHO-COMAC/BME task group report 3. Tor Vergata Medical Physics Monograph Series. University of Rome, Rome, pp 14–17

Visser AG, Deurloo IKK, Levendag PC, Ruifrok ACC, Cornet B, van Rhoon GC (1989) An interstitial hyperthermia system at 27 MHz. Int J Hyperthermia 5: 265–276

Visser AG, Kaatee RSJP, Levendag PC (1993) Radiofrequency techniques for interstitial hyperthermia. In: Seegenschmiedt MH, Sauer R (eds) Interstitial and intracavitary thermo-radiotherapy. Springer, Berlin Heidelberg New York, pp 35–48

Vora N, Forell B, Joseph C, Lipsett J, Archambeau J (1982) Interstitial implant with interstitial hyperthermia. Cancer 50: 2518–2523

Waldow SM, Hendersow BW, Dougherty TY (1985) Potentiation of photodynamic therapy by heat: effect of sequence and time interval between treatments in vivo. Lasers Surg Med 5: 83–94

Walker AE, Burton CV (1966) Radiofrequency telethermocoagulation. JAMA 197: 108–112

Wilkinson DA, Saylor TK, Shrivastava PN, Werts ED (1990) Calorimetric evaluation of antennas used for microwave interstitial hyperthermia. Int J Hyperthermia 6: 655–663

Wong TZ, Strohbehn JW, Jones KM, Mechling JA, Trembly BS (1986) SAR patterns from an interstitial microwave antenna array hyperthermia system. IEEE Trans Microwave Theory Tech 34: 560–567

Wong TZ, Trembly BS (1994) A theoretical model for input impedance of interstitial microwave antennas with choke. Int J Radiat Oncol Biol Phys 28: 673–682

Wu A, Watson ML, Sternick ES, Bielawa RJ, Carr KC (1987) Performance characteristics of a helical microwave interstitial antenna for local hyperthermia. Med Phys 14: 235–237

Yeh MM, Trembly BS, Douple EB et al. (1994) Theoretical and experimental analysis of air cooling for intracavitary microwave hyperthermia applicators. IEEE Trans Biomed Eng 41(9): 874–882

Zhang Y, Dubal NV, Hambleton RT, Joines WT (1988) The determination of the electromagnetic field and SAR pattern of an interstitial applicator in a dissipative dielectric medium. IEEE Trans Microwave Theory Tech 36: 1438–1444

Zhang Y, Joines WT, Oleson JR (1990) Microwave hyperthermia induced by a phased interstitial antenna array. IEEE Trans Microwave Theory Tech 38: 217–221

Zhang Y, Joines WT, Oleson JR (1991a) Heating patterns generated by phase modulation of a hexagonal array of interstitial antennas. IEEE Trans Biomed Eng 38: 92–96

Zhang Y, Joines WT, Oleson JR (1991b) Prediction of heating patterns of a microwave interstitial antenna array at various insertion depths. Int J Hyperthermia 7: 197–207

Zhu XL, Gandhi OP (1988) Design of RF needle applicators for optimum SAR distributions in irregularly shaped tumors. IEEE Biomed Eng 35: 382–388

14 Intracavitary Heating Technologies

D.I. Roos, M.H. Seegenschmiedt, and B. Sorbe

CONTENTS

14.1 Introduction

There is growing interest in combining radiotherapy or chemotherapy with hyperthermia in the treatment of cancer since it has been shown that hyperthermia in the range of 43°C applied for about 60 min enhances the effect of both radiotherapy and chemotherapy. Clinical work has been focused on combined local hyperthermia treatment and radiotherapy of, for example, malignant melanoma and neck nodes (Overgaard and Overgaard 1987; Valdagni et al. 1988). The main techniques utilised for inducing external localised hyperthermia involve the use of microwave antennas in various forms (hyperthermia applicators), but radiofrequency applicators coupled to the tissue inductively or capacitively are also used extensively. Another field of interest is deep heating, where microwaves, radiofrequency or ultrasound techniques have been used to reach various target volumes inside the body. Deep local heating of small target volumes can be performed using microwave antennas or ultrasound transducers in the form of phased arrays or scanning or focusing devices. Deep hyperthermia of larger target volumes (regional hyperthermia) has also been used in the clinic, with annular microwave or radiofrequency applicators. Occasionally conductive methods, and rarely perfusion with extracorporeal heated blood, are used. Whole-body hyperthermia can be achieved, for example, by conductive heat transfer (e.g., infrared light exposure or immersion in hot water) to raise the body temperature. However, many tumours are localised to the walls of body cavities and therefore can be reached using intracavitary techniques, where the energy is guided to the tumour site and delivered there. Intracavitary hyperthermia applicators are designed to be inserted through the body orifices to be positioned at the tumour site. Intracavitary hyperthermia is often combined with radiotherapy, mainly administered by brachytherapy. The purpose of intracavitary hyperthermia (as with brachytherapy) is to limit the treatment to only the tumour volume and to spare normal tissue.

14.2 Intracavitary Hyperthermia Techniques in General

Mendecki et al. (1978) were among the first to discuss intracavitary hyperthermia and to mention treatment sites such as the bladder, the oesophagus and the rectum. Various applicators and results from heat mapping experiments were presented, both from simulated body cavities and from in vivo measurements in animals, demonstrating some characteristics of these applicator types. After this a lot of theoretical as well as experimental reports were published. Many papers described tissue phantom material measurements of the power deposition pattern or the specific absorption rate (SAR) distribution, often also making reference to animal experiments. Reports on preliminary clinical trials, frequently

D.I. Roos, PhD, Department of Gynecological Oncology, Örebro Medical Center Hospital, S 701 85 Örebro, Sweden
M.H. Seegenschmiedt, MD, Department of Radiation Oncology, University of Erlangen-Nürnberg, Universitätsstraße 27, D-91054 Erlangen, FRG
B. Sorbe, MD, Department of Gynecological Oncology, Orebro Medical Center Hospital, S-70185 Örebro, Sweden

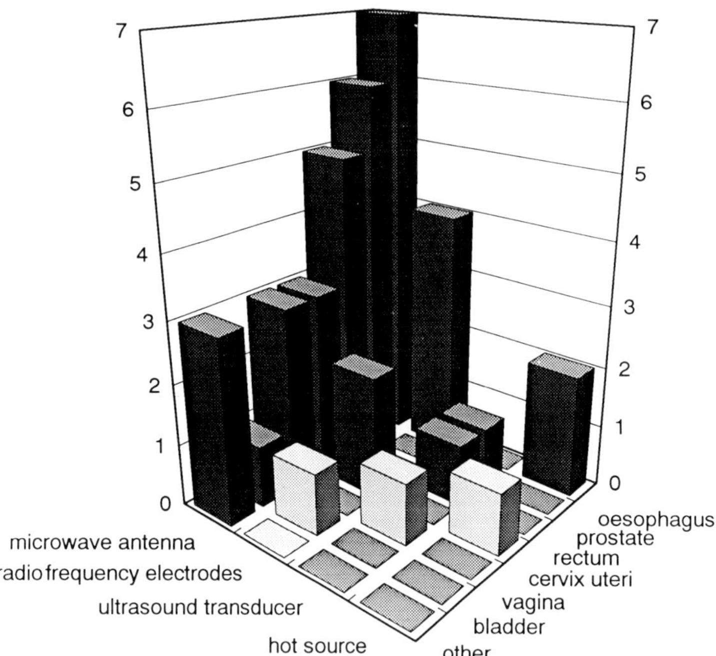

Fig. 14.1. Numbers of published papers on specific heating techniques and treatment sites. A few papers mentioned several possible treatment sites for the technique in question. A single paper dealt with two different techniques for the same treatment site

with a few case reports, showed encouraging results, and clinical phase II studies have since confirmed these preliminary results.

In the literature, various techniques are described to reach treatment sites in different body cavities with the purpose of inducing hyperthermia of the cavity tumours. The oesophagus is the treatment site most frequently reported on, followed by the prostate, the rectum, the cervix uteri, the vagina and the bladder. Less frequently mentioned treatment sites are the trachea, the bile duct and the nasopharynx (Fig. 14.1).

The applicator design should be adapted to the specific anatomy of the treatment site. Access to the tumour site, thickness and extension of the tumour along the cavity walls, and the presence of critical organs in the proximity of the exposed tumour are parameters to be taken into consideration in the design of the applicators. A specific technique cannot be expected to be appropriate for all possible tumour sites, and consequently there will be a number of different techniques for different types of treatment. Techniques variously entail the use of microwave antennas, radiofrequency electrodes, ultrasound transducers and hot sources, all of which will be described in more detail below. Microwave antenna techniques are those most commonly used, followed by radiofrequency electrodes. The use of ultrasound transducers is not yet very frequently reported on, and for hot source techniques only a few reports are available. It can be noted that microwave antennas have been used in most treatment sites and that radiofrequency electrodes are mostly used in the oesophagus.

14.2.1 Microwave Antenna Techniques

A microwave antenna in tissue emits microwave power into the surroundings and, due to the absorption, there will be a temperature increase. The distribution of the microwave power is the SAR distribution which is acting as the heat source. To obtain an efficient emission of the microwave power, the length of the antenna should be in the range of half a wavelength. The wavelength of the antenna is determined by the antenna diameter, the insulation diameter, the tissue dielectric properties, the insulation dielectric properties and the frequency. Antennas of lengths in the range of a few centimetres will be optimally operating at a frequency of 915 MHz in muscle tissue. Other frequencies can be used but the selection of microwave frequency is also guided by the equipment at hand. Since many commercial microwave hyperthermia systems operate at 915 MHz, this is often the frequency used because components are easily available.

The SAR pattern produced by a typical microwave antenna is shown in Fig. 14.2. According to

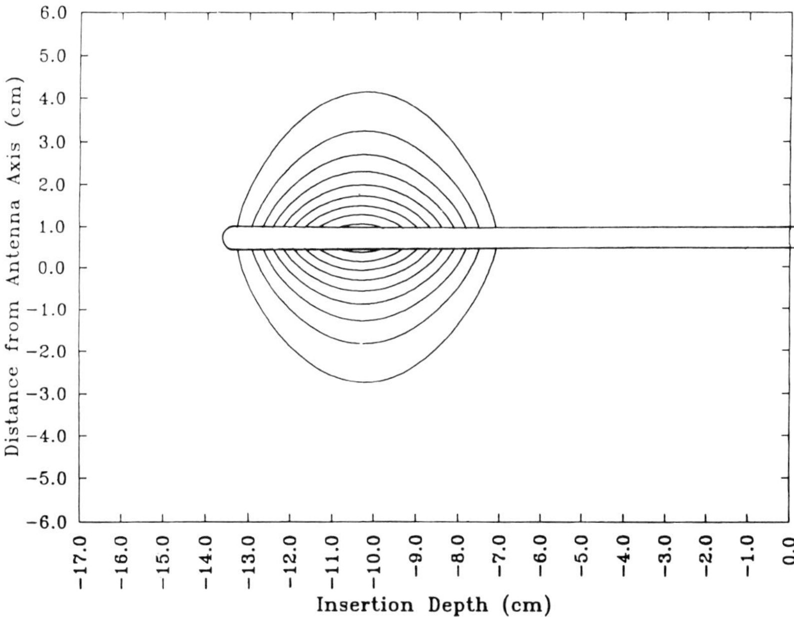

Fig. 14.2. SAR distribution at 915 MHz microwave antenna measured in phantom. The ISO-SAR lines are shown in steps of 10% in the range 90%–10% of the maximal measured SAR value

theory (KING and SMITH 1981; BROCHAT et al. 1988), the total electrical field (E field) generated by an insulated linear coaxial antenna consists of two components: the axial E field (along the antenna axis) and the radial E field (perpendicular to the antenna axis). Within the insulation the radial E field is predominant, whereas in the surrounding tissue region the axial E field is dominant. At the antenna end, however, the radial E field component can be significant, especially very close to the antenna surface. The SAR value at each point is proportional to the square of the amplitude of the vectorial sum of the two E field components. The size of the volume enclosed by, for example, the 50% ISO-SAR contour is in the range of 3 ml for an antenna operating at 915 MHz. The length of the 50% ISO-SAR contour in the longitudinal plane is typically 50% of the antenna length. Recent results (VRBA et al. 1992) have shown that the radial penetration of the SAR is limited by the cavity radius (Fig. 14.3) so that it is not possible to obtain a radial penetration larger than the cavity radius. The same situation is found for waveguide applicators where both the aperture size and frequency set the penetration depth (HAND 1987).

An intracavitary microwave applicator consists of an antenna and, depending on the clinical situation, an additional outer casing in the form of a plastic catheter or tube. The antenna can be either centred in the outer casing or eccentrically positioned to achieve directed heating (SORBE et al. 1991; MANRY et al. 1992). Within the outer casing circulating cooling water can be utilised to prevent the tissue close to the surface of the applicator from being overheated. The cooling water acts as a conductive heat transfer and has a very limited effect on the temperature level at a depth of more than a few millimetres from the surface of the applicator. As a result there is a peak temperature at a radial distance of about 1 cm from the surface of the applicator. Theoretical calculations have been performed (BIFFI-GENTILI et al. 1991) for the SAR distribution as well as for the resulting temperature distribution at steady state which confirm experimental data. Internal water cooling has also been included in the calculations.

Clinically this technique has been used in the preoperative treatment of advanced carcinoma of the rectum (BERDOV and MENTESHASVILI 1990; YOU et al. 1993), prostatic carcinoma (BICHLER et al. 1990) and carcinoma of the oesophagus (LI et al. 1982; PETROVICH et al. 1988). Besides the linear coaxial microwave antennas, helical structures terminating coaxial cables have been designed

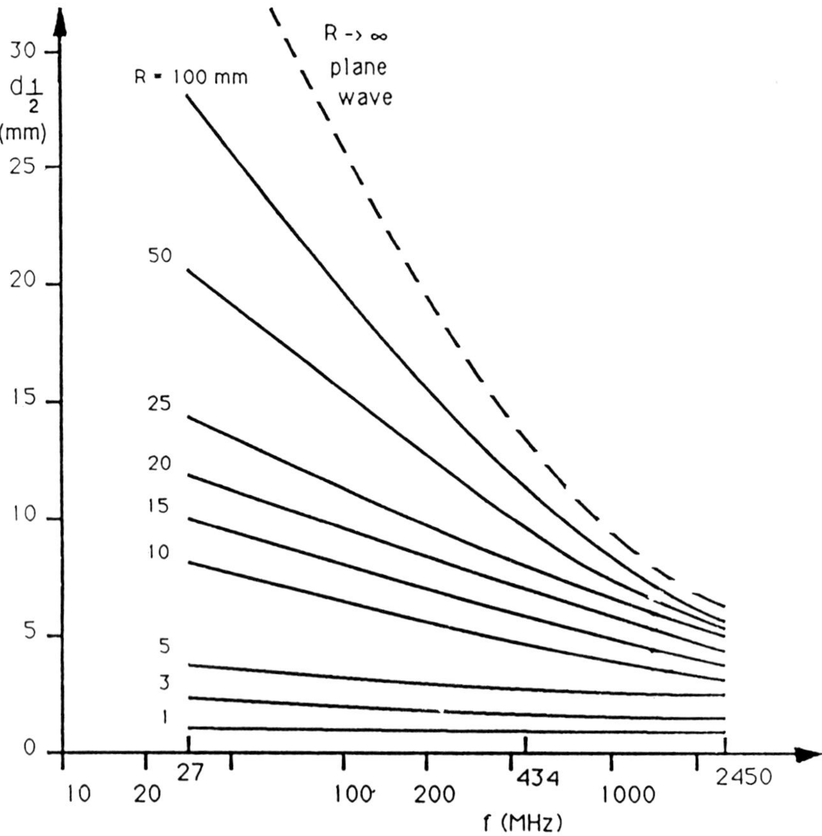

Fig. 14.3. The radial penetration ($d_{1/2}$) as a function of frequency and different cavity radius (R). (Redrawn from Vrba et al. 1992)

(Satoh and Stauffer 1988; Astrahan et al. 1991) and used in transurethral treatment of, for example, benign prostatic hyperplasia.

14.2.2 Radiofrequency Electrodes

Hyperthermia by radiofrequency intracavitary electrodes is accomplished by a high-frequency (typically 13.56 MHz or 27.12 MHz) electrical field distribution between two electrodes: one in the body cavity and one on the outside of the body. The electrical field drives a conductive radiofrequency current between the electrodes and due to the resistivity of the tissue ohmic losses will cause a temperature increase. Because of the small area of the internal electrode, the electrical field strength and thereby the current density is high here. The external electrode has a larger area and the electrical field strength is much less at this site. Consequently a concentrated heating will occur close to the inner electrode.

The radial SAR distribution declines roughly exponentially going outwards from the inner electrode surface but there is a more or less even SAR distribution along the surface of the inner electrode. The heat distribution can be influenced by the position of the external electrode. If a circumferential heating is desired, the external electrode should also be circumferential or rotated (Sugimachi et al. 1990). A good electrical contact for the external electrode is critical to avoid concentration of the electrical current, causing undesired heating of the skin. Special care should also be taken to avoid interference with equipment for monitoring physiological parameters.

The internal electrode is positioned inside a catheter at the distal end, providing a means of reaching the treatment site in the body. As for the microwave technique, the catheter often contains circulating cooling water. A balloon filled with water is utilised at the distal end enclosing the electrode (Fig. 14.4). Thermocouples are usually fixed at the surface of the applicator to register

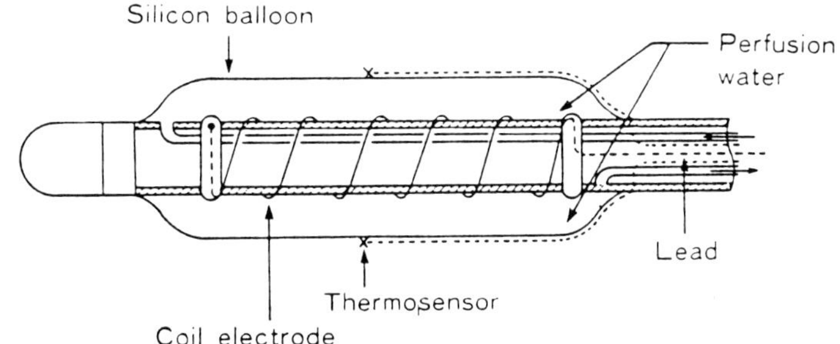

Fig. 14.4. Internal electrode of a radiofrequency hyperthermia device. (Redrawn from SUGIMACHI and MATSUDA 1990)

the temperature of the surface. However, the balloon material should be selected carefully so that no radiofrequency energy is absorbed in the balloon material.

This technique has been used clinically in the treatment of oesophageal carcinoma (SUGIMACHI and MATSUDA 1990) and bladder tumours (BICHLER et al. 1990).

14.2.3 Ultrasound Transducers

An ultrasonic transducer can be made of a disc or tube of ceramic material with a specific resonance frequency determined by the dimensions of the material. It is driven at resonance at frequencies typically in the range of 0.5–4 MHz. Intracavitary ultrasound transducers are normally of cylindrical shape and the ultrasonic pressure wave is emitted from the surface radially into the surrounding tissue. The absorbed acoustic power distribution is then acting as the heat source. The wavelength in tissue is small compared to the radius of the emitting applicator surface. This makes it possible to focus the power deposition with relatively good penetration by using linear multi-element arrays (DIEDRICH and HYNYNEN 1990).

The radial penetration of ultrasonic applicators is in the range of a few centimetres and is significantly larger than corresponding penetration of microwave or radiofrequency applicators. The rotational power distribution is uneven but this is probably smoothed out by the heat transfer of the blood flow and thermal conduction in the tissue when the technique is used in vivo. Directed heating is feasible by means of sectorial cylindrical transducers. The power distribution can be controlled by individual electrical feed signals to each element. Recently, HAND et al. (1993) simulated SAR distributions of a 25-element array, demonstrating the possibility of focusing the power to a volume at a depth of 6 cm (Fig. 14.5).

The outer casing of an intracavitary ultrasonic applicator also includes some form of cooling system, which normally is circulating degassed water. In this case, too, there will be a temperature peak at a certain radial distance. The position of the peak is dependent on the radius of the transducer, the frequency and the temperature of the cooling water and is typically located about 20 mm from the surface (DIEDRICH and HYNYNEN 1989). Preclinical phase I studies using non-focused intracavitary ultrasound are in progress for the treatment of tumours of the rectum and the vagina (LEWIS et al. 1992).

Further technical details of ultrasound intracavitary hyperthermia may be found elsewhere in this volume (Chap. 12, Sect. 12.5.3).

14.2.4 Hot Source Techniques

Intracavitary hyperthermia by hot source techniques was first discussed by the Swedish gynaecologist F. Westermark almost a century ago. A device for hyperthermia treatment of cervical tumours using a vaginal spiral copper tube containing circulating hot water was presented (WESTERMARK 1898). In modern times hot source intracavitary hyperthermia is achieved by infusing hot water in the range of 60°C into an oesophageal tube or balloon positioned at the oesophageal tumour site (SUGIMACHI et al. 1983). The hot water can be changed continuously to keep the temperature at the desired level during the treatment.

By this method the heat is transferred from the surface of the applicator into the tissue. A radial penetration of the temperature field of a few millimetres is achieved due to both conduction and the active heat transport by blood perfusion. A treatment depth (temperature level >43°C) in the range of a few millimetres can be expected but is highly dependent on the rate of the blood

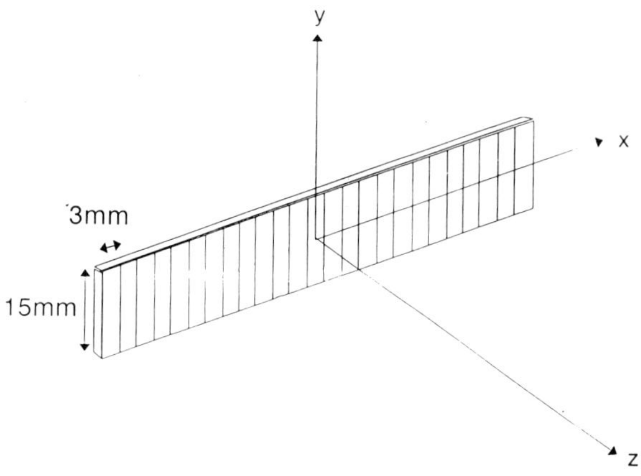

Fig. 14.5. Simulated SAR distribution in the plane $y = 0$ for an array focused on a spot 6 cm distant. The contour intervals are 10% of the maximum SAR. (Redrawn from HAND et al. 1993)

perfusion. The longitudinal heat distribution is relatively even provided that the flow rate of hot water within the applicator is sufficiently high. The method is relatively simple to use and could possibly be performed simultaneously with radiotherapy. A significant advantage of this method is that an upper limit to the maximum tissue temperature is always known.

This technique has been used in the preoperative treatment of oesophageal tumours (KOCHEGAROV et al. 1981; SUGIMACHI et al. 1983).

14.3 Thermometry in Intracavitary Hyperthermia

14.3.1 Invasive Techniques

Careful thermometry is essential in all kinds of hyperthermia treatments for treatment control and for documentation. In the case of intracavitary hyperthermia, temperature measurements on the surface of the applicator are generally performed by means of built-in temperature probes. The common types of temperature probes are thermocouples, thermistors and fiberoptic probes. When microwave or radiofrequency techniques are used, self-heating of thermocouples and thermistor probes when positioned close to the applicator surface is a problem. An electrically conductive probe such as thermocouple or thermistor picks up microwave or radiofrequency energy and will be self-heated. There are two ways of minimising this effect: positioning of the probe perpendicular to the E field of the antenna or measuring when the microwave power is temporarily off. The first can be realised if the probe leads are wound around the applicator a few turns since the major E field component at the surface is parallel to the applicator axis. The second is easily realised but compensation for the tissue cooling during power off must be made to obtain the correct reading of the temperature.

Temperatures should also be recorded at least in the centre and at the periphery of the tumour. Thereby we are confronted with a problem of thermometry in intracavitary hyperthermia for all treatment sites: the tumour is not easily accessible for thermometry with the applicator in position. This is probably the reason why intratumoral temperature levels are rarely reported in the literature. However, in the treatment of vaginal tumours, intratumoral temperature measurements can be performed using an interstitial template technique (SORBE et al. 1990).

14.3.2 Non-invasive Techniques

From the above one can easily understand that non-invasive thermometry is urgently needed, especially in intracavitary hyperthermia. Several non-invasive methods for obtaining information about the temperature distribution can be considered: computer tomography (CT), magnetic resonance imaging (MRI), active microwave imaging, electrical impedance tomography (EIT) and microwave radiometry. CT and MRI techniques are not practical simultaneously with hyperthermia treatments and the microwave imaging technique is not yet ready for use in the clinic. Consequently, two techniques remain: EIT and microwave radiometry.

The EIT technique is well suited to intracavitary hyperthermia since measurements are performed externally by placing a ring of electrodes on the skin around the part of the body where the treatment is given internally. The method is based on measurement of the electrical conductivity distribution in the plane formed by the annular electrodes (CONWAY 1987; BLAD et al. 1992). When the hyperthermia treatment is started, the conductivity will change at a rate of about 2%/°C, which is large enough to be measurable. The spatial resolution of existing EIT systems is in the range of 5% of the largest dimension of the plane of measurement and the temperature resolution is about 0.5°C. The resolutions have to be improved to a level of approximately 1% and 0.2°C, respectively. Equally important, however, is extension of the peripheral spatial resolution of today's systems to the area around the applicator, which is often the central region. Today's systems have the best resolution just below the skin and around the periphery of the plane of measurement, which is unnecessary in intracavitary applications. Since we do have the applicator located in the body, preferably in the plane of measurement and often in the central region, there will be a marked conductivity change in the distribution at the location of the applicator even without any heating. This should be used to modify computer algorithms and optimise measurement sequences so that the best spatial resolution is moved towards this area.

The microwave radiometer technique is based on the emission of electromagnetic energy from the heated volume. Due to reciprocity of a microwave applicator the same applicator in theory could be used as a receiving antenna in a radiometer. The antenna will then collect the microwave energy from the same volume as it was delivered, making the technique highly useful in intracavitary and interstitial hyperthermia. Unfortunately the received microwave power is very low, in the range of a few pW. This might be solved by the use of a suitable high-gain low-noise amplifier. Another problem is the spatial resolution, i.e., how each infinitely small volume, with different temperatures, will contribute to the total received power level. To help solve this, multifrequency radiometers are under development (MIZUSHINA et al. 1992, FABRE et al. 1993).

Further technical details of multifrequency microwave radiometry may be found elsewhere in this volume (Chap. 16, Sect. 16.3).

14.4 Summary

- Among the intracavitary heating techniques discussed above, microwave antenna techniques are the most frequenctly used to date. It cannot be expected, however, that one single technique will be appropriate for all treatment sites since there are limitations to all the techniques presented. In the case of microwave antennas the radial penetration can be insufficient when tumours are more than 1 cm in thickness.
- Radiofrequency electrodes and hot source techniques have less penetration than the microwave technique and treatment sites and tumour sizes should be selected with this in mind.

- The ultrasound technique seems from measurements in phantoms and theory to have deeper penetration and additonal possibilities for controlling the power deposition pattern. However, the technique is still in a developmental phase.
- Non-invasive thermometry is urgently needed in intracavitary hyperthermia in order to obtain more information about intratumoral temperature distributions. The EIT technique and microwave radiometer techniques might provide us with this possibility in the future.

References

Astrahan M, Imanaka K, Jozsef G et al. (1991) Heating characteristics of a helical microwave applicator for transurethral hyperthermia of benign prostatic hyperplasia. Int J Hyperthermia 7: 141–155

Berdov B, Menteshasvili G (1990) Thermoradiotherapy of patients with locally advanced carcinoma of the rectum. Int J Hyperthermia 6: 881–890

Blad B, Persson B, Lindström K (1992) Qualitative assessment of impedance tomography for temperature measurements in hyperthermia. Int J Hyperthermia 8: 33–43

Bichler K, Strohmaier W, Steimann W, Fluchter S (1990) Hyperthermia in urology. In: Gautherie M (ed) Interstitial, endocavitary and perfusional hyperthermia: methods and clinical trials. Springer, Berlin Heidelberg New York, p 43

Biffi-Gentili G, Gori F, Leoncini M (1991) Electromagnetic and thermal models of a water-cooled dipole radiating in a biological tissue. IEEE Trans Biomed Eng 38: 98–103

Brochat S, Chou C-K, Luk K, Guy A, Ishimaru A (1988) An insulated dipole applicator for intracavitary hyperthermia. IEEE Trans Biomed Eng 35: 173–178

Conway J (1987) Electrical impedance tomography for thermal monitoring of hyperthermia treatment: an assessment using in vitro and in vivo measurements. Clin Phys Physiol Meas 8 (Suppl A): 141–146

Diedrich C, Hynynen K (1989) Induction of hyperthermia using an intracavitary multielement ultrasonic applicator. IEEE Trans Biomed Eng 36: 432–438

Diedrich C, Hynynen K (1990) The development of intracavitary ultrasonic applicators for hyperthermia: a design and experimental study. Med Phys 17: 626–634

Fabre J, Chive M, Dubois L, Camart J et al. (1993) 915 MHz microwave interstitial hyperthermia. Part 1: theoretical and experimental aspects with temperature control by multifrequency radiometry. Int J Hyperthermia 9: 433–444

Hand J (1987) Electromagnetic applicators for non-invasive local hyperthermia. In: Field S, Franconi C (eds) Physics and techniques of hyperthermia. Martinus Nijhoff, Dordrecht, pp 189–210

Hand J, O'Keeffe D, Israel D, Mohammadtaghi S (1993) SAR Distributions from ultrasound linear arrays suitable for endocavitary hyperthermia applicators. 24 Wissenschaftliche Tagung der Deutschen Gesellschaft fur Medizinische Physik e.V. 20–23 October 1993. Erlangen, Germany

King R, Smith G (1981) Antennas in matter. MIT Press, Cambridge, Chap. 8

Kochegarov A, Muratkhodzhaev N, Alimnazarov S (1981) Hyperthermia in the combined treatment of oesophageal cancer patients. J Soviet Oncol 2: 17–22

Lewis L, Stea B, Hynynen K, Hatch K, Fosmire H, Villar H (1992) Feasibility and toxicity of intracavitary ultrasound hyperthermia in the treatment of locally advanced pelvic malignancy. In: Gerner E (ed) Hyperthermic oncology 1992. Summary papers. Proceedings of the 6th International Congress on Hyperthermic Oncology (ICHO), Tucson, Arizona, April 27–May 1, Taylor & Francis, London and Philadelphia, vol 1, p 474

Li D-J, Wang C-Q, Qiu S-L, Shao L-F (1982) Intraluminal microwave hyperthermia in the combined treatment of oesophageal cancer: a preliminary report on 103 patients. Natl Cancer Inst Monogr 61: 419–421

Manry C, Brochat S, Chou CK, McDougall J (1992) An eccentrically coated asymmetric antenna applicator for intracavitary hyperthermia treatment of cancer. IEEE Trans Biomed Eng 39: 935–942

Mendecki J, Friedenthal E, Botstein C, Sterzer F, Paglione R, Nowogrodski M, Beck E (1978) Microwave-induced hyperthermia in cancer treatment: apparatus and preliminary results. Int J Radiat Oncol Biol Phys 4: 1095–1103

Mizushina S, Shimizu T, Sugiura T (1992) Precision of non-invasive temperature profile measurement using a multi-frequency microwave radiometric technique. In: Gerner E (ed) Hyperthermic oncology 1992. Summary papers. Proceedings of the 6th International Congress on Hyperthermic Oncology (ICHO), Tucson, Arizona, April 27–May 1, Taylor & Francis, London and Philadelphia, vol 1, p 212

Overgaard J, Overgaard M (1987) Hyperthermia as an adjuvant to radiotherapy in the treatment of malignant melanoma. Int J Hyperthermia 3: 483–501

Petrovich Z, Astrahan M, Lam K, Tilden T, Luxton G, Jepson J (1988) Intraluminal thermoradiotherapy with teletherapy for carcinoma of the oesophagus. Endocurietherapy/Hyperthermia Oncol 4: 155–161

Satoh T, Stauffer P (1988) Implantable helical coil microwave antenna for interstitial hyperthermia. Int J Hyperthermia 4: 497–512

Sorbe B, Roos D, Karlsson L (1990) The use of microwave-induced hyperthermia in conjunction with afterloading irradiation of vaginal carcinoma. Acta Oncol 29: 1029–1033

Sugimachi K, Matsuda H (1990) Experimental and clinical studies of hyperthermia for carcinoma of the oesophagus. In: Gautherie M (ed) Interstitial, endocavitary and perfusional hyperthermia: methods and clinical trials. Springer, Berlin Heidelberg New York, p 59

Sugimachi K, Inokuchi K, Kai H, Kuwano H, Matsuzaki K, Natsuda Y (1983) Hyperthermo-chemo-radiotherapy for carcinoma of the oesophagus. Jpn J Surg 13: 101–105

Valdagni R, Amichetti M, Pani G (1988) Radical radiation alone versus radical radiation plus microwave hyperthermia for N3 (TNM-UICC) neck nodes: a prospective randomized clinical trial. Int J Radiat Oncol Biol Phys 15: 13–24

Vrba J, Franconi C, Lape M (1992) Theoretical limits of intracavitary applicators. In: Gerner E (ed) Hyperthermic oncology 1992. Summary papers. Proceedings of the 6th International Congress on Hyperthermic Oncology (ICHO) Tucson Arizona April 27–May 1, Taylor & Franics, London and Philadelphia, vol 1, p 275

Westermark F (1898) Über die Behandlung des ulcerirenden Cervixcarcinom mittels konstanter Wärme. Centralbl Gyn 22: 1335–1339

You Q-S, Wang R-Z, Suen G-Q et al. (1993) Combination of preoperative radiation and endocavitary hyperthermia for rectal cencer: long term results of 44 patients. Int J Hyperthermia 9: 19–24

15 Invasive Thermometry Techniques

F.M. Waterman

CONTENTS

15.1 Introduction

Several reviews of invasive thermometry for clinical hyperthermia have previously appeared in the literature (Cetas et al. 1980; Cetas 1982, 1985, 1987, 1990; Fessenden et al. 1984; Hand 1985; Martin 1986; Samulski 1988; Samulski and Fessenden 1990). Since the latest reviews appeared, there has been little advancement in the development of thermometers for invasive thermometry, but several papers have appeared which focus on improving the quality and standardization of thermometry (Dewhirst et al. 1990; Emami et al. 1991; Sapozink et al. 1991; Waterman et al. 1991). These papers report the Radiation Therapy Oncology Group (ROTG) task force's recommendations for improving thermometry for multi-institutional trials, but many of the general concepts and guidelines presented are applicable to nonprotocol treatments. In general, there has been an impetus to obtain more temperature data during therapy to describe more completely the three-dimensional temperature field and for evaluation of thermal descriptors which have been found to be of prognostic significance. Measurements of temperature at a few fixed points are no longer considered adequate. Instead, it is recomnended that catheters and thermal mapping techniques be used in connection with standardized catheter placement strategies.

Highly developed nonperturbing thermometers are available for microwave or RF hyperthermia which are capable of measuring temperature to within ±0.2°C, or better. However, equivalent thermometers do not yet exist for ultrasound, where temperature cannot be measured as accurately.

Thermocouples which are generally used for ultrasound are prone to measurement errors due to absorption and/or viscous heating and the conduction of heat along the wire leads. Several papers have recently been published which either point out problems in ultrasound thermometry or describe advancements in overcoming these problems (Hynynen and Edwards 1989; Waterman 1990, 1992; Waterman and Leeper 1990; Waterman et al. 1990; Greig et al. 1992; Anhalt and Hynynen 1992).

This review contains much of the same basic information on thermometers as is included in prior reviews. However, in general, there is less emphasis on hardware and more emphasis on the clinical use of invasive thermometers, including the thermometry guidelines and strategies developed by the RTOG task force for quality assurance for hyperthermia. Special attention is also given to defining the problems associated

---

F.M. Waterman, PhD, Professor of Medical Physics, Department of Radiation Oncology, Thomas Jefferson University Hospital, 111 South 11th Street, Philadelphia, PA 19107-5097, USA

with the use of thermocouples in both electromagnetic and ultrasound fields.

15.2 Thermometers for Hyperthermia

15.2.1 General Specifications

Thermometers used for invasive thermometry should be miniaturized to the greatest extent possible, accurate, stable, and able to function in intense electromagnetic or ultrasonic fields. Ideally, they should be immune to such fields. They should have adaquate spatial resolution to measure temperature in the steep thermal gradients frequently encountered in the clinic and be free of measurement errors caused by the conduction of heat along the probe.

Thermometer specifications for invasive thermometry have been recommended by several authors (Shrivastiva et al. 1989; Dewhirst et al. 1990; Cetas 1987, 1990; Samulski 1988). Although there are some differences in the specifications recommended by the different authors, there is general agreement on the following parameters.

1. *Diameter*. The diameter of the thermometer probe should not exceed 1.1 mm. A probe with a diameter of 1.1 mm will just fit into a 16-gauge catheter. Smaller diameters are desirable in that they introduce less trauma.
2. *Accuracy*. The thermometer should be accurate to within ±0.2°C at the time of calibration. Greater accuracy is desirable and achievable with some types of thermometry.
3. *Drift*. The calibration of some thermometry units is prone to drift with time. The drift should not be greater than 0.1°C/h so that large errors do not occur during the course of 60 min of heating.
4. *Insensitivity to moisture*. Some early fiberoptic probes were sensitive to moisture. Insensitivity to moisture is important because some catheters are permeable to moisture.
5. *Response time*. This is the time required for the sensor to respond to a step change in temperature. The response time is an important consideration when the thermometer probe is used for thermal mapping. The temperature should not be recorded until the probe has remained in the new position for a time interval equivalent to 3 time constants (Waterman 1985). The time constant of most bare probes is 1 s, or less. However, when these probes are inserted into a catheter the time constant is typically increased by a factor of 2 or more.
6. *Precision*. Precision is the uncertainty in the temperature reading due to "noise." The precision can be measured by recording ten readings with the sensor in a constant temperature enviroment and computing the standard deviation of the mean temperature recorded. This value should be ±.01°C, or less.
7. *Passivity*. The thermometer should be passive. That is, it should not be perturbed by the heat source, nor should it perturb the heating pattern. The probe should not experience self-heating by either electromagnetic or ultrasound fields.

15.2.2 Thermocouples

Thermocouples are commonly used to monitor temperature during hyperthermia. They are attractive because they are commercially available at relatively low cost and can even be fabricated in-house. However, thermocouples also have some distinct disadvantages. They are perturbed by both electromagnetic and ultrasonic fields, resulting in measurement errors or temperature "artifacts." Also, certain types of thermocouples, such as copper-constantan, are particularly prone to a measurement error due to the conduction of heat along the copper wire. This type of error is commonly referred to as "thermal smearing" or as the "conduction error." The problems associated with the use of thermocouples in electromagnetic fields can be circumvented by using nonperturbing thermometers; however, this is not possible with ultrasound because a nonperturbing probe has not been developed for this modality.

The principle of operation of a thermocouple is detailed in several reviews of thermometry for hyperthermia (Carnochan et al. 1986; Cetas 1987, 1990; Samulski and Fessenden 1990; Hand 1985). Therefore, only an overview of the principle is given here, with a greater emphasis placed on problems associated with the use of thermocouples in the clinic.

The principle of the thermocouple is based on the Seebeck effect, the discovery that when two wires composed of dissimilar metals are joined at both ends, and one of the ends is heated, a continuous current flows through the circuit formed by the wires. If this circuit is broken by unjoining the unheated end, the net open circuit voltage is a function of the temperature of the heated junction. For small changes in temperature, this voltage is linearly proportional to the temperature difference between the two junctions. However, when the leads of a voltmeter are connected to the ends of the two wires to measure the voltage, two additional junctions are created.

A basic diagram of a copper-constantan thermocouple is shown in Fig. 15.1. Note that one of the junctions created by the voltmeter leads is copper-to-copper, which creates no thermal electromotive force (emf). Therefore, the number of junctions is effectively reduced to the two which are labeled J_1 and J_2. The resultant voltmeter reading is proportional to the difference $(T_1 - T_2)$ in temperature at these two junctions. Thus, to determine the temperature T_1 at junction J_1, it is necessary to know the temperature T_2 at J_2, the junction formed by the constantan wire and the copper voltmeter lead. Historically, this was accomplished by immersing J_2 in an ice bath at 0°C, as shown in the upper half of Fig. 15.1. The configuration used in most thermocouple readout

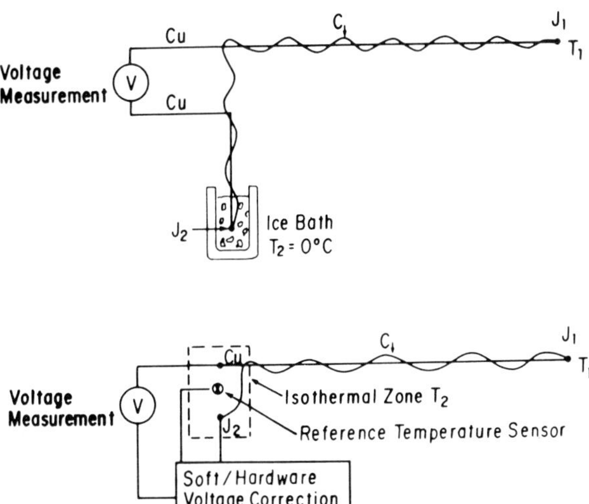

Fig. 15.1. Basic diagram of a copper-constantan thermocouple. In the *upper diagram* the reference junction J_2 is inserted in an ice bath. In the *lower diagram*, J_2 is bonded to a thermally isolated copper block at temperature T_2, which is corrected back to the ice point by computer software (software compensated) or by an electronic circuit (hardware compensated). (From SAMULSKI and FESSENDEN 1990)

units employed for clinical use is illustrated in the lower half of Fig. 15.1. The junction J_2 is bonded to a thermally isolated copper block, the temperature of which is monitored by a reference temperature sensor. Since T_2 is known, it is possible to correct T_2 back to the ice point (0°C) by adding or subtracting an offset voltage. This correction can be made by computer software (software compensated) or by an electronic circuit (hardware compensated).

Thermocouples are rarely used for hyperthermia in the United States, except for ultrasound. When thermocouples are used, they tend to be copper-constantan because this is the type of thermocouple supplied with most commercial ultrasound hyperthermia units. Thermocouples are more widely used in many other parts of the world, but not necessarily copper-constantan thermocouples. In Europe, the ESHO protocols specify that manganin-constantan thermocouples be used (HAND et al. 1989). A Canadian group utilizes chromel-alumel (type K) thermocouples (GREIG et al. 1992). This is an important point because copper-constantan thermocouples are more prone to thermal smearing errors than some other types, such as manganin-constantan and chromel-alumel thermocouples.

Thermocouples are commonly configured as multisensor probes containing as many as ten junctions (CARNOCHAN et al. 1986). To reduce the diameter, these thermocouples are often constructed using a common wire. They are then usually encased in a metal needle or sheathed in plastic. The needle probes are sterilized and inserted directly into tissue. Plastic-sheathed thermocouples are sometimes implanted directly into tissue (ANHALT and HYNYNEN 1992), but are more commonly inserted into indwelling catheters. However, if catheters are used, considerable care must be exercised to ensure that the plastics employed do not create unacceptably large temperature artifacts due to the higher absorption of ultrasonic power in plastic compared to tissue.

15.2.3 Thermistors

A thermistor consists of a bead of semiconductor material which may be made from a variety of sintered oxides. Its usefulness as a thermometer stems from the fact that its electrical resistance is a function of temperature. Two pairs of leads

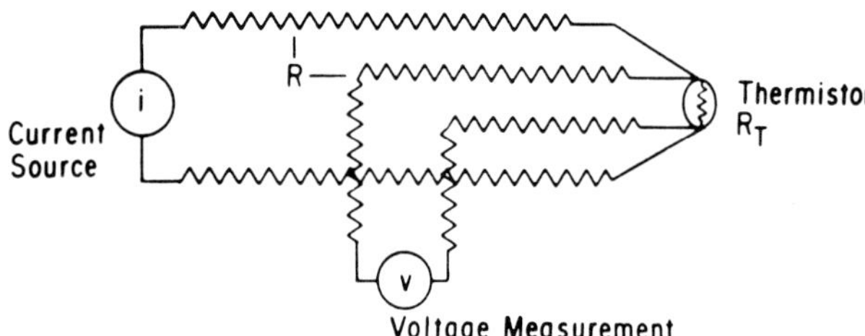

Fig. 15.2. Schematic of a thermistor resistance measurement circuit. A small constant current is driven through the thermistor (R_T) and the voltage drop which is proportional to the thermistor resistance is measured at contact points adjacent to the thermistor sensor. (From SAMULSKI and FESSENDEN 1990)

are generally connected to the thermistor, as illustrated in Fig. 15.2. One pair is connected to a constant current source which is kept small (typically 10 μA) to avoid self-heating of the thermistor. The other pair is used to measure the voltage drop across the thermistor. The resistance is determined from the current and resulting voltage drop.

Conventional thermistors with metallic leads can be used to monitor temperature during either electromagnetic or ultrasound hyperthermia, but are not as widely used as thermocouples. Like thermocouples, they are perturbed by both electromagnetic and ultrasound fields and are prone to measurement errors due to the conduction of heat along the copper leads. An advantage of a thermistor is its sensitivity. The resistance of the thermistor decreases exponentially with temperature, typically at the rate of 4% per °C. Partly because of this sensitivity, a thermistor can be made quite small, which provides good spatial resolution and enables the thermistor to be encased in a small-diameter needle or plastic sheath. Still another advantage of a thermistor is that its calibration is more stable than that of other thermometry systems available for invasive thermometry. The calibration of a thermistor has been known to remain within specifications for years (CETAS 1990).

The so-called Bowman probe is a nonconventional thermistor probe which was developed for use in radiofrequency (RF) fields (BOWMAN 1976). The field perturbation and self-heating problems which occur with conventional thermistors are virtually eliminated by using leads which have a resistance similar to tissue. The probe consists of high-resistance carbon-impregnated Teflon leads connected to a small high-resistance thermistor. The high resistance of the leads prevents the induction of large currents which are the source of the field perturbations and self-heating artifacts. A thermistor probe utilizing this concept was initially marketed under the trade name of Vitek, but became more widely known as the "Bowman probe" supplied by BSD Medical Corporation (Salt Lake City, Utah), with their microwave and RF hyperthermia units. These probes are accurate and stable, but have a relatively large diameter (1.1 mm) which requires a 16-gauge catheter. Multisensor probes of this type are not available, although BSD Medical Corporation does offer a thermal mapping system which allows multiple temperature measurements along each catheter track.

15.2.4 Fiberoptic Thermometers

Fiberoptic thermometers offer two distinct advantages over conventional thermocouples and thermistors. Because the probes have no metallic components, they are essentially nonperturbing in microwave or RF fields, and they produce no thermal smearing. Hence, artifact-free temperature measurements can be made while the power is on. Several different systems have been proposed or developed (CETAS 1990), but only the two described below have gained widespread use in clinical hyperthermia.

15.2.4.1 Gallium Arsenide Crystal

A fiberoptic probe which is nonperturbing in an electromagnetic field was developed (CHRISTENSEN 1977; VAGUINE et al. 1984) based on the temperature dependence of the transmission efficiency of infrared light through a gallium arsenide crystal. The probe is fabricated by optically coupling a gallium arsenide crystal, in the form of a prism, to the ends of two optical fibers. A narrow band of infrared light emitted from a light-emitting diode (LED) travels down one optical fiber, passes through the crystal, and returns through the second optical fiber to a photo detector. The relative transmission is determined by comparing the intensity of the emitted and returning light. Temperature is determined from a look-up table of temperature versus transmission efficiency established at the time of calibration. The relative transmission of the narrow band of infrared light through the crystal at 25° and 40°C is shown in Fig. 15.3. Note the 25% difference (drop) in transmission efficiency over this temperature range.

Fiberoptic probes based on the gallium arsenide crystal technology were originally marketed by Clini-Therm, Inc. (Dallas, Tex.) as part of their TS-1200 thermometry system. They are currently available from The Tex-L Company (Arlington, Tex.). Probes are available with both single and multiple sensors. The single-sensor probe has a diameter of approximately 0.7 mm and can be inserted into a 19-gauge catheter. The multisensor probe has four sensors, which are typically spaced 1 cm apart, and a diameter of 1.1 mm, which requires a 16-gauge catheter.

The gallium arsenide thermometry system is sufficiently stable for a 60-min hyperthermia treatment, but lacks long-term stability and needs to be recalibrated frequently. The maximum temperature is limited to 55°C and the probes are susceptible to strain artifacts. Early versions of the probe were not sufficiently waterproof and were sensitive to the moisture which often permeates the catheter walls. Water strongly absorbs the narrow band infrared light, which reduces the transmission efficiency, resulting in an error in the temperature measurement.

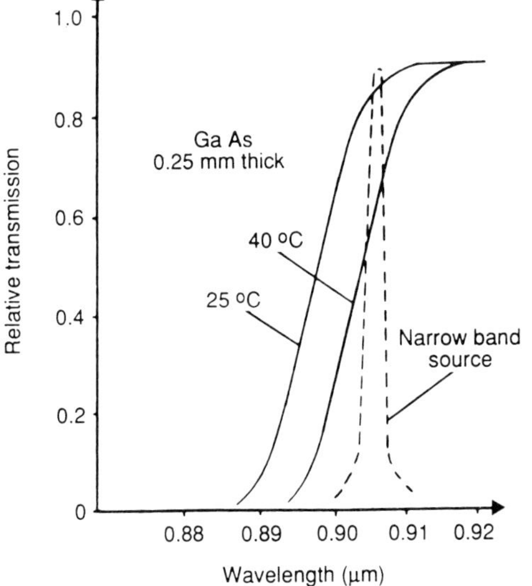

Fig. 15.3. The relative optical transmission of a GaAs crystal as a function of wavelength for a 0.25-mm sample at 25° and 40°C. (From VAGUINE et al. 1984)

15.2.4.2 Photoluminescent Thermometry

A fiberoptic thermometry system based on a different principle is the Luxtron Model 3000 (WICKERSHEIM and ALVES 1979) marketed by Luxtron Corporation (Santa Clara, California). This system is based on the technology of SAMULSKI and SHRIVASTAVA (1980) and of SCHOLES and SMALL (1980). The sensor a manganese-activated magnesium fluorogermanate phosphor mounted on the tip of an optical fiber. The phosphor is excited by a light pulse from a xenon flash lamp which causes it to exhibit a deep red fluorescence. The principle of operation is based on the temperature dependence of the fluorescence decay time, which is shown in Fig. 15.4. Temperature is determined by comparing the time taken for the fluorescence to decay from one intensity level to another to data stored in a calibration table. Because the temperature is determined from a decay time interval, and not from differences in the intensity of the fluorescent light, problems with light losses due to bends in the fiber or drifts in the light source are eliminated.

Since only one optical fiber is required per sensor, the diameter of the probes can be made quite small. The single-sensor probe is approximately 0.5 mm in diameter and the four-sensor probe is 0.8 mm in diameter. The Model 3000 is much more stable than the earlier Luxtron Models 1000 and 2000. There is no detectable system drift during a 60-min period and the long-term (14 day) stability is <0.25°C (SAMULSKI and LEE 1986).

15.3 The Role of Indwelling Catheters

15.3.1 Advantages of Catheters

At many institutions, closed-end catheters are inserted prior to the first treatment session and left in place for the duration of hyperthermia therapy, which may be several weeks. Indwelling catheters offer distinct advantages to both the patient and the physician. The benefit to the patient is that the invasive procedure must be endured only once, instead of prior to each treatment. The physician benefits by saving the time which would be required to insert invasive thermometry probes prior to each treatment. It can also be argued that the quality of the

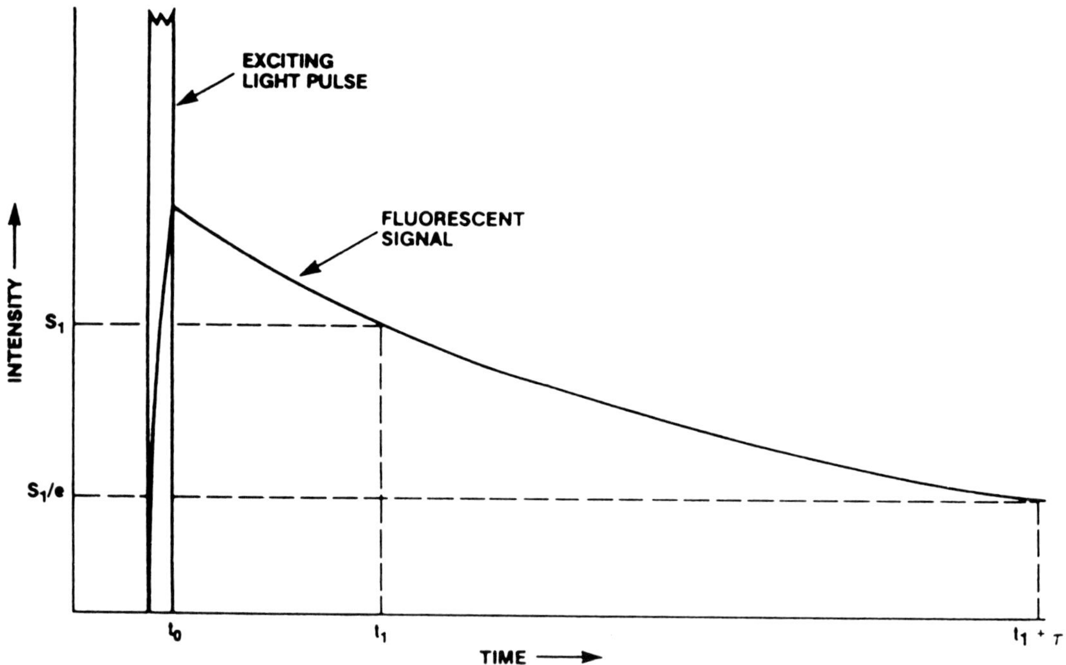

Fig. 15.4. The process by which temperature is determined in the photoluminescent thermometry system. A short high-intensity light pulse excites the sensor which causes it to emit fluorescent light with an intensity which decays with time. The time required for the light to decay from an intensity S_1 to S_1/e is temperature dependent. This parameter is measured, as shown, to determine temperature. (From WICKERSHEIM 1986)

thermometry is improved when indwelling catheters are used because it is feasible to allocate more time and resources to the probe placement when it is done only once. For example, it becomes feasible to use CT guidance when inserting deep catheters and for documenting catheter placement. The cost of these procedures would be prohibitive if carried out in conjunction with each hyperthermia treatment.

Although many institutions use indwelling catheters, there is little information in the literature pertaining to complications caused by leaving catheters in place for several weeks. However, the Rotterdam Radio-therapeutic Institute (VAN DER ZEE et al. 1987) has reported the problems and complications which they encountered with 180 indwelling catheters inserted in 74 treatment sites over a period of 2½ years. The most serious problems were infection and the loss of catheters. Infection was observed in 16% of the catheters, necessitating the removal of 6% of them. Another 6% were lost, primarily because they were not sutured or glued in place. The authors report that their complication rate decreased with increasing experience and that the catheters were well tolerated by the patients. In additions, this group (VAN DER ZEE et al. 1992) separately reported a case study in which tumor growth occurred at the insertion site of a catheter which was outside the treatment field. This finding indicates that catheters should not be placed outside the treatment volume in any locally curative treatment. In general, complications arising from the use of indwelling catheters appear to be relatively minor and tolerable in view of the advantages which they offer.

15.3.2 Types of Catheter

Closed-end catheters for hyperthermia can be made in-house (VAN DER ZEE et al. 1987) by melting closed one end of a plastic tube. However, because catheters designed specifically for hyperthermia are commercially available, it is usually more convenient to procure them. Unfortunately, there has been only one vendor and this vendor has changed three times during the last decade. These catheters were originally designed for invasive thermometry by BSD Medical Corporation and marketed by Deseret Medical (Sandy, Utah) until the late 1980s. They

STYLET INSERTION TYPE CATHETER

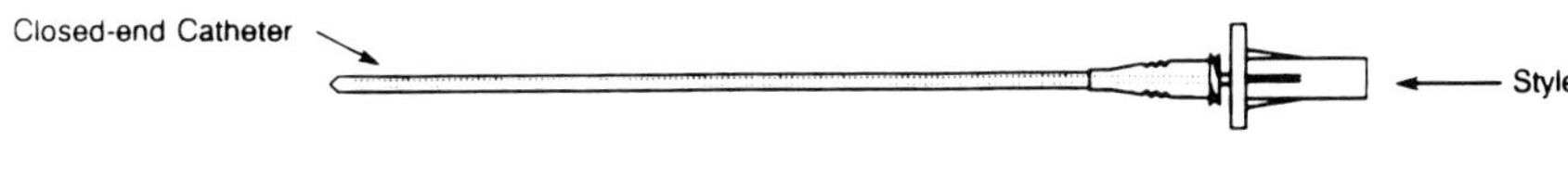

Skin is punctured with scalpel and penetration is made with catheter itself supported by a stainless steel stylet. Catheter is fitted with a female luer lock.

STANDARD NEEDLE INSERTION CATHETER

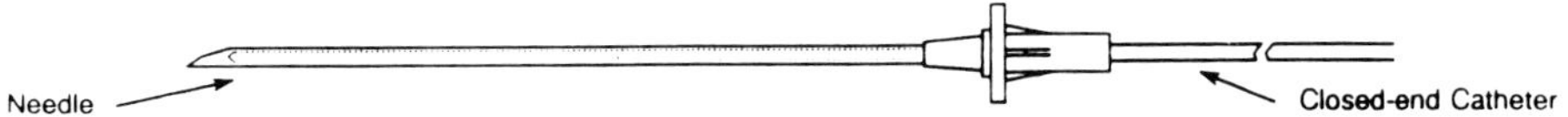

Penetration is made with a standard B-bevel needle (14 ga. thin wall needle for 16 ga. catheters and 17 ga. thin wall needle for 19 ga. catheters). The needle is then withdrawn over the catheter. There is <u>no</u> luer fitting on the catheter to interfere with needle removal.

SPLITTABLE NEEDLE INSERTION CATHETER

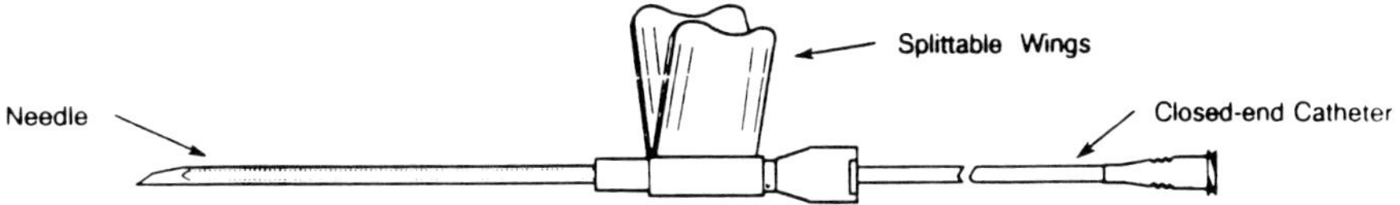

Penetration is made with a splittable needle (14 ga. extra thin wall needle for 16 ga. catheters and 17 ga. extra thin wall needle for 19 ga. catheters). The needle is then withdrawn and split to allow for removal over the female luer adapter on the catheter.

Fig. 15.5. Commercially available closed-end catheters for invasive thermometry

were subsequently marketed by Valley Medical Research, Inc. (Fruit Heights, Utah) for a period of time and are currently available from Delta Research Inc. (Murray, Utah).

Thermometry catheters are presently available in the three different configurations shown in Fig. 15.5. The uppermost diagram shows a catheter which uses a stylet for insertion. The skin is punctured with a scalpel and penetration is made with the catheter itself supported by a stainless steel stylet. The center diagram shows the standard needle insertion catheter without a Luer adapter. Penetration is made with a standard B-bevel needle which fits over the catheter. Once the catheter is fully inserted, the needle is withdrawn over the catheter. The lower diagram shows the splittable needle insertion catheter, which has a Luer adapter. Penetration is made with the splittable needle which fits over the catheter. When the catheter is fully inserted, the needle is withdrawn over the catheter to a point where the tip is out of tissue. The needle is then split to remove it, leaving the Luer adapter in place. The stylet insertion catheter is available only in 16 gauge, but the other two types are available in either 16 or 19 gauge.

15.3.3 Insertion Techniques

Techniques used to insert indwelling catheters have been described in detail in the literature (van der Zee 1987; Samulski and Fessenden 1990). It is apparent that some details of the procedure vary from institution to institution depending upon physician preference and the products available, but the tasks which must be performed are universal. The insertion technique used at Thomas Jefferson University Hospital in Philadelphia is described below.

The intended catheter tracks and insertion points are first drawn on the skin with a marking pen. The skin is then cleansed with a Bedadine® solution and local anesthesia is achieved using

1% lidocaine solution. The needle and catheter are then inserted. It is frequently necessary to temporarily remove the catheter from the needle and infiltrate the tissue ahead of the needle with lidocaine solution. After the catheter is fully inserted, the needle is withdrawn over the catheter while it is held in place. The catheter is then sutured in place. To further prevent slippage, the catheter is cemented to the suture and skin with colostomy cement. Finally, a piece of adhesive is affixed over the suture and cement. Flexible plastic rods are insertet into the catheters between treatments to help prevent the catheter from kinking.

It is often advantageous to insert the catheters under CT guidance, particularly when there is a risk to critical structures. The catheter depth and orientation are first planned on the CT image. The needle is then partially inserted along the intended track and a CT image is obtained to assess progress toward the intended goal. The ability to monitor progress with the CT scanner gives the physician confidence to insert catheters deeper than he or she would generally be willing to do based on clinical palpation alone. Problems associated with 141 CT-guided catheter insertions into deep-seated or half-deep-seated tumors in 95 treatment areas were reported by FELDMAN et al. (1993). Although there were a few problems, the procedure and the catheters were generally well tolerated. Eight catheters had to be removed due to infection. One patient developed acute pancreatitis and two patients had an inflammatory response. No metastases were observed in the catheter tracks.

15.3.4 Impact on Temperature Measurements

Although catheters offer distinct advantages, they can affect the temperature measurement in several different ways. When used in an ultrasound field, absorption heating of the catheter can produce an overestimation of the temperature (FESSENDEN et al. 1984; HENYNEN and EDWARDS 1989; WATERMAN and LEEPER 1990). Catheters also enhance thermal smearing (SAMULSKI et al. 1985, GREIG et al. 1992) and perturb the microwave heating pattern slightly (CHAN et al. 1988b).

Catheters increase the response time of the thermometer probe. The catheter can be viewed as an insulating material separating the sensor from the surrounding medium. Because heat must flow through the catheter wall to reach the sensor, it takes longer for the sensor to attain thermal equilibrium with the surrounding medium whenever its temperature changes. The presence of the catheter affects the measurement of heating and cooling rates which are used to determine the specific absorption rate (SAR) and effective blood flow, respectively. The measured rate of temperature change lags the true rate of change immediately after a transient, but the sensor will record the correct rate of temperature change after an interval equivalent to three time constants. Reliable values of the SAR and effective blood flow can be obtained if the data recorded within three time constants of the transient are ignored (WATERMAN 1985).

15.4 Measurement Errors with Thermocouples

15.4.1 Temperature Artifacts (Electromagnetic Field)

Temperature measurement errors caused by the presence of an electromagnetic field are commonly referred to as temperature artifacts. Three different types of artifact may occur: (a) interference with the thermometry electronics which causes an error in the indicated temperature; (b) reradiation of the electromagnetic energy by the thermocouple leads, which causes a perturbation in the heating pattern; and (c) self-heating of the thermocouple wires. These artifacts have been described by a number of authors, including; CETAS and CONNER (1987), CETAS (1982), CHAKRABORTY and BREZOVICH (1982), GAMMAMPILA et al. (1982), DUNSCOMBE and MCLELLAN (1986), CHAN et al. (1988a), CONSTABLE et al. (1987), and DUNSCOMBE et al. (1988).

The first of these artifacts, interference with the thermometry electronics, can be reduced significantly by filtering and shielding. It has become standard procedure to turn off the power for up to 1 s before recording the temperature to eliminate any residual artifact. This procedure completely eliminates this type of artifact, but may not completely eliminate the other two types, a fact which is not always appreciated. Care is also required in extrapolating back in time to the true temperature at power off.

The second type of artifact, reradiation of the electromagnetic energy produces a perturbation of the heating pattern which cannot be eliminated

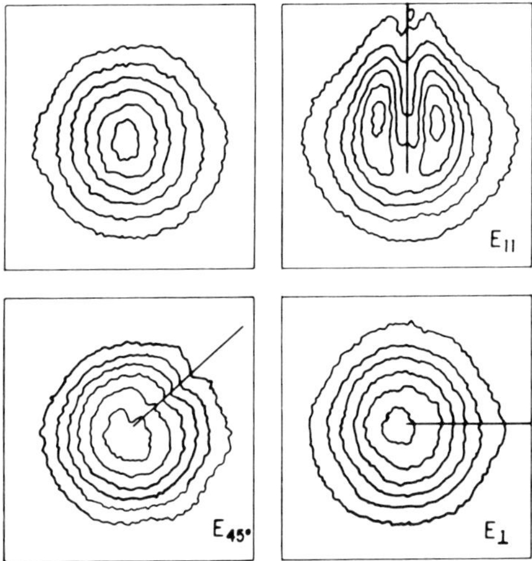

Fig. 15.6. Thermographic images of the perturbation of the microwave heating pattern by a thermocouple probe inserted parallel, perpendicular, and at an angle of 45° with respect to the electric field. The unperturbed heating pattern is shown in the *upper left*. (From CHAN et al. 1988a)

by turning off the power. Perturbation of a 915-MHz microwave heating pattern by a thermocouple oriented in different positions with respect to the electric field is shown in Fig. 15.6 (CHAN et al. 1988a). A thermographic image of the unperturbed heating pattern is shown in the upper left. The perturbations that occur when a thermocouple is inserted parallel, at an angle of 45°, and perpendicular to the electric field are shown in the other images. The perturbation is greatest when the probe is parallel to the field. Hence, this type of artifact can be minimized by orienting the leads perpendicular to the field, if the applicator has a defined electric field direction.

The third type of artifact, self-heating of the thermocouple wires, is more complex. The thermoocouple junction becomes hotter than the adjacent tissue, resulting in an overestimation of the temperature. However, this is not the only consequence of the self-heating artifact. The excess heat generated in the wires is conducted to the surrounding tissue, thereby elevating its temperature above what it would be if the probe were not there.

The self-heating artifact can be resolved into two distinct components (DUNSCOMBE et al. 1988) as:

$$\Delta T = \Delta T_p + \Delta T_h, \tag{15.1}$$

where ΔT is the total artifact due to self-heating, ΔT_p is the elevation in the temperature of the tissue immediately adjacent to the probe due to the conduction of heat from the probe, and ΔT_h is the difference between the temperature of the themocouple and that of the adjacent tissue.

The component ΔT_h is a result of the thermal insulation provided by the thermocouple sheath, the catheter, and any air gaps which may exist between the wires and the adjacent tissue. These materials allow a thermal gradient to become established between the hot wires and the adjacent tissue. When the power is turned off, ΔT_h decays rapidly as the excess heat in the wires flows through the insulating material to the adjacent tissue. The time required for this portion of the artifact to dissipate depends on the time constant of the probe. To eliminate it, the power should be turned off for an interval equivalent to three time constants of the probe (plus catheter) before the temperature is recorded (WATERMAN 1985). Note that this is longer than the time required to eliminate the interference artifact. The power-off interval which will eliminate both artifacts can be reduced by reducing the time constant of the probe. An effective means of accomplishing this is to eliminate the air gaps by replacing the air with water (DUNSCOMBE et al. 1988).

When the power is turned off, ΔT_h decays very rapidly, but ΔT_p does not. The time constant of ΔT_p is approximately two orders of magnitude greater than that of ΔT_h and is similar to that of perfused tissue. Thus, ΔT_p which can be as much as 1°–2°C, cannot be eliminated by turning off the power for a few seconds before reading the thermocouple. No satisfactory technique has been identified for dealing with the tissue heating artifact, $\Delta T_p'$. This artifact is generally overlooked because its presence is not readily apparent.

In summary, artifacts can be minimized by reducing the coupling of the electric field by orienting the thermocouple wires perpendicular to the electric field and by reducing the heat generated by use of high-resistance wires (GAMMAMPILA et al. 1982; DUNSCOMBE and MCLELLAN 1986). The interference artifact can be reduced by filtration and eliminated altogether by reading the temperature with the power off. The adoption of these procedures will significantly reduce, but not completely eliminate, the measurement error due to artifacts.

15.4.2 Temperature Artifacts (Ultrasound Field)

Thermocouples are ordinarily used to monitor temperature during hyperthermia induced by ultrasound. These probes are prone to measurement errors commonly referred to as "temperature artifacts." However, it should be noted that this problem is not restricted to thermocouples. All of the thermometry systems currently available produce artifacts in an ultrasound field; fiberoptic probes, which are nonperturbing in an electromagnetic field, offer no advantage here.

Artifacts are a result of viscous and/or absorption heating of the probe. Viscous heating arises from the relative movement of the surrounding tissue with respect to the probe, thereby causing shear forces and local energy absorption at the probe surface (Fry and Fry 1954a,b; Dunn 1962; Goss et al. 1977; Hynynen et al. 1982, 1983; Carnochan et al. 1986). Absorption heating occurs in probes which have plastic materials exposed to the ultrasound beam. Absorption heating can be caused by something as seemingly insignificant as a plastic coating on the junction (Hand 1984), but is generally associated with the use of catheters or plastic-sheathed thermocouples. An artifact occurs because plastic has a larger coefficient of ultrasonic power absorption than tissue (Hynynen et al. 1983; Martin and Law 1983; Hand and Dickinson 1984; Carnochan et al. 1986). Hence, the probe becomes hotter than the surrounding tissue.

Absorption heating can be eliminated by encasing the thermocouple in a steel needle which is then inserted directly into tissue. However, the temperature artifact cannot be eliminated completely because viscous heating may still occur. Thermocouples encased in steel needles are generally recommended for ultrasound hyperthermia to minimize the artifact. However, this approach has a number of disadvantages. Most notably, it is necessary to reinsert the probes prior to each treatment and the advantages of indwelling catheters cannot be realized. For these reasons, some investigators are willing to accept a potentially larger artifact in return for the advantages of using indwelling catheters. However, this step should be taken with caution because the absorption artifact can become very large, on the order of several degrees (Fessenden et al. 1984), if the wrong plastics are used (most notably Teflon) or if high power levels are employed. These points are explained more fully in the following paragraphs.

The magnitude of the viscous or absorption artifact is directly proportional to the ultrasound intensity (Fry and Fry 1954a,b; Hynynen et al. 1983; Dunscombe and McLellan 1986; Waterman and Leeper 1990). Thus, the artifact obtained with any probe, with or without a catheter, is a dynamic variable which increases with the power level. For this reason, it is necessary to distinguish between thermometry recommendations for planar ultrasound, where the intensity is relatively low, and scanned focused ultrasound, where the intensity may be an order of magnitude greater. For example, a catheter which produces an acceptable artifact with planar ultrasound would probably produce a totally unacceptable artifact at the power levels used for scanned focused ultrasound.

The magnitude of the absorption artifact depends upon the type of plastic employed (Martin and Law 1983; Hand and Dickinson 1984; Kuhn and Christensen 1986; Hynynen and Edwards 1989). Figure 15.7 shows the relative heating of various sheathing materials (Kuhn and Christensen 1986). In this work, a thermocouple was inserted in the plastic to be tested, which was immersed in a water bath. It was then exposed to a 1-MHz ultrasound beam with an intensity of about 5 W/cm^2 and heated until an equilibrium temperature was attained. The temperature scale in Fig. 15.7 indicates the temperature elevation attained. Note that the temperature elevation attained with fused silica and polyethylene tubing was significantly less than with Teflon. Hence, catheters fabricated from these materials would be expected to produce a smaller artifact than Teflon. Care must be exercised to assure that catheters are fabricated from a plastic which will minimize the absorption artifact. In particular, Teflon should be avoided.

Fortunately, the commercially available catheters (Delta Research, Inc., Murray, Utah) which are widely used for hyperthermia are made from polyurethane, not Teflon. The artifacts produced by these catheters were evaluated at 72 different sensor locations in ten different tumor sites heated by use of planar ultrasound transducers operated at 1 and 3 MHz (Waterman et al. 1990). The ultrasound intensity used during these treatments was typically 1 W/cm^2. Histograms of the artifacts observed in these patients are shown in Fig. 15.8. Most of the data were obtained with multisensor thermocouples inserted into 16-gauge polyurethane catheters, as can be seen by the larger number of samples in the histogram in the

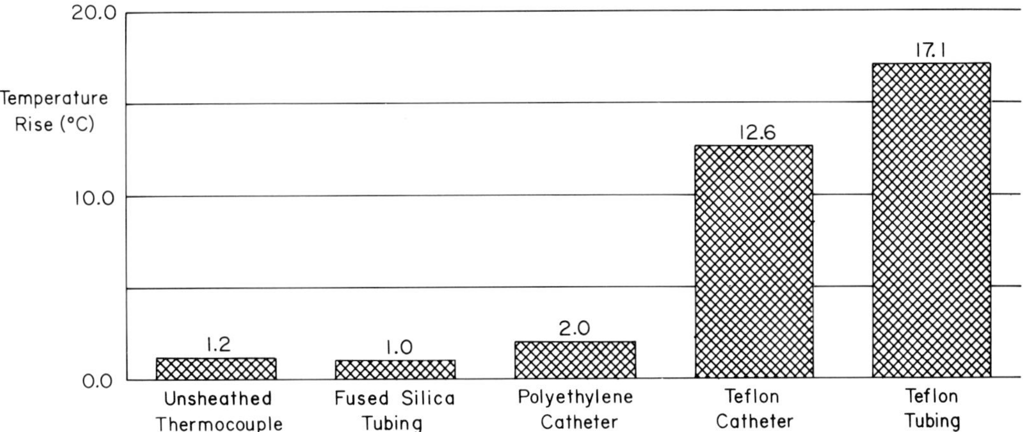

Fig. 15.7. Bar graph illustrating the relative magnitude of the ultrasonic-induced temperature artifact for different thermocouple sheathing materials. (From KUHN and CHRISTENSEN 1986)

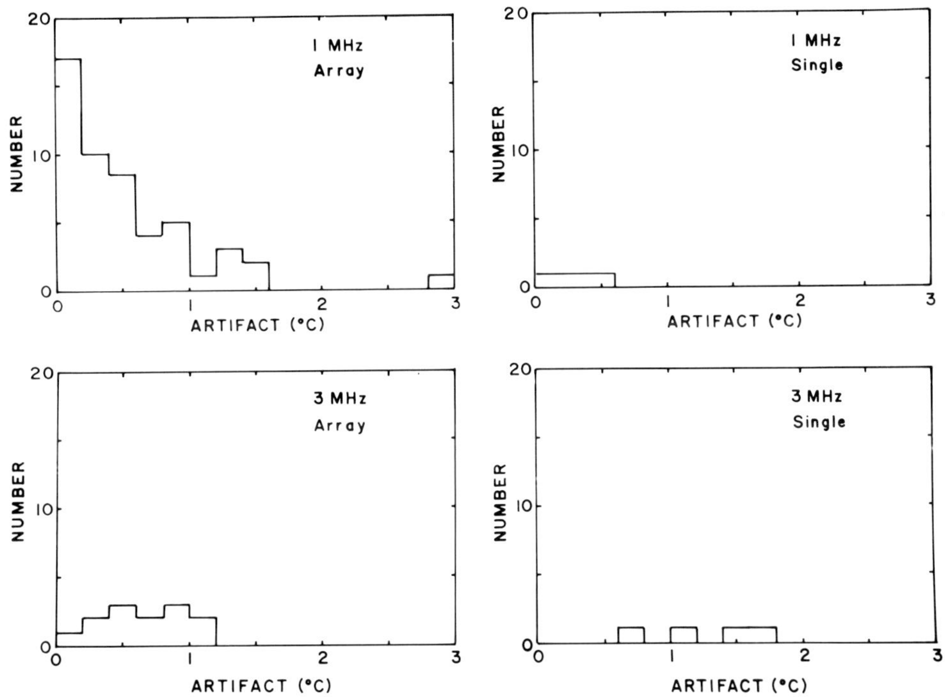

Fig. 15.8. Frequency distribution of temperature artifacts observed in human tumors by (**a**) multisensor thermocouples in 16-gauge polyurethane catheters at 1 MHz, (**b**) single-sensor thermocouples in 19-gauge polyurethane catheters at 1 MHz, (**c**) multisensor thermocouples in 16-gauge polyurethane catheters at 3 MHz, and (**d**) single-sensor thermocouples in 19-gauge polyurethane catheters at 3 MHz. (From WATERMAN et al. 1990)

upper left. The mean artifact was 0.6°C and only 15% of the artifacts exceed 1°C. The largest artifact observed was 3.0°C. These results indicate that the magnitude of the artifact which occurs in clinical data when the ultrasound intensity is on the order of 1 W/cm^2 is generally less than 1°C. If higher ultrasound intensities are used, the artifacts will be proportionally greater.

The magnitude of the artifact also depends on the orientation of the probe relative to the direction of the ultrasound beam. According to the theory of FRY and FRY (1954a), the maximum and minimum artifacts occur when the wires are perpendicular and parallel to the direction of the beam, respectively. The angular dependence of the artifact is shown in Fig. 15.9 (HYNYNEN and

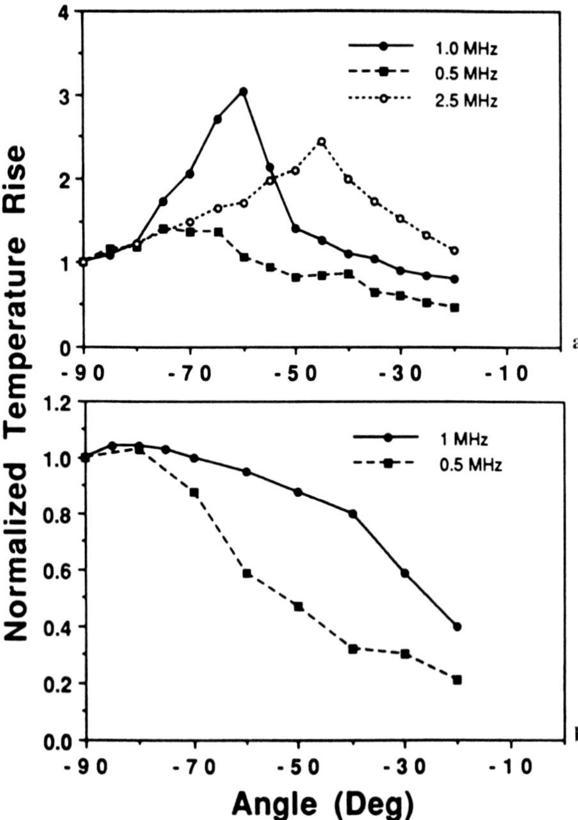

Fig. 15.9. Relative artifact as a function of the angle between the probe and the central axis of the ultrasound beam. These measurements were carried out in water with the thermocouple (**a**) in a 0.7-mm O.D. fused silica tube at three different frequencies and (**b**) in a 0.96-mm O.D. polyethelene tube at two different frequencies. (From HYNYNEN and EDWARDS 1989)

EDWARDS 1989) for a fused silica probe (upper half of figure) at three different ultrasound frequencies and for a polyethylene-sheathed thermocouple (lower half of figure) at two frequencies. The angle plotted is the angle between the probe and the beam axis. For the fused silica probes, the maximum artifactual heating appears to be at an angle smaller than 90°, contrary to the theory of FRY and FRY (1954a). However, the artifactual heating of the polyethylene-sheathed probe decreases with the angle in accordance with theory. This result demonstrates the potential for reducing the temperature artifact by aligning the thermocouple probe as closely as possible to the direction of the ultrasound beam.

HYNYNEN and EDWARDS (1989) describe a third type of artifact caused by scattering of the ultrasound beam by the probe. They found that probes with diameters equal to or greater than one-half the square root of the wavelength scatter and reflect the waves, and thus distort the heating pattern. This scattering can increase the power density around the probe, resulting in artificially high temperature readings.

The presence of viscous or absorption heating is apparent from the shape of the temperature rise curve, as illustrated in Fig. 15.10. In this figure, the temperatures recorded by a polyurethane-sheathed thermocouple in a polyurethane catheter and by a thermocouple in a steel needle are plotted versus time as the power is turned on for 90 s and then turned off. The circles depict the recorded temperatures and the straight line represents an approximation of the actual phantom temperature. The artifact is the difference between the solid line and the data. Immediately after the ultrasound power is turned on, the probe temperature increases more rapidly than that of the surrounding medium due to viscous and absorption heating. As the temperature difference between the probe and the surrounding medium increases, thermal energy is conducted from the probe to the medium, eventually reaching an equilibrium after which time the probe temperature increases at approximately the same rate as that of the surrounding medium. The abnormal abrupt rise in temperature immediately after the power is turned on is the signature of the temperature artifact.

The presence of the artifact is also evident in the temperature decay curves shown in Fig. 15.10. Immediately after the power is turned off, the probe temperature decays very rapidly because the source of artifactual heating is no longer present to maintain the temperature differential between the probe and the surrounding medium. This abrupt drop in temperature is another signature of the artifact which is evident in both clinical and phantom data.

The artifact can be determined from the temperature decay curve, as illustrated in Fig. 15.11. The linear portion of the temperature decay curve is extrapolated back to the time the power was turned off. The artifact is the difference between the extrapolated temperature and the temperature recorded by the probe at that time. In perfused tissue, the temperature elevation (T − 37°C) should be plotted on semilog paper as a function of time after the power is turned off to perform the extrapolation (assuming 37°C is indeed the baseline). The

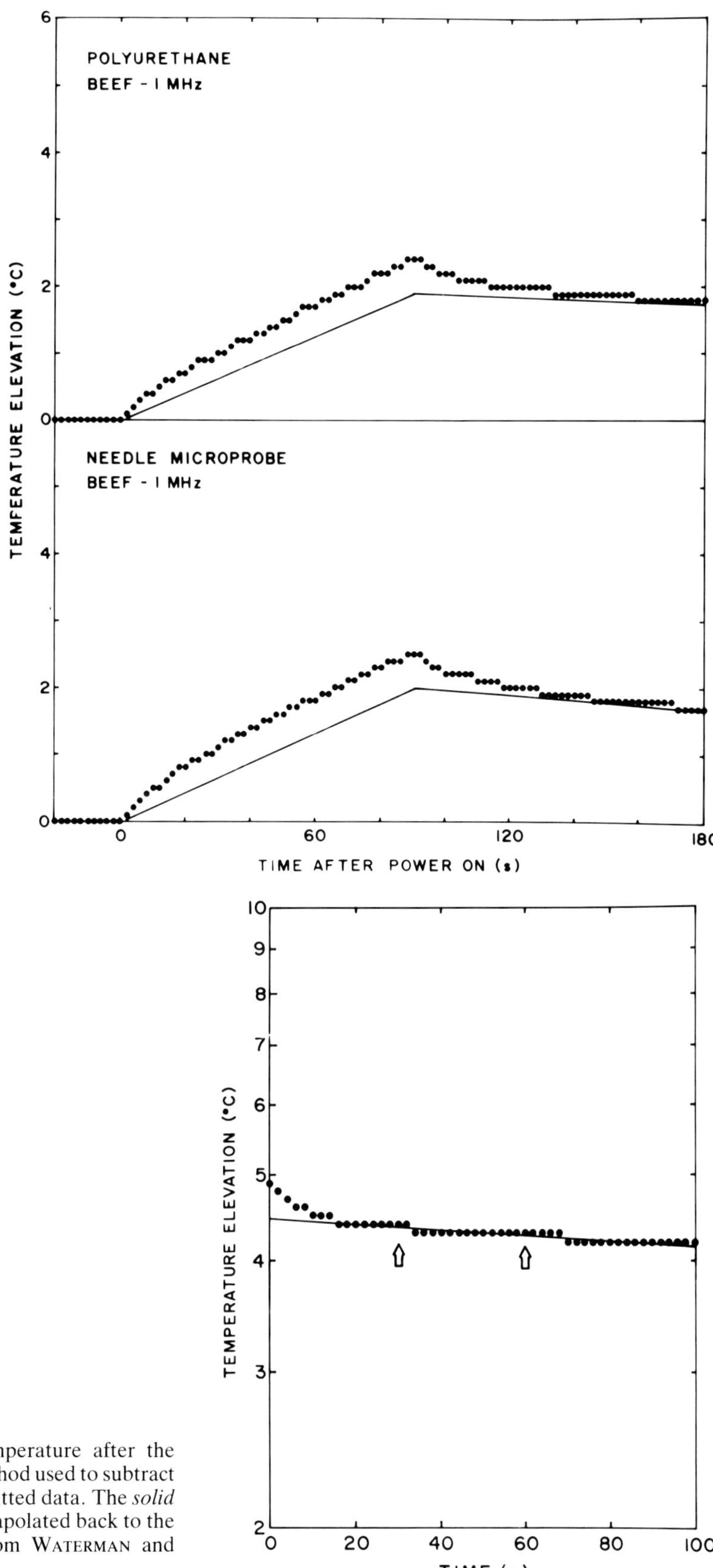

Fig. 15.10. Temperature versus time recorded by a polyurethane-sheathed thermocouple in a 19-gauge polyurethane catheter and a 23-gauge needle probe in a beef phantom heated for 90 s by 1-MHz planar ultrasound at an applied power of 40 W. (From WATERMAN and LEEPER 1990)

Fig. 15.11. Plot of the decay of temperature after the power is turned off, illustrating the method used to subtract the artifact. The *arrows* designate the fitted data. The *solid line* is the fit to these data which is extrapolated back to the time the power was turned off. (From WATERMAN and LEEPER 1990)

artifact should not be determined from data recorded immediately after the power is turned on by extrapolating the linear portion of the temperature rise curve backward. The slope of the temperature rise curve decreases continuously with time as the temperature increases due to the increasing rate of heat dissipation by perfusion and conduction. As a result, the artifact may be underestimated (WATERMAN 1990).

Viscous and absorption heating of the probe affects the temperature of the surrounding tissue in a manner similar to that described in Sect. 15.4.1 due the self-heating of a thermocouple in a microwave field. The probe essentially becomes a linear heat source and heat is conducted from the probe to the surrounding tissue, thereby raising its temperature above what it would be if the probe were not there. This artifactual elevation in the tissue temperature is not obviously evident in either the temperature rise oı decay curves, nor is it easily removed by backward extrapolation of the temperature decay curve (WATERMAN 1992). Furthermore, it is very difficult, if not impossible, to demonstrate the presence of this artifact experimentally because almost any instrument inserted to measure the temperature in the absence of the probe would itself produce an artifact. Because this artifact is not evident, it is generally overlooked and often not accounted for. However, the presence of the artifact can be demon-

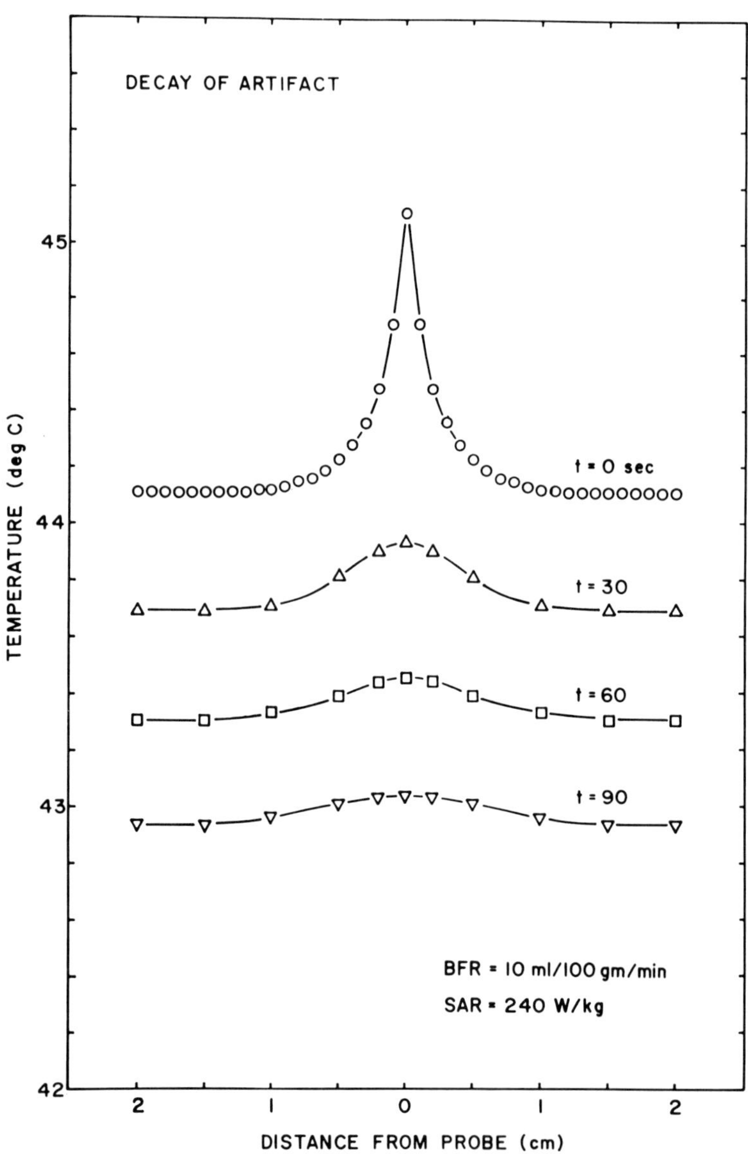

Fig. 15.12. Simulation of the decay of the artifact at the location of the probe and in the surrounding tissue as a function of cooling time. Temperature profiles are shown at the time the power was turned off and after 30, 60, and 90 s of cooling. (From WATERMAN 1990)

strated by use of a computer model (WATERMAN 1990).

Figure 15.12 shows the results of a computer simulation of artifactual heating of the tissue adjacent to the probe. This figure shows the distribution of temperature along a line which runs through the probe perpendicular to its axis, and includes 2 cm of tissue on each side. In this example, the tissue is assumed to have a uniform blood flow of 10 ml/100 g/min. The upper curve, labeled $t = 0$ sec, shows the temperature profile at the moment the ultrasound power is turned off. An artifact of approximately 1°C is clearly evident at the location of the probe (0 cm). Note that there is also an elevation in the temperature of tissue within 1 cm from the probe. However, at a distance of 1.5 cm, or greater, there is no elevation in temperature as result of heat conducted from the probe. Hence, in the absence of the probe, the profile would be a straight line equivalent to the temperature 1.5 cm from the probe. The lower curves show the profiles 30, 60, and 90 s after the power was turned off. Note that the temperature of the probe and adjacent tissue is still slightly elevated 90 s after the power is turned off.

Figure 15.13 shows how the temperature decayed when the power was turned off at two points: at the location of the probe (triangles) and at a point in tissue 1.5 cm from the probe (circles). The artifact is generally determined by extrapolating the decay curve recorded by the probe backward to the time the power was turned off, as illustrated by the dashed line. The difference between the extrapolated line and the temperature recorded by the probe at $t = 0$ is normally taken to be the artifact. However, the total artifact is actually the difference between the temperature recorded by the probe and the lower curve, which

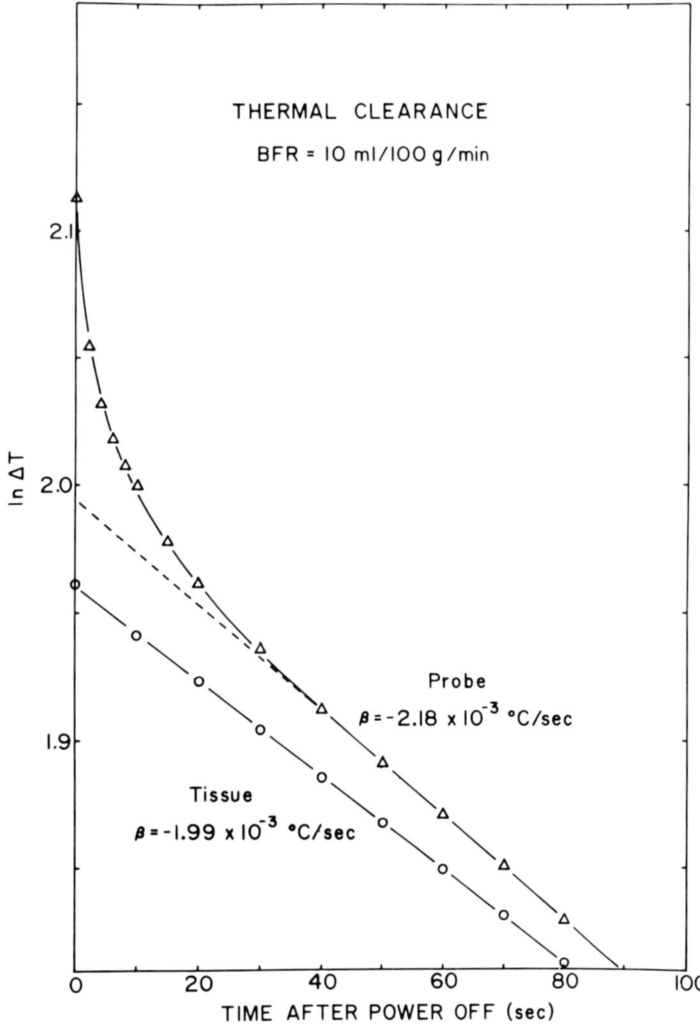

Fig. 15.13. Calculated decay of temperature at the location of the probe and at a point in tissue at 1.5 cm distance. This temperature represents the temperature that would exist at the location of the probe, if it were not there. This figure illustrates the underestimation of the artifact by backward extrapolation of the linear portion of the decay curve recorded by the probe

represents what the temperature would be at the probe location if the probe were not there. It is apparent that in the technique of removing the artifact by backward extrapolation the decay curve removes only a portion of it. In terms of the nomenclature defined in Sect. 15.4.1, ΔT_p is removed, but ΔT_h is not. The computer simulation (WATERMAN 1990) indicates that the artifact may be underestimated by as much as 40% by this subtraction technique.

At least 60 s of thermal clearance data are required to determine the artifact by the extrapolation technique. Therefore, it is generally not feasible to determine the artifact in this manner during the therapy because repeatedly turning off the power for this period of time could compromise the patient's treatment. It has been shown that it is also possible to determine the artifact from a 10-s interruption in power (WATERMAN 1992). Turning off the power for such a short period would not compromise the patient's treatment and would allow essentially on-line subtraction of the artifact. However, this technique has not yet been tested in the clinic.

The temperature artifact is an even greater problem for scanned focused ultrasound because the intensity is an order of magnitude greater; however, the situation is improved somewhat by the fact that the scanning beam only impinges on the probe intermittently. Hence, artifactual heating is more confined to the probe with less heating of adjacent tissue and there is an opportunity for the artifact to dissipate between scans. It has been found that a good estimate of the tissue temperature can be attained by turning off the power for up to 3 s before reading the thermocouples (HYNYNEN and EDWARDS 1989). When ultrasound absorbing probes are used, there are several different techniques which can be used to reduce the artifact. One is to turn off the scanning beam as it moves over the probe. Another is to record the minimum temperature between scan cycles (HYNYNEN and EDWARDS 1989). Still another approach is to insert flexible plastic-sheathed thermocouples directly into tissue without a catheter (ANHALT and HYNYNEN 1992). The advantage of this approach is that the artifact is lowered as a result of the improved thermal contact between the thermocouple junction and the surrounding medium. Other techniques have been devised by covering the plastic probe at the location of the sensors with a high- (or low-) acoustic impedance material which would scatter the sound around the probe, thus preventing energy absorption in the plastic (HYNYNEN and EDWARDS 1989).

15.4.3 Thermal Conduction Errors

Thermocouples and thermistors having metal leads are prone to a temperature measurement error caused by the conduction of heat along the wires (SINGH and DYBBS 1976; ANDERSON et al. 1984; DICKINSON 1985; LYONS et al. 1985; SAMULSKI et al. 1985; GREIG et al. 1992). This problem is particularly acute for copper-constantan thermocouples due to the high thermal conductivity of copper. Unfortunately, this type of thermocouple is supplied with most commercial ultrasound hyperthermia units. The conduction error associated with copper-constantan thermocouples can often be 1°C, or greater, yet this source of error has received relatively little attention in comparison to the temperature artifact. This is probably because the conduction error is not apparent in the data and can only be detected by remeasuring the temperature with a fiberoptic probe, something which is seldom done, especially in the clinic.

The existence of a conduction error can be demonstrated in the laboratory by sequentially mapping a thermal step with a thermocouple and a fiberoptic probe, as shown in Fig. 15.14. A plastic-sheathed thermocouple with six junctions spaced at 0.5-cm intervals and a common constantan wire was inserted into a 16-gauge polyurethane catheter for this test. The measurements were made by pulling the probe through a 10°C thermal step from left to right. The first curve on the right shows the thermal step mapped by a fiberoptic probe which has a negligible conduction error. Note that the profiles recorded by the thermocouples become increasingly more distorted with each successive junction from the tip. This test reveals the existence of a significant conduction error which increases with each successive junction from the tip, as reported by DICKINSON (1985).

The pronounced dip in the profiles of the thermal step recorded by the first three junctions is evidence of another type of measurement error which can occur with multijunction thermocouples having a common wire when the thermal gradient is so steep that a temperature differential exists over the dimensions of the junction (ANDERSEN et

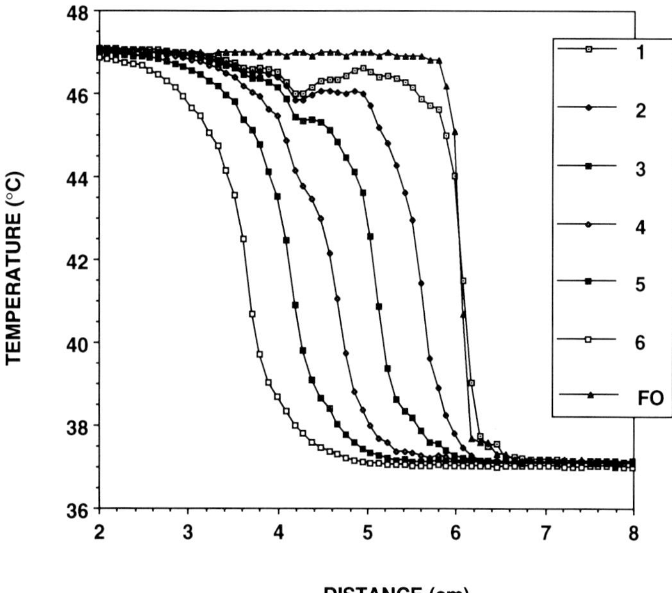

Fig. 15.14. Temperatures recorded by a six-sensor copper-constantan thermocouple having a common constantan wire and by a fiberoptic probe (*FO*) in mapping a 10°C thermal step. Sensor 1 is at the tip of the thermocouple

al. 1984), generating a thermal emf within the junction. This effect is small for each individual junction, but the emfs are cumulative and can result in errors on the order of a degree. This type of error is not of as much concern because the gradients encountered in the clinic are seldom steep enough to cause a significant error of this type. This error can be minimized by reducing the diameter of the junction, so as to reduce the gradient across it.

The performance of a thermocouple in mapping a step function can be quantitated in terms of an error length (DICKINSON 1985) or thermal smearing length (SAMULSKI et al. 1985). It has been recommended that probes or probe – catheter combinations having a thermal smearing length greater than 1.5 mm not be used in the clinic (SAMULSKI and FESSENDEN 1990). Copper-constantan thermocouples do not meet this criterion (SAMULSKI et al. 1985), and it is strongly recommended that this type of thermocouple not be used in the clinic. Further evidence of the large conduction error which can occur in clinical data was obtained by testing the ability of a single-junction copper-constantan thermocouple to map a thermal peak having an amplitude of 6°C with a full-width at half-maximum of 3.5 cm (WATERMAN and HOH 1992). This peak constitutes a modest test with a maximum gradient of only 3°C/cm. However, the average error in mapping this profile was ±0.6°C. This error is defined as the average value of the absolute difference between the true and measured profiles, evaluated at 0.5-cm intervals over the entire span of the peak.

The condution error can be significantly reduced by replacing copper-constantan thermocouples with manganin-constantan thermocouples. Manganin has essentially the same thermoelectric emf as copper at 40°C (copper 42 μV/°C; manganin 41 μV/°C) but a much lower thermal conductivity (copper 385 W m/K; manganin 22 W m/K) (DICKINSON 1985). Figure 15.15 shows a 10°C thermal step mapped with a manganin-constantan thermocouple having five junctions spaced at 1-cm intervals with separate wires to each junction. The dramatic reduction in thermal smearing is evident by comparing Figs. 15.14 and 15.15. Other types of thermocouples, such as chromel-alumel, have been shown to provide a similar reduction in the conduction error (GERIG et al. 1992).

Although manganin-constantan thermocouples are required for ESHO protocols (HAND et al. 1989), most institutions in the United States continue to use copper-constantan thermocouples. The reasons for this are twofold: manganin-constantan thermocouples are not commercially available and the thermometry units supplied by the Labthermics and Clini-Therm ultrasound hyperthermia units were designed for copper-constantan thermocouples. Institutions in the United States which do use manganin-constantan

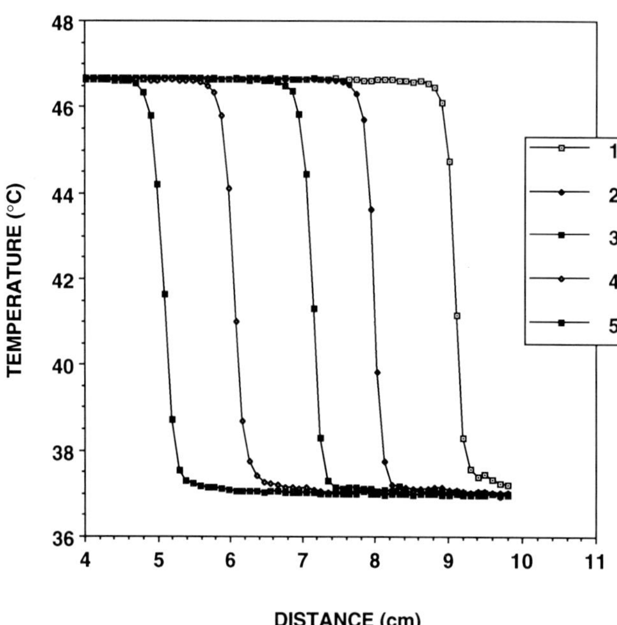

Fig. 15.15. Temperatures recorded by a five-sensor manganin-constantan thermocouple in mapping a 10°C thermal step. Sensor 1 is at the tip. The thermocouple has separate wires to each junction

thermocouples fabricate them in-house from materials which are commercially available. The experience of the University of Arizona group in fabricating and using such thermocouples is detailed in the literature (Anhalt and Hynynen 1992). Because of the similarity of the thermoelectric emf of copper and manganin, manganin-constantan thermocouples can be used in the Labthermics LT-100 (Labthermics Technologies, Inc., Champaign, Ill.) and Clini-Therm TS-1200/TM-100 thermocouple thermometry units without loss of accuracy if appropriate calibration procedures are followed (Hoh and Waterman 1994).

Finally, it should be pointed out that there are factors other than the thermal conductivity of the thermocouple wires which affect the magnitude of the conduction error. In order for thermal smearing to occur, a temperature gradient must exist between the junction and the surrounding medium. When the junction is surrounded by insulating materials, such as plastic or air gaps, such a gradient is more readily established. Thus, reducing or eliminating these materials is a key factor in minimizing the conduction error (Greig et al. 1992). Air gaps, in particular, should be eliminated because the thermal conductivity of air is much less than that of plastic. The conduction error can also be reduced by decreasing the diameter of the wire leads.

15.5 Thermal Mapping

Insertion of a few static thermometer probes generally provides too few samples of temperature to provide a reliable determination of descriptors, such as T_{min}, T_{90}, or T_{50}, which have been found to have prognostic significance (Oleson et al. 1989; Kapp et al. 1992; Leopold et al. 1992, 1993). As pointed out by Corry (1988), the observed minimum temperature tends to decrease as the number of samples increases. Multisensor probes provide more data per catheter than single-sensor probes, but usually have no more than four sensors which span a total length of 3 cm, or less. The only practical means of sampling temperature over the dimensions of the heat field, and thereby providing the data necessary to provide meaningful descriptors, is to employ manual or automated thermal mapping. For this reason, thermal mapping is a requirement of the thermometry guidelines developed for RTOG (Dewhirst et al. 1990). Manual thermal mapping is a tedious procedure. However, thermal mapping can be facilitated by automated systems designed to index one or more thermometer probes under computer control.

Gibbs (1983) reported the first system of this type which was developed for use with the BSD annular phased array. This mapping system indexed three probes in unison by means of a stepper-motor driven actuator which was con-

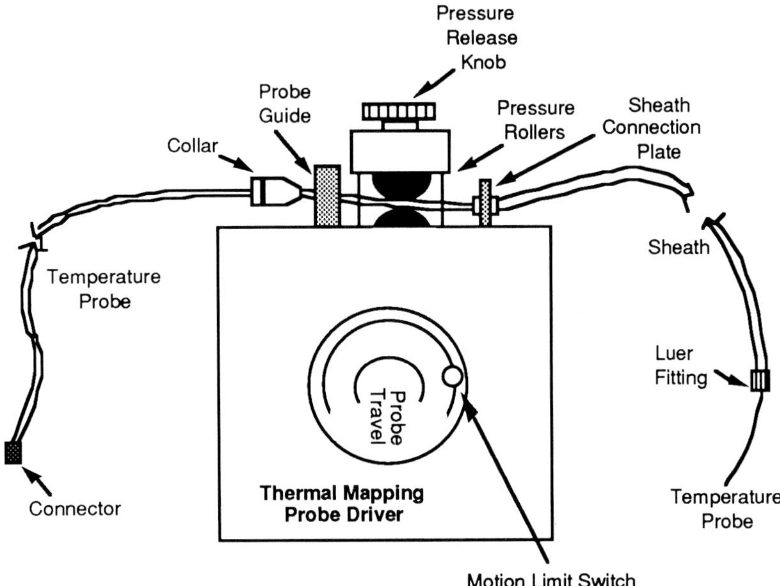

Fig. 15.16. Diagram of the BSD Medical Corporation's thermal mapping probe driver and accessory parts. (From BSD Medical Corp.)

trolled by a microprocessor in the control console. This system was later refined by BSD Medical and marketed as an option to their hyperthermia units. It is also available as a "stand alone" thermal mapping system (TMS-480) which is the only commercially available system. The BSD system, shown in Fig. 15.16, is designed for use with the Bowman probe and uses a pinch roller technique to index the probe. It can index up to eight probes simultaneously with a length of travel of 0–30 cm, stopping at intervals of 0.5–30 cm for a minimum of 6 s to measure temperature. The positioning accuracy stated by the manufacturer is ±0.2 cm.

Noncommercial automated thermal mapping systems have been reported by ENGLER et al. (1987) and TARCZY-HORNOCH et al. (1992). The system developed by Engler et al. is shown in Fig. 15.17. In this approach, each probe is driven by a separate device. Translation of the probe is achieved by use of a rotational stepping motor with a threaded armature shaft which screws into the nonrotational actuator. Each rotation of the armature shaft indexes the probe 0.005 cm. The probe lead is fixed to the actuator, but in such a manner that it would slip if the probe accidentally struck the end of the catheter or some other obstruction. An advantage of driving each probe separately is that the length of travel and interval between readings can be tailored to each catheter. The hysteresis and positioning error of this device appears to be smaller than that of devices which utilize a roller to move the probe because the probe is not as likely to slip when it encounters

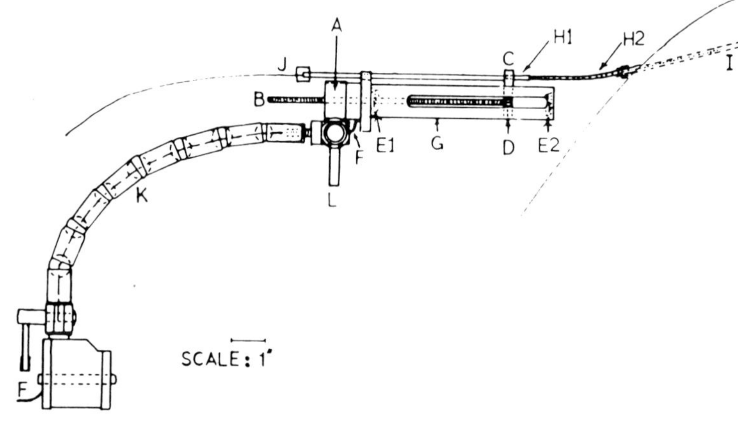

Fig. 15.17. Schematic of the thermal mapping device showing the actuator (*A*), shaft (*B*), plug (*C*), magnet (*D*), reed switches (*E1*, *E2*), cable (*F*), outrigger (*G*), outer tube (*H1*), inner tube (*H2*), fitting for thermometry catheters (*I*), junction of thermometry leads and tube (*K*), and cylindrical motor clamp (*L*). (From ENGLER et al. 1987)

frictional resistance in the catheter. ENGLER et al. (1987) report a positional accuracy of less than 0.005 cm.

TARCZY-HORNOCH et al. (1992) reported four different thermal mapping devices which were developed and tested at Stanford University. Two of the devices were designed to map a single sensor, while the others were designed to map parallel arrays of sensors. All four devices employ a stepper motor actuated roller and idler wheel drive to move the probes. Two of the devices incorporate positive positioners to obtain higher positioning accuracy when there is a significant amount of friction between the probe and catheter. Figure 15.18 shows one of these devices, a multiprobe mapping device utilizing a rotary position defining cylinder. This device has two stepper motors working in unison. One drives the positioning cylinder around which the probe leads are wound. This cylinder limits the maximum outward travel of the probes and provides the primary force for withdrawing the probes from the catheters. The drive cylinder and idler provide the motion drive for insertion of the probes into the catheters. The drive software utilizes two procedures to maximize positioning accuracy. To eliminate backlash, all probes are driven past the desired location and then withdrawn to their final location. Second, the relative rates of rotation of the positioner and driver cylinders are adjusted to keep the probes under constant controlled tension during operation. This device can move the probes at a speed of 20 cm/s with a positional accuracy of 0.1 cm.

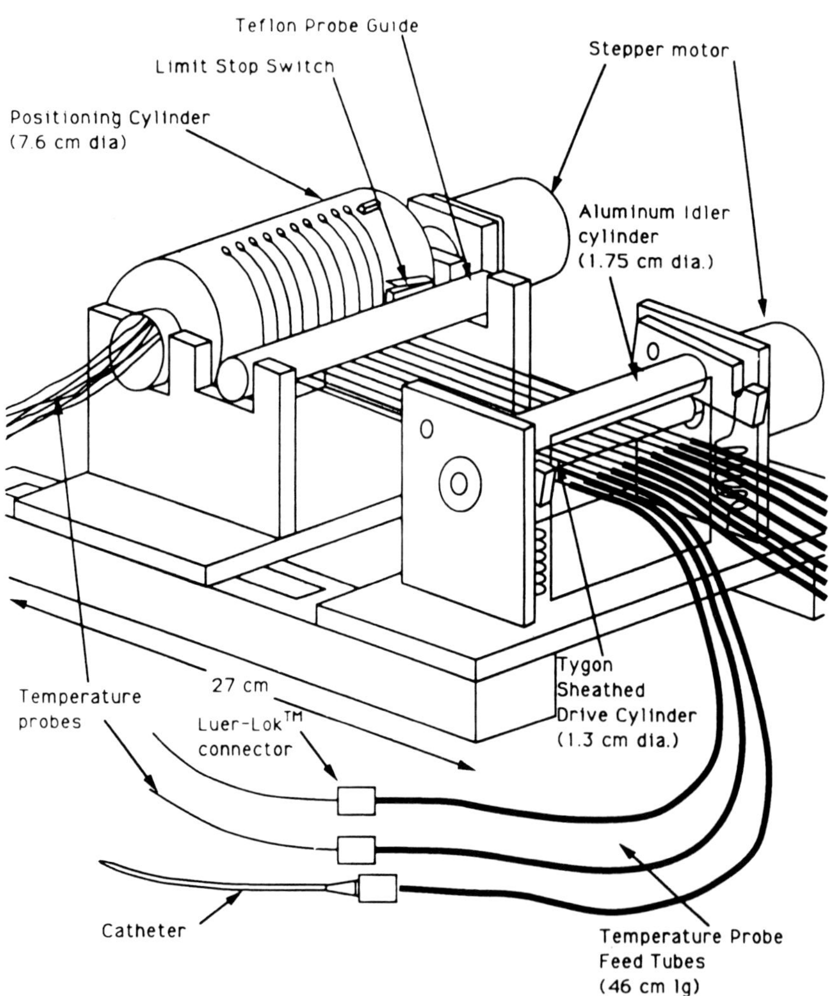

Fig. 15.18. Functional diagram of a multiprobe mapping device utilizing a rotary position defining cylinder. (From TARCZY-HORNOCH et al. 1992)

15.6 Application to the Clinic

15.6.1 Surface Measurements

Surface measurements are commonly used to monitor temperature at points at risk. With the advent of multichannel applicators, surface measurements may also be used to monitor the relative power output of the different channels. However, exactly what is being measured by a thermometer sandwiched between the skin surface and the coupling bolus of an applicator has never been very clear. This is particularly true when the bolus temperature is very different from the skin temperature.

The interpretation of surface measurements was clarified considerably by a recent investigation of the influence of the water bolus temperature on skin surface and intradermal temperatures using human subjects (LEE et al. 1994). Microwave applicators with circulating bolus water set at 21°C and 41°C were placed on the skin surface, but no microwave energy was applied. Thermocouples were inserted interstitially at a shallow depth intended to be at the layer of epidermal cells just beneath the stratum corneum. Single-sensor Luxtron fiberoptic temperature probes were placed on the surface. The temperatures recorded by the surface probes in contact with both the bolus and the skin were compared to those recorded by the interstitial probes. The results obtained with a mechanically scanned two-element microstrip spiral antenna applicator (without microwave power on) are shown in Fig. 15.19. The upper half of the figure shows the data obtained in the three human subjects when the water bolus was approximately 41°C. The lower half of the figure shows the results obtained when the water bolus was approximately 21°C. The bar graphs for each subject show the water bolus temperature, the average skin temperature, and the average interstitial temperature. Note that the surface temperature is closer to the interstitial temperature than to the temperature of the water bolus. Several applicators were tested. The overall results indicated that the average measurement offset with the bolus at 41°C was 15% of the difference between the interstitially measured skin temperature and the coupling bolus temperature, towards the temperature of the coupling bolus. The corresponding offset with coupling boluses set near 21°C was 32%. The offset errors varied with the type and volume of the water bolus. The significance of these results is that they show that surface measurements do provide a reasonable measure of the subcutaneous temperature. The difference between the surface and interstitial temperatures was typically less than 1°C, even when the bolus temperature was 21°C.

15.6.2 Catheter Placement Strategies

15.6.2.1 Mathematical Models

The use of indwelling catheters allows temperature to be measured at a relatively large number of points, especially if automated thermal mapping is employed. However, these points lie along the catheter tracks and are not dispersed throughout the tumor volume. As a result, temperature is actually sampled over a small fraction of the tumor volume and the distribution obtained may not be representative of the three-dimensional temperature distribution (DEWHIRST et al. 1987). The challenge is to place the catheters such that several one-dimensional temperature distributions will provide a reasonable representation of the three-dimensional temperature distribution.

The key questions are, "How many catheters are needed and how should they be placed?" These questions have been studied by use of mathematical models (DEWHIRST et al. 1987; EDELSTEIN-KESHET et al. 1989). The latter investigation used a three-dimensional temperature distribution which could be readily calculated to test various schemes of catheter placement. The schemes were evaluated by comparing thermal descriptors calculated from the temperatures along the catheter tracks with the same descriptors calculated from the three-dimensional temperature distribution. These studies served as the foundation for the thermometry strategies devised by an RTOG Task Force for clinical trials of hyperthermia (DEWHIRST et al. 1990). In formulating these strategies it was recognized that descriptors obtained in a few linear tracks will inevitably have a geometric bias when this information is extrapolated to three dimensions. Because there is no straightforward way to eliminate this bias, the emphasis was placed on standardizing the thermometry so that the biases would at least be equivalent. The thermometry strategies devised for different modes of heating and different tumor sites are summarized below.

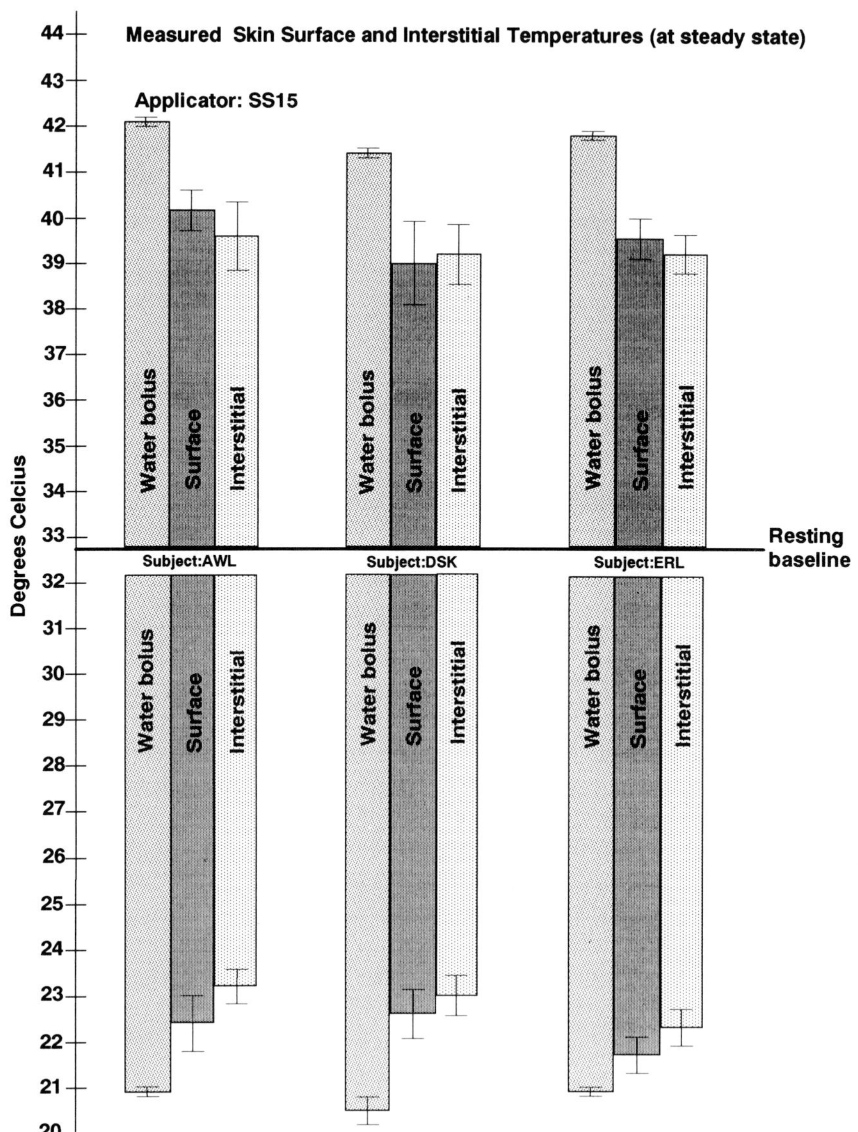

Fig. 15.19. Bar graphs showing a comparison of the water bolus, skin, and interstitial temperatures in three human subjects. The data in the upper and lower halves of the figure were obtained with bolus temperatures of 41° and 21°C, respectively. (From LEE et al. 1994)

15.6.2.2 Superficial Tumors

Superficial tumors treated by use of external microwave applicators can be subdivided into four categories: (a) superficial bulky malignancy, (b) multiple small nodules, (c) an isolated single nodule, (d) diffuse erythematous dermal infiltration. Each of these types of tumor requires a somewhat different thermometry strategy which is described below.

Superficial bulky malignancies extending between 1.5 and 3.0 cm depth require a minimum of three thermometry catheters placed in accordance with one of the strategies illustrated in Fig. 15.20. It is recommended that two catheters be inserted orthogonal to each other so as to intersect at the center of the tumor. This may be accomplished by inserting the catheters parallel to the mid plane, as shown in the uppermost diagram and the one on the right. The catheters can also be inserted at oblique angles, as shown in the diagram on the left, provided they are orthogonal to each other and cross at the mid plane. The two orthogonal catheters should cross the entire tumor and include

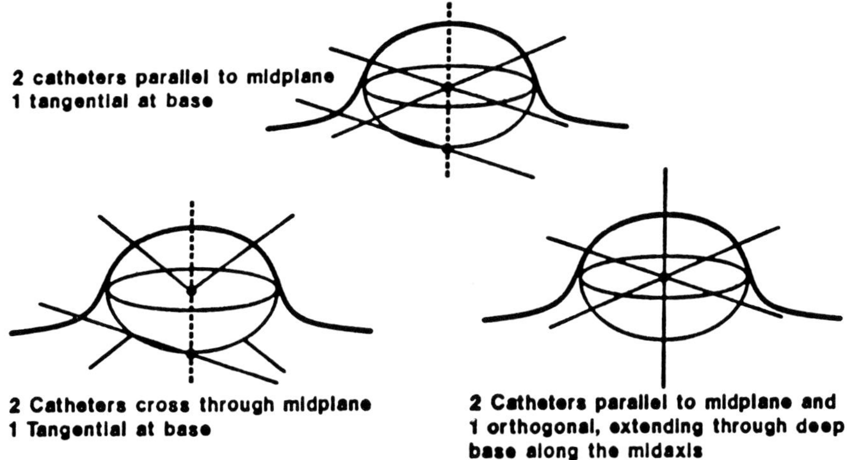

Fig. 15.20. Optimal strategies for catheter locations in superficial bulky malignancies. (From DEWHIRST et al. 1990)

margins of normal tissue. The third catheter should be inserted to the base of the tumor by approaching either tangentially, as shown in the uppermost and left diagrams, or inserted vertically, as shown in the diagram on the right. Tumors extending less than 1.5 cm depth (and less than 1.5 cm in diameter) should have thermometry inserted in the manner recommended for multiple small nodules.

Multiple small nodules ranging from 0.5 to 1 cm in diameter should be instrumented by inserting catheters, fully interstitially, but at the bases of the nodules such that a maximum number of the nodules are intersected, as shown in Fig. 15.21. The number of catheters which should be inserted depends on the area encompassed by the disease. A 25 cm^2 area requires at least one catheter, 25–100 cm^2, at least two, and an area greater than 100 cm^2, three or more catheters. Single nodules which are greater than 1.5 cm in diameter should be instrumented in the manner described for bulky superficial lesions.

Diffuse erythematous dermal infiltration with no discrete nodules should be instrumented by inserting catheters interstitially at 0.5–1.0 cm depth across the field, as shown in Fig. 15.22. The number of catheters needed depends on the area of disease and the criteria defined above for multiple small nodules should be applied. With this type of disease it is not clear whether the catheter is in tumor or normal tissue, but it should be regarded as being in tumor when

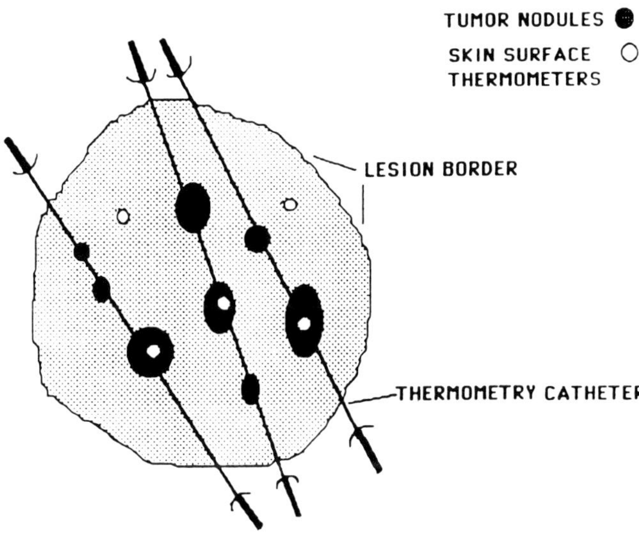

Fig. 15.21. Optimal strategy for locating catheters and surface probes in treatment sites consisting of multiple small nodules. (From DEWHIRST et al. 1990)

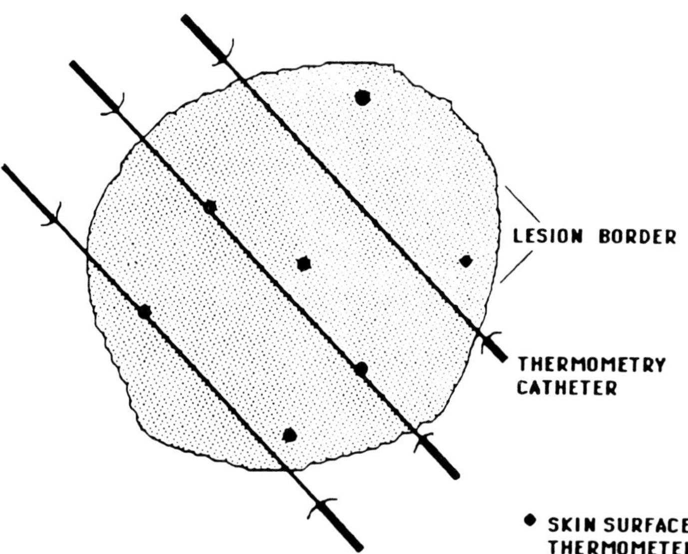

Fig. 15.22. Optimal strategy for locating catheter and surface probes in treatment sites consisting of an inflammatory pattern or plaque of breast carcinoma on the chest wall. (From DEWHIRST et al. 1990)

within the visible margins of the erythematous infiltration.

The guidelines outlined above include only the catheters which are inserted interstitially. In addition, there is a need to monitor multiple skin surface sites. Sites which definitely should be sampled are scars, skin flaps, the tops of discrete nodules, and regions where high temperatures are expected because of maxima in the heating pattern of the applicator.

The strategies adopted for treatment of bulky superficial malignancies with ultrasound are essentially the same as for microwaves except that it is recognized that ultrasound is capable of heating larger tumor volumes because of its deeper penetration, in which case, additional thermometry is needed. For tumors with depths of 3–6 cm, the catheters should be inserted at an oblique angle, crossing in the mid plane of the tumor in close proximity to each other (<0.5 cm). It is recommended that at least three such catheters be inserted in order to obtain an adequate sampling of the larger volume (WATERMAN et al. 1991). An additional catheter should be inserted to measure the temperature at the deepest margin of the tumor compatible with patient safety. Insertion of the catherters at oblique angles is helpful for reducing the artifact due to viscous and absorption heating (HYNYNEN and EDWARDS 1989).

15.6.2.3 Regional Hyperthermia

Instrumentation of deep-seated malignancies is more difficult, but no less important than for superficial malignancies. Optimal thermometry strategies have been devised for RF capacitive heating techniques and for RF annular phased array devices (DEWHIRST et al. 1990; SAPOZINK et al. 1991). These strategies are device dependent to the extent that it is recommended that the catheters be inserted parallel to and perpendicular to the direction of the electric field.

The optimal thermometry placement for RF capacitive heating devices is shown in the uppermost diagram in Fig. 15.23. With parallel plate RF capacitive devices the dominant electric field is usually oriented transaxially. One catheter should extend from the deep tumor margin to the surface parallel to the electric field. A second catheter should be inserted to monitor temperature in a direction perpendicular to the electric field. The optimal thermometry placement for the annular phased array devices is shown in the uppermost diagram of Fig. 15.24. Here, the dominant electric field is oriented along the cranial–caudal body axis. One catheter should extend from the deep tumor margin to the surface along the longitudinal axis. A second catheter should extend from a deep tumor margin to the surface oriented to be radially perpendicular to

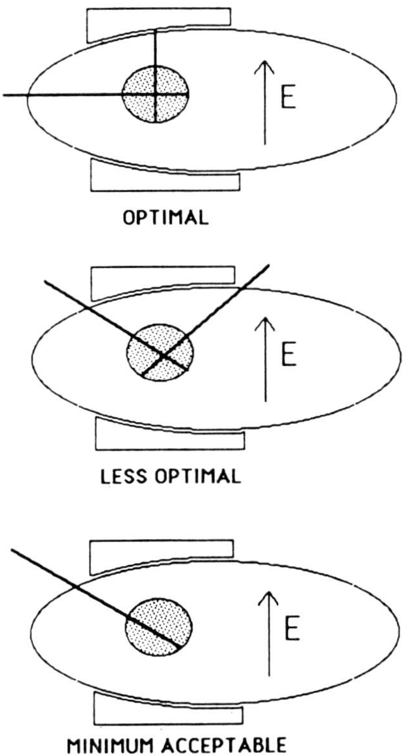

Fig. 15.23. Strategies for catheter placement in association with RF capactive heating techniques. (From DEWHIRST et al. 1990)

the longitudinal axis. A third catheter should be inserted to monitor temperature along a tumor margin. Intracavitary thermometry should be used for sites near or around cavities such as the rectum, bladder, or vagina.

Whenever possible, interstitial catheters should also be inserted to traverse necrotic or low radiographic density areas, the tumor/normal tissue interface, and tumor adjacent to regions with suspected high blood flow. Other areas, such as surgical scars, which are expected to experience significant heating as a result of compromised blood flow, should be monitored through separate thermometry catheters (SAPOZINK et al. 1991). It is also important to monitor the patient's systemic temperature during regional heating.

Unfortunately, it is often impossible to implement the optimal strategies because insertion of the catheters in the required directions would present an unacceptable risk to the patient. For example, in the thorax, transpleural placement risks pneumothorax and longitudinal mediastinal placement requires direct visualization to avoid great vessels. In the abdomen or pelvis, transbowel placement presents risks of perforation or peritonitis and transhepatic or transrenal placement risks hemorrhage. A more comprehensive discussion of the problems associated with placing catheters in the thorax, abdomen, pelvis, and the extremities and axial connective tissue is available in the literature (SAPOZINK et al. 1991; FELDMANN et al. 1993).

Because the optimal thermometry strategies often cannot be implemented, it is important to define the minimum acceptable thermometry. In general, at least one catheter should be placed interstitially through the normal epithelial surface and connective tissue, extend through the tumor center, and traverse as much of the tumor as possible. Examples of less optimal and minimal acceptable thermometry for RF capacitive heating and RF annular phased arrays are illustrated in Figs. 15.23 and 15.24, respectively.

15.6.2.4 Interstitial Hyperthermia

Interstitial hyperthermia includes several different modes of heat delivery: microwave antenna, RF local current field (RF-LCF), ferromagnetic seeds, and hot water or hot wire sources have all been used clinically. Each of these heating modes presents somewhat different requirements for thermometry. A summary of the strategies devised (DEWHIRST et al. 1990; EMAMI et al. 1991) for each of these modes of heating is given below.

15.6.2.4.1 Microwave Antennas. Microwave antennas are usually powered in groups of two to four antennas. To provide adequate feedback for power control, it is recommended that a thermometry catheter be inserted at the center of each group of antennas parallel to the antennas. In addition, it is recommended that at least one catheter be inserted on the periphery of the implant and that another be inserted at the center. Because of the large variation in power deposition along the length of the antenna, it is particularly important to map the temperature in these catheters. It is also recommended that a catheter be inserted through the center of the implant orthogonal to the antenna and that another catheter be inserted into adjacent normal tissue.

The thermometry for microwave interstitial hyperthermia is sometimes carried out using thermometer probes inserted into the heating catheters together with the antenna. At least one manufacturer (BSD Medical Corporation) supplies

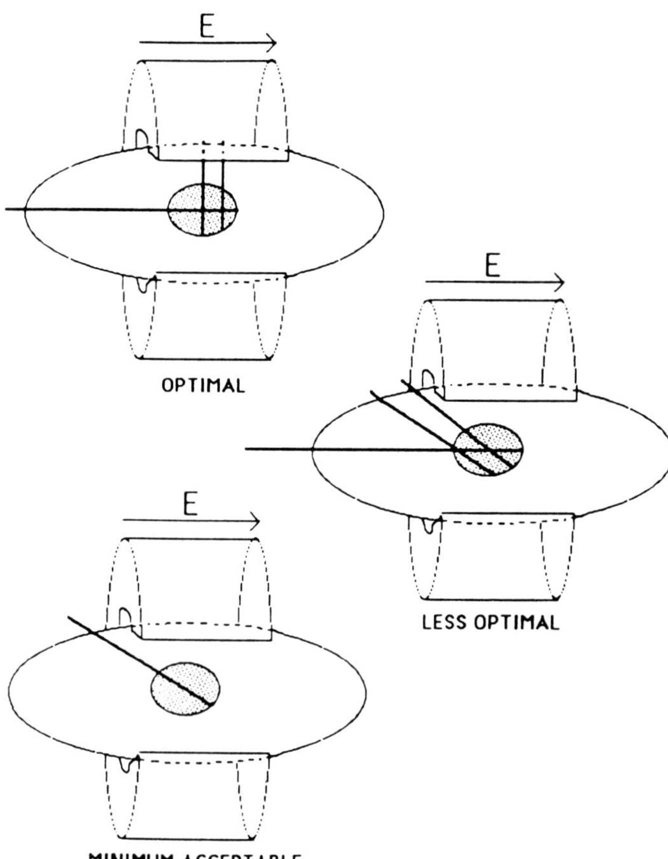

Fig. 15.24. Strategies for catheter placement in association with annular microwave or RF array devices. (From DEWHIRST et al. 1990)

microwave dipole antennas with miniature thermistor sensors embedded inside the coaxial cable dielectric near the hottest part of the antenna. This approach eliminates the trauma associated with the insertion of additional catheters for thermometry, but provides incomplete and sometimes erroneous information. It is assumed that the temperature recorded in the heating catheter is equal to the temperature of the tissue immediately adjacent to the antenna. However, it has been demonstrated (ASTRAHAN 1988) that this assumption is not valid when plastic catheters are employed. Another disadvantage is that there is no knowledge of the minimum temperatures in the field nor data to determine thermal descriptors. It is strongly recommended that temperatures measured in the catheters containing microwave antenna not be used for treatment evaluation (ASTRAHAN 1988; DEWHIRST et al. 1990). However, such data do provide useful feedback information for balancing the power supplied to each antenna.

15.6.2.4.2 RF-LCF Electrodes. RF-LCF heating is normally performed using arrays of needle electrodes connected in pairs to an RF power source. The thermometry strategy for RF-LCF electrodes (DEWHIRST et al. 1990; EMAMI et al. 1991) is essentially the same as for microwave antennas. However, because the needle electrodes are normally spaced closer than microwave dipole antennas, it becomes impractical to place a catheter between each pair of electrodes. The thermometry can be supplemented by placing multisensor probes snugly in the needle electrodes. Because the needles are metal, these probes give a reliable indication of the temperature of the tissue in contact with the electrode, but they do not give reliable estimates of the minimum tumor temperature.

15.6.2.4.3 Ferromagnetic Seeds. With Curie point thermoregulating ferromagnetic seeds, tissue heating occurs only by the conduction of heat from the seeds which are the points of highest temperature. Therefore, the tumor volume does not need to be probed to locate local maxima, as in the case of electromagnetic heating. Ideally, the temperature of all the seeds should be equal and predictable; however, it is required that the temperature of at least one seed be verified. It is recommended tht the temperature be mapped in the regions of expected minimum temperatures, namely along the axis of each square array of four sources.

15.6.2.4.4 Hot Water or Hot Wires. Thermometry recommendations for implants using tubes of flowing hot water or DC resistance wire heaters are essentially the same as for ferromagnetic seeds. The tissue temperature cannot become hotter than the sources; however, the high temperatures used may present a risk to poorly perfused normal tissue (e.g., fat) adjacent to the sources. Therefore, additional thermometry is required to monitor temperature at the surface entrance and exit points in normal tissue when this condition occurs.

Additional discussion of temperature probe placement may be found elsewhere in this volume (Chap. 21, Sect. 21.6).

15.6.3 Localization of Thermometers

It is extremely important to document the location of thermometry catheters and the type of tissue adjacent to the catheter at each point of temperature measurement. Otherwise, it is impossible to properly evaluate thermal descriptors or the adequacy of heating. Locating catheters only by clinical palpation is unreliable. When catheters are inserted by clinical palpation, followed by a CT scan to document their location, they are frequently not in the intended location. Furthermore, the catheter sometimes misses the tumor altogether (SAMULSKI and FESSENDEN 1990; ENGIN et al. 1992), as illustrated in the example shown in Fig. 15.25. In this case, the catheter transects the muscle, but misses the tumor which is behind it. Without the CT scan, the temperatures obtained in this catheter would have been assumed to be in tumor. Documentation by use of radiographs is also inadequate because the tumor cannot be visualized. In the case shown in Fig. 15.25, a radiograph would not have revealed that the catheter was not in tumor.

The thermometry strategies developed by the RTOG Task Force (DEWHIRST et al. 1990) require CT verification to the catheter placement whenever the tumor depth exceeds 1.5 cm. This information is essential for determining whether the

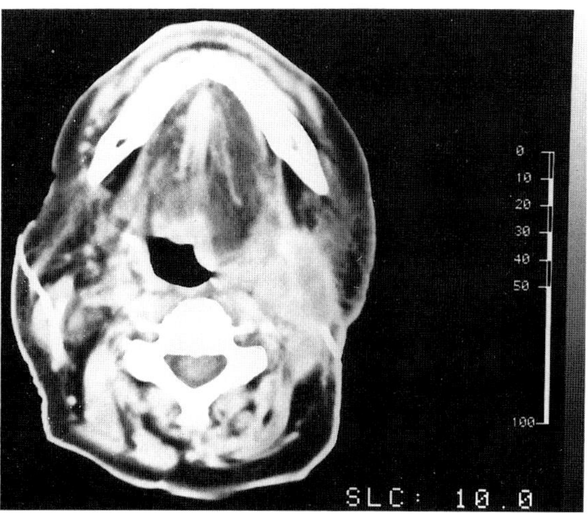

Fig. 15.25. CT documentation of the catheter placement in a patient. In this example, the catheter insertion was guided only by clinical palpation and it missed the tumor entirely

catheters are in the intended locations and for defining which portion of the catheter track traverses tumor. The CT scan is also helpful in defining the extent of the disease, especially the depth below the surface. The depth of disease often cannot be assessed reliably by clinical palpation alone. If a prior CT scan of the tumor site is not available, and the catheters are inserted by clinical palpation, the catheter intended to be at the base of the tumor is often inserted too superficially. As a result, the temperature at the deepest extent of the tumor is not adequately sampled.

It is recognized that obtaining CT verification is both expensive and time consuming. Furthermore, it is sometimes difficult to interpret the films. Tumor boundaries may be poorly defined and it is often difficult to determine the location of each temperature measurement in catheters which do not lie in the plane of the scan. Sections of these catheters may appear in several adjacent CT images and require multiplanar reconstruction in order to visualize the entire catheter length (MONGE et al. 1990). Nevertheless, CT or MRI documentation is essential for proper evalution of the effectiveness of hyperthermia therapy.

15.7 Summary

There has been an impetus to improve the standards of invasive thermometry during the past several years. The state-of-the-art can be summarized as follows:

- Nonperturbing thermometers are available for microwaves and RF hyperthermia, but not for ultrasound.
- Temperature can be measured to within ±0.2°C in microwave fields, but measurements in ultrasound fields with thermocouples are probably seldom more accurate than ±0.5°C due to viscous and absorption heating artifacts, as well as the conduction of heat along the wires leads.
- Thermometry strategies have been devised which provide more complete descriptors of the temperature field.
- Measurements of temperature at a few fixed points is no longer considered acceptable.
- Thermal mapping by use of multisensor probes or automated mapping devices is essential.

Acknowledgements. The author would like to thank Joy McFarlane for her help in preparing this manuscript and Larry Hoh for his help in generating the date shown in two of the figures.

References

Andersen JB, Baun A, Harmark K, Heintzl L, Rasmark P, Overgaard J (1984) A hyperthermia system using a new type of inductive applicator. IEEE Trans Biomed Eng 31: 21–27

Anhalt D, Hynynen K (1992) Thermocouples – the Arizona experience with in-house manufactured probes. Med Phys 19: 1325–1333

Astrahan MA, Luxton G, Sapozink MD, Petrovich Z (1988) The accuracy of temperature measurements from within an interstitial microwave antenna. Int J Hyperthermia 4: 593–607

Bowman R (1976) A probe for measuring temperature in radiofrequency heated material. IEEE Trans Microwave Theory Tech 24: 43–45

Carnochan P, Dickinson RJ, Joiner MC (1986) The practical use of thermocouples for temperature measurement in clinical hyperthermia. Int J Hyperthermia 2: 1–19

Cetas TC (1982) Invasive thermometry. In: Nussbaum GH (ed) Physical aspects of hyperthermia. American Institute of Physics, New York, pp 231–265

Cetas TC (1985) Thermometry and thermal dosimetry. In: Overgaard J (ed) Hyperthermic oncology 1984, vol 2. Taylor and Francis, London, pp 91–112

Cetas TC (1987) Thermometry. In: Field SB, Franconi C (eds) Physics and technology of hyperthermia. Martinus Nijhoff, Dordrecht, pp 470–508

Cetas TC (1990) Thermometry. In: Field SB, Hand JW (eds) An introduction to the practical aspects of clinical hyperthermia. Taylor and Francis, London, pp 423–477

Cetas TC, Conner WG (1978) Thermometry considerations in localized hyperthermia. Med Phys 5: 79–91

Cetas TC, Conner WG, Manning MR (1980) Monitoring of tissue temperature during hyperthermia. Ann NY Acad Sci 335: 281–297

Chakraborty DP, Brezovich IA (1982) Error sources affecting thermocouple thermometry in RF electromagnetic fields. J Microw Power 17: 17–28

Chan KW, Chou CK, McDougall JA, Luk KH (1988a) Changes in heating patterns due to perturbations by thermometer probes at 915 and 434 MHz. Int J Hyperthermia 4: 447–456

Chan KW, Chou CK, McDougall JA, Luk KH (1988b) Perturbations due to the use of catheters with nonperturbing thermometry probes. Int J Hyperthermia 4: 699–702

Christensen DA (1977) A new non-perturbing temperature probe using semiconductor band edge shift. J Bioeng 1: 541–545

Constable RT, Dunscombe P, Tsoukatos A (1987) Perturbation of the temperature distribution in microwave irradiated tissue due to the presence of metallic thermometers. Med Phys 14: 385–388

Corry PM, Jabboury K, Kong JS, Armour EP, McCraw FJ, Leduc T (1988) Evaluation of equipment for hyperthermic treatment of cancer. Int J Hyperthermia 4: 53–74

Dewhirst MW, Winget JM, Edelstein-Keshet L et al. (1987) Clinical application of thermal isoeffect dose. Int J Hyperthermia 2: 165–178

Dewhirst MW, Phillips TL, Samulski TV et al. (1990) RTOG quality assurance guidelines for clinical trials using hyperthermia. Int J Radiat Oncol Biol Phys 18: 1249–1259

Dickinson RJ (1985) Thermal conduction errors of manganin-constantan thermocouple arrays. Phys Med Biol 13: 445–453

Dunn F (1962) Temperature and amplitude dependence of acoustic absorption in tissue. J Acoust Soc Am 34: 1545–1547

Dunscombe PB, McLellan J (1986) Heat production in microwave-irradiated thermocouples. Med Phys 13: 457–461

Dunscombe PB, Constable RT, McLellan J (1988) Minimizing the self-heating artifacts due to the microwave irradiation of thermocouples. Int J Hyperthermia 4: 437–445

Edelstein-Keshet L, Dewhirst MW, Oleson JR, Samulski TV (1989) Characterization of tumour temperature distributions in hyperthermia based on assumed mathematical forms. Int J Hyperthermia 5: 757–777

Emami B, Stauffer P, Dewhirst MW et al. (1991) RTOG quality assurance guidelines for interstitial hyperthermia. Int J Radiat Oncol Biol Phys 20: 1117–1124

Engin K, Tupchong L, Waterman FM, Nerlinger RE, Leeper DB (1992) Optimization of hyperthermia with CT scanning. Int J Hyperthermia 8: 855–864

Engler MJ, Dewhirst MW, Winget JM, Oleson JR (1987) Automatic temperature scanning for hyperthermia treatment monitoring. Int J Radiat Oncol Biol Phys 13: 1377–1382

Feldmann HJ, Hoederath A, Molls M, Sack H (1993) Problems associated with CT-guided catheter insertions. Int J Hyperthermia 9: 219–225

Fessenden P, Lee ER, Samulski TV (1984) Direct temperature measurement. Cancer Res 44 (Suppl): 4799s–4804s

Fry WJ, Fry RB (1954a) Determination of absolute sound levels and acoustric adsorption coefficients by thermocouple probes – theory. J Acoust Soc Am 26: 294–310

Fry WJ, Fry RB (1954b) Determination of absolute sound levels and acoustic absorption coefficients by thermocouple probes – experiment. J Acoust Soc Am 26: 311–317

Gammampila K, Dunscombe PB, Southcott BM, Stacey AJ (1982) Thermocouple thermometry in microwave fields. Clin Phys Physiol Meas 2: 285–292

Gibbs FA (1983) Thermal mapping in experimental cancer treatment with hyperthermia: description and use of a semi-automatic system. Int J Radiat Oncol Biol Phys 9: 1057–1063

Goss SA, Cobb JW, Frizzell LA (1977) Effect of beam width and thermocouple size on the measurement of ultrasonic absorption using thermoelectric technique. IEEE ultrasonics symp proc 82CH1823–4. IEEE, New York, pp 745–749

Greig LH, Szanto J, Raaphorst GP (1992) On the spatial resolution of clinical thermometers. Med Phys 19: 679–684

Hand JW (1984) Linear thermocouple arrays for in vivo observation of ultrasonic hyperthermia fields. Br J Radiol 57: 656

Hand JW (1985) Thermometry in hyperthermia. In: Overgaard J (ed) Hyperthermic oncology 1984, vol 2. Taylor and Francis, London, pp 299–308

Hand JW, Dickinson (1984) Linear thermocouple arrays for in vivo observation of ultrasonic hyperthermia fields. Br J Radiol 57: 656

Hand JW, Lagendijk JW, Bach Anderson J, Bolomey JC (1989) Quality assurance guidelines for ESHO protocols. Int J Hyperthermia 5: 421–428

Hoh LL, Waterman FM (1995) Use of manganin-constantan thermocouples in thermometry units designed for copper-constantan thermocouples Int J Hyperthermia 11: 131–138

Hynynen K, Edwards DK (1989) Temperature measurements during ultrasound hyperthermia. Med Phys 16: 618–626

Hynynen K, Watmough DJ, Fuller M, Mallard JR (1982) Temperature distributions during local ultrasound induced hyperthermia in vivo. IEEE ultrasonic symp proc 82CH1823–4. IEEE, New York, pp 745–749

Hynynen K, Martin CJ, Watmough DJ, Mallard JR (1983) Errors in temperature measurement by thermocouple probes during ultrasound induced hyperthermia. Br J Radiol 56: 969–970

Kapp DS, Cox RS, Fessenden P, Meyer JL, Prionas SD, Lee ER, Bagshaw MA (1992) Parameters predictive for complications of treatment with combined hyperthermia and radiation therapy. Int J Radiat Oncol Biol Phys 22: 999–1008

Kuhn PK, Christensen DA (1986) Influence of temperature probe sheathing materials during ultrasound heating. IEEE Trans Biomed Eng 33: 536–538

Lee ER, Kapp DS, Lohrbach AW, Sokol JL (1994) The influence of water bolus temperature on measured skin surface and intradermal temperatures. Int J Hyperthermia 10: 59–72

Leopold KA, Dewhirst M, Samulski T et al. (1992) Relationships among tumor temperatrue, treatment time, and histopathological outcome using preoperative hyperthermia with radiation in soft tissue sarcomas. Int J Radiat Oncol Biol Phys 22: 989–998

Leopold KA, Dewhirst MW, Samulski TV et al. (1993) Cumulative minutes with T_{90} greater than $Temp_{index}$ is predictive of response of superficial malignancies to hyperthermia and radiation. Int J Radiat Oncol Biol Phys 25: 841–847

Lyons BE, Samulski TV, Britt RH (1985) Temperature measurements in high thermal gradients. I. The effects of conduction. Int J Radiat Oncol Biol Phys 11: 951–962

Martin CJ (1986) Temperature measurement in tissues by invasive and non-invasive techniques. In: Watmough DJ, Ross WM (eds) Hyperthermia. Blackie, Glasgow, pp 154–179

Martin CJ, Law ANR (1983) Design of thermistor probes for measurement of ultrasound intensity distributions. Ultrasonics 21: 85–90

Monge OR, Lindskold L, Lyng H, Sager EM (1990) Positioning of temperature measurement points using multiplanar computed tompography. Int J Hyperthermia 6: 957–960

Oleson JR, Dewhirst MW, Harrelson JM, Leopold KA, Samulski TV, Tso CY (1989) Tumor temperature distributions predict hyperthermia effect. Int J Radiat Oncol Biol Phys 16: 559–570

Samulski TV (1988) Current technologies for invasive thermometry. In: Paliwal BR, Hetzel FW, Dewhirst MW (eds) Biological, physical and clinical aspects of, hyperthermia. American Institute of Physics, New York, p 168

Samulski TV, Shrivastava PN (1980) Photoluminescent thermometer probes: temperature measurements in microwave fields. Science 208: 193–194

Samulski TV, Lee ER (1986) Premedical evaluation of a Luxtron 3000. In: Kondraske GV, Robinson CJ (eds) Proceedings of 8th Annual Conference IEEE-EMB. IEEE, New York, pp 1493–1495

Samulski TV, Fessenden P (1990) Thermometry in theraputic hyperthermia. In: Gautherie M (ed) Clinical thermology, Springer Berlin Heidelberg New York (subseries thermotherapy) pp 1–34

Samulski TV, Lyons BE, Britt RH (1985) Temperature measurements in high thermal gradients. II Analysis of conduction effects. Int J Radiat Oncol Biol Phys 11: 963–971

Samulski TV, Grant WJ, Oleson JR, Leopold KA, Dewhirst MW, Vallario P, Blivin J (1990) Clinical experience with a multi-element ultrasonic hyperthermia system: analysis of treatment temperatures. Int J Hyperthermia 6: 909–922

Sapozink MD, Corry PM, Kapp DS et al. (1991) RTOG quality assurance guidelines for clinical trials using hyperthermia for deep-seated malignancy. Int J Radiat Oncol Biol Phys 20: 1109–1115

Scholes RR, Small JG (1980) Fluorescent decay thermometer with biological applications. Rev Sci Inst 51: 882–884

Shrivastave P, Luk K, Oleson J et al. (1989) Hyperthermia quality assurance guidelines. Int J Radiat Oncol Biol Phys 16: 571–587

Singh BS, Dybbs A (1976) Error in temperature measurements due to conduction along the sensor leads. J Heat Trans 98: 491–494

Tarczy-Hornoch P, Lee ER, Sokol JL, Prionas SD, Lohrbach AW, Kapp DS (1992) Automated mechanical thermometry probe mapping systems for hyperthermia. Int J Hyperthermia 8: 543–554

Vaguine VA, Christensen DA, Lindley JH, Walston TE (1984) Multiple sensor optical thermometry for application in clinical hyperthermia. IEEE Trans Biomed Eng 31: 168–172

van der Zee J, van Rhoon GC, Broekmeijer-Reurink MP, Reinhold HS (1987) The use of implanted closed-tip catheters for the introduction of thermometry probes during local hyperthermia treatment series. Int J Hyperthermia 3: 337–345

van der Zee J, Veeze-Kuijpers B, Wiggers T, van de Merwe SA, Treurniet-Donker AD (1992) Risk of tumour growth along thermometry catheter trace: a case report. Int J Hyperthermia 8: 621–624

Waterman FM (1985) The response of thermometer probes inserted into catheters. Med Phys 12: 368–372

Waterman FM (1990) Determination of the temperature artifact during ultrasound hyperthermia. Int J Hyperthermia 6: 131–142

Waterman FM (1992) Estimation of the temperature artifact from a short interruption in ultrasonic power. Int J Hyperthermia 8: 395–400

Waterman FM, Leeper JB (1990) Temperature artifacts produced by thermocouples used in conjunction with 1 and 3 MHz ultrasound. Int J Hyperthermia 6: 383–399

Waterman FM, Hoh LL (1992) Error in temperature measurement caused by thermal conduction when copper-constantan thermocouples are used for hyperthermia. Med Phys 19: 805

Waterman FM, Nerlinger RE, Leeper JB (1990) Catheter induced temperature artifacts in ultrasound hyperthermia. Int J Hyperthermia 6: 371–381

Waterman FM, Dewhirst MW, Fessenden P et al. (1991) RTOG quality assurance guidelines for clinical trials using hyperthermia administered by ultrasound. Int J Radiat Oncol Biol Phys 20: 1099–1107

Wickersheim (1986) A new fiberoptic thermometry system for use in medical hyperthermia. SPIE Proceedings SPIE Bellingham, Washington, vol 713, pp 150–157

Wickersheim KA, Alves RB (1979) Recent advances in optical temperature measurement. Ind Res Dev 21: 82–89

16 Recent Trends in Noninvasive Thermal Control

J.C. Bolomey, D. Le Bihan, and S. Mizushina

CONTENTS

16.1 Introduction

Owing to its evident possible impact on the development of hyperthermia treatments, noninvasive thermometry (NIT) is in clinical demand, especially for deep-seated and/or large tumors. A recent International Consensus Meeting on Hyperthermia (1989) pointed out that (a) measuring the temperature distribution and (b) comparing it to a specified standard are essential to validate the results obtained from clinical trials. As is well known, these problems cannot yet be considered completely solved. Invasive techniques are now regarded as sufficiently accurate (except for ultrasound), but they only indicate the temperature at a limited number of points and are considered traumatic for patients. For approximately a decade, several noninvasive techniques have been considered and presented as potential candidates for clinical use, but as yet none has achieved a marked impact on clinical practice. For this reason, there is now a need to update previous attempts at a systematic comparison of these techniques (e.g., Bolomey and Hawley 1989; Cetas 1984; Hand 1984; Mizushina 1987).

The NIT techniques can be grouped into two main classes. Radiometric techniques are based on the measurement of the electromagnetic or acoustic radiation spontaneously transmitted by a body at a given temperature. Microwave radiometry is the most illustrative example of such "passive" approaches, which require no interrogating radiation. In fact, it is still the only technique to be implemented effectively on heating equipment. Quite different is the "active" imaging approach consisting of deducing temperature data from the response of the heated region to interrogating radiation. This indirect approach consists in (a) producing temperature-sensitive images and (b) calibrating these images in terms of temperature (Fig. 16.1). Well-established imaging modalities such as x-ray tomodensitometry, ultrasound echotomography and magnetic resonance imaging (MRI) constitute representative examples of candidate techniques for which equipment and technology are available. Other imaging techniques such as electrical impedance tomography and microwave imaging are less developed but must not be neglected.

During the last few years, significant research has been devoted to NIT, and the resultant findings have been reported at different workshops. Two of these workshops have been organized within the framework of the European COMAC-BME program on hyperthermia

J.C. Bolomey, PhD, Professor, Electromagnetic Department, SUPELEC, University of Paris XI Plateau du Moulon, F-91190 Gif-sur-Yvette, France
D. Le Bihan, MD, Department of Health and Human Services, National Institutes of Health, The Warren G. Clinical Center, Building 10, Room 1C660, Bethesda, MD 20892, USA
S. Mizushina, PhD, Professor, Research Institute of Electronics, Shizuoka University, 3-5-1 Johoku, Hammamatsu 432, Japan

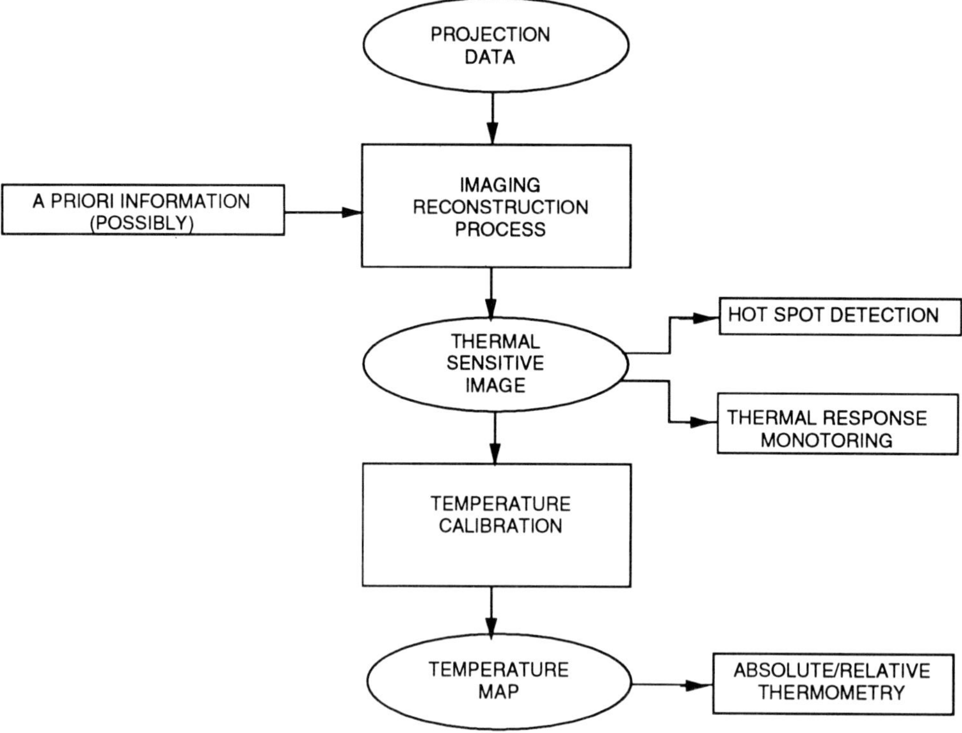

Fig. 16.1. Principle of the active imaging approach to NIT

(COMAC-BME 1989; COMAC-BME 1991). More recently, a special session was devoted to noninvasive thermal control at the concluding COMAC-BME workshop, in Utrecht (COMAC-BME 1992). Furthermore, another workshop on NIT was organized in Tucson in 1992 during the 6th International Conference on Hyperthermic Oncology. Also of importance, though less recent, are the results obtained after the completion of a Japanese National Research and Development Program for Medical and Welfare Apparatus aiming to incorporate noninvasive control systems in deep-heating equipment. This effort was supported by the Agency of Industrial Science and Technology (AIST). All these events, as well as other results in the literature, make it possible to assess the state of the art in NIT and to try to predict future milestones that will be achieved within the next few years. Indeed, the quite significant recent achievements are of assistance in answering the questions (how? and when?) asked by the clinical community about NIT.

The object of this chapter is not to explain again the basics of NIT techniques, which have already been presented in previous papers, but rather to report on the results obtained and to point out major trends. The chapter is organized as follows. In Sect. 16.2, the evolution of NIT specifications is analyzed. One of the most significant developments over the past few years has been the change in attitude of the clinical community with respect to NIT. While absolute NIT is still the ultimate goal, noninvasive control is recognized as a potentially useful intermediate step. In the following two sections, the two main approaches used in NIT are discussed. The evolution in microwave radiometry, which is the only technique to be integrated in available commercial equipment, is analyzed in Sect. 16.3, while new advances in MRI are discussed in Sect. 16.4. Although MRI remains an expensive technique, it has attractive specific advantages which may ultimately make it the modality of choice for real-time noninvasive temperature imaging. Section 16.5 deals with other techniques based on x-ray and ultrasound tomography, as well as on dielectric imaging in the low and microwave frequency ranges via electrical impedance tomography and active microwave imaging. Finally, in Sect. 16.6, as a conclusion, several questions concerning the future of NIT are addressed.

16.2 Evolution in NIT Needs and Specifications

Consideration needs to be given to both NIT specifications stricto sensu and noninvasive control (NIC) or monitoring, two aspects that are, in fact, intimately related. The change of emphasis from NIT to NIC has resulted mainly from the difficulties encountered in the practice of deep hyperthermia and from the difficulties in developing perfect NIT providing temperature and only temperature.

The specifications for NIT equipment required for clinical purposes now seem to have stabilized at reasonable levels. By reasonable, we mean more realistic in terms of (a) clinical usefulness (taking into account what can be achieved today) and (b) the expected performance of NIT candidate techniques. In all cases, the objective is to obtain a thermal image, the specifications of which may be summarized by a resolution voxel in the space, temperature, and time domains (Fig. 16.2). Even if the ultimate goal should consist in 1 mm spatial and 0.1°C temperature resolutions, with 25 images per second to achieve real-time display, it is recognized that "degraded" performances could be very valuable for clinical usefulness. For instance, tracking temperature gradients on the order of 1°C, extending over 1 cm, in less than 1 min should provide a very significant improvement and accommodate the most commonly encountered variations in these gradients.

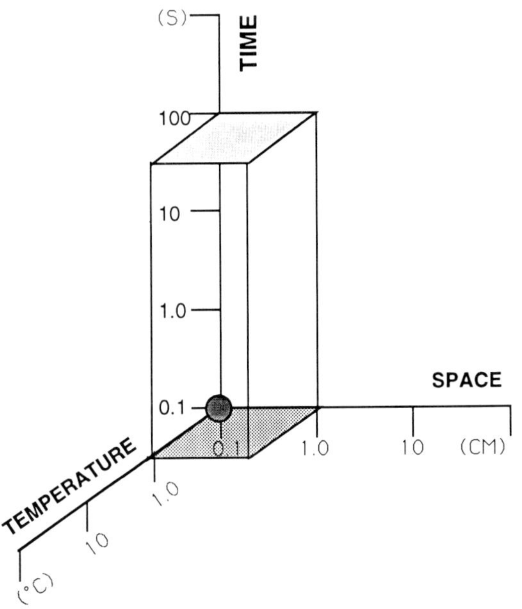

Fig. 16.2. Temperature/space/time resolution voxel for NIT purposes

It is worth noting that the resolution voxel dimension is not completely sufficient for comparing different NIT approaches. Indeed, for some techniques the intrinsic voxel dimensions may be affected by different factors such as the anatomical structure and related contrasts, the location of the area under investigation, the amount of a priori available information, and the clinical context. More particularly, special attention has to be paid to the artifacts related to patient movement. Many available imaging techniques make use of subtraction processes to achieve the required sensitivity, but it has been observed that thermal imaging performance is significantly reduced by patient movements. More generally, it is clear that too rapid conclusions, based only on results concerning resolution, could lead to the premature rejection of some techniques which, in other respects to be detailed later, appear promising. In addition, very good resolution results achieved with phantoms in laboratory environments are not always clinically relevant.

Independently of the NIT problem stricto sensu, a new orientation is emerging which extends the debate. Besides temperature itself, in terms of which the treatment efficacy can be assessed via the thermal dose concept, it appears that the global thermal response of the tissues could provide interesting clinical information. The global thermal response includes both direct and indirect effects of heat delivery such as vascular thermoregulatory processes, edema formation, and burns. As will be shown later, the global thermal response can be rendered visible by means of imaging modalities. One of the major advantages of this approach could be that it will allow some discrimination between healthy and tumoral tissues. Furthermore, the availability of the global thermal response could provide useful information on the evolution of the tissues, session after session or during the same session. For instance, in the case of tumor cells, analysis of the global thermal response could indicate whether they have been sufficiently heated and may be killed. This approach is further supported by the development of new techniques such as focused ultrasound "surgery," which effectively aims to destroy tumoral tissues. Another important aspect of NIC concerns the need for the adjustment of multiapplicator equipment before heat delivery.

To summarize, the following four levels of requirement have now been recognized, as acknowledged at the final COMAC-BME (1992) workshop in Utrecht:

1. Hot spot detection
2. Monitoring of the global thermal response
3. Differential temperature measurements
4. Absolute temperature measurements

Points 1–3 would find their immediate application in routine deep hyperthermia treatments. By contrast, absolute temperature measurements are ultimately needed to assess the efficacy of hyperthermia treatments, but also represent the most difficult objective.

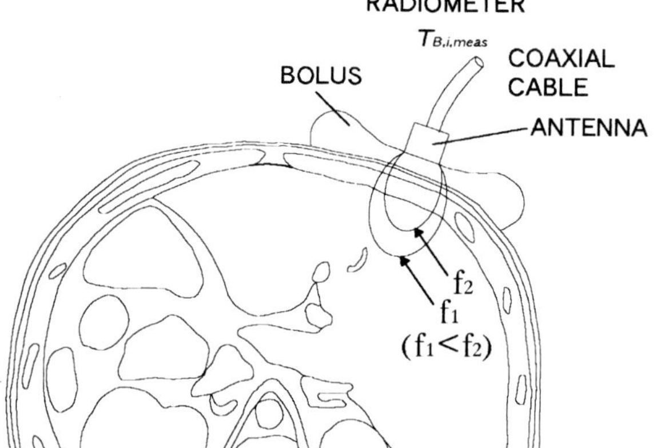

Fig. 16.3. Typical multifrequency microwave radiometric measurement situation in hyperthermia

16.3 Microwave Radiometry

16.3.1 Introduction

Microwave radiometry has been investigated for noninvasive monitoring and control of hyperthermia for more than 10 years (NGUYEN et al. 1979), and perhaps is the only technique that has been used clinically in combination with heating equipment (PLANCOT et al. 1987; CHIVE 1990; DUBOIS et al. 1993). During the last few years there has been a trend toward exploitation of the capabilities of multifrequency schemes for the reconstruction of temperature profiles and thermal images.

16.3.2 Framework of Multifrequency Radiometry

In a typical microwave radiometric measurement situation in hyperthermia, an antenna is held in contact with a bolus filled with distilled water, as depicted in Fig. 16.3. The thermal radiation from subcutaneous tissues and the bolus is measured as a brightness temperature $T_{B,i,meas}$ over a frequency-band centered at f_i; f_i is typically in the range from 1 to 6 GHz due to the electrical properties of tissues. The lowest frequency is limited by the diffraction of microwaves by the antenna aperture and the highest frequency by the penetration distance of microwaves in tissue, which decreases rapidly with frequency. $T_{B,i,meas}$ is a weighted average of temperatures over a view field of the antenna. Since the depth of the antenna view field decreases as f_i increases at these frequencies, a set of $T_{B,i,meas}$ measured at multifrequencies f_i ($i = 1, 2, \ldots, n$) contains information with regard to temperature-depth distribution in the object. It is then possible to retrieve a temperature distribution from $T_{B,i,meas}$ ($i = 1, 2, \ldots, n$).

The first step in the temperature distribution retrieval is to analyze the near-field coupling between the antenna and the object with the aid of a model to derive weighting functions $W_i(r)$. Plane-parallel layered models have been analyzed with one-dimensional treatments (BARDATI 1987a,b; CHIVE 1990; MIZUSHINA 1993) and more recently with three-dimensional treatments (NIKITA et al. 1989; MAMOUNI et al. 1991; BOCQUET et al. 1993; BARDATI et al. 1993). Once $W_i(r)$ are obtained, the brightness temperatures for the model $T_{B,i,model}$ can be calculated by:

$$T_{B,i,model} = \int W_i(r)T(r)dv \quad (i = 1, 2, \ldots, n), \tag{16.1}$$

where $T(r)$ is the physical temperature of an incremental volume dv at a position r, provided that electrical characteristics of the tissues are known (FOSTER et al. 1979, 1981; JOHNSON et al. 1972; REDDY and SAHA 1984; SCHEPPS and FOSTER 1980; SCHWAN and PIERSOL 1954; STEEL and SHEPPARD 1985; STUCHLY and STUCHLY 1980, 1990). Then, Eq. 16.1 is to be solved for $T(r)$ from a set of $T_{B,i,model}$ ($i = 1, 2, \ldots, n$) under the constraints:

$$T_{B,i,model} = T_{B,i,meas} \text{ at } f_i \ (i = 1, 2, \ldots, n). \qquad (16.2)$$

The number of independent measurements or the discrete data n is limited in practice, for example $n = 2$–7. The upper limit is set approximately by the ratio $(6\,\text{GHz} - 1\,\text{GHz})/(B + B_{sep})$ where B $(= B_i)$ is the bandwidth and B_{sep} is a reasonable frequency separation between adjacent frequency bands. In addition, the radiometric data $T_{B,i,meas}$ fluctuates randomly with a standard deviation σ_i, which is given by the resolution of f_i band of the radiometer:

$$\sigma_i = \Delta T_{B,i,min} = \frac{2(T_{B,i,meas} + T_{rec,i})}{(B_i\tau)^{1/2}} = \frac{2(310 + T_{rec,i})}{(B_i\tau)^{1/2}}(\text{K}), \qquad (16.3)$$

where $T_{rec,i}$, B_i, and τ are the equivalent noise temperature of the radiometer receiver, bandwidth of the f_i band and signal integration time, respectively. In Eq. 16.3 Dicke radiometer theory is assumed (Ulaby 1981).

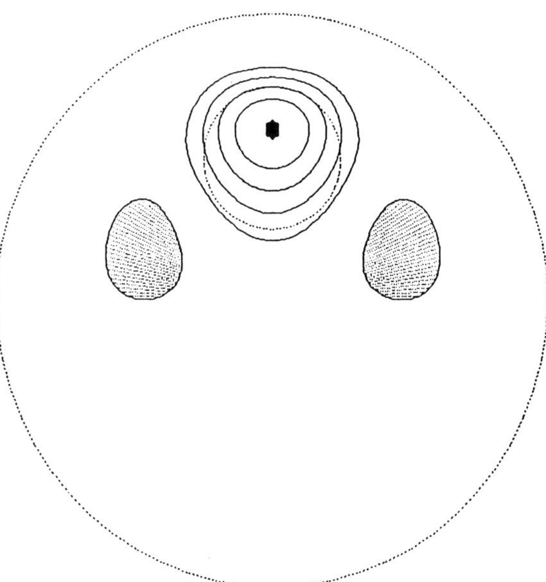

Fig. 16.4. Tomographic thermal image retrieved by the singular system method from radiometric data measured on a cylindrical phantom containing muscle-equivalent saline solution by a four-channel radiometer. Outer cylinder diameter: 11.8 cm. Inner tube diameter: 3 cm. $\Delta T = +5°\text{C}$. *Shading*, negative portions. (Courtesy of F. Bardati)

16.3.3 Methods of Temperature Retrieval

Equations 16.1–16.3 constitute an inverse problem whose solutions are prone to instability or poor precision. However, during the last few years interesting developments have been reported with respect to the inversion process based on three different approaches, as discussed below.

16.3.3.1 Singular System Analysis

Bardati et al. have developed a method of solving Eq. 16.1 based on singular system analysis, where temperature fields to be retrieved are expanded in terms of suitable basis functions (Bardati et al. 1987a,b, 1993). The regularity of the temperature field is accommodated in the basis functions. This method enables one to reconstruct a two-dimensional thermal image. The method was tested by an experiment in which the radiometric measurements were taken by a four-channel radiometer (f_i = 1.1, 2.5, 4.5, 5.5 GHz) via four waveguide antennas mounted flush, 90° apart on a 11.8-cm-diameter cylindrical phantom containing muscle-equivalent saline solution. An inner tube with the same saline solution at an elevated temperature was revolved through 360° at a fixed distance from the wall of the outer cylinder. Two-dimensional temperature images were successfully obtained to demonstrate the potential of the method. A two-dimensional thermal image for a ΔT = +5°C case is reproduced in Fig. 16.4 from Bardati et al. (1993). The isothermal contours are separated by 20% of the maximum postive value of the retrieved temperature. The black shaded area corresponds to the region where the retrieved temperature is not less than 98% of the maximum value.

16.3.3.2 Combined Model Fitting and Monte Carlo

Mizushina et al. have developed a method (Hamamura et al. 1987; Mizushina et al. 1992, 1993) in which use is made of a temperature profile model function:

$$T(z) = T_{model}(z; \text{model parameters}), \qquad (16.4)$$

where z is the depth. The model function must have an appropriate form to describe temperature profiles that would be expected under given heating conditions using only a limited number of model parameters m, for example, $m = 3$–7. The rational for this approach is that the use of a priori knowledge would improve the precision at the expense of generality of solution. Substituting the model function into Eq. 16.1 and integrating, one obtains a set of algebraic equations containing m model parameters. Of the m model parameters, the bolus water and body surface temperatures are determined by direct probe measurements, and $m - 2$ unknown model parameters are determined by fitting the model to the radiometric measurements, i.e., by seeking a combination of the model parameters that minimizes the error function:

$$\sum_{i=1}^{n} (T_{B,i,model} - T_{B,i,meas})^2 = F_{error}(\text{model parameters}), \qquad (16.5)$$

with $n > 2m - 2$.

The above procedure permits one to find a temperature profile $T(z)$ that fits a particular set of $T_{B,i,meas}$ data. However, $T_{B,i,meas}$ fluctuate randomly, resulting in random fluctuations in $T(z)$. The spreading in $T(z)$ at a value of z can be taken as a measure of the precision of tissue temperature at that depth. A Monte Carlo technique has been developed to calculate the confidence interval of $T(z)$ (MIZUSHINA et al. 1992, 1993). The model-fitting/Monte Carlo method was tested by a phantom experiment. The radiometric measurements were taken on a muscle equivalent agar phantom through a 1-cm layer of distilled water via a single waveguide antenna using a five-band radiometer operating at f_i = 1.2 GHz (0.074°K), 1.8 GHz (0.067°K), 2.5 GHz (0.056°K), 2.9 GHz (0.065°K), 3.6 GHz (0.075°K), where the numbers in parentheses are measured values of $\Delta T_{B,i,mim}$ at $\tau = 5$ s. A typical result is presented in Fig. 16.5, where the area bounded by $+\sigma$ and $-\sigma$ shows the evolution of 2σ interval with depth. The 2σ interval increases with z, as is to be expected for a homogeneous medium, and is 1.8°K at $z = 4$ cm. It is desirable to reduce the 2σ intervals, particularly at deeper locations. A numerical simulation study has shown that an improvement in the radiometer resolution $\Delta T_{B,i,min}$ is quite effective: $\Delta T_{B,i,min} = 0.03$°K ($i = 1, 2, \ldots, 5$) will have a 2σ interval of 0.8°K at $z = 4$ cm. The simulation has also shown that the use of tighter constraints on Eq. 16.5, i.e., $n > m - 2$ rather than $n = m - 2$, is effective in reducing the 2σ intervals. $\Delta T_{B,i,min} = 0.03$°K can be achieved by a radiometer that employs a modern low-noise microwave amplifier and low loss microwave components at $\tau = 8$ s.

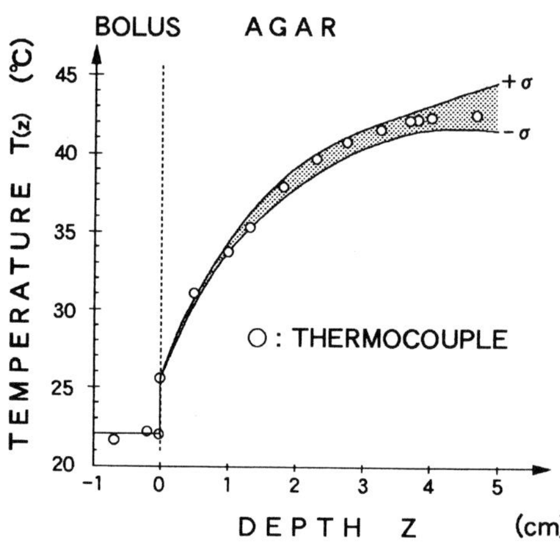

Fig. 16.5. Temperature-depth profile 2σ values retrieved by the model-fitting/Monte Carlo method from radiometric data measured on a muscle-equivalent agar phantom by a five-channel radiometer. σ = standard deviation. *Open circles*, temperatures by thermocouple probes for comparison

16.3.3.3 Radiometry-Matched Bio-heat Transfer Analysis

Chive developed a method in which a temperature profile $T(z)$ is first calculated by solving the bio-heat transfer equation (PENNES 1948) in one-dimensional form under 915-MHz heating conditions (CHIVE 1990; DUBOIS et al. 1993):

$$d(z)c(z)\frac{\partial T(z,t)}{\partial t} = \frac{\partial}{\partial z}\left[K_a(Z)\frac{\partial T(z,r)}{\partial Z} + B(z,t) + P_a(z,t) + Q_m(z)\right] \qquad (16.6)$$

where $T(z)$, z, t are the tissue temperature, space, and time variables; $d(z)$, the tissue density; $c(z)$, tissue-specific heat; K_a, the tissue thermal conductivity; $B(z, t)$, the rate of heat exchange with blood; $P_a(z, t)$, the rate of energy input due to microwave heating; and $Q_m(z)$, the rate of metabolic heat generation. The $B(z, t)$ term is assummed to be given by:

$$B(z,t) = V_s[T_a - T(z,t)], \qquad (16.7)$$

where T_a is the arterial blood temperature and V_s the product of flow and heat capacity of blood.

The heat conduction at the body surface is given by:

$$K_a \frac{\partial T(O, t)}{\partial Z} = h[T(O, t) - T_e], \qquad (16.8)$$

where h is the heat conductance between the skin and the bolus, T_e is the temperature external to the body and O refers to the body surface. A temperature profile $T(z)$ at a given time t is calculated from Eqs. 16.6–16.8 for a set of V_s and h. $T(z)$ thus obtained is substituted into Eq. 16.1 to compute $T_{B,i,model}$ at 1 GHz and 3 GHz. The computation is repeated with variable V_s and h until $T_{B,i,model}$ and $T_{B,i,meas}$ at 1 GHz and 3 GHz match within ±0.2°C. A hyperthermia system that combines 1-GHz and 3-GHz radiometers with 434-MHz or 915-MHz heating equipment has been built, tested, and used in the clinic (Chive 1990; Dubois et al. 1993). A feature of the system is that the same applicator, which is a microstrip–microslot applicator, is used for both heating and radiometry. A temperature profile obtained after 1 h of heating of a cervical node is reproduced in Fig. 16.6 from Chive (1990). The above method has recently been extended to obtain the two-dimensional thermal profile (Dubois et al. 1993). It is anticipated that the two-dimensional thermal profile may permit reasonably accurate estimation of thermal dose in a heated volume.

16.3.4 Conclusion

Advances in microwave radiometry for non-invasive monitoring and control of hyperthermia during the last few years have been reviewed. It is now possible to obtain temperature-depth profiles with 2σ intervals, and two-dimensional temperature profiles or tomographic temperature images, using multifrequency microwave radiometry employing three different techniques of inversion from the radiometric data to tissue temperatures. Among these, the technique based on the combination of two-channel radiometry and the bio-heat transfer equation has been used in the clinic to treat superficial tumors. This technique appears to permit reasonably accurate estimation of thermal dose in a heated volume for some situations. With these recent developments, it has been shown that microwave radiometry is useful for hyperthermia treatments of superficial tumors. However, further improvements in the accuracy and the depth of measurement sensitivity are needed for wider clinical applications. This calls for further studies to develop (a) a radiometer with high sensitivity and stability (Eq. 16.3), (b) weighting functions with improved accuracy for various anatomical sites (Eq. 16.1), and (c) inversion processes that permit solutions with a sufficient degree of precision (Eqs. 16.1–16.3); in addition it is necessary to compile extensive data on the electrical properties of normal and tumorous tissues (Eq. 16.1). It is important to recognize that no factors other than the weighting functions are involved in connecting tissue temperatures to radiometric data in Eq. 16.1, which is the basis of microwave radiometry, and that all progress on the aforementioned points is bound to improve capabilities of microwave radiometry for non-invasive thermal control and dosimetry.

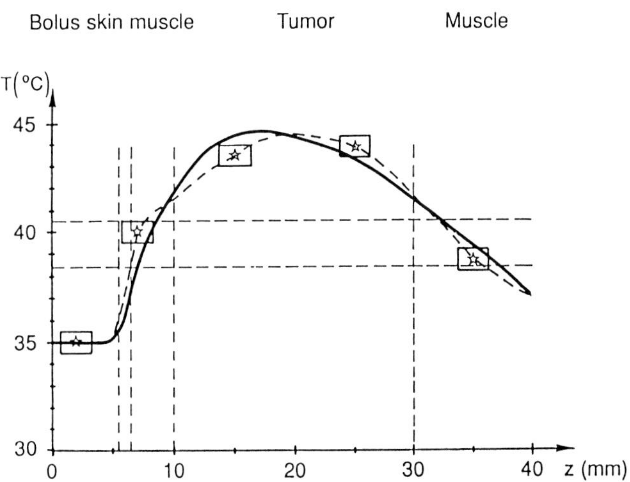

Fig. 16.6. Temperature-depth profile obtained by the two-channel radiometry/bio-heat transfer equation method on a cervical node. (Courtesy of M. Chive)

16.4 Nuclear Magnetic Resonance Imaging

16.4.1 MRI and NIT Requirements

Magnetic resonance imaging offers a safe approach since no ionizing radiation isinvolved. Tomographic images may be acquired in any part of the body in any orientation. Multiple slices and even a three-dimensional data set can be obtained. Ultrafast imaging techniques now provide images with a millimeter spatial resolution in a few tens of milliseconds. These achievements have largely resulted from the significant progress recently made in MRI technology, especially in radiofrequency and gradient system hardware stability. Suitable gradient coil sets have been designed which allow strong gradient pulses to be switched quickly without significant eddy current problems and with reasonable power amplifiers. These coils permit fast imaging, such as echo-planar imaging (EPI), to be performed. Fast imaging is required to monitor physiological changes in temperature of other physiological parameters at a subsecond time scale. Furthermore, fast scanning limits effects of motion artifacts. The concept behind EPI is to acquire the data corresponding to a whole image from a single echo signal, hence the nickname "single-shot" imaging (Stehling et al. 1991). To achieve this goal, the main signal (echo, either spin-echo or gradient-echo) is split in a series of 64, 128, or 256 gradient-echoes according to desired image resolution, each encoding for a separate line in Fourier space. Such fast scanning requires fast switching (typically in less than 200 ms) of large gradient pulses (typically 20 mT/m), which is a difficult technical challenge. Among compromises made are the use of long acquisition sampling times (about 50 ms) which make EPI very sensitive to chemical shift and field inhomogeneity artifacts. Nevertheless, EPI is probably one of the best techniques available when acquisition time is a premium, e.g., in order to acquire motion artifact-free multiple data in a reasonable time, as for diffusion imaging. EPI is now being implemented on clinical MRI systems by manufacturers.

Magnetic resonance imaging may also have a significant impact on the evaluation of important parameters other than temperature during hyperthermia. For instance, blood flow, which is the dominant factor in bioheat transfer, cannot be evaluated routinely during hyperthermia procedures. Monitoring and, perhaps more importantly, active control of blood flow should play a determinant role in hyperthermia treatment. In this respect, MRI has recently been shown to be a very promising technique for evaluating blood flow with high spatial and temporal resolution (Le Bihan 1992). In addition, metabolic parameters (e.g., metabolite concentrations, metabolic process rates, oxygenation status, and production of radicals) which change upon heating may be suitable indicators of the success of hyperthermia treatment. Theoretically, at least, these parameters are measurable by nuclear magnetic resonance imaging or spectroscopy.

16.4.2 Current Achievements and Limitations

Several MRI parameters have been suggested for the evaluation of temperature. Using MR spectroscopy techniques temperature may be evaluated in samples with extremely high accuracy by observing the chemical shift of particular molecular groups of specific compounds introduced into the sample as tracers (Knuttel and Juretschke 1986). Unfortunately, the potential toxicity of these compounds, in combination with the rather poor sensitivity of localized MR spectroscopy, precludes their clinical use at present. Looking indirectly at chemical shift of water through phases effects may be an interesting alternative. The relaxation time, T1, of water has also bee proposed (Parker et al. 1983; Dickinson et al. 1986; Hall et al. 1990). However, the sensitivity of T1 to temperature seems low and tissue dependent. Deviation from linearity has been seen in some biological tissues when temperature reaches 40°C. Furthermore, measuring T1 with good accuracy from MRI images is difficult. The most recently suggested candidate for MRI-based temperature imaging has been the diffusion coefficient of water, D (Le Bihan et al. 1989a). This approach has so far been the most successful. Diffusion is not per se an MRI parameter and its relationship with temperature (T) was empirically established in liquids long before the age of MRI as D exp $(-Ea/kT)$, where Ea is the activation energy for diffusion a, and k is the Boltzman constant. In the physiological temperature range, the sensitivity of diffusion to temperature is about 2.4%/°C, which is about twice as high as that of T1. MRI pulse sequences can generate maps of diffusion coefficients. From these maps, images of temperature changes may be

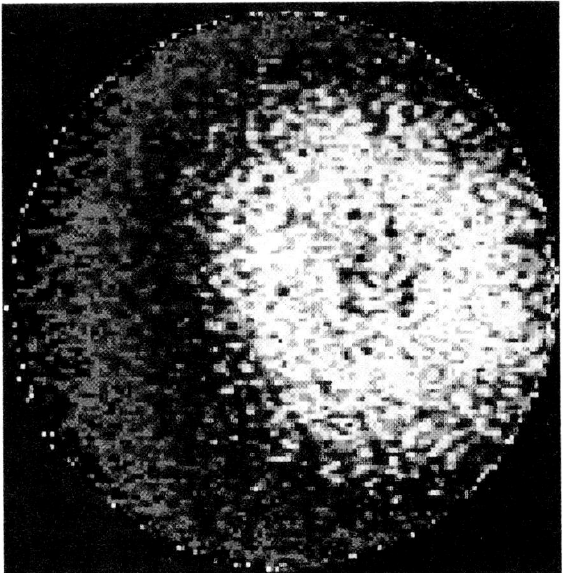

Fig. 16.7. Temperature image obtained by diffusion MRI. A gel phantom was heated inside the MRI unit using a radiofrequency annular phased-array (MAPA) clinical hyperthermia device made compatible with the MRI unit. Brightness in the image directly reflects temperature. Maximum heating was achieved off-center, due to the position of the phantom within the MAPA. The periphery of the phantom was cooled using a cold water bath

calculated. MR temperature imaging based on diffusion has good potential for application in hyperthermia. Phantom results demonstrate resolution on the order of 0.2°C over 0.3-cm^3 regions (ZHANG et al. 1992) (Fig. 16.7). Although diffusion images may require ultrafast acquisition schemes, such as EPI, to avoid motion artifacts and particularly stable hardward (TURNER et al. 1990), diffusion measurements from images are usually faster, more robust, and more accurate than T1 measurements.

Thus, there is little doubt that this technique can meet the desired requirement for temperature, spatial, and temporal resolution in vitro. In this respect, the technique might be a useful nondestructive, noninvasive research tool for acquiring temperature distributions in complex media, for instance to characterize the absorbed energy distribution pattern of a heating device or to verify numerical models of energy absorption and heat transfer.

The future of this methodology for in vivo and clinical applications is less clear, although diffusion MR imaging is actively proceeding toward routine clinical use (LE BIHAN et al. 1992). First, diffusion imaging requires good signal-to-noise ratios in raw images, since diffusion images are calculated and not directly acquired (LE BIHAN et al. 1988; SOUZA 1992). Achievement of such good signal-to-noise ratios is relatively easy in brain tissues where spin-spin relaxation is slow and background field inhomogeneities are low, but becomes problematic in other parts of the body. Effects of blood flow and perfusion, which may mimic diffusion effects (LE BIHAN et al. 1989a), also have to be considered, in particular in the context of hyperthermia, given the role of blood flow in tissue thermal clearance. On the other hand, preliminary results have shown that *Ea* is identical in brain, muscle, and liver tissue, but variations, and, thus, the need for local calibration, may not yet be completely ruled out. Also, changes in tissue intrinsic diffusion properties as a result of hyperthermia could exist, as shown in brain white matter (LE BIHAN et al. 1989b). Such changes might be helpful in understanding or detecting lethal effects of heat at the cellular level, but would severely affect temperature measurements.

16.4.3 Coupling of Heating and MRI

To use MRI to monitor hyperthermia, however, it is necessary to combine a hyperthermia device with an MRI unit. This is not a priori trivial since each device might be functionally disturbed, if not damaged, by the presence of the other. Compatibility problems may be expected to arise mainly from the interaction of the strong magnetic field and the radiofrequency fields used by MRI with the applicator of the hyperthermia system. The hyperthermia device must be able to work under such conditions and must also be physically compatible, e.g., must fit inside the MRI transmitter and receiving coils. The most difficult challenge, however, is to assure the correct operation of the MRI unit in the presence of the heating device. The magnetic field of the MRI unit should not be distorted by the presence of any ferromagnetic parts. Also, the hyperthermia device must not include large metallic parts that could be the origin of eddy currents when the gradient pulses used for MRI are switched. Finally, and perhaps most importantly, the MRI signal, which is on the order of nanowatts, must be purged of any radiofrequency pollution emanating from the hyperthermia applicator. This is especially true for electromagnetic applicators which are operating in a close frequency range at the level of several hundred watts. (Current clinical MRI systems use frequencies from 4 to 85 MHz.) Even if frequencies seem well separated, one should always fear some leakage out of the expected frequency range. A possible solution is to process in a time-sharing manner between heating and MRI signal collection (DELANNOY et al. 1990).

Interstitial techniques requiring metallic electrodes may result in severe artifacts, but laser interstitial thermotherapy, with Nd:YAG lasers for instance, using optic fibers to deliver energy to tissues should not pose any compatibility problems. This approach has been successfully used in phantoms and animal models (HIGUCHI et al. 1992; BLEIER et al. 1991) in combination with T1 and diffusion echo-planar MRI to monitor thermal effects in real time. Clinical applications of MRI-guided interstitial laser therapy have begun in neurosurgery. However, the size of laser-induced lesions is limited by optical absorption and thermal diffusion, so that multiple fibers would be required to treat large tumors.

The specific merits of each noninvasive heating technique have not yet been systematically examined. Noninvasive heating techniques employing ultrasound, microwaves, or radiofrequency waves may be adapted to function simultaneously or nearly simultaneously with MRI. Initial trials have been conducted using radiofrequency capacitive heating operating at 27 MHz in an MRI system operating at 6.68 MHz (DICKINSON et al. 1986). More recently, the approach based on an annular array of radiofrequency heating antennas (mini annular phased array, MAPA) has been demonstrated to be feasible in phantoms (Delannoy et al. 1990). Moreover, it is possible to integrate in a single device the annular arrays of antennas and the MRI gradient and imaging coils (DELANNOY et al. 1990). This particular approach has clinical relevance since the annular array heating technique is routinely used in hyperthermia (Fig. 16.8).

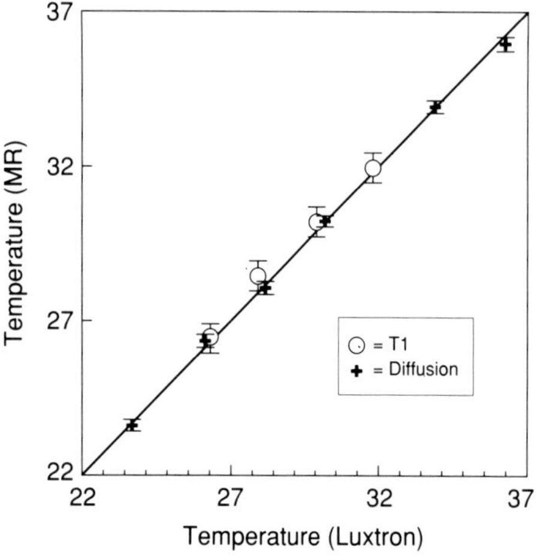

Fig. 16.8. Correlation of temperature, as measured with diffusion and T1-weighted MRI, and optic fiber probes (Luxtron) in a polyacrylamide gel phantom positioned inside the modified MAPA applicator. The predicted temperatures were found to be within 0.2°C and 0.5°C of the probe measurements using D and T1, respectively

The most promising approach, however, relies on the use of focused ultrasound beams that provide minimally invasive therapy of large irregularly shaped tumors in any region of the anatomy where the path to focus is free of bone or air interfaces. The use of short high-intensity pulses which elevate almost instantaneously the temperature at the focus to the range of 60°–70°C until tissue is destroyed by coagulation necrosis reduces the effects of variable perfusion. It is well known that with conventional hyperthermia, blood vessels can create cold spots that interfere with therapy. This focused ultrasound "surgery" technique has been successfully combined with MRI and applied to in vivo animal models (CLINE et al. 1992; see also Chap. 12, Sect. 12.5.6). Temperature measurement is not a significant issue with this technique, but both T1 and diffusion MRI have been used to visualize induced lesions.

16.4.4 Conclusion

Noninvasive temperature mapping with MRI is feasible and potentially fulfills clinical requirements regarding safety, temperature accuracy, and spatial/temporal resolution. Several parameters may be used, but molecular diffusion seems the most accurate. Accurate, artifact-free measurements would require the use of ultrafast acquisition schemes, such as EPI. Coupling of MRI and heating is a difficult challenge but has been shown to be feasible, for instance using radiofrequency heating (capacitor systems and annular phased-arrays). Important developments are expected in the field of "interventional MRI," mainly using laser or focused ultrasound beams. At this time, however, the potential of MRI to monitor interventional procedures and temperature remains to be evaluated in vivo and in a clinical environment.

16.5 Other Imaging Techniques

16.5.1 X-rays

In 1988, x-rays [computerized tomography (CT) scanners] were considered to be probably very close to operational performance in terms of space and time resolutions – such were the conclusions at the end of the Symposium on Equipment for cancer therapy. This Symposium has been organized in Tokyo 1988, jointly by the Agency for Industrial Science and technology (AIST), the Association of Medical and Welfare Apparatus and the Ministery for International Trade and Industry (MITI). At that time, very encouraging results were presented (Saito et al. 1988) by the Shimadzu company, which was developing heating equipment combining (a) 4 or 6 E-polarized waveguide applicators in the 80- to 90-MHz frequency range and (b) an x-ray scanner devoted to noninvasive thermometry. Measurements were performed on complex phantoms consisting of water and pig organs. By using image substraction and spatial averaging techniques, a temperature resolution of 1°C over 1 cc was typically achieved after a smoothing process to eliminate motion artifacts. From the most recent information (T. Marume, personal communication, 1993), it appears that this program is now suspended without preclinical or clinical assessment of the prototype. The main difficulties were (a) subtraction artifacts due to patient movements, especially those resulting from patient translation between the heating equipment and the x-ray scanner, and (b) poorly known temperature coefficients of the density of living tissues. The basic question concerning the possible use of x-rays for noninvasive thermometry, despite their ionizing effects, has been analyzed by G. Gaboriaud (personal communications, 1993) on the following basis. Temperature measurements are assumed to be performed every 5 min, the patient being moved on each occasion from the heating equipment into an x-ray scanner. Typically, the duration of the hyperthermia session is 1 h and the total hyperthermia treatment consists of ten sessions. Accordingly, the patient is subjected to 120 scanner sessions. For imaging an abdomen slice, the irradiation dose ranges between 8 and 20 mGy, according to the desired image quality. Consequently, an estimation of the total dose required for x-ray NIT would be between 0.96 and 2.4 Gy. It should be expected to be larger due to the high sensitivity required by temperature measurements. If this dose is compared to the therapeutic dose for the first couse of treatment of a tumor in the abdomen – typically between 40 and 55 Gy – it is seen that the latter is approximately 20 times larger than the dose required by NIT. However, decreasing the temperature measurement interval to 1 min leads to comparable doses for treatment and measurements. This estimation illustrates the limits of using x-rays in NIT during hyperthermia sessions.

16.5.2 Ultrasound

As is well known, the acoustic parameters of living tissues depend on temperature. With available ultrasound equipment, the echoes on temperature. With available ultrasound equipment, the echoes are processed on the basis that the ultrasound velocity is constant over the whole tissue volume. The time resolution is usually not better than 50 ps and the temperature change cannot be measured. More sophisticated processing techniques have been considered. Despite very encouraging phantom experiments, no real implementation associated with heating equipment has been reported. However, it is worth observing that there is some renewed interest in techniques which had been abandoned. This is the case for the diffraction tomography approach (Duchêne and Tabbara 1985; Nadi et al. 1992), which is, in principle, only valid for low-contrast imaging and which is limited by bone or air shadowing.

Greater success has been achieved with the nonlinear approach to NIT. This approach consists in superimposing probe and pump pulse waves (Fukukita et al. 1987; Ueno et al. 1989). The acoustic parameters, and hence temperature changes, can be derived with the help of simple equations from the spectral response of the echoes. However, despite the fabrication of an advanced prototype by Matsushita (Ueno et al. 1990) and preliminary assessments on animals, the development program is now completed. Figure 16.9 shows the equipment and some results obtained during a hyperthermia session on a

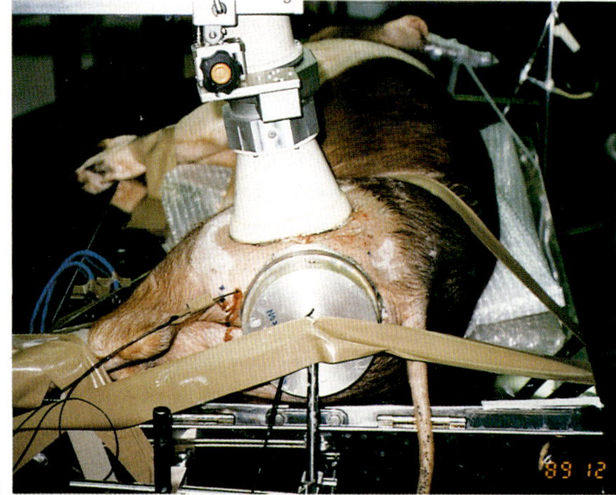

a

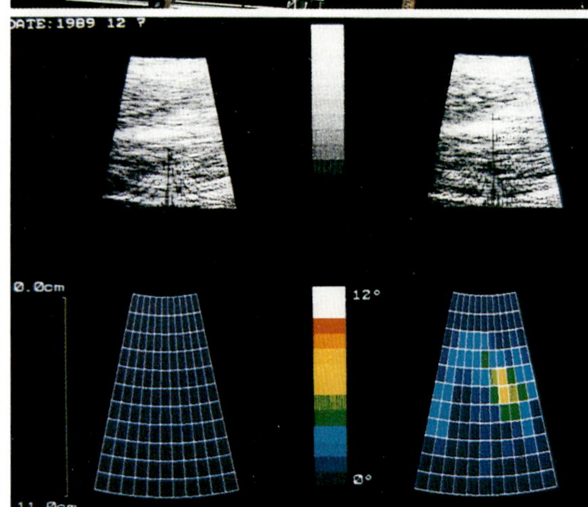

b

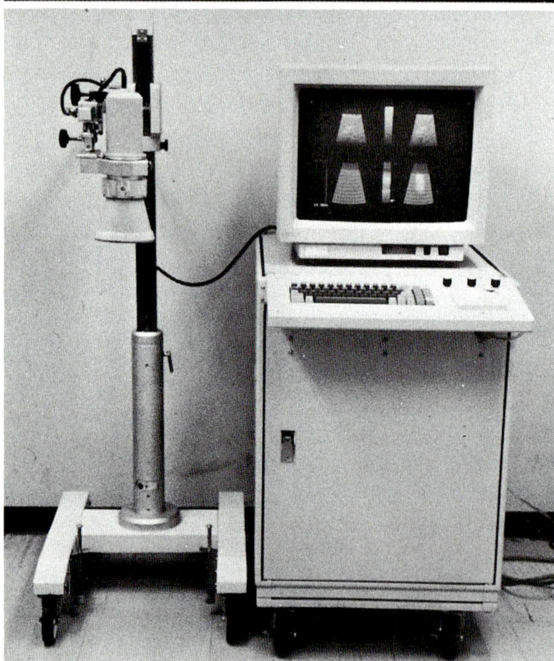

c

pig. One of the recognized major difficulties in developing this measurement technique was in preparing a data base for the temperature dependence of acoustic properties for various living tissues; a further difficulty has been the time required to develop a commercial product (T. YANO, personal communication, 1993).

It is expected that ultrasound-NIT could be very much stimulated over the next few years by taking advantage of the technological developments in ultrasound lithotripsy and in the emerging focused ultrasound surgery field.

16.5.3 Electrical Impedance Tomography

Electrical impedance tomography (EIT) aims to retrieve the conductivity of the tissues under observation and, accordingly, provides images which are dependent on temperature via the conductivity of these tissues. Low-frequency EIT, which is widely used in industrial process tomography (XIE 1993), exhibits very attractive features in terms of NIT. Basically, the conductivity temperature coefficient is significantly high. Secondly, the process is rapid and the equipment is cheap. However, the images provided by such equipment suffer from certain weaknesses. The spatial resolution is limited to approximately one-tenth of the radius of the ring of electrodes that encircles the body part, and the sensitivity is significantly decreased at the center of the ring. Furthermore, the reconstruction algorithms are not linear and are very sensitive to the contrrast of the tissues.

Some assessment of EIT equipment on phantoms has been organized within the framework of the COMAC BME program. The Sheffield equipment, which operates at 50 kHz, has been combined with a 27-MHz capacitive ring applicator (CONWAY et al. 1992a,b; HAWLEY et al. 1992). For this study, a leg phantom was used consisting of a 127-mm muscle equivalent cylinder with foam inserts. The EIT ring of electrodes was located in the middle plane between the two capacitive ring electrodes (Fig. 16.10a).

Fig. 16.9. a Measurement configuration for anesthetized pig; *1*, focused ultrasound applicator at 0.8 MHz; *2*, nonlinear ultrasound probe; *3*, optic fiber sensors. **b** B-mode image and temperature increase distribution in pig's thigh. **c** General view of the nonlinear ultrasound thermometry equipment. (Courtesy of T. Yano)

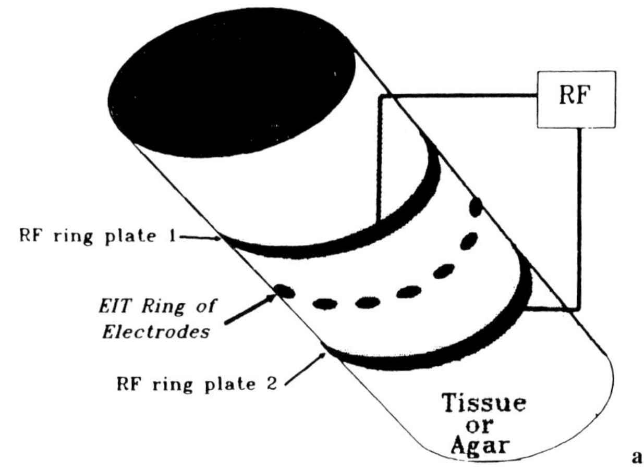

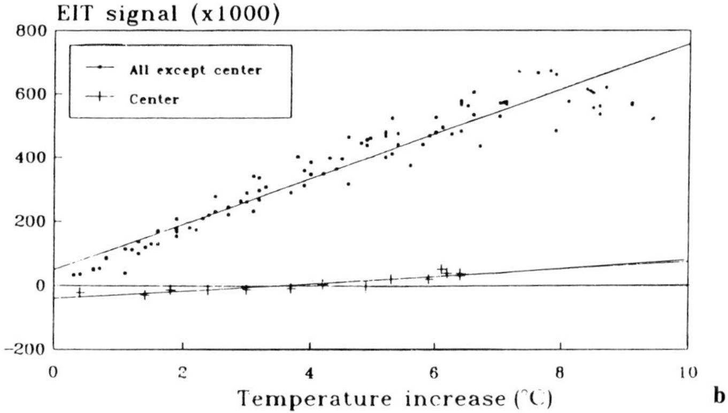

Fig. 16.10. **a** Schematic representation of an RF ring capacitor applicator heating a cylindrical tissue phantom during EIT imaging of the central plane. **b** Correlation between temperature increase and EIT signals at all sensor sites. (Courtesy of J. Conway)

Comparison between fiberoptic invasive temperature measurements and EIT regional analysis has demonstrated a good correlation between measured temperature increase and EIT signal (Fig. 16.10b), except at the center, where the agreement is less good. The temperature resolution was about 0.75°C. The same trends have been observed on a human thigh, though with much lower sensitivity (GRIFFITHS and AHMED 1987).

From a practical point of view, past trials have shown some difficulties in integrating an EIT system into heating equipment. For example, for the purposes of electromagnetic compatibility, it is recommended that a "power-off protocol" be used. Such a protocol entails collecting EIT data during pauses in the treatment. Off-pauses are expected to be on the order of 30 s, incorporating delays for transient decay and EIT data collection. Such a sequence protects against interference between heating and imaging equipment, and, more particularly, RF currents circulating on EIT equipment wiring. Such induced currents have been shown to be decreased by suitable materials and orientation.

Furthermore, in vivo measurements over long periods of time show some artifacts and drifts in the measured impedance. Such drifts probably result from changes in electrode contact impedance. These changes are due to the deterioration of the electrodes or to skin modifications, such as sweating. In addition, in vivo measurements demonstrate a far lower signal to noise ratio than phantom measurements. As a result, the temperature resolution seems to be at least one order of magnitude poorer than what is required in ESHO protocols (HAND et al. 1984).

A potential way to compensate for EIT drawbacks could be to integrate EIT data with other external complementary data (HENRIKSON 1993, private communication). External images, consisting of a 64 × 64 matrix, can be imported from x-ray or MRI systems. Such a high-resolution image can be used to identify reference points where temperature is measured with high accuracy, for instance with fiberoptic or thermistor

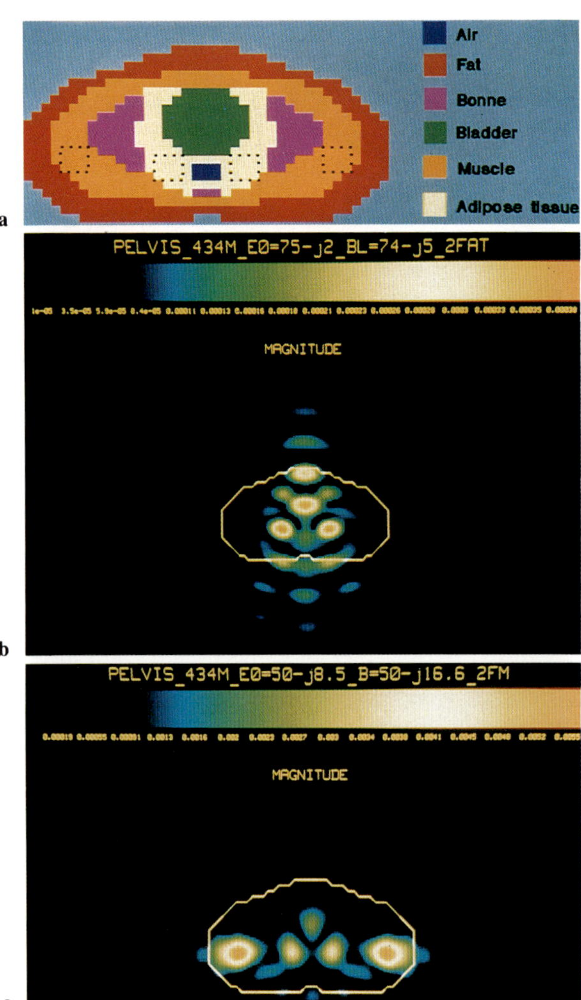

Fig. 16.11. a Pelvis phantom permittivity. The *dashed lines* show the contours of the heated regions. **b** Differential imaging of dielectric contrast reconstructed when two zones of adipose tissue surrounding the bladder in the pelvic phantom are heated 5°C above normal temperature. **c** Differential imaging of dielectric contrast reconstructed when two muscle regions in the pelvic phantom are heated 5°C above normal temperature, in addition to those of **b**. (Courtesy of A. Broquetas)

probes. If these points do not correlate with the imported image, then the image can be corrected. If the object is nonhomogeneous, the imported image can be used to identify different areas with different temperature coefficients. Furthermore, in the event of movement, the absolute EIT image can be used to keep track of the movements. This partial list of examples illustrates that a lot of possibilities exist for combining EIT and an imported image. However, it is clear that the best way of combining them in clinical situations is still to be found: an interesting area of investigation for the next few years.

16.5.4 Active Microwave Imaging

Active microwave imaging is expected to provide convenient basic sensitivity, i.e., the temperature coefficient of the complex dielectric constant. However, it suffers from the need for complex nonlinear reconstruction algorithms. Such algorithms are required to compensate for the diffraction of microwave beams. Furthermore, the spatial resolution may change significantly within the field of investigation according to the complexity of anatomical structures. Linearized forms of the reconstruction process, such as spectral diffraction tomography, have shown difficulties in processing highly contrasted structures. In situ assessments of a 2.45-GHz planar microwave camera have been conducted within the framework of the COMAC BME Hyperthermia program, in Amsterdam on a dual-waveguide applicator (Joisel et al. 1991) and at the Institut Curie on the ring capacitive applicator developed by the Rotterdam group (Gaboriaud et al. 1991). Such assessments have clearly shown major difficulties resulting from the need for a water bolus. The bolus results in leakage around the patient larger than the signal propagating in the patient. At 2.45 GHz, the losses in tissues are very significant and the maximal depth of investigation proved to be limited to around 26 cm to maintain a convenient signal to noise ratio. In such circumstances, reconstruction via diffraction tomography is useless. Additional simulations have been performed on a cylindrical microwave scanner (Martin et al. 1991). The objective was to investigate the possible use of lower frequencies in order to achieve better sensitivity. However, decreasing the operating frequency decreased the spatial resolution, which is on the order of half a wavelength in tissues. Two-dimensional numerical modeling of abdominal or pelvic configurations at 434 MHz has shown that the spatial resolution is low but sufficient to record the main hot spots produced in the heated region (Mallorqui et al. 1992) (Fig. 16.11). Some attempts have been devoted to reducing artifacts by (a) improving microwave penetration through the use of immersion media approximating living tissue characteristics and (b) making more valid the assumptions involved in the reconstruction process, namely the uniformity of the illuminating field in inhomogeneous targets, which is responsible for image distortions (BROQUETAS et al. 1993).

More recently, studies have been devoted to nonlinear iterative processes aiming to quantitate imaging, i.e., to retrieve the value of the complex permittivity (JOACHIMOWICZ et al. 1991; CHEW and WANG 1990). Currently these algorithms are very time consuming and their sensitivity to noise or systematic errors has to be more extensively assessed. Taking into account a prior information has been shown to yield a valuable decrease in the computation time. A promising feature of such algorithms is the fact that, for instance, the spatial resolution should not be limited by diffraction to one-half of a wavelength but could be significantly smaller, as shown by preliminary simulations.

Another "hardware" solution to compensate for diffraction effects is based on time domain spectroscopy (LARSEN and JACOBI 1986; MIYAKAWA 1991; MIYAKAWA et al. 1992). The selection of the shortest path contribution between the transmitting and the receiving antenna is a means of eliminating the effect of multiple scattering, and this allows the use of classical x-ray tomographic algorithms.

16.6 Discussion and Conclusion

In recent years significant advances have been made with respect to NIT and NIC. The most significant points with respect to the various modalities are as follows:

1. Improved performance of microwave radiometry can be expected from more sophisticated multiprobe and/or multifrequency data collection procedures. Both model and imaging approaches are worthy of further consideration for tumor configurations that are not too deep.

2. MRI is undoubtedly the technique which has realized the most important step, namely a drastic reduction in the measurement duration. At present, MRI equipment is probably the closest fit to clinical requirements in terms of sensitivity and spatial resolution. However, extensive assessment is still needed to validate its clinical usefulness, taking into account the key points of mechanical and electromagnetic compatibility.

3. X-rays seem to have been abandoned during recent years, despite good results obtained on phantoms. The resulting global dose would have been a major problem for time resolutions of less than 1 min.

4. One can observe renewed interest in ultrasound, but the best approach has not yet been identified. It is expected that technological advances stimulated by focused ultrasound surgery will contribute to the maintenance of research efforts in this area.

5. In the case of EIT, only a few attempts have been devoted to exploitation of existing equipment with advanced software. Both algorithmic and technological difficulties remain to be resolved before the technique will become very attractive clinically. The fusion of EIT data with other imported images as well as with local temperature measurements is probably a way of achieving adequate performance for hot spot detection and qualitative assistance during deep hyperthermia treatment. The technology developed for industrial applications is also expected to have a positive impact on EIT development.

6. In the case of active microwave imaging, studies using existing microwave cameras have revealed difficulties related to both equipment and algorithms. These difficulties may be overcome with a new generation of equipment which is being developed for incorporation into the coaxial TEM applicator of the Utrecht clinical group (LAGENDIJK and DE LEEUW 1986). This new equipment uses integrated microwave antennas and quantitative algorithms.

These observations call for some comments.

Firstly, the possible role of the global thermal response in assessing the efficacy of hyperthermia treatments needs to be more thoroughly investigated, modality by modality. The most important challenge would then be to produce temperature-sensitive images and to correlate these images with the treatment efficacy. Such a global approach eliminates the need for specific tissue temperature calibration, which was one of the reasons for the abandonment of x-rays and nonlinear ultrasound. This difficulty will have to be overcome for the remaining imaging techniques if the ultimate goal of absolute thermometry is to be realized.

Secondly, the past years are rich in very promising phantom experiments that have not been successfully extended to in vivo and/or clinical situations. Taking into account realistic environments is now of essential importance, and the decisive improvement in MRI imaging performance awaits clinical validation. All NIT or NIC techniques face the same problem with respect to validation: validation can be relatively easily considered using phantoms, but in vivo the situation is more difficult. There is a need to ascertain the most convenient references for demonstrating that the technique being tested achieves the expected performance.

The cost aspect is not, for prototype systems, of prime importance. Indeed, the problem is not at the moment to disseminate MRI controlling setups to every hyperthermia site. Rather, it is to answer the basic question of whether deep hyperthermia can be achieved via noninvasive heating and monitoring modalities, or whether equipment inadequacies, hostile physiological factors, etc. will result in only local interstitial or endocavitary modalities being efficient. The compatibility of NMR equipment with focused ultrasound surgery should provide a powerful therapeutic tool.

Mechanical and electromagnetic compatibility has proven very important. Off-pause protocols, consisting in alternatively heating and imaging, are probably one feasible approach as long as the duration of the imaging phase is short enough not to perturb the heating process.

Dielectric imaging, even if faced with more complex reconstruction processes, should be continued. Indeed, in addition to noninvasive thermal imaging, dielectric imaging is, by essence, probably the most convenient modality to obtain the complex permittivity distribution inside the patient. The knowledge of the permittivity distribution is expected to allow significant improvement in the prediction of the specific absorption rate (SAR) which is performed via numerical modeling. Finally, it is worth observing that even the most advanced prototypes previously reported have not been commercialized. It would be interesting, but difficult, to establish the reasons why the requisite research and development and commercial efforts have not been made. Was the technology inappropriate in terms of performance? Or was the market too uncertain to justify these efforts? It is clear that, to demonstrate proper efficiency, both NIT and NIC systems need to be integrated into heating equipment. But, conversely, the market offered to hyperthermia equipment is evidently proportional to its expected efficiency. There is some kind of vicious circle to be broken.

16.7 Summary

- Noninvasive thermal control constitutes a key issue for the development of deep hyperthermia. Even if none of the candidate techniques is now fully recognized as operationally effective for clinical applications, significant advances have been reported in the literature.
- This chapter summarizes the most recent results with special emphasis on microwave radiometry, the only modality to be already integrated in hyperthermia equipment, and magnetic resonance imaging which appears to be today the most advanced technique and very close to fit clinical requirements.
- The evolution of other imaging modalities, including x-rays, ultrasounds and dielectric imaging, is also adressed. All these approaches are compared and expected future developments are discussed.

References

Bardati F, Bertero M, Mongiardo M, Solimini D (1987a) Singular system analysis of the inversion of microwave radiometric data: applications to biological temperature retrieval. Inverse Problems 3: 347–370

Bardati F, Bertero M, Mongiardo M, Solimini D (1987b) Singular system analysis for temperature retrieval in microwave thermography. Radio Science 22(6): 1035–1041

Bardati F, Brown VJ, Tognolatti P (1993) Temperature reconstructions in a dielectric cylinder by multifrequency microwave radiometry. J Electromagn Waves Appl 7: 1549–1571

Bleier AR, Jolesz FA, Cohen MS et al. (1991) Real-time magnetic resonance imaging of laser heat deposition in tissue. Magn Reson Med 21: 132–137

Bocquet B, Dehour P, Mamouni A, Van de Velde JC, Leroy Y (1993) Near field microwave radiometric weighting functions for multilayered materials. J Electromagn Waves Appl 7: 1497–1514

Bolomey JC (1988) Diffraction tomography and the possibility of temperature measurements, Symposium on equipment for cancer therapy, AIST/MITI/JETRO, Tokyo, March 1st 1988

Bolomey JC, Hawley MS (1989) Non-invasive control of hyperthermia. In: Gautherie M (ed) Methods of hyperthermia control. Clinical Thermology Subseries Thermotherapy, Springer, Berlin, pp 35–111

Bolomey JC, Gaboriaud G, Broquetas A, van Dijk J, Cottis P (1989) Note on microwave imaging capabilities for non-invasive thermometry. COMAC-BME Hyperthermia Workshop on NIT, Vitterbo (I), 24–25 November 1989

Broquetas A, Mallorqui JJ, Rius JM, Cardama A (1993) Active microwave sensing of highly contrasted dielectric bodies. J Electromagn Waves Appl 7: 1439–1453

Cetas C (1984) Will thermometric tomography become practical for hyperthermia treatment monitoring? Cancer Res 44 (Suppl): 4805s–4808s

Chive M (1990) Use of microwave radiometry for hyperthermia monitoring and as a basis for thermal dosimetry. In: Gautherie M (ed) Methods of hyperthermia. Springer, Berlin Heidelberg New York, pp 113–128

Christensen DA (1982) Current techniques in non-invasive thermometry. In: Nussbaum GH (ed) Physical aspects of hyperthermia. Medical Physics Monograph no 8. American Institute of Physics, New York, pp 266–279

Cline HE, Schenck JF, Hynynen K, Watkins RD, Souza SP, Jolesz FA (1992) Magnetic resonance imaging guided focused ultrasound surgery. J Comput Assist Tomogr 16: 956–965

COMAC-BME Hyperthermia Workshop on Non-Invasive Thermometry in Clinical Hyperthermia, (1989) Viterbo, Italy, 24–25 November

COMAC BME Hyperthermia Workshop on Non-Invasive Thermometry (1991) Sitges Spain, 16–18 May

COMAC-BME Hyperthermia Final Workshop (1992), Utrecht, The Netherlands, September

Conway J, Hawley M, Mangnall YF, Amasha H, van Rhoon GC (1992a) Experimental assessment of electrical impedance imaging for hyperthermia monitoring. Clin Phys Physiol Meas 13 (Suppl A): 185–189

Conway J, Whitaker AJT, van Rhoon GC (1992b) Investigation of means to reduce the sensitivity of the electrical impedance tomography to RF-interference. COMAC-BME Hyperthermia, EOS#49, Dpt Med Phys Clinical Eng., Weston Park Hospital, Sheffield

Delannoy J, Le Bihan D, Hoult D, Levin R (1990) Hyperthermia system combined with a MRI unit. Med Phys 17: 855–860

Dicke RH (1946) The measurement of thermal radiation at microwave frequencies. Rev Sci Instr 17: 268–175

Dickinson RJ, Hall AS, Hind AJ, Young IR (1986) Measurement of changes in tissue temperature using MR imaging. J Comput Assist Tomogr 10(3): 468–472

Dubois L, Pribetich J, Fabre J-J, Chive M, Moschetto (1993) Non-invasive microwave multifrequency radiometry used in microwave hyperthermia for bidimensional reconstruction of temperature patterns. Int J Hyperthermia 9(3): 415–431

Duchêne B, Tabbara W (1985) Tomographie ultrasonore par diffraction. Rev Phys Appl 20: 299–304

Foster KR, Schepps JL (1981) Dielectric properties of tumor and normal tissues at radio through microwave frequencies. J Micro Power 16(2): 107–119

Foster KR, Schepps JL, Stoy RD, Schwan HP (1979) Dielectric properties of brain tissue between 0.01 and 10 GHz. Phys Med Biol 24(6): 1177–1187

Fukukita H, Ueno S, Yano T (1987) Application of non-linear effect to ultrasound pulse reflection method, Jpn J Appl Phys, 26 1 (Suppl 26): 49–51

Gaboriaud G, Joisel A, Van Rhoon GC (1991) Evaluation of the performance and the compatibility of a microwave camera on a ring capacitive heating system, COMAC-BME Hyperthermia Report EOS#01, Laboratoire des Signaux etSystèmes (CNRS/Supélec)

Geffrin JM, Joisel A, Bolomey JC, Pichot C (1993) Electromagnetic field distribution in a 434 MHz circular microwave scanner for non-invasive control of deep hyperthermia. ESHO-93, Brussel, June 16–19, p 7

Griffiths H, Ahmed A (1987) Applied potential tomography for non-invasive temperature mapping in hyperthermia. J Phys Physiol Meas 8 (Suppl A): 147–153

Hall AS, Prior MV, Hand JW, Young IR, Dickinson RJ (1990) Observation by MR imaging of in vivo temperature changes induced by radio frequency hyperthermia. J Comput Assist Tomogr 14: 430–436

Hamamura Y, Mizushina S, Sugiura T (1987) Non-invasive measurement of temperature-versus-depth profile in biological systems using a multiple-frequency-band microwave radiometer system. Automedica 8: 213–232

Hand JW (1984) Thermometry in hyperthermia. In: Overgaard J (ed) Hyperthermic oncology, vol 2. Taylor and Francis, London, pp 299–308

Hand JW, Lagendijk JJW, Bach Anderson JB, Bolomey JCh (1989) Quality control assurance guidelines for ESHO protocols, Int Journ Hyperthermia 5: 421–428

Hawley MS, Conway J, Amasha H, Mangnall YF, van Rhoon GC (1992) Electrical impedance tomography: prospects for non-invasive control of deep hyperthermia treatments. Front Med Biol Eng 4(2): 119–128

Henrikson H (1993) A combined EIT and thermistor thermometry system, private communication

Higuchi N, Bleier AR, Jolesz FA, Colucci VM, Morris JH (1992) Magnetic resonance imaging of the acute effects of interstitial neodymium: YAG laser irradiation on tissues. Invest Radiol 27: 814–821

International consensus meeting on hyperthermia (1989), Trento, Int J Hyperthermia 6(5): 839–877

Joachimowicz N, Pichot C, Hugonin JP (1991) Inverse scattering: an iterative numerical method for electromagnetic imaging, IEEE Trans Ant Prop 39: 1742–1752

Johnson CC, Guy AW (1972) Nonionizing electromagnetic wave effects in biological materials and systems. Proc IEEE 60: 692–718

Joisel A, Franchois A, Bolomey JC (1991) Active microwave imaging and control of hyperthermia: first trials at Utrecht and Amsterdam. COMAC-BME Hyperthermia Report EOS#05/EOS#06, Laboratoire des Signaux et Systèmes (CNRS/Supélec)

Joisel A, Bolomey JC, Gaboriaud G, Lagendijk J, van Dijk J, van Rhoon G (1992) The impact of active microwave imaging on the control of deep hyperthermia treatments. 6th International Conference on Hyperthermic Oncology, Tucson (USA), E.W. Gerner Ed, 206, Arizona Board of Regents

Kosterich JD, Foster KR, Pollack SR (1983) Dielectric permittivity and electrical conductivity of fluid saturated bone. IEEE Trans Biomed Eng 30(2): 81–86

Knuttel B, Juretschke HP (1986) Temperature measurements by nuclear magnetic resonance and its possible use as a means of in vivo noninvasive temperature measurement and for hyperthermia treatment assessment. Recent Results Cancer Res 101: 109–118

Larsen EL, Jacobi JH (1986) Linear FM pulse compression radar techniques applied to biological imaging. In: Larsen EL, Jacobi JH (eds) Medical application of microwave imaging. IEEE Press, New York, pp 138–147

Lagendijk J, de Leeuw ACC (1986) The development of applicators for deep-body hyperthermia. In: Bruggmoser G, Hinkelbein W, Engelhardt R, Wannenmacher M (eds) Locoregional high-frequency hyperthermia and temperature measuerement, Recent results in cancer research series. Springer, Berlin Heidelberg New York, 101: 19–35

Le Bihan D (1992) Theoretical principles of perfusion imaging. Invest Radiol 27: S6–S11

Le Bihan D, Breton E, Lallemand D, Aubin ML, Vignaud J, Laval-Jeantet M (1988) Separation of diffusion and perfusion in intravoxel incoherent motion (IVIM) MR Imaging. Radiology 168: 497–505

Le Bihan D, Delannoy J, Levin RL (1989a) Temperature mapping with MR imaging of molecular diffusion: application to hyperthermia. Radiology 171: 853–857

Le Bihan D, Delannoy J, Levin R, Pekar J, Le Dour O (1989b) Temperature dependence of water molecular diffusion in brain tissue. In: Book of abstracts of the 8th Annual Meeting, Society of Magnetic Resonance in Medicine, Berkeley, p 141.

Le Bihan D, Turner R, Moonen CTW, Pekar J (1991) Imaging of diffusion and microcirculation with gradient sensitization: design, strategy and significance. JMRI 1: 7–28

Le Bihan D, Turner R, Douek P, Patronas N (1992) Clinical diffusion magnetic resonance imaging. AJR 159: 591–600

Lewa CJ, Majeska Z (1980) Temperature relationships of proton spin-lattice relaxation time T1 in biological tissues. Bull Cancer (Paris) 67: 525–530

Mallorqui JJ, Broquetas A, Jofre L, Cardama A (1992) Non-invasive active thermometry with a microwave tomographic scanner in hyperthermia treatments. Applied computational electromagnetics Society Journal 7(2): 121–127

Mamouni A, Leroy Y, Bocquet B, Van de Velde JC, Gelin P (1991) Computation of near-field microwave radiometric signals: Definition and experimental verification. IEEE Trans. Microwave Tech 39: 124–132

Martin J, Broquetas A, Jofre L (1991) Dynamic active microwave thermography applied to hyperthermia monitoring. J Photogr Science 39: 146–148

Miyakawa M (1991) Tomographic imaging of temperature change in a phantom of human body using of chirp radar-type microwave tomograph. Med & Biol Eng Comput 29(2): 745

Miyakawa M, Watanabe D, Hayashi T, Saitoh Y (1992) Improvement of the chirp radar-type microwave CT for non-invasive thermometry. 6th International Conference on Hyperthermic Oncology, Tucson (USA), E.W. Gerner Ed, 213, Arizona Board of Regents

Mizushina S (1987) Non-invasive temperature measurement. Aspects of medical technology. Series of monographs and conference proceedings. Gordon and Breach, New York

Mizushina S, Shimizu T, Sugiura T (1992) Non-invasive thermometry with multi-frequency microwave bradiometry. Front Med Biol Eng 4: 129–133

Mizushina S, Shimizu T, Suzuki K, Kinomura M, Ohba H, Sugiura T (1993) Retrieval of temperature-depth profiles in biological objects from multi-frequency microwave radiometric data. J Electromagn Waves Appl 7: 1515–1548

Nadi M, Kourtiche D, Marchal C, Hedjiedj A, Kontaxakis G, Rouane A, Prieur G (1992) Ultrasound thermography: theoretical aspects and feasibility. Ultrasonics 30(2): 131–134

Nguyen MT, Faust U (1992) Possibilities and limitations of temperature monitoring using ultrasound techniques. Ultrasonics 30(2): 128–131

Nguyen DD, Mamouni A, Leroy Y, Constant E (1979) Simultaneous microwave local heating and microwave thermography. Possible clinical applications. J Micro Power 14(2): 135–137

Nikita K, Uzunoglu A (1989) Analysis of the power coupling from a waveguide hyperthermia applicator into a three-layered tissue model. IEEE Trans Microwave Theory Tech 37: 1794–101

Ozyar MS, Koÿmen H (1992) Non-invasive method for in-situ estimation of intensity using non-linear effects in ultrasound hyperthermia. Ultrasonics 30(2): 123–124

Parker DL, Smith V, Sheldon P, Crooks LE, Fussel L (1983) Temperature distribution measurements in two-dimensional NMR imaging. Med Phys 10(3): 321–325

Pennes HH (1948) Analysis of tissue and arterial blood temperature in resting human forearm. J Appl Physiol 1: 93

Plancot M, Prevost B, Chive M, Fabre JJ, Ledel L, Giaux G (1987) A new method for thermal dosimetry in microwave hyperthermia using microwave radiometry for temperature control. Int J Hyperthermia 3(1): 9–19

Reddy GN, Saha S (1984) Electrical and dielectric properties of wet bone as a function of frequency. IEEE Trans Biomed Eng 31(3): 296–302

Saito M, Sano T, Itoh T (1988) Possibility of temperature monitoring by x-ray CT. Symposium on equipment for cancer therapy, AIST/MITI/JETRO, Tokyo, March 1st 1988

Schepps JL, Foster KR (1980) The UHF and microwave dielectric properties of normal and tumor tissues: variation in dielectric properties with tissue water content. Phys Med Biol 25(6): 1149–1159

Schwan HP, Piersol GM (1954) The absorption of electromagnetic energy in body tissues. Am J Phys Med 33: 371–404

Souza SP (1992) Uncertainties in temperature imaging via diffusion imaging. In: Book of abstracts of the 11th Annual Meeting, Society of Magnetic Resonance in Medicine, Berkeley, pp 1214–1219

Stehling MK, Turner R, Mansfield P (1991) Echo-planar imaging: magnetic resonance imaging in a fraction of a second. Science 254: 43–50

Steel MC, Sheppard RJ (1985) Dielectric properties of mammalian brain tissue between 1 and 18 GHz. Phys Med Biol 30(7): 621–630

Stuchly MA, Stuchly SS (1980) Dielectric properties of biological substances – tabulated. J Microw Power 15(1): 19–23

Stuchly MA, Stuckly SS (1990) Electrical properties of biological substances. In: Gandhi OP (ed) Biological effects and medical applications of electromagnetic energy. Prentice-Hall, Englewood Cliff, NJ, pp 75–112

Turner R, Le Bihan D, Maier J, Vavrek R, Hedges LK, Pekar J (1990) Echo-planar imaging of intravoxel incoherent motion. Radiology 177: 407–414

Ueno SI, Furuya N, Fukukita H, Yano T (1989) Application of nonlinear ultrasonic pulse reflection method–measurement of acoustic parameters. Jpn J Appl Phys 28 (Suppl 28-1): 191–193

Ueno S, Fukukita H, Yano T, Miyakawa M, Kanai H, Egawa S (1990) Non-invasive thermometry system using ultrasound nonlinear pheomena. Jpn J Hyperthermic Oncol 6(4): 402–411

Ulaby FT, Moore RK, Fung AK (1981) Microwave remote sensing: active and passive, vol 1. Microwave remote sensing fundamentals and radiometry. Addison-Wesley, Reading Mass., p 379 and pp 394–395

Xie CG (1993) Review of image reconstruction methods for process tomography. In: Beck MS, Campogrande E, Morris M, Williams WA, Waterfall RC (eds) Process Tomography 1993, UMIST, Manchester, pp 114–119

Zhang Y, Samulski TV, Joines WT, Mattiello J, Levin RL, Le Bihan D (1992) On the accuracy of noninvasive thermometry using molecular diffusion magnetic resonance imaging. Int J Hyperthermia 8: 263–274

17 Phantom Design: Applicability and Physical Properties

C.J. SCHNEIDER, R. OLMI, and J.D.P. VAN DIJK

CONTENTS

17.1 Introduction

The interest in phantoms patients emanates from different viewpoints: a clinical interest in simulating a patient undergoing a treatment, a practical interest regarding technical maintenance of a clinical device, or a more technical interest in research and development.

C.J. SCHNEIDER, PhD, Department of Radiotherapy, Amsterdam University Hospital, Academisch Medisch Centrum, Meibergdreef 9, NL-1105 AZ Amsterdam, The Netherlands
R. OLMI, PhD, IROE – National Research Council, Via Panciachiti 64, I-50127 Firenze, Italy
J.D.P. VAN DIJK, PhD, Department of Radiotherapy, Amsterdam University Hospital, Academisch Medisch Centrum, Meibergdreef 9, NL-1105 AZ Amsterdam, The Netherlands

Most of the clinical hyperthermia systems are RF systems, of which the heating capabilities strongly depend on the dielectric characteristics of the patient's or the phantom's tissue. In the range of radio and microwave frequencies applied for hyperthermia, the dielectric properties of different biological tissues show a variation of at least a factor of 10 both in the permittivity, determining wavelength and diffraction, and in the conductivity, i.e., absorption (STUCHLY and STUCHLY 1980). Besides their dependency on tissue type, the dielectric characteristics also vary with frequency of the applied EM field and with temperature: for biological tissues the dielectric constant decreases with increasing temperature, whilst the conductivity increases with temperature (SCHWAN 1965). As a consequence, the description of the electric field distribution throughout the heterogeneous tissue composition inside a patient is a complex problem (PAULSEN 1990). The fact that different patients represent different loads for the system is one reason for the difficulty in the control and the description of especially a deep body hyperthermia system. Applying a phantom as a stable load, the performance of a system can be determined under standardized, repeatable conditions, with a reduced number of variables (AAPM 1987). Nevertheless, in RF multiapplicator systems the number of variables already inherent in the device is great, e.g., the relations of phases and amplitudes of the applicators or the frequency (TURNER 1984). For experimental verification a great diversity of tissue substitutes and phantom designs are reported in the literature (GUY 1971; CETAS 1982; CHOU 1987; BINI et al. 1984; HARTSGROVE et al. 1987).

The objectives of phantom experiments fall into two main categories: understanding of the physical processes inside the phantom and understanding of the behavior and control of the power-delivering RF equipment, e.g., impedance of the applicators, cross-coupling, and interference control. These objectives can be further divided into applicator characterization, comparative studies of applicators, improvement and development, and quality assurance.

In this chapter we will discuss the different objectives of phantom experiments, the diversity of phantoms designed for various purposes, the different application of phantoms, and the reliability of measuring techniques. While the discussion is focused on the application of phantoms in RF deep-body hyperthermia systems, it generally covers most of the subjects inherent to the other hyperthermia techniques.

17.2 Standard Phantoms and Objectives of Experiments

Depending on the objectives of experiments, phantoms have to fulfill different demands: quality assurance phantoms have to be practical and easy to use in rapid checks, whereas phantoms for improvement and development of hyperthermia systems have to provide data which are as precise as possible.

17.2.1 Standard Phantoms

In 1988 the CDRH phantom, made of a 1-cm fat-equivalent shell and filled with muscle-equivalent gel (Durney et al. 1986), was developed as a standard phantom for RF deep body hyperthermia (Allen et al. 1988). Furthermore, in the consensus report of the COMAC-BME workshop on quality assurance (QA) in hyperthermia (September 1990, Sabaudia, Italy), guidelines concerning the three main fields of clinical hyperthermia (superficial, deep body, and interstitial) were prepared. As an extension to the European Society of Hyperthermic Oncology (ESHO) guidelines, the use of a layered (fat – muscle) polyacrylamide phantom (Bini et al. 1984; Bini and Olmi 1990) was proposed for QA in superficial hyperthermia (Hand and Fessenden 1991). The Amsterdam phantom with a light-emitting diode (LED) matrix, filled with a saline solution of 3 g NaCl per liter of water at 22°–26°C, was recommended as a standard phantom for deep body hperthermia (Lagendijk and Molls 1991). At the same workshop, liquid crystal plate (LCP) thermography in transparent phantoms was proposed for QA in interstitial hyperthermia devices (Seegenschmiedt and Visser 1991).

17.2.2 Applicator Characterization

The power deposition pattern of a hyperthermia applicator is an essential part of QA and needs to be defined prior to its introduction in clinical practice, as advised in the QA guidelines of the RTOG (Dewhirst et al. 1990) and the ESHO (Hand et al. 1989). In the ESHO guidelines on superficial hyperthermia a phantom setup in which the applicator is to be measured is described as constructed from muscle-equivalent material according to Chou et al. (1984) and covered by a 1-cm layer of a fat equivalent.

In RF multiapplicator deep body systems the degrees of freedom (phase and amplitude settings, frequency, patient positioning, patient size, and dielcetric properties) are numerous. Up to now, there is no consensus on which setups have to be used to achieve sufficient characterization of a deep body device. For practical reasons a consensus will have to be a compromise in terms of the number of setups, the time needed to conduct experiments, and the required spatial data density throughout the irradiated volume.

17.2.3 Comparative Studies of Applicators

Guy (1971) and Chou (1987) investigated the heating patterns of different applicators operating at frequencies between 433 and 2450 MHz by means of a thermographic camera and various splittable, layered phantoms. A first study comparing three different units of a commercially available RF deep body system was done by Allen et al. (1988) using the CDRH phantom together with a high-precision thermometry system. Lamaitre et al. (1992) measured the effective field size at 1 cm depth in saline and the penetration depth of various types of RF superficial applicators in a program involving site visits to several institutes in Europe. For this study, a flat phantom covered with a 1-cm-thick fat-equivalent plate (Guy 1971) was used according to the ESHO guidelines, and filled with saline solution of 6 g NaCl per liter of water. A first QA study on different RF deep body systems was carried out applying the Amsterdam phantom with an LED matrix (Schneider et al. 1994a).

17.2.4 Improvement and Development

Experimental data are essential for the improvement and development of applicators and the control of parameters such as power and phase settings. They are also necessary for the development and evaluation of computer models describing power deposition and temperature distribution, leading to clinical hyperthermia planning systems. While the knowledge of SAR patterns in homogeneous phantoms is the minimal knowledge required to characterize a hyperthermia applicator, scientists who have gathered profound experience in these experimental setups continue their investigations by designing new phantoms which are closer to the anatomical reality of patients (SULLIVAN et al. 1992).

17.2.5 Quality Assurance

Necessary contributions to QA are performance evaluation of the hyperthermia equipment (AAPM report no. 26, 1989), including applicator characterization, checks on RF disturbance [especially on the registration system acquiring data from the patient or the phantom (thermometry, E-field probes)], and recognition of potential sources of perturbations and artifacts, e.g., in phase and amplitude monitoring. The aim is to provide a standard means of describing the physical properties, as opposed to clinical effectiveness, of a particular hyperthermia device during the course of time or in a comparison of various heating modalities or applicators.

17.3 Phantom Tissue Characterization

17.3.1 General Requirements

The quantity of electromagnetic (EM) energy absorbed by biological tissues depends on their dielectric characteristics. The microscopic interactions of the EM field with tissue molecules can be described at a macroscopic level by the complex permittivity, i.e., by dielectric constant ε and conductivity σ, which gives the amount of displacement of molecular dipoles and conduction current of ions in the biological material.

General requirements for a phantom material are:

1. *Reproducibility and reliability of preparation*. Dielectric characteristics must be reproducible and the preparation procedure must be reliable, since only a few institutes have the facilities to measure the complex permittivity by themselves. Moreover, the phantom should not have hysteresis: ε and σ should revert to their original values after heating and cooling. The procedure must guarantee that ε and σ are constant throughout the volume of a prepared mixture.

2. *Stability*. Dielectric characteristics and thermophysical properties, i.e., specific heat, thermal conductivity, and density, must not change for a reasonable time, e.g., by evaporation, which means at least from the time of preparation to that of experiments. Phantoms should have a lifetime long enough to allow repetition of experiments. Also, the low viscosity of gels or other semiliquid materials necessary to avoid convection in measurements of the temperature increase should not be lost during heating up, e.g., due to SAR peaks in the vicinity of interstitial applicators.

Other requirements are associated specifically with the type of technique used to construct the SAR distribution. For example, electric field probe techniques require liquid phantoms, a phantom for the LED matrix method must be liquid and transparent, and LCP dosimetry needs a transparent, solid phantom. A phantom must not be toxic, although its constituents can be, and its preparation procedure should not be too complex.

17.3.2 Classification of Phantom Types

Phantoms can be classfied with regard to their volume and shape, and with regard to the treatment technique they are used for:

1. *Interstital/superficial hyperthermia*. These phantoms are of medium size. Their borders are outside the irradiated volume with the exception of the contact surface of superficial applicators, and thus their size does not influence the irradiated volume. Their shape is often that of a flat block or cylinder, either whole or in slices (LEYBOVICH and NUSSBAUM 1984; SUROWIEC et al. 1992), and for superficial applicators covered with a fat layer or a very thin plate.

2. *Deep body hyperthermia*. These phantoms are of human scale, i.e., their size is similar to the irradiated volume and therefore influences the irradiation pattern. Phantoms with a circular (MYERSON et al. 1991) or square cross-section feature symmetry with respect to all four applicators, whereas phantoms with an elliptical cross-

section are symmetric with respect to opposing applicators. The filling is usually homogeneous, but phantoms have been described in which a "permittivity contrast object" is inserted by blocks (LAGENDIJK and DE LEEUW 1986), a cylinder (PAULSEN and ROSS 1990), or a composition of two halves of a cylinder and a block with a hole, e.g., the Utah phantom (SULLIVAN et al. 1992). There are also human-shaped phantoms such as the BSD mannequin, or anthropomorphic phantoms such as the Franconi mannequin (RICCI et al. 1991).

The wall material of phantoms is assumed to influence the RF irradiation conditions. However, experiments comparing an elliptical phantom with a 2-mm PVC wall, an elliptical phantom with a 1-cm wall of fat-equivalent material, and a square phantom with a 2-mm PVC wall showed only minor differences (SCHNEIDER et al. 1993). For this experiment, the irradiation efficiency was defined as the ratio of power delivered to an applicator, to the square of the electric field at a predefined point in the phantom. The power was supplied to a 70-MHz waveguide radiator, on which three types of phantoms were fixed at various bolus thickness. Then the power level was adjusted in order to keep the signal on a dipole, which was positioned at 12 cm invasive depth in the phantom, i.e., the center of the elliptical phantoms, at a constant level. The experiment revealed the bolus thickness to be an important parameter (Fig. 17.1), but not the wall material or the shape of the phantom.

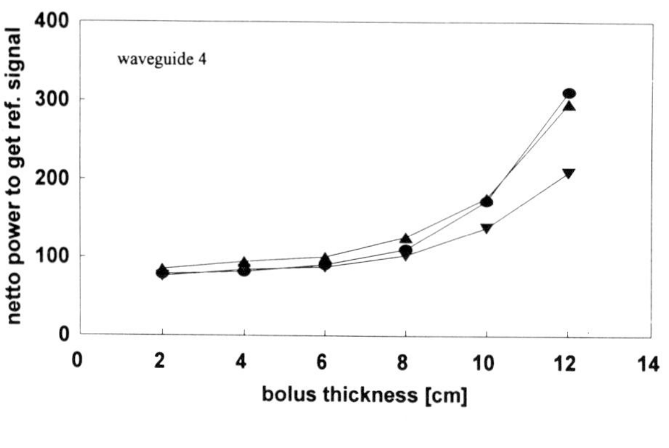

Fig. 17.1. Irradiation efficiency as a function of bolus thickness, for three phantoms with different shapes and wall materials. The power supplied to a 70-MHz waveguide radiator on the phantoms was adjusted in order to keep the signal on a dipole, positioned at 12 cm invasive depth, i.e., the center of elliptical phantoms, at a constant level. -●-, elliptical phantom with 2-mm PVC wall; -▼-, elliptical phantom with 10-mm fat-equivalent wall; -▲-, square phantom with 2-mm PVC wall

Regarding the type of measuring technique, phantoms can be classified as follows:

1. Liquid phantoms to scan an E-field probe or to visualize the E field by an LED matrix
2. Semisolid and solid phantoms to measure the temperature increase:
   a) Saline-equivalent phantoms, designed to match E-field scans in saline phantoms
   b) Tissue-equivalent phantoms, designed to match dielectric properties and to model thermal effects of microvascularization in biological tissue
   c) Real tissue phantoms (excised animal organs), used with artificial vessel perfusion to simulate heat sinks in biological tissue.

17.3.3 Techniques of Complex Permittivity Measurement

The measurement of the dielectric properties of materials can be performed by means of several different techniques, which can be broadly classified into three main subgroups based on the frequency range of interest: (a) lumped constant, (b) transmission line, and (c) fringing-field methods. These techniques are usually performed in the frequency domain, but recently time-domain techniques using short pulses have been introduced as a fast alternative. The presence of both a high value of permittivity ε and conductivity σ causes several problems in the measurement of the dielectric characteristics of various biological substances and their tissue-equivalent materials.

17.3.2.1 Lumped Constant Technique

Lumped constant methods are especially suitable up to short wave frequencies, i.e., approximately 100 MHz, where the dimensions of the measuring cell are such that it represents a lumped capacitor. The parallel plates or cylinder capacitor (GRANT et al. 1978) is filled with the dielectric under study. At low frequencies, for example below 1 MHz, bridge techniques are generally used, while for higher frequencies vector-impedance meters are usually preferred. The frequency limit for lumped constant operations is also determined by the filling dielectric, with a maximum of about 100 MHz for muscle-like materials and about twice that limit for fatty tissues, for reasonable cell sizes.

By measuring the conductance G and a capacitance C of the filled cell, ε_r (the relative permittivity) and σ can be obtained by the following expressions:

$$\sigma = \varepsilon_0 G/C_0 \tag{17.1}$$

$$\varepsilon_r = C/C_0, \tag{17.2}$$

where C_0 is the capacitance of the empty cell.

17.3.2.2 Transmission Line Technique

Above a few hundred MHz, transmission lines are employed. Depending on the type of line, whether it is coaxial or waveguide, techniques having different characteristics can be implemented. Below 3 GHz, in the frequency range of interest for hyperthermia applications, coaxial line cells and reflection methods are most commonly used.

The dielectric sample can completely or partially fill the transmission line, giving rise to somewhat different measuring procedures (Von Hippel 1966). Complex permittivity is finally obtained by measuring the reflection coefficient at a reference plane usually coincident with the interface of the dielectric under test. In the past, when slotted line methods were used for these measurements, minima and maxima of RF voltage had to be sought manually by means of a probe inserted in the line (Chou 1987). With network analyzers having high phase precision, these measurements can now be automated.

One of the most used configurations is that in which the measuring cell consists of a section of coaxial line, short-circuited at one end, with the sample material filling a length d starting from the shorted end (Von Hippel 1966). In this case, the impedance Z_m of the filled coaxial part, referred to the interface of the dielectric sample, can be easily shown to be:

$$Z_m = jZ_c/\sqrt{\varepsilon_r}\tan(k_0\sqrt{\varepsilon_r}d), \tag{17.3}$$

where k_0 is the free-space wave number and Z_c is the characteristic impedance of the empty coaxial line. Solution of the above equation, which is in implicit form, is obtained by standard iterative methods.

The lumped constant and transmission line techniques are both volume techniques, in that the information on the dielectric sample is averaged on the whole volume it occupies. They both allow very good precision, well above the needs for phantom applications: proper sample dimensions lead to a measurement accuracy better than 1%. The major drawback of these methods stems from the necessity of "filling" the measuring cell with the sample material, which is done during phantom preparation. Dielectric measurements on an existing solid phantom, such as checks on material properties during the course of time, are generally not allowed with the lumped constant and transmission line methods.

17.3.2.3 Fringing-Field Technique

In the range of frequencies between about 100 MHz and more than 10 GHz the fringing-field technique represents a valid alternative to those described above. The measuring probe consists of an open-ended coaxial line, sometimes with the inner conductor protruding for a short length (short monopole probe). The dielectric properties of the material under test are in this case determined by measuring the terminal impedance of the probe (Burdette et al. 1980).

The "lumped equivalent circuit" method is commonly adopted: the terminal impedance is seen as a parallel combination of the radiation conductance of the open coaxial (or short monopole) and a fringe complex capacitance including a part resulting from the electric field lines crossing the sample material (C_s), and a part due to the fringing field in the dielectric of the coaxial line (C_d). C_s and C_d are determined from measurements on reference liquids. Finally, if the measured terminal admittance of the open coaxial is $Y_m = G_m + j\omega C_m$, complex permittivity $\varepsilon' - j\varepsilon''$ can be calculated as follows:

$$\varepsilon' = (C_m - C_d)/C_s \tag{17.4}$$

$$\varepsilon'' = G_m/\omega C_s. \tag{17.5}$$

With this last method, good precision can be achieved using suitable calibration techniques, generally by making use of reference liquids of known permittivity. A commercially available system for nondestructive measurements (HP 85070A) has a typical accuracy of ±5% in dielectric constant measurements and of ±0.05% in loss tangent measurements, as reported on the manufacturer's data sheets. The closer the permittivity of the reference liquid to that of the sample material, the higher the accuracy/precision. An analysis of the uncertainties in permittivity measurements with reference liquid calibration has been performed by NYSHADHAM et al. (1992).

The most attractive characteristic of the fringing-field technique is the possibility of nondestructive measurements on solid and semisolid materials. The main drawback of open-ended coaxial methods is related to their character as surface techniques. In fact, the principal contribution to the terminal impedance comes from a region very close to the discontinuity: a poor contact with the surface of the dielectric, when measuring solids, or a slightly inhomogeneous superficial condition, e.g., due to evaporation of water, greatly reduces the accuracy of the measurement.

A brief mention should be made of the very promising class of time-domain (TD) techniques, based on TD reflectometric measurements. This type of technique, which is based on cumbersome algorithms and usually requires powerful computers and long computation times, has the attractive property of allowing in principle a complete determination of the dispersion curve of the test dielectric from only a single measurement. In this case, a short steep pulse is passed through the sample material: comparing in time the input and output pulses and taking their Fourier transforms, the dielectric properties of the material are finally obtained.

17.3.4 Recipes for Phantom Materials

More than 20 years of research on hyperthermia have produced a large number of different phantom materials. This section gives an up-to-date list of references on the subject.

Table 17.1 shows a selection of some commonly used phantom materials, together with main components, consistency, and frequency range as the principal characteristics. The reader is referred to the reference citations in the table for extensive information about the phantom recipes.

Overviews on phantom recipes have been provided by STUCHLY and STUCHLY (1980), CETAS (1982), and CHOU (1987). A gelatin phantom for the frequency range 10–50 MHz has been proposed by MARCHAL et al. (1989), while a technique for SAR reconstruction based on a multilayer polyacrylamide phantom has recently been proposed by SUROWIEC et al. (1992).

Saline solutions with a proper NaCl concentration are commonly used as phantoms associated

Table 17.1. A selection of some materials used for RF phantoms

Simulated tissue	Main components	Consistency	Frequency range (MHz)	Reference
Muscle	TX150 (Superstuff), NaCl solution, polyethylene powder	Moist gel	13.56–2450	GUY (1971)
Muscle	Acrylamide, NaCl solution	Solid gel	10–2450	BINI et al. (1984) ANDREUCCETTI et al. (1988)
Muscle	Eudispert (R)	Gel	13.56–2450	GAUTHERIE et al. (1988)
Muscle	Natrasol (R)	Semiliquid	10–2450	HARTSGROVE et al. (1987)
Bone/fat	Laminac polyester resin	Solid	200–2450	GUY (1971)
Bone/fat	Acrylamide, ethylene glycol	Solid gel	13.56–2450	BINI et al. (1984) ANDREUCCETTI et al. (1988)
Bone/fat	Flour, oil, saline	Solid	433	LAGENDIJK (1984)
Bone/fat	Epoxy resin, KCl solution	Solid	100–1000	HARTSGROVE et al. (1987)
Bone/fat	Microemulsion	Liquid	100–1000	HARTSGROVE et al. (1987)
Mix	Saline (NaCl)	Liquid	60–100	This chapter
Mix	Methylcellulose, saline (NaCl)	Semiliquid	60–100	This chapter

with E-field probe techniques. The concentration of salt needed to obtain the target absorption σ is often extrapolated using the formulas given by STOGRYN (1971); a direct measurement of these solutions with the methods reported in Sect. 17.3.3 is, however, recommended because the dielectric constant varies a little in the RF frequency range. The dielectric constant can be adjusted: it can be reduced by adding glycerin or other low-permittivity liquids, or increased by substances producing a dielectric increment such as glycine or other amino acids.

17.3.5 Measured Permittivity of Saline and Saline Gel

A new semiliquid phantom, based on saline gel made of wallpaper paste (WPP) dissolved in saline solution, has been developed by the authors.

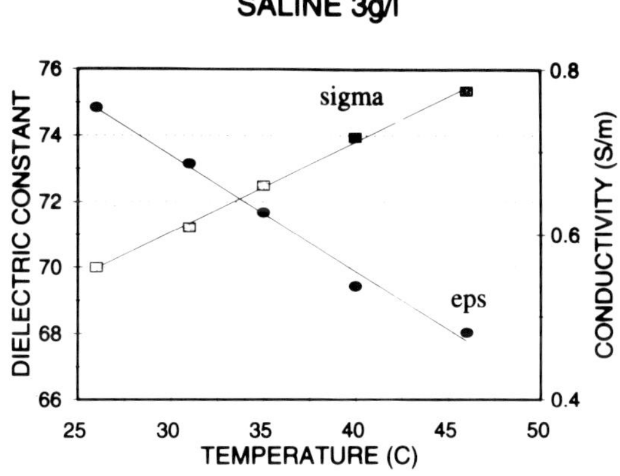

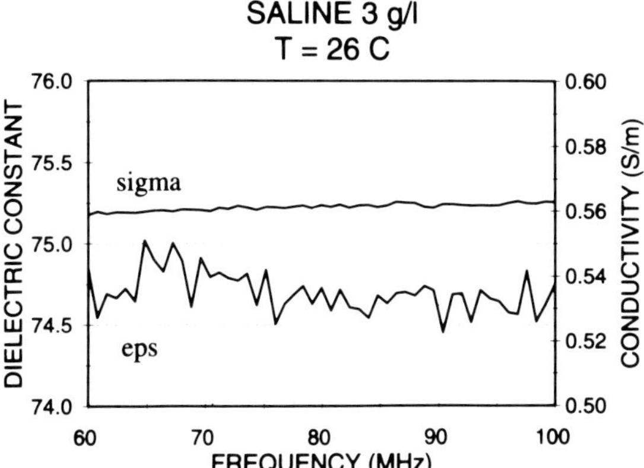

Fig. 17.2. Measured dielectric constants (Olmi, IROE, Florence) of saline, with 3.0 g NaCl per liter distilled water, as a function of temperature and frequency

Various recipes have been prepared to simulate the conductivity of muscle and fat/muscle tissues at the frequency of 70 MHz and 433 MHz (the dielectric constant equals that of saline). As an example, a gel phantom was obtained with dielectric characteristics measured to be equivalent to those of saline (Fig. 17.2), by mixing 27 g/l of WPP in a saline solution with 3 g/l of NaCl. The phantom is low cost, readily available, and of simple preparation. It can be used for the characterization of deep body systems, both with short-pulse thermal techniques and with E-field probe techniques. At 70 MHz, the interpolation functions for ε' and σ are, with T in °C (Fig. 17.2):

Saline: $\varepsilon(T) = 84.002 - 0.3531T$
$\sigma(T) = 0.2754 + 0.0109T\,[\mathrm{S/m}]$
$\varepsilon(25°\mathrm{C}) = 75$
$\sigma(25°\mathrm{C}) = 0.55\,[\mathrm{S/m}]$

WPP: $\varepsilon(T) = 81.82 - 0.2595T$
$\sigma(T) = 0.3273 + 0.008895T\,[\mathrm{S/m}]$
$\varepsilon(25°\mathrm{C}) = 75$
$\sigma(25°\mathrm{C}) = 0.55\,[\mathrm{S/m}]$.

This phantom was used for the comparison between ΔT-measurements and E-field scans in saline in the Amsterdam deep body hyperthermia system (see Fig. 17.3).

17.4 Phantom Application in SAR Measurements

For a rapid qualitative and even limited quantitative check on system performance the LED matrix is the most efficient tool. Its real-time visualization is especially convenient for the monitoring of interference fields. E-field scans offer the highest resolution along scanned paths and under certain conditions can reveal the three orthogonal components of the electric field, which are of particular interest for the investigation of multiapplicator interference systems. These techniques, applied in liquid phantoms, offer the advantage that the phantom temperature and its dielectric characteristics are constant throughout the phantom with proper mixing. It is easily stabilized by circulating the liquid through a thermostatically controlled cooling unit, even if the RF irradiation lasts for hours. On the other hand, measuring the temperature increase in solid or semisolid phantoms with small temperature sensors offers the advantage of high spatial resolution, or of full plane monitoring if thermographic imaging is applied. These techniques are the typical approach for experiments applying heterogeneous phantoms, e.g., studies on interfaces between muscle and fat or bone (LAGENDIJK and DE LEEUW 1986; SAMULSKI et al. 1987; SULLIVAN et al. 1992).

Generally, hyperthermia phantoms do not necessarily require that dielectric and thermal properties are as close as possible to real biological tissue. Any type of phantom is more or less a marked simplification of the anatomy and physiology of a patient. However, attention should be paid to making a choice of phantom material that is appropriate to the result which is sought in experiments. For example, in a deep body phantom filled with a material of which the absorption is as high as that of muscle, there may exist no focus of SAR. However, a lower absorption leads to an interference pattern with a relative focus, i.e., a local maximum of electric field strength surrounded by minima, which are highly sensitive to the interference from phase and amplitude relations (see Fig. 17.4).

17.4.1 Measurement of the Electric Field

17.4.1.1 LED Matrix

The phantom with LED matrix is accepted as a QA tool for rapid checks of the system performance (LAGENDIJK and MOLLS 1991; SATHIASEELAN et al. 1992) and it is used in ten institutes in Europe and the United States. It has also been applied for a study on the qualitative behavior of various RF deep body hyperthermia systems in clinical use (SCHNEIDER et al. 1994). Power stepping, i.e., a series of photographs of the increasing light pattern on the LED matrix at increasing power delivered to the system, offers the possibility of evaluating SAR patterns quantitatively, as well (SCHNEIDER et al. 1992a).

Another improvement of this visualization technique was the arrangement of LEDs with their dipoles oriented in the aperture midplane. In this way, radial components of the electric field, e.g., the fringing fields at the edges of the boli, also became visible (SCHNEIDER et al. 1992b). Similarly, the radial distribution of the electric field in capacitive hyperthermia systems was investigated (VAN DIJK et al. 1992).

17.4.1.2 Antenna-sensor and Read-out Equipment

For the direct measurement of the electric field, which provides SAR values via SAR $= \frac{1\sigma}{2\rho} E^2_{Rms}$, with ρ being the mass density, various combinations of antenna-sensors and read-out transmission lines have been described: a monopole or dipole connected to a coax cable, a diode dipole read out by high-resistance leads or by an optical fiber, and isotropic sensors made of three orthogonal dipoles. An example of E-field scans with an LED dipole and fiberoptic read-out is shown in Fig. 17.3.

A monopole or dipole connected to a coax cable (GAJDA et al. 1979; LUMORI et al. 1990) offers the advantage of reading the local RF signal in phase and amplitude, e.g., by a vectorvoltmeter or network analyzer. These coax sensors are unfortunately only reliable for measurements of superficial or interstitial applicators at frequencies of typically 433 MHz or higher. For experiments in deep body systems operating at lower frequencies where the penetration depth is greater, a coax cable leading through the irradiated volume acts as a parasitic antenna. Therefore the local RF signal of the sensor has to be transformed into another signal type: a DC voltage rectified by a diode and read out by high-resistance leads, which transmit no RF signals (DE LEEUW et al. 1987), or a DC current transformed into a light signal by an LED and read out by an optical fiber (SCHNEIDER et al. 1991). The LED-dipole probe is the cheapest type of probe, the components of which are widely available.

As a consequence of the stray fields of deep body systems the data acquisition has to be remote, e.g., outside the Faraday cage and carried by an optical fiber, which is either directly connected to an LED-dipole or by a voltage-to-light transformer to the high-resistance leads. A disadvantage of the undisturbed read-out of a DC voltage is that the signal is no longer linearly dependent on the E field. As a consequence, the sensor has to be calibrated and all measured signals have to be processed to represent E-field values or SAR. Furthermore, the rectification of the RF signal results in the loss of the phase information.

Recently, high-tech designs of E-field probes have been presented, which are capable of measuring both phase and amplitude in deep body phased arrrays, i.e., at frequencies between 60

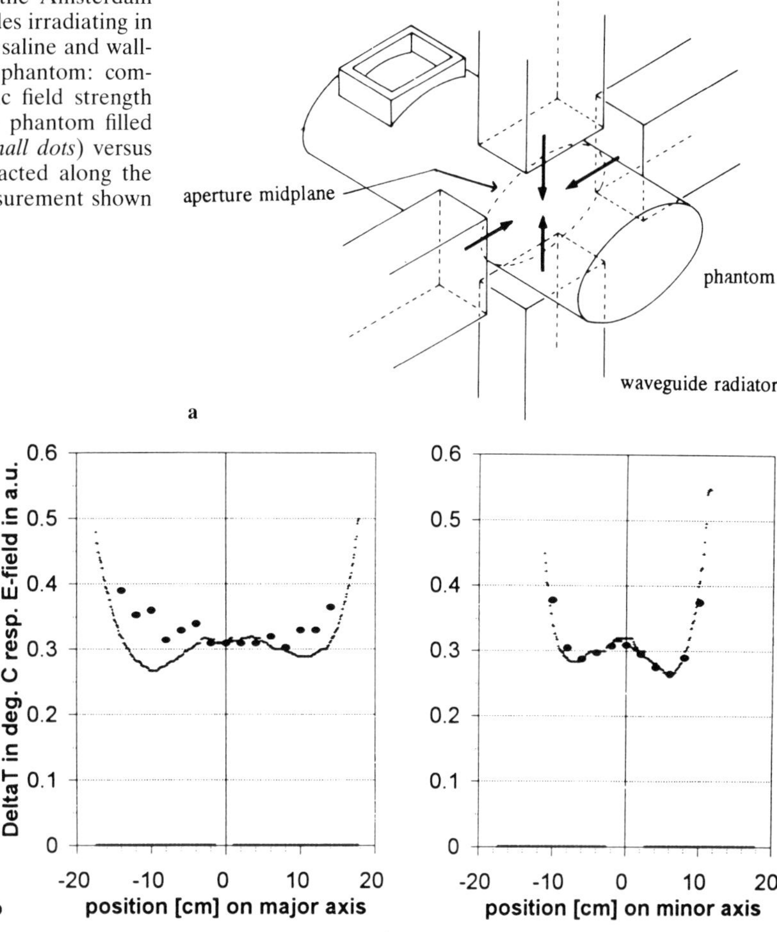

Fig. 17.3. **a** Experimental setup in the Amsterdam matched phased array: four waveguides irradiating in the Amsterdam phantom, filled with saline and wallpaper paste. **b** Liquid versus solid phantom: comparison of the square of the electric field strength measured with a 2-cm dipole in the phantom filled with saline (3.0 g NaCl per liter) (*small dots*) versus ΔT measurements (*large dots*), extracted along the major and minor axes from the measurement shown in Fig. 17.4

and 120 MHz. First applications have included the measurement of phase and amplitude in the annular bolus of a BSD-2000 phased array (Wust et al., this volume), and the measurement of the incident field of individual applicators inside a phantom (Schneider et al. 1995). Once the incident fields of individual applicators are measured, the applicators are completely characterized. Furthermore, these individual fields can be easily superposed to realize any interference pattern (Fig. 17.4).

E-field scanning is rather time-consuming, especially if all three orthogonal components of the electric field vector have to be measured. The application of isotropic sensors (Stuchly et al. 1984) built from three orthogonal dipoles, reduces this problem. E-field sensors share some general problems, notably:

1. The dependence of the sensor performance on σ and ε of the surrounding material and on frequency (Mousavinezhad et al. 1978)
2. The nonisotropic spatial resolution of a dipole: the spatial resolution in the direction of the dipole is much worse than in the plane perpendicular to the dipole
3. The possible perturbation of the local E field by the sensor carrier, especially if the dipole is fixed inside an air-filled tube (Paulsen and Ross 1990), or by metallic read-out cable as coaxial cable.

17.4.2 Measurement of the Temperature Increase

The thermal method to determine SAR consists in the measurement of the changes in temperature at known points in the phantom following a brief period of heating at high power. With this procedure, which involves short periods for the power pulse as well as for the measurement of the temperature increase, effects of thermal conductivity within the phantom are relatively small and SAR can be inferred from:

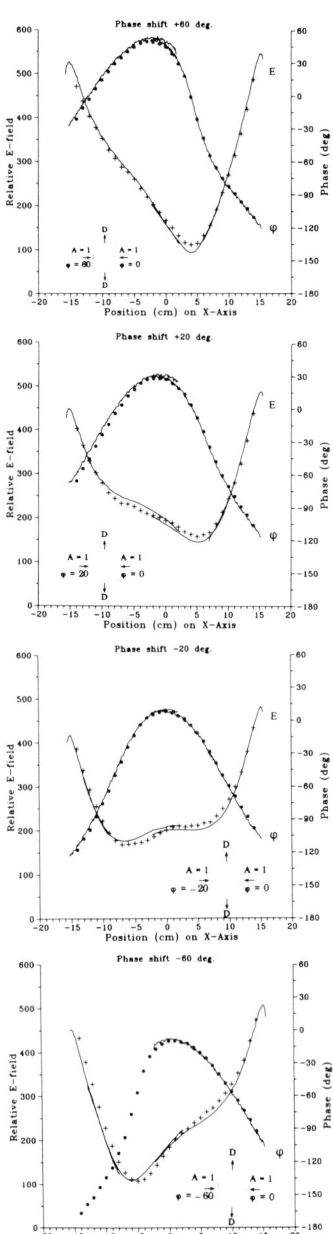

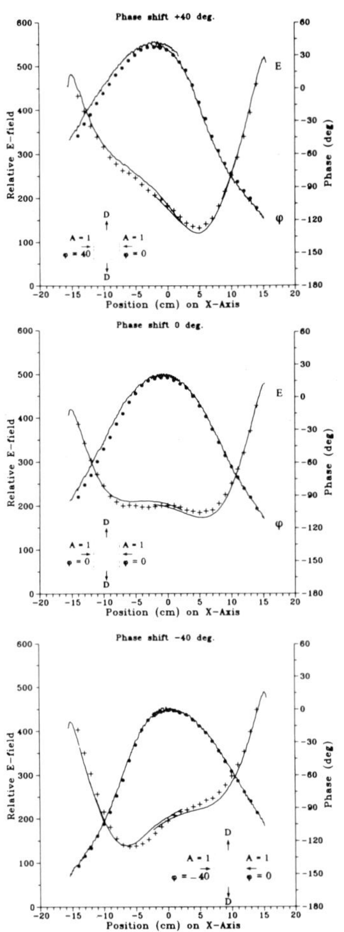

Fig. 17.4. Amplitude and phase scans along the horizontal x-axis in a square phantom. The left and right applicator of the AMC phased array are radiating with equal amplitude and phase shifts of −60°, −40°, −20°, 0°, 20°, 40°, and 60° for the left applicator with respect to the right one. The *crosses* indicate the amplitude and the *dots*, the phases derived by superposition of individually measured incident fields. The *lines* indicate the phase and amplitude measured in the interference field

$$\mathrm{SAR}(r) = c(r) \times \Delta T(r)/\Delta t, \qquad (17.6)$$

where c is the specific heat of the phantom material and $\Delta T(r)/\Delta t$, the temperature increase at point r.

The temperature inside the phantom can be measured by two types of technique: multiple point measurement, i.e., by thermocouples, thermistors, or fiberoptic sensors, or thermographic imaging, i.e., surface imaging by a thermographic camera or imaging at depth by liquid crystal plates. Examples of the measurement of the temperature change with thermocouples are shown in Figs. 17.3, 17.5, and 17.6.

17.4.2.1 Thermal Condition of the Phantom

A constant temperature throughout the phantom before a heating pulse is advised. In experiments irradiating small volumes by interstitial or superficial applicators it does not take much time to find a constant temperature in the phantom again,

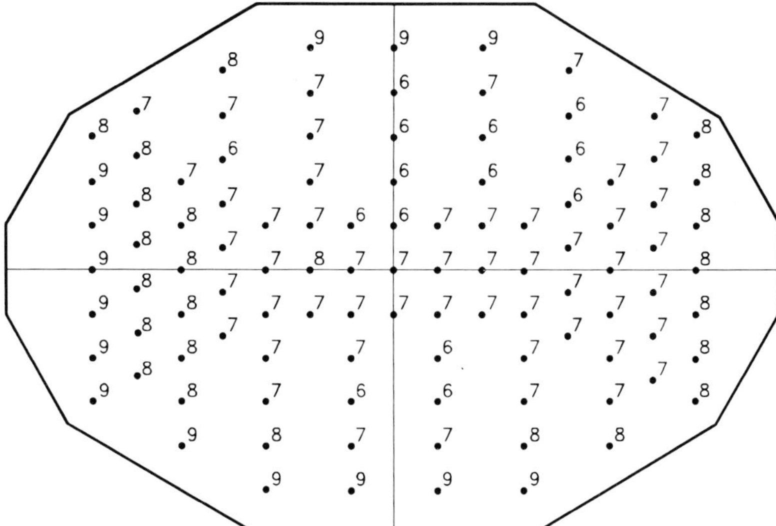

Fig. 17.5. 2D SAR distribution, measured by temperature increase with 105 thermocouples in the Amsterdam phantom, with the maximum increase of 0.42°C normalized to be 10. The applied power was 400 W for 100 s, and the increased temperature was measured 5 s after power off. The phantom was filled with wallpaper paste and saline with 3.0 g NaCl per liter distilled water

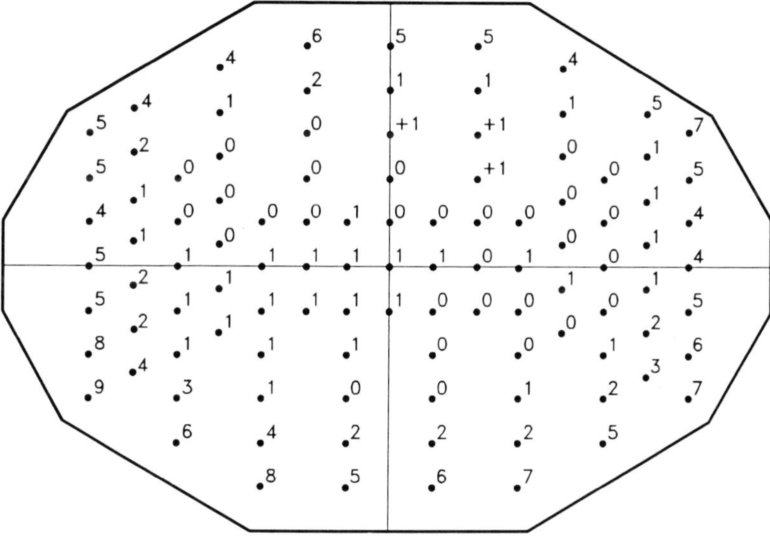

Fig. 17.6. Normalized temperature decrease in the Amsterdam phantom filled with wallpaper paste. After a series of numerous power pulses (see Fig. 17.5), the temperature in the phantom showed an overall rise in temperature of approximately 10°C. Then the heat conduction was measured during a measuring cycle of 100 s with power off. Except for the three positive values (+1), which represent an increase of 0.01°C, all ΔT values are negative. The maximum value of 0.17°C temperature decrease is normalized to be 10

but in large deep body phantoms the large heat capacity results in long cooling periods. Furthermore the thermal situation is different for large-volume irradiations: the contribution of the boli can become a dominant factor. For example, the thermal conduction to a large bolus of at least 100 l of water, in which convection occurs, can be much higher than the thermal conduction inside the solid phantom.

An excessively long cooling period between successive pulses prohibits long experimental series investigating a greater number of setups with, for example, different relations of phases and amplitudes. The need to realize a significant

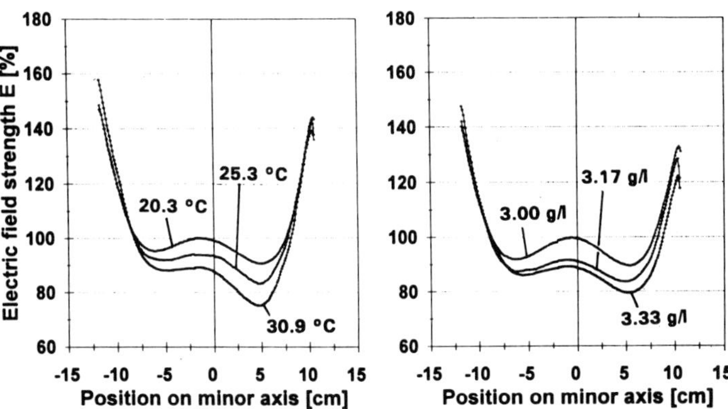

Fig. 17.7. Comparison of E-field scans in saline: with a constant salt concentration of 3.00 g/l at different temperatures (*left*), and with different salt concentrations at a constant temperature of 20.3°C (*right*). With increasing temperature or salt concentration (conductivity) the absorption increases (see Sect. 17.3.4) in both situations from 0.50 S/m (*upper lines*) to 0.55 S/m and 0.60 S/m (*lower lines*)

thermal increase in order to gain a good signal to noise resolution makes this problem even worse. An increase of 5°C in phantom temperature also increases the electrical conductivity, which significantly alters the SAR pattern, as can be seen in the experimental result shown in Fig. 17.7. Scans in the Amsterdam phantom, irradiated with only the top and bottom applicator, demonstrate the decrease in the electric field strength with increasing temperature or salinity. If series of experiments are carried out with short time intervals between heating pulses, the heat conduction throughout the phantom should be measured, e.g., by registration of the temperature change after a measuring cycle with zero power (Myerson et al. 1991; Fig. 17.6).

17.4.2.2 Temperature Sensors and Thermal Mapping

Temperature sensors in hyperthermia are typically thermocouples, thermistors, and fiberoptic thermometers. To avoid RF disturbance, thermocouples are usually read out in power-off periods, whereas thermistors and fiberoptic thermometers are free of interference with the RF field and thus can be used during power on. Thermocouples offer a fast acquisition rate after a waiting period of a few seconds for the RF disturbance to be suppressed. The spatial resolution depends on the number of thermocouple points and the spacing along a string as well as on the number of thermometry channels. Thermal mapping has the advantage of high spatial resolution along the catheter track, but suffers from a slow acquisition rate due to the waiting period for thermal equilibrium at every point of measurement. Furthermore, the number of motorized mapping channels limits the number of catheter tracks available for a measurement. For experiments in the "Utah deep body phantom," Sullivan (1992) mentions a step size of 1 cm together with a waiting period of 4 s, i.e., a measuring time as long as 2 min for 30 cm across the long axis of the phantom. This is a period during which thermal conduction inside a phantom and to the bolus might alter the temperature profile (Myerson et al. 1991).

17.4.2.3 Liquid Crystal Plate Dosimetry

Liquid crystal plate (LCP) dosimetry allows a fast and accurate determination of the SAR on a plane inside a phantom. It presents some advantages over other techniques like the infrared thermographic camera and E-field probe techniques, and it has proven to be one of the most reliable methods. This is especially true for the characterization of applicators for superficial hyperthermia. This technique can be used with any solid, convection-free transparent phantom.

The phantom commonly used for LCP dosimetry is a gel of polyacrylamide, obtained by a polymerization process (see Sect. 17.3.3). A liquid crystal foil, consisting of a plastic film over which a thin layer of thermochromic liquid crystals is deposited, is embedded in the phantom

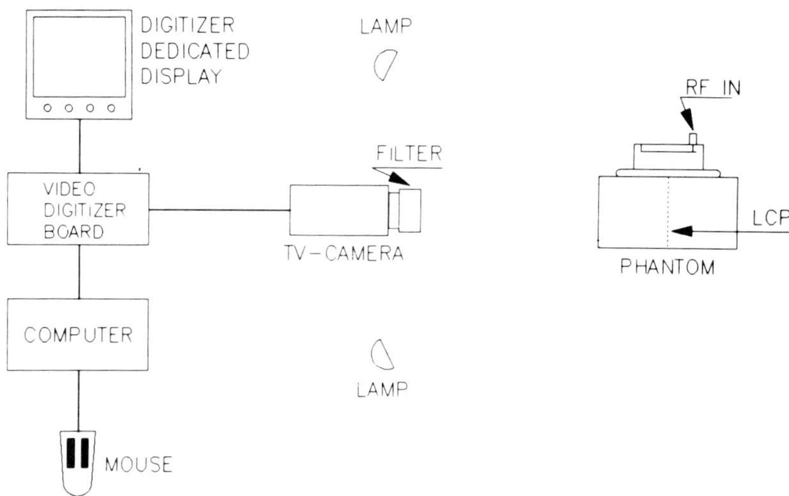

Fig. 17.8. Computerized setup for liquid crystal plate dosimetry

material before polymerization. The property of thermochromic LCPs to reflect different light wavelengths depending on their temperature is the basic principle of LCP dosimetry. A typical setup for LCP dosimetry is depicted in Fig. 17.8. The data acquisition system consists in a TV CCD camera connected to a computer via a video digitized board. The LCP inside the phantom is illuminated by two lamps placed behind the CCD camera.

Two procedures based on LCP dosimetry by a CCD camera are principally used at present. The first, developed by ANDREUCCETTI et al. (1991), consists in using a professional black and white CCD camera with an infrared blocking filter mounted in front of the CCD sensor in order to enhance the camera resolution. A narrow band interference filter is mounted in front of the lens to select a single color from the LCP thermochromic palette. The time evolution of the selected color curve is recorded to allow SAR reconstruction in the plane of the LCP. The second procedure, developed by CRISTOFORETTI et al. (1993), is based on a measurement of the hue by means of a color TV camera, After a proper calibration of the LCP, hue can be converted into temperature and finally, considering the time increment and σ, the SAR distribution in the plane of the LCP is obtained.

17.4.2.4 Thermographic Camera

The use of a thermographic camera to determine the SAR profile produced by an EM applicator was originally proposed by Guy and has been successfully adopted by several researchers, especially in the United States. In this method a solid, splittable phantom is heated by a short EM pulse; after the exposure the phantom is quickly opened and the temperature pattern is recorded by means of a thermographic camera. SAR is finally obtained, knowing the initial temperature in the phantom, by means of Eq. 17.6 of Sect. 17.4.2.

The thermographic method has the favorable characteristic of being very fast. The major drawbacks are the necessity of very high powers (especially for the heating of large phantoms) and the unknown error introduced by the deterioration of the temperature distribution in the period between the end of the iradiation and the acquisition of the thermographic image. The QA guidelines for ESHO protocols (HAND et al. 1989) recommend a maximum time of 60 s between the start of the pulse and the measurement of the temperature distribution to minimize the artifacts due to thermal conduction within the phantom. The time limit comes from experience with the thermographic camera, and it should not be considered an exact figure: the maximum time allowed before significant errors take place clearly depends on the temperature resolution and on the precision of the thermographic camera, as well as on the intensity of the power pulse and on the thermal characteristics of the phantom surface environment.

Additional technical discussion concerning SAR measurements with phantoms may be found in Chap. 21, Sect. 21.5.

17.5 Reliability of Experimental Outcome

The precision and reliability of experimental results can be determined by internal checks, i.e., tests on reproducibility, signal resolution, and spatial resolution, by the scientists running the experiment, and by external checks with respect to the adequacy of the description of the applied material and of the experimental setup, which should enable other scientists to repeat an experiment. Besides precision and accuracy, the spatial data density determines the conclusion which can be drawn from experimental outcomes.

17.5.1 Accuracy and Precision

17.5.1.1 Reproducibility

When the first experiment of a series is repeated at the end of a series, the similarity of the results indicates the stability of the entire setup. Changes in an SAR pattern arise from changes in absorption due to heating of material, and possibly the sensitivity of a temperature-dependent LED dipole as E-field sensor (SCHNEIDER et al. 1991). With regard to the reliability of a measured signal, particularly crossing E-field scan paths or thermometry catheters offer the opportunity to check the equality of measured data on the common points.

17.5.1.2 Recognized Signal Resolution

There are two approaches to "recognize" the signal resolution for E-field scans:

1. Stepping through a phantom while sampling a number of signals at each step during a short period (GROSS and RASKMARK 1989). This results in a mean value and standard deviation for an E-field value at every particular point.
2. Scanning with continuous sampling of signals providing, for example, one sample per millimeter. If the data points are dense even in a strong E-field gradient, then the "noise band" of the signal gives information similar to the mean value and the standard deviation.

A recognized signal resolution for ΔT measurements can be determined by:

1. A ΔT-measurement with 0 W to determine the ratio of ΔT noise at 0 W to the maximum ΔT measured with a high power pulse
2. Immediate repetition of a power pulse
3. Comparison of E-field scans with ΔT measurements (PAULSEN and ROSS 1990; Fig. 17.3).

17.5.1.3 Spatial Resolution of the Sensors

The resolution of dipoles depends on their size. It is good in a direction orthogonal to the dipole, but moderate in the direction of the dipole. The small size of temperature probes results in a good spatial resolution, but artifacts are possible in SAR measurements due to poor heat conduction through the catheter, heat conduction in the phantom as a consequence of the slow acquisition rate characteristic for thermal mapping, or crosstalk and limited isolation of the channels in multipoint/multichannel thermocouple systems (see also Chap. 15).

17.5.1.4 Spatial Resolution in Thermographic Imaging

Liquid crystal plate dosimetry and the thermographic camera/splittable phantom techniques both offer high spatial resolution. With splittable phantoms as well as with slab phantoms, however, care has to be taken that the contact surfaces present neither a dielectric discontinuity for the incident electric field nor a discontinuity in thermal characteristics (e.g., due to thin air layers).

17.5.2 Spatial Data Density

The relationship between the greatest SAR gradients and the greatest distance between adjacent data points indicates the reliability of values interpolated in between, e.g., by contour plots. For the different measuring techniques this has different implications:

1. *LED matrix*. The LED matrix visualizes E-field patterns in a complete plane with the data density determined by the spacing between the LEDs, which is typically 1 cm for superficial phantoms and 2 cm for deep body phantoms.

2. *E-field scans*. A general technical limit, which defines the spatial data density for E-field scans, is the user-friendliness of the scanning mechanics.

3. *ΔT measurements*. The spatial data density is defined by the choice of catheter tracks in the

phantom and further limited by either the number of thermocouples or, for thermal mapping, the time needed for thermal equilibrium at each point of measurement. On the other hand, liquid crystal plates and thermographic phtographs supply data on a complete plane.

4. *3D measuring*. For 3D SAR measurements in homogeneous phantoms, several planes have to be measured either by moving an LED matrix or a scanning plane through the phantom, or by multilayer phantoms (LEYBOVICH and NUSSBAUM 1984; SUROWIEC et al. 1992). In inhomogeneous phantoms, where thermometry catheters fixed in three directions (SULLIVAN et al. 1992) allow SAR measurements along preselected lines, the limited number of measuring points causes a further decrease in spatial data density. However, E-field scanning in inhomogeneous phantoms is a complex problem due to mechanical considerations, the availability of adequate soft material, and variations in the sensitivity of E-field probes in materials with different dielectric characteristics (MOUSAVINEZHAD et al. 1978).

17.5.2.1 Measured Data and Fit Routines Applied for Graphic Presentation

The number of spatial points at which data are measured in the irradiated volume is often limited, with liquid crystal plate and thermographic imaging giving the highest data density at least in a plane. Nevertheless, a complete presentation of the SAR distribution is often desired and realized in lines connecting data points or in contour plots. The fit techniques applied for graphic presentations are general fit algorithms which are not based on physical theories describing hyperthermia power deposition. Therefore a clear presentation of the original measured data points indicates the reliability of contour plots (TURNER 1984; MYERSON 1991).

17.6 Summary

- Today, a great diversity of hyperthermia phantoms and various techniques to measure the power deposition exist. These available combinations of phantoms and techniques differ in their ease of application, the time needed for experiments or performance checks, and the value of information and reliability of conclusions. Therefore, prior to phantom experiments, a proper choice of phantom should be made on the basis of a clear definition of the aim of an experiment. Furthermore, a complete description of the experimental setup, including all applied technical materials as well as an unequivocal description of the phantom material, is necessary for the repetition of experimental outcomes in other institutes and with other devices.
- The validity of experimental results depends on checks regarding possible sources of random error, such as noise and RF disturbance on the signal, and sources of systematic errors such as heat conduction to a bolus. A clear indication of the spatial distribution of the measured signals aids in the interpretation of the graphical presentation of experimental outcomes.
- For experiments in deep body hyperthermia devices, saline phantoms filled with 3 g NaCl per liter distilled water are advisable as reliable standard phantoms. This type of phantom offers the advantage that saline is certainly identical from one experiment to another, its temperature and dielectric characteristics can be stabilized for unlimited numbers of experimental runs, and results can be checked independently in comparison with qualitative results observed on an LED matrix.
- As yet, standard phantoms and appropriate measuring equipment are not available at every institute active in clinical hyperthermia. The aim of phantom techniques able to measure a sufficient data set as input for hyperthermia planning systems, which characterizes the treatment device and is similar to a QA standard in radiotherapy, demands even more progress and development.

Acknowledgements. The research and development at the Academic Medical Center in Amsterdam is financially supported by the Dutch Cancer Society Koningin Wilhelmina Fonds.

References

AAPM report no. 26 (1989) Performance evaluation of hyperthermia equipment, report of hyperthermia committee task group no. 1. American Association of Physicists in Medicine

Allen S, Kantor G, Bassen H, Ruggera P (1988) CDRH RF phantom for hyperthermia systems evaluation. Int J Hyperthermia 4: 17–23

Andreuccetti D, Bini M, Ignesti A, Olmi R, Vanni R (1988) Use of polyacrylamide as a tissue-equivalent material in the microwave range. IEEE Trans Biomed Eng 35: 275–277

Andreuccetti D, Bini M, Ignesti A, Olmi R, Priori S, Vanni R (1991) Characterization of hyperthermia applicators by semi-automatic liquid crystal dosimetry. Phys Med VII: 145–151

Bini M, Ignesti A, Millanta L, Olmi R, Rubino N, Vanni R (1984) The polyacrylamide as a phantom material for electromagnetic hyperthermia studies. IEEE Trans Biomed Eng 31: 317–322

Bini M, Olmi R (1990) Phantom materials for hyperthermia. IROE technical report TR/POE/90.13

Burdette EC, Cain FL, Seals J (1980) In vivo probe measurement technique for determining dielectric properties at VHF through microwave frequencies. IEEE Trans Microwave Theory Tech 28: 414–427

Cetas TC (1982) The philosophy and use of tissue-equivalent phantoms. In: Nussbaum GH (ed) Physical aspects of hyperthermia. AAPM Monogr 8: 441–461

Chou CK (1987) Phantoms for electromagnetic heating studies. In: Field SB, Franconi C (eds) Physics and technology of hyperthermia. Nijhoff, Dordrecht, 294–318

Chou CK, Chen GW, Guy AW, Luk KH (1984) Formulas for preparing phantom muscle tissue at various radiofrequencies. Bioelectromagnetics 5: 435–441

Cristoforetti L, Pontalti R, Cescatti L, Antolini R (1993) Quantitative colourimetric analysis of liquid crystal films (LCF) for phantom dosimetry in microwave hyperthermia. IEEE Trans Biomed Eng 40: 1159–1165

De Leeuw AAC, Lagendijk JJW (1987) Design of a clinical deep-body hyperthermia system based on the "Coaxial TEM" applicator. Int J Hyperthermia 3: 413–421

Dewhirst MW, Phillips TL, Samulski TV et al. (1990) RTOG quality assurance guidelines for clinical trials using hyperthermia. Int J Radiat Oncol Biol Phys 18: 1249–1259

Durney C, Massoudi H, Iskander M (1986) Radiofrequency radiation dosimetry handbook, 4th edn. SAM-TR-85-73, USAF, Brooks AFB, TX 78235, 7.28–7.29

Gajda G, Stuchly MA, Stuchly SS (1979) Mapping of the near-field pattern in simulated biological tissues. Electronic Letters 15: 120–121

Gautherie M, El Akoum H, Johnsen A (1988) Experimental hyperthermia. Guidelines for phantom studies using thermosensitive liquid crystal foils and transparent muscle-equivalent gels. Röhm Pharma, Weiterstadt, Deutschland.

Grant EH, Sheppard RJ, South GP (1978) Dielectric behaviour of biological molecules in solution. Clarendon Press, Oxford

Gross EJ, Raskmark P (1989) Phased array hyperthermia: an experimental investigation. In: Sugahara T, Saito M (eds) Hyperthermic oncology 1988, vol 1. Summary papers. Taylor & Francis, London, 724–725

Guy AW (1971) Analysis of electromagnetic fields induced in biological tissues by thermographic studies on equivalent phantom models. IEEE Trans Microwave Theory Tech 19: 205–214

Guy AW, Lehmann JF, Stonebridge JB (1974) Therapeutic applications of electromagnetic power. Proc IEEE 62: 55–75

Hand JW, Fessenden P (1991) QA for superficial heating. COMAC-BME workshop. Quality assurance in hyperthermia. Hyperthermia bulletin 5

Hand JW, Lagendijk JJW, Bach Andersen J, Bolomey JC (1989) Quality assurance guidelines for ESHO protocols. Int J Hyperthermia 5: 421–428

Hartsgrove G, Kraszewski A, Surowiec A (1987) Simulated biological materials for electromagnetic absorption studies. Biolectromagnetics 8: 29–36

Lagendijk JJW, Nilsson P (1984) Hyperthermia dough: a fat and bone equivalent to test microwave/radiofrequency hyperthermia heating systems. Phys Med Biol 30: 709–712

Lagendijk JJW, De Leeuw AAC (1986) The development of applicators for deep-body hyperthermia. Recent Results Cancer Res 101: 18–35

Lagendijk JJW, Molls M (1991) Conclusions: deep body quality assurance. COMAC-BME Bulletin 5: 95–96

Lamaitre G, Postma A, Van Dijk JDP (1992) COMAC-BME site visit program for superficial devices: preliminary results. In: Gerner EW (ed) Proceedings of the 6th ISHO, vol 1. Tuscon, Arizona, p 28

Leybovich LB, Nussbaum GH (1984) A practical, modular hyperthermia phantom. Med Phys 11: 207–208

Lumori ML, Bach Andersen J, Gopal, MK, Cetas TC (1990) Gaussian beam representation of aperture fields in layered, lossy media: simulation and experiment. IEEE Trans Microwave Theory Tech 38: 1623–1630

Marchal C, Nadi M, Tosser AJ, Roussey C (1989) Dielectric properties of gelatine phantoms used for simulations of biological tissues between 10 and 50 MHz. Int J Hyperthermia 5: 725–732

Mousavinezhad SH, Chen KM, Nyquist P (1978) Response of insulated electric field probes in finite heterogeneous biological bodies. IEEE Trans Microwave Theory Tech 26: 599–607

Myerson RJ, Leybovich L, Emami B, Straube L (1991) Phantom studies and preliminary clinical experience with the BSD 2000. Int J Hyperthermia 7: 937–951

Nyshadham A, Sibbald CL, Stuchly SS (1992) Permittivity measurements using open-ended sensors and reference liquid calibration – an uncertainty analysis. IEEE Trans Microwave Theory Tech 40, no. 2

Paulsen KD (1990) Calculation of power deposition patterns in hyperthermia. In: Galltherie M (ed) Thermal dosimetry and treatment planning. Springer, Berlin Heidelberg New York, 57–117

Paulsen KD, Ross MP (1990) Comparison of numerical results with phantom experiments and clinical measurements. Int J Hyperthermia 6: 333–349

Ricci A, Chiariello L, Bordi F et al. (1991) An upper trunk anatomic phantom for low RF frequency lung and liver tumor hyperthermia. Abstract, 12th ESHO conference, Bergen. Strahlenterapie 167: 338

Samulski TV, Kapp DS, Fessenden P, Lohrbach A (1987) Heating deep seated eccentrally located tumours with an annular array system: a comparative clinical study using two annual array operating configurations. Int J Radiat Oncol Biol Phys 13: 83–94

Sathiaseelan V, Mittal BB, Taflove A, Reuter C, Piket-May MJ, Pierce MC (1992) Strategies for improving sigma-60 deep hyperthermia applicator performance. In: Gerner EW (ed) Proceedings of the 6th ISHO, vol 1, Tuscon, Arizona, p 247

Schneider CJ, Van Dijk JDP (1991) Visualization by a

matrix of light emitting diodes of interference effects from a radiative four-applicator hyperthermia system. Int J Hyperthermia 7: 355–356

Schneider CJ, Engelberts N, Van Dijk JDP (1991) Characteristics of a passive RF field probe with fibre-optic link for measurements in liquid hyperthermia phantoms. Phys Med Biol 36: 461–474

Schneider CJ, De Leeuw AAC, Van Dijk JDP (1992a) Quantitative determination of SAR profiles from photographs of the light-emitting diode matrix. Int J Hyperthermia 8: 609–619

Schneider CJ, Van Dijk JDP, Sijbrands J et al. (1992b) Visualization of interfering RF-electric fields in a lossy liquid simulating patient's body in hyperthermia treatment by a LED-matrix. In: Morucci JP, Plonsey R, Coatrieu JL, Laxminarayan S (eds) Proceedings of the 14th Annual Int Conf IEEE EMBS, Paris, vol 1. IEEE, Piscataway NJ, pp 256–257

Schneider CJ, Van Dijk JDP, Sijbrands J, Van Os RM, Van Stam G, Zum Vörde Sive Vörding PJ (1993) Evaluation of the shape of the water bolus as a critical parameter for the amplitude ratios of applicators in a radiative deep body hyperthermia system. Abstracts of the 14th ESHO, Brussels, June 16–19 1993

Schneider CJ, Van Dijk JDP, De Leeuw AAC, Wust P, Baumhoer W (1994) Quality assurance in various radiative hyperthermia systems applying a phantom with LED-matrix. Int J Hyperthermia 5: 733–747

Schneider CJ, Kuijer JPA, Colussi LC, Schepp CJ, Van Dijk JDP (1995) Performance evaluation of annular arrays in practice: the measurement of phase and amplitude patterns of RF deep body hyperthermia applicators. Medical Physics. 22, June 1995

Schwan H (1965) Biophysics of hyperthermia. In: Licht S (ed) Therapeutic heat and cold. Waverly Press, Baltimore, 63–125

Seegenschmiedt MH, Visser AJ (1991) QA for interstitial hyperthermia. COMAC-BME workshop. Quality assurance in hyperthermia. Hyperthermia Bulletin 5

Stogryn A (1971) Equation for calculating the dielectric constant of saline water. IEEE Trans Microwave Theory Tech 19: 733–736

Stuchly MA, Stuchly SS (1980) Dielectric properties of biological substances – tabulated. J Microw Power 15: 19–26

Stuchly MA, Kraszewski A, Stuchly SS (1984) Implantable electric-field probes – some performance characteristics. IEEE Trans Biomed Eng 31: 526–531

Sullivan DM, Buechler D, Gibbs FA (1992) Comparison of measured and simulated data in an annular phased array using an inhomogeneous phantom. IEEE Trans Microwave Theory Tech 40: 600–604

Surowiec A, Shrivastava PN, Astrahan M, Petrovich Z (1992) Utilization of a multilayer polyacrylamide phantom for evaluation of hyperthermia applicators. Int J Hyperthermia 8: 795–807

Turner PF (1984) Regional hyperthermia with an annular phased array. IEEE Trans Biomed Eng 31: 106–114

Van Dijk JDP, Schneider CJ, Di Palma M, Nagi M, Lamaitre G, Sidi J, Hand JW (1992) Visualization by a double LED-matrix of electric field distributions in a three-plate capacitive deep-body hyperthermia system. In: Gerner EW (ed) Proceedings of the 6th ISHO, Tusco, Arizona, vol 1, A22

Von Hippel AR (1966) Dielectric materials and applications. M.I.T. Press, Cambridge

18 Principles of Power Deposition Models

K.D. PAULSEN

CONTENTS

18.1 Introduction

One interpretation of the mixed clinical results that have been reported over the last decade (e.g., see CURRAN and GOODMAN 1992) on the therapeutic benefits of hyperthermia as an adjuvant cancer therapy is that consistently heating tumors is a difficult task which remains problematic. A tracking of the device development for hyperthermic delivery that has occurred over this time frame lends support to this view. While some relatively simple methods are being used with success (e.g., BREZOVICH et al. 1989; DEFORD et al. 1991), for the most part hyperthermia systems have become increasingly complex. Multiapplicator devices which rely on an intricate interplay among excitation sources are now commonplace (e.g., HYNYNEN et al. 1987; CAIN and UMEMURA 1986; EBBINI and CAIN 1991; TURNER and SCHAEFERMEYER 1989; GOPAL et al. 1992).

The development of devices with many degrees of freedom has become necessary because of the complex conditions under which the heating of tumors must take place. Anatomical complexity creates geometry and heterogeneity effects that nonintuitively shape the power deposition in tumor and surrounding tissues, which ultimately leads to temperature rise. Further, vascular complexity confounds the understanding of the temperature elevation realized in tumors for any given power deposition pattern. This makes power deposition adjustment at both the pre- and concurrent stages of treatment an essential capability of any hyperthermia therapy system. Methods to expedite the development, operation, and control of such systems are critical to the realization of hyperthermia equipment that can consistently elevate tumor temperatures to a predefined set of treatment goals.

Of particular interest since the early 1980s has been the use of computational models to serve this purpose (e.g., STROHBEHN and ROEMER 1984). The underlying hypothesis has been that computational models would advance clinical treatment through both enhanced understanding of the physical processes involved during therapy and improved ability to design, develop, and evaluate hyperthermia equipment. The expectation is that good numerical modeling will provide the therapist with more information about the type of device to use for a particular tumor site, where thermometry probes should be placed to extract the most information from a given treatment, where pain-limiting hot spots are likely to occur as a result of localized power deposition peaks, what kind of temperature distributions can be expected for specific assumptions about blood flow, etc. Based on this type of rationale, high hopes exist for utilizing computational models as important contributors in the quest to clarify the confusing and conflicting results that have been reported on the efficacy of hyperthermia (e.g., PEREZ et al. 1991; PHILLIPS 1993).

The problem of simulating hyperthermic treatment has traditionally been divided into two

K.D. PAULSEN, PhD, Thayer School of Engineering, Dartmouth College, Hinman Box 8000, Hanover, NH 03755, USA

components: (a) the deposition of power or SAR (specific absorption rate in units of power per unit mass) in tissue and (b) the redistribution of this energy due to the heat transfer mechanisms at work in vivo, namely thermal conduction and blood flow, While these two components are closely linked physically in that the deposited power is the "driving force" for subsequent temperature rise, the complexity of the processes taking place in tissue has demanded specialization in these two facets of hyperthermic treatment modeling. In fact, two separate chapters (18 and 19) in this monograph have been devoted to each of these topics, their merging being discussed in yet a third chapter (20) under the general heading of Treatment Planning.

Because power must be absorbed before any temperature rise (above normothermia) can occur, the power deposition problem is usually discussed first and this will be the topic of the present chapter. It will begin with a historical overview starting with the early 1980s and will trace the evolution of power deposition modeling to the present day. This presentation will be followed by a review of the basic principles and a highlighting of the computational advances that have been necessary to achieve the state of the art in the field. Results that are representative of power deposition models that are or have been used in treatment simulations will be included. Since the two primary sources of thermal energy that have been used in hyperthermia therapy are electromagnetic (EM) and ultrasonic (US) radiation, attention will be limited to these two modalities. Where appropriate, an effort will be made to unify the discussion of EM and US power deposition models, since they possess a number of common features. This chapter will conclude with a section devoted to an assessment of the state of the art and the needs of and future directions in power deposition modeling.

18.2 Historical Perspective

Two general thrusts in power deposition modeling seem to have emerged. One has been aimed at performing the requisite calculations under clinical conditions with the goal of providing the heat source input to subsequent thermal modeling. The other has focused on computing SAR patterns of specific applicator configurations as they radiate into homogeneous or layered tissue geometries. In the former case, a chronology of advancement is relatively easy to trace. Models in this arena must deal with issues of dimensionality, geometry, and heterogeneity – items which are common to all applicators in that they are more concerned with the computational domain than the heating device itself. Further, a natural progression in the complexity with which these items are modeled readily exists. For example, model complexity escalates significantly as the dimensionality of the computational domain increases from one to three dimensions. A logical path to the realization of a fruitful 3D model is to first implement it in one and two dimensions, respectively, and to gain experience and insight into its behavior under these simpler scenarios prior to full 3D implementation.

Applicator modeling, on the other hand, does not have a chronological path of advancement that can be pointed to so easily. For the most part, the details of the particular device at hand have driven the modeling effort in this area of SAR computation. As a result, only a modest amount of work has attempted to develop general modeling principles for hyperthermia applicators (e.g., Lumori et al. 1990a,b) upon which a foundation for future advancement could be built. There has been advancement in the sense that the applicators being modeled have become more complex over time. However, from the point of view of the inherent capabilities of the computational method used, it is more difficult to argue that one applicator model is superior to another in the same way that a 2D model is superior to a 1D model or a CT-based anatomical representation is better than a symmetrically layered geometry. As a result, this section will primarily trace the evolution of patient-based SAR modeling; however, some indications will be given of the status of applicator modeling as well.

18.2.1 Early to Mid 1980s

Some of the first SAR modeling work was reported in the early 1980s and corresponded with the appearance of the commercial hyperthermia device known as the Magnetrode (Young et al. 1980; Hill et al. 1983a; Halac et al. 1993). These modeling efforts were one- and two-dimensional and utilized ideal geometrical representations of the body anatomy. The work of Hill et al. was particularly noteworthy at that time. It utilized a

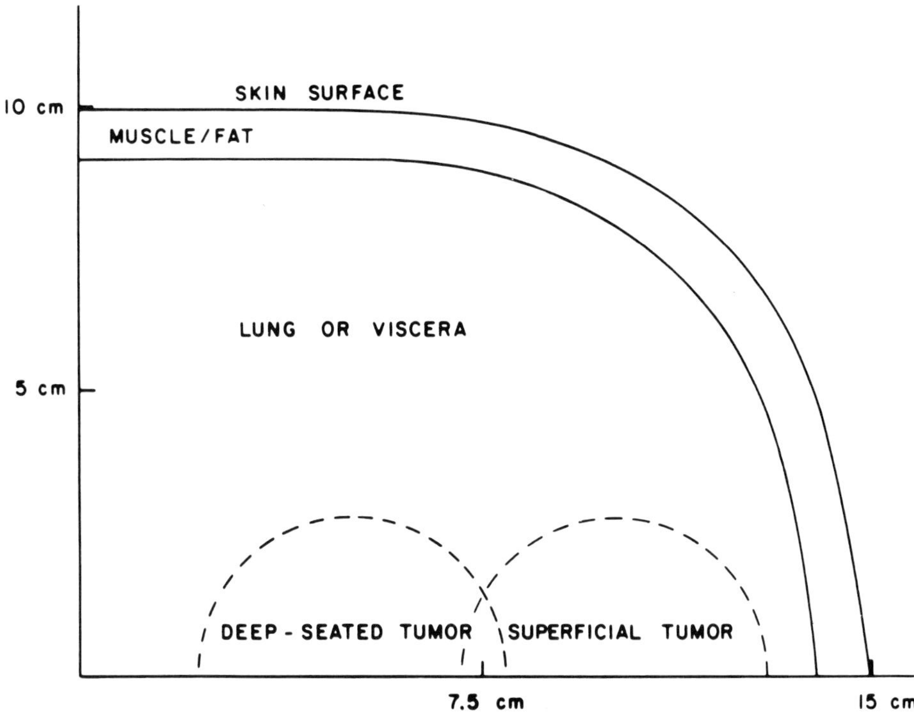

Fig. 18.1. Early 1980s anatomical model developed by HILL et al. (1983a) to simulate magnetically induced power deposition. (From PAULSEN et al. 1984a)

moment method solution of a low-frequency approximation to Maxwell's equations (HILL et al. 1983b). The computational domain was two-dimensional with quadrant symmetry where each quadrant consisted of a tumor area embedded in lung tissue which was surrounded by a subcutaneous layer. Figure 18.1 shows a schematic of the anatomical model.

It is important to recognize that prior to this Magnetrode modeling there had been some pioneering work in the computation of SAR in biological tissues (e.g., LIVESAY and CHEN 1974; HAGMANN et al. 1979). In fact, this work was three-dimensional and utilized heterogeneous block models of the human body and thus could be viewed as far more advanced than the early Magnetrode modeling that was emerging in the hyperthermia field circa 1983. However, the emphasis in the 3D block model effort was to study potential health hazards resulting from SAR deposited in the body due to various environmental EM sources. As such, it was more concerned with full-body exposures and gross levels of SAR over large regions of the body. The hyperthermia SAR modeling, on the other hand, was seeking to compute the fine details of the absorbed power over localized portions of the body anatomy. The early 3D block models in the health hazards research field were far too crude to yield this type of information.

At approximately the same time as modeling interest in the Magnetrode was peaking, a second commercial device, the APAS (TURNER 1984; GIBBS et al. 1984) emerged and a significant amount of interest in simulating the performance of this system immediately arose. Perhaps one of the most important contributions to APAS simulation was that of ISKANDER et al. (1982). They utilized a moment method approach, but rather than limiting their calculations to an idealized body geometry, they incorporated CT-based anatomy into their model. While the model used by Iskander et al. did not contain any tumor region, others followed suit (e.g., VAN DEN BERG et al. 1983; PAULSEN et al. 1984b) and by the mid 1980s, CT-based, two-dimensional modeling of the power deposition patterns produced by the Magnetrode and APAS in actual cancer patient tumors was the norm within the modeling community.

The most complete set of studies in this vein were those of PAULSEN et al. (1985). They chose a

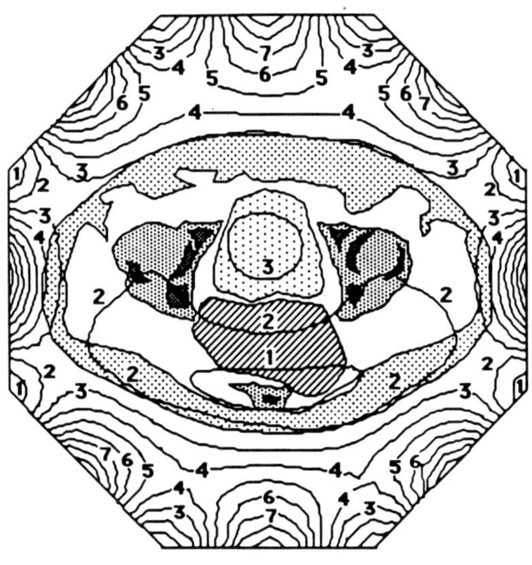

Fig. 18.2. Mid 1980s anatomical model based on CT data showing a computed field pattern for an annular array type device. (From STROHBEHN et al. 1986)

variety of anatomical tumor sites and subjected 2D CT-based anatomical models to heat treatments with the Magnetrode and APAS systems. Figure 18.2 shows a representative 2D model constructed from CT data. This work was successful in comparing the relative performance of hyperthermia devices and for predicting general trends observed with these systems during clinical treatments (STROHBEHN et al. 1986). It, along with the efforts of others, contributed the initial support for the hypothesis that computational models improve clinical treatment. It also provided proof for the concept that calculations of this type would be possible in the hyperthermia context.

Not surprisingly, clinically based power deposition modeling has its roots in noninvasive regional heating. Such treatments are more difficult to plan, control, and evaluate because access to temperature and SAR measurements is limited (SAPOZINK et al. 1991). Recent clinical studies have borne out the fact that noninvasive deep heating devices are capable of delivering enough energy to achieve therapeutic temperature elevation, but treatments are often limited due to pain (e.g., SAPOZINK et al. 1990; EMANI et al. 1991; Samulski et al. 1990; FESSENDEN et al. 1984). Use of aggressive sedation has been precluded to date because of lack of knowledge of the heating patterns produced in the clinical setting. It was recognized very early in the evolution of noninvasive deep heating systems that resolution of power limiting pain problems would represent a major advance for this therapy and that treatment simulation offered a means for obtaining the needed information about the heating patterns to be expected clinically. This information could be used to diminish the number of pain-limiting episodes by highlighting potential "hot spots," providing alternate treatment plans that might diminish their severity and allowing clinicians to prescribe deeper levels of sedation based on greater confidence in device operation.

In applicator specific modeling, a core of initial interest centered around interstitial EM radiators. The theory and ensuing computation were worked out for a linear dipole housed within a catheter embedded in a homogeneous infinite extent of lossy tissue (KING et al. 1983). Investigations were carried out on the heating patterns and subsequent temperature distributions for arrays of interstitial antennas (STROHBEHN et al. 1982). Modeling of implantable RF needles (e.g., STROHBEHN 1983) and ferromagnetic seeds (e.g., MATLOUBIEH et al. 1984) under similar circumstances was also performed very early in the evolution of power deposition simulation in hyperthermia. Two-dimensional simulation studies comparing the relative performance of interstitial methods began to appear in the mid 1980s (e.g., MECHLING and STROHBEHN 1986) at about the same time as clinically based modeling efforts were reporting similar comparative analyses of the Magnetrode and APAS. Because it was reasonable to assume (at least initially!) that interstitial devices deposit power over length scales where tissue properties and geometry are relatively uniform, modeling efforts concentrated on capturing the details of the energy source rather than the surrounding medium.

Ultrasonic power deposition models began in much the same way. With this modality, the operating assumption was that ultrasound propagates largely undisturbed in many soft tissues; hence, it is reasonable to assume that power absorption can be computed by representing the details of the applicator as it radiates into a typical soft tissue. These models have their origins in the diagnostic ultrasound field; however, for hyperthermia treatment simulation attenuation effects due to tissues have been added. Early simulation results appeared in the literature, first for planar (e.g., CHAN et al. 1974) and later for focused ultrasound systems (e.g., MADSEN et al. 1981;

SWINDELL et al. 1982), but it was clear that as of the mid 1980s considerably more attention had been devoted to EM SAR models, both clinical and applicator-based, than their US counterparts. A comprehensive review of the state of the art in hyperthermia treatment simulation until approximately 1984 can be found in STROHBEHN and ROEMER (1984).

18.2.2 Mid 1980s to Early 1990s

The ensuing years saw increased interest in power deposition models and it readily became apparent that 2D calculations would be insufficient for clinical treatment planning and analysis (e.g., DEWHIRST et al. 1987; HAGMANN 1987). The thrust to develop 3D models of power absorption began in approximately 1986 and has continued to gain momentum as more data demonstrating the inadequacy of 2D models have been reported (e.g., WUST et al. 1991; FELDMANN et al. 1991; PAULSEN and ROSS 1990; PIKET-MAY et al. 1992). For example, Fig. 18.3 shows a recent result comparing the SAR distribution computed in a 2D and 3D patient-specific model of the thigh irradiated by an external 915-MHz waveguide applicator. Interestingly, the 3D model predicts a higher SAR maximum for the same normalized incident field and a deeper overall penetration of the power deposition than its 2D counterpart. This is a nonintuitive result because of the overall complexity of the problem. Figure 18.3 illustrates the magnitude of the importance of the results for effective therapy delivery. External heating models with anatomically based patient geometries received the largest amount of sustained effort and had the goal of reaching the level of sophistication illustrated by the calculations shown in Fig. 18.3. By contrast, many of the earlier applicator-based models of SAR were already 3D, for example interstitial dipole antennas (KING et al. 1983); hence, the need to "three-dimensionalize" computed results was not felt nearly so strongly for these types of simulations.

Major strides were made when the potential of the finite-difference time-domain method (FDTD) for computing power deposition patterns in anatomically complex, full-scale body models was realized (e.g., SULLIVAN et al. 1988). The 3D FDTD charge was led by several investigators (e.g., SULLIVAN 1990; LAU and SHEPPARD 1986; WANG and GANDHI 1989) and has continued to gain support since that time (e.g., PIKET-MAY et al. 1992). Some of the most recent SAR modeling with FDTD has been very exciting (e.g., BEN YOSEF et al. 1992; TAYLOR and LAU 1992) in that not only have patient-specific simulations been achieved in a pretreatment planning mode, but it also appears that hot spots predicted with 3D SAR analysis do correlate with observed patient pain symptoms. This work has provided the first real clinical evidence that SAR models can be important treatment planning aids.

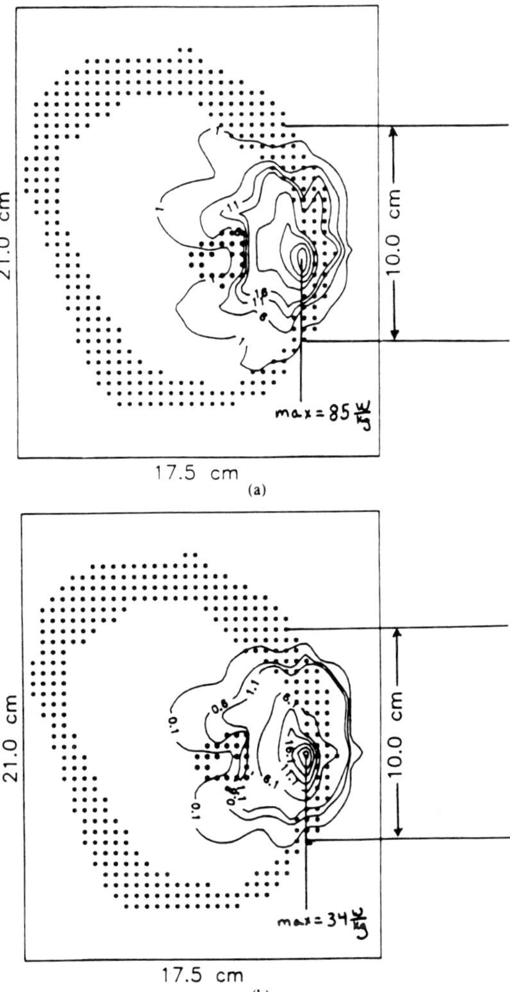

Fig. 18.3. Computed SAR distributions in a 3D (**a**) and 2D (**b**) patient-specific model of the thigh exposed to external waveguide heating. The difference in the power level contours between the two models is clear and suggests that a more favorable heating pattern is obtained in this case when 3D effects are modeled. (From PIKET-MAY et al. 1992)

Efforts involving other techniques, most notably finite element and integral equations, also began the quest for achieving 3D SAR simulation on realistic anatomical models of the body in the late 1980s. By 1988 homogeneous conforming and crude (in terms of spatial resolution) heterogeneous block models of three-dimensional bodies were in existence for finite element and integral equation techniques (e.g., HAGMANN and LEVIN 1986; PAULSEN et al. 1988a,b) but these lagged the degree of detail that was being achieved with FDTD at the time. Nonetheless, interesting findings did emerge from these studies, for example, the concept of aberrant heating, which is the deposition of significant energy levels outside the body region of direct exposure, was put forward (HAGMANN and LEVIN 1986) and independently verified (PAULSEN et al. 1988a). However, throughout the remainder of the 1980s and early 1990s it remained the case that the most significant progress in SAR modeling in 3D was achieved with FDTD. While the reasons for this become more clear in the remainder of this chapter, the essential difficulties with advancing these other techniques were twofold: (a) they both lacked the computational efficiency afforded by FDTD and (b) the ability to generate conforming unstructured 3D meshes was not readily available.

Recent advances indicate that the computational efficiency question with finite element and integral equations is rapidly vanishing. In fact, 3D simulations with these techniques which rival the impressive FDTD models that emerged in the late 1980s and early 1990s have now appeared (e.g., ZWAMBORN et al. 1992; PAULSEN et al. 1992a, 1993; CLEGG et al. 1993a). On the unstructured mesh generation front, significant progress has also been made (PAULSEN et al. 1993; JOHNTSON and SULLIVAN 1993; DAS et al. 1993; SEEBASS et al. 1992). While this problem has not been completely solved to date, it does appear to be solvable and will allow another level of detail to be employed in investigations of tissue interface and body curvature effects which seem to be critical determinants of the SAR patterns induced in patients. An example of a 3D patient model which is representative of those that are presently in use is shown in Fig. 18.4. Given that at least three computational techniques are now available which can compute power deposition patterns on models such as that displayed in Fig. 18.4, clinical SAR modeling can be expected to be entering a new era of rapid proliferation of 3D computed results that should lead to new insights into hyperthermia delivery.

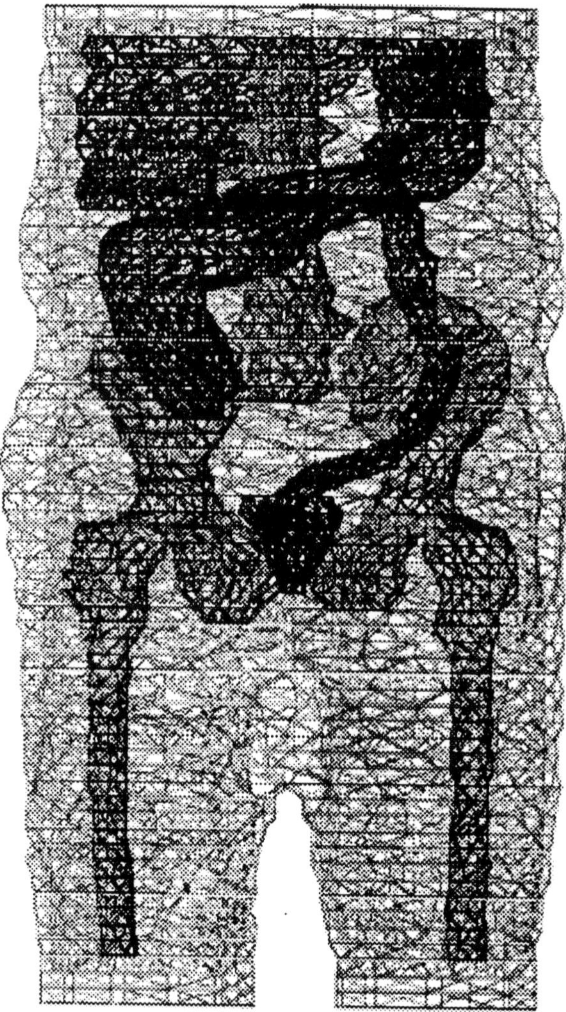

Fig. 18.4. Early 1990s anatomical mesh based on CT data which is representative of current capabilities

Since the mid 1980s important milestones have also occurred in simulation of ultrasonic power deposition and specific applicator modeling. However, these advances have not been computational in that the basic techniques have remained largely status quo, but rather the types of devices being modeled have advanced in degree of complexity. For example, the emergence of the sector-vortex ultrasound array (CAIN and UMEMURA 1986) has resulted in a number of interesting simulation studies that have highlighted the potential payoffs in terms of SAR focus and control that should be achievable (e.g., EBBINI and CAIN 1991). Further, the clinical spiral antenna which has been used successfully for a number of years has just recently been modeled for the first time (ZHANG et al. 1993). While advances such as these have been forthcoming, it has continued to be true through the late 1980s and early 1990s that US power deposition modeling has received considerably less attention than the EM case and that applicator modeling efforts have remained distinct from clinically based patient simulations in that they have focused on device-specific investigations in idealized geometries. This suggests that there is a significant opportunity to advance the state of the art in applicator modeling and general US power deposition calculations.

As evidenced by a cursory scanning of Figs. 18.1–18.4, SAR models have advanced dramatically over the last 10–12 years. To appreciate the present capabilities in this area, it is instructive to review a few basic principles and to discuss in some detail the current status of SAR modeling. These are the topics of the next two sections of this chapter.

18.3 Basic Principles

In this section the basic principles of power deposition modeling are discussed. The focus is on the nature of the techniques that are being used and their associated computational implications. Discussion of the state of the art and the recent advances that have allowed 3D computations to become possible are reserved for the next section. For presentation purposes, it is convenient to consider the two classes of problems identified earlier: (a) those which intend to model the tissue geometry and heterogeneity and (b) those which center on the details of the hyperthermia applicator as it radiates into idealized tissue structures. A further consideration is the fact that within each of these two categories, two modalities – electromagnetic and ultrasonic heating – need to be addressed. Clearly the merging of patient modeling with applicator modeling is essential for the most realistic simulation of clinical power deposition patterns in patients; however, the historical overview given in the previous section indicates that they have remained distinct in many respects. The complexity associated with either modeling of 3D anatomical effects or modeling of the details of the excitation sources has delayed their confluence. Because of space limitations a complete discussion of patient and applicator modeling for both EM and US heating is not possible. Where appropriate, analogies between categories will be drawn and the discussion streamlined to focus on the central points. The reader may also wish to consult other rather recent reviews of these areas (e.g., PAULSEN 1990a,b; HYNYNEN 1990; SATHIASEELAN et al. 1992).

18.3.1 Patient Modeling

18.3.1.1 Electromagnetic

There has been tremendous interest in modeling the effects of anatomical structure and composition on the EM fields induced in tissue. It has been known for some time (e.g., ISKANDER 1982) that even simple planar interfaces between tissues can dramatically alter the electric field and resulting power deposition simply based on field polarization and the electrical contrast between the two tissues forming the interface. Because electrical properties vary significantly as a function of both tissue type and excitation frequency (JOINES 1984), interfaces with substantial electrical contrast are prevalent within the body. As a result, knowledge of the details of power absorption within the treatment field is difficult to gain and computational models are viewed as a way to obtain the needed information.

To compute SAR, the spatial and temporal behavior of the EM field must be calculated in the presence of spatially varying electrical properties. As a first approximation, the electrical properties of tissues can be assumed to be uniform within a given tissue type, but variable from tissue to tissue. This gives rise to the so-called electromagnetic jump conditions (PAULSEN 1990a) which act to influence the field and resulting SAR dramatically. These jump conditions require continuity in all EM field components at tissue boundaries except for the normally directed electric field, which is discontinuous at the interface by an amount equal to the ratio of the complex permittivities of the two tissues forming the interface.

Hence, solution of the EM power deposition problem must satisfy the basic Maxwell relations subject to the jump conditions and driving sources, which must obey conservation properties. Since the sources typically do not encircle the entire treatment site, boundaries (either real or imaginary) which envelop the region of interest where some EM behavior can be dictated do not exist. As a result, propagation of EM energy cannot be a priori confined to the treatment region and must be allowed the degree of freedom to travel far from the area of interest. In formal mathematical terms, the enclosing boundary necessary to accommodate the far-field behavior of the EM field is at an infinite distance from the region of interest (unless, for example, the treatment is carried out in a shielded room in which case enough of the behavior of the EM field can be specified on the walls of the treatment room for it to act as a suitable enclosing boundary). Thus, in addition to satisfying the basic Maxwell relations, jump conditions, and excitation source conservation, the far-field behavior must also be captured appropriately. The details of the necessary mathematical framework can be found elsewhere (e.g., PAULSEN 1990a).

Three methods – (a) finite differences, (b) finite elements, and (c) integral equations – have proved to be the most useful in computing SAR patterns in anatomically complex models of the body. These techniques possess a number of similarities and differences which affect their suitability for 3D power deposition calculations in this context. They are all similar in that they attempt to solve the mathematical framework described above by dividing the region of interest into a finite set of points or nodes which are grouped together in an orderly fashion to form small subvolumes (often referred to as cells or elements) that comprise the computational domain. The complete collection of nodes and elements is termed the mesh (or grid). The construction of the mesh and how best to determine the connectivity of the nodes to form elements is a research topic itself (e.g., GEORGE 1991), especially in the emerging area of unstructured meshing and adaptive refinement thereof (e.g., SHEPARD and WEATHERILL 1991), which is beyond the scope of this chapter. Figure 18.5 shows a simple unstructured mesh where a node and element have been highlighted.

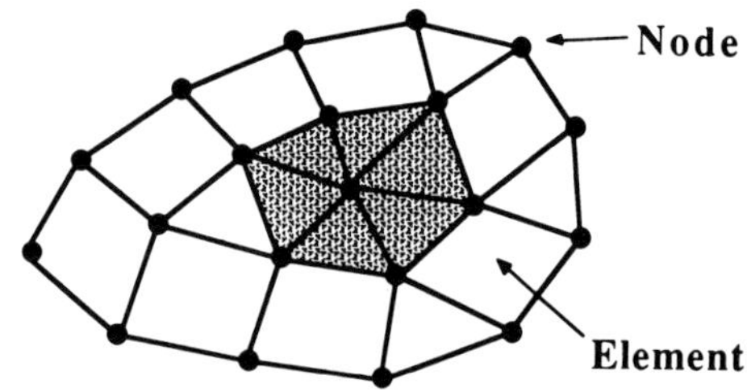

Fig. 18.5. An unstructured 2D mesh illustrating the concept of a node and element. (From PAULSEN et al. 1990a)

Once the mesh or discretization has been chosen, the strategy behind these numerical methods is to convert the functional equations and boundary conditions into an algebraic set of relations the solution of which approximates that of the functional form. Note that once a particular method has been selected, certain choices about the nature of the mesh have also already been made as a result of practical implementation issues. For example, finite difference methods are almost exclusively used on uniformly structured meshes, since they are naturally represented on such discretizations, but are cumbersome on highly unstructured nodal positions. In many instances the algebraic relationships generated are coupled, which necessitates matrix solution (e.g., ZWAMBORN et al. 1992; PAULSEN et al. 1992a). The properties of the matrix, including its size, affect the solvability of the problem. In certain cases, the algebraic relations can be decoupled, which has potential computational advantages in that a costly matrix solution can be avoided (e.g., LYNCH and PAULSEN 1990; SULLIVAN et al. 1988).

The differences between finite difference, finite element, and integral equation methods can be understood in terms of trade-offs between computational efficiency and computational accuracy (PAULSEN 1990b). In 3D simulations involving complex body anatomy, computational efficiency has been an overriding concern in that without it, solutions to most problems of interest in hyperthermia treatment simulation are simply not possible. The viability of algorithms in this context, at least for present-day computing power, is dependent on achieving essentially linear growth in computational costs as the size of the problem increases (i.e., as the number of nodes increases). In this regard all three techniques have realized linear scaling relations, though not with equal ease. The way in which this has been achieved is method dependent and understanding the approaches taken involves analyses of operation count trade-offs between various matrix solution techniques as well as nonmatrix methods. For example, in the case of the finite element method the interested reader may wish to consult PAULSEN et al. (1992b) for some insights into the important issues. Because the computational efficiencies of these three methods can now be placed more or less on an equal footing, each is capable of computing solutions on meshes with enough nodes to reasonably represent 3D body anatomy. This has not always been the case and as recently as 3 or 4 years ago, 3D SAR calculations were dominated by finite differences largely due to its computational efficiency edge over competing methods. As evidenced by the most current results, this efficiency gap between competing methods has closed dramatically (e.g., compare JAMES and SULLIVAN 1992; ZWAMBORN et al. 1992; PAULSEN et al. 1992a).

As a result of the advances in computational efficiency, issues of computational accuracy are now moving to the forefront. In this arena, several points merit consideration. They of course center around how well the mathematical framework is being approximated, which consists of the basic Maxwell equations, the boundary and interface conditions, and the excitation source description. While the implementation details are different, the ability of these techniques to satisfy the basic relations given by the Maxwell equations, themselves, is not of concern. In the absence of tissue heterogeneity and unbounded wave propagation, the influence of which is felt through the boundary and/or interface relations, solution of the Maxwell equations is relatively simple and all three techniques are more than adequate (arguments for choosing one over the other falling back to only computational efficiency considerations). For the anatomical modeling considered in this subsection, source details have been largely neglected, since the emphasis has been on representing the computational domain (i.e., the patient anatomy), rather than the source. In this context the source acts to drive the computed solution. Thus, any changes in source assumptions can be viewed as changing the solution itself, not the inherent accuracy of that solution; that is, given equivalent source assumptions all three methods should produce the same solution within the accuracy bounds of the method. It should be noted that no uniformity exists with respect to source assumptions and that the approaches taken have tended to be those which are amenable to implementation within a given technique and not necessarily based on the most realistic physical considerations.

Hence, issues of computational accuracy for geometric modeling center on treatment of the boundary and interface conditions. The nature of the discretization (i.e., the mesh) plays a role in this regard. Uniform Cartesian meshing creates a "staircasing" effect on curved boundaries (PAULSEN 1990a; CANGELLARIS and WRIGHT 1992) which can be minimized through "over resolution" (i.e., resolution at the imaging pixel level) of the computational domain. Finite difference methods almost exclusively use such meshes as do the integral equation schemes showing the most promise in terms of large model sizes. The integral equation methods need not do this (e.g., WUST et al. 1993), but they become significantly less competitive from a computational efficiency standpoint when implemented on completely unstructured meshes. The finite element method, on the other hand, is well suited to unstructured meshes and can be viewed as having this advantage without loss of its inherent computational efficiency.

Further, the finite element method can implement discrete forms of the EM jump conditions at the conforming boundaries that are made possible on an unstructured mesh (YUAN et al. 1991). The finite difference technique as commonly practiced in this context seeks to satisfy continuity requirements on individual electric and magnetic field components which are positioned at distinct spatial locations (TAFLOVE and UMASHANKAR 1990). By doing so, the jump condition on the electric field, which is an important determinant of hot spots in highly heterogeneous anatomical locations, is not strictly enforced. As a result of the strategy taken with finite difference methods, some ambiguities also can arise in the tangential interface relations (PAULSEN 1990a). Integral equation approaches are similar to the finite element method in that interface jump conditions can be enacted (e.g., see WUST et al. 1993); however, they are not amenable to the most efficient implementation of an integral equation approach. It should be recognized that the impact of Cartesian versus conforming meshes and strong versus weak constraint of the solution to obey the EM jump conditions may constitute "second order" effects. Nonetheless, in terms of the overall accuracy of the computed solution at interfaces, it does seem clear that the finite element method retains an advantage, here (the "size" of this advantage is yet to be determined), over the other methods in that it completely maintains computational efficiency while also achieving a high level of computational integrity at such locations.

Satisfaction of far-field propagation characteristics is the other area where computational accuracy may be compromised. In this situation, finite difference and finite element methods both have shortcomings that are absent in integral equation methods. Integral equation techniques in defining their governing relations establish the correct far-field behavior at the outset. In essence, the computational domain includes all space so no artificial truncation of the computational domain is needed. Finite difference and finite element techniques do not possess this attribute. The termination of the mesh represents the end of the computational domain; hence, short of meshing out to the walls of a shielded treatment room, some approximate conditions must be applied at the outer boundary of the mesh which do not adversely alter the interior solution. Such conditions are known as radiation or absorbing boundary conditions and have been the subject of active research (e.g., MITTRA and RAMAHI 1990). They are localized in order that the finite difference and finite element methods maintain computational efficiency, but they are also approximate. In the hyperthermia treatment simulation context, there has been little systematic study of the effects of artificial mesh termination on computed SAR patterns, so the overall importance of this issue remains unknown. It should be noted that exact mesh terminations do exist for finite difference and finite element methods, but they result in global relationships which severely compromise the computational efficiency of these techniques, especially in 3D (LYNCH et al. 1986; PAULSEN et al. 1988b; ZIOLKOWSKI et al. 1983). It should also be recognized that 3D anatomical models must often be truncated due to lack of complete imaging data. The effects of this type of model termination would be present in all computational techniques. Its importance and the best approaches for minimizing artificial influences on the computed fields in the region of interest are largely undocumented at the present time.

18.3.1.2 Ultrasonic

Because ultrasound can be described mathematically via the propagation of pressure waves through tissues, many of the same principles that are used to compute EM SAR patterns also apply to this modality (HYNYNEN 1990). In fact, under assumptions of linearity (i.e., small particle displacements), the ultrasound field obeys a governing equation of very similar form to that of EM fields. Hence, the same numerical techniques should be applicable to computing SAR in geometry-based anatomical models that results from ultrasonic excitation. Even in cases where nonlinearities are included, finite difference and finite element methods can be brought to bear and have been used successfully in other circumstances where nonlinear wave phenomena are present. While similarities exist which suggest that anatomically based ultrasonic power deposition modeling is exactly analogous to its EM counterpart, several important distinctions also exist which make it considerably less feasible with standard techniques on today's computer workstations.

One significant difference which works in favor of the computability of ultrasound fields is the fact that they are scalar in nature. Hence, for each node in the mesh only a single quantity (which may be complex-valued) needs to be found. This is in contrast to the EM case, where the quantities are vector in nature and thus require three values (which may be complex-valued) to be computed at each node within a three-dimensional mesh. Since for a linear system to have a unique solution, one equation is needed for each unknown, EM field calculations involve three equations that need to be enforced at each node to balance the number of unknown variables that exist. Assuming that all three unknowns are involved in all three equations, this results in a factor of 9 escalation in computational overhead for EM relative to US fields.

While the scalar versus vector nature of the fields to be computed has major computational implications, the overriding factor which makes US power deposition difficult to compute on geometric models of the body is the very small wavelengths of ultrasound relative to typical body dimensions. Experience in discretization of propagating equations by finite difference, finite element and integral equations has suggested that for linear field variation between nodes in a mesh, approximately 20 samples (or nodes) are needed per wavelength to maintain highly accurate solutions (e.g., LYNCH et al. 1985). This rule of thumb can be understood in the context of piece-

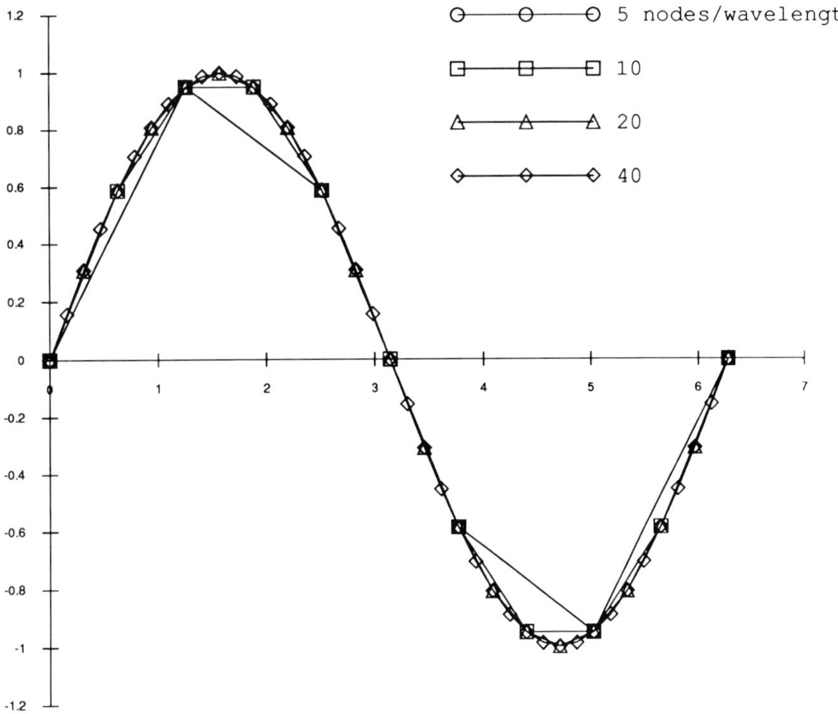

Fig. 18.6. Linear interpolation of one period of a sinusoidal function sampled at various rates

wise linear interpolation of one cycle of a sinusoidal wave, where it takes about 20 points to manufacture a smooth rendering of this function. Ten samples per wavelength have also been used as a sampling criterion for wave propagation problems, but this resolution should be viewed as being at the margin of acceptability. Figure 18.6 shows a piecewise linear interpolation of a sinusoidal function for various sampling rates from 5 to 40 samples per wavelength. The coarseness of the rendering of this function is apparent for sampling rates below 20. Thus, for ultrasonic fields which may penetrate over many wavelengths, the number of nodes in the mesh increases dramatically. For example, in soft tissue at 0.5 MHz the ultrasonic wavelength is approximately 3 mm, whereas the distance over which 50% or more of the power can be propagated may be 10–15 cm or more than 30 wavelengths (Hunt 1990). Using a conservative sampling rate of only 10 per wavelength in each Cartesian direction results in 27 million nodes, and this is only to the point where half of the ultrasonic power has been lost. The situation may be even worse since there is evidence that sampling rates must increase significantly as the number of wavelengths traversed is increased in order to maintain accuracy in discrete wave propagation problems (Cangellaris and Lee 1992). Hence, it becomes clear why no ultrasound power deposition calculations of this type have been performed. One 2D study using finite elements with an anatomical model of the body has appeared but the frequency used was very low (0.1 MHz) in order to keep the wavelength long enough so that a quasi-realistic but complete 2D cross-section could be discretized with reasonable computational costs (Kagawa et al. 1986).

One possibility for making US calculations on realistic heterogeneous anatomies would be to expand the unknown solution in a higher order basis. In particular, a spectral representation of the spatial variation of the solution may hold some promise (Patera 1984). This approach would significantly reduce the number of degrees of freedom needed to represent the field variation over each wavelength. Similar techniques have been used effectively in fluid dynamics problems where highly accurate solutions are desired and conventional low-order polynomial representations fail miserably due to the excessive computational costs (e.g., Maday and Ronquist 1990; Maday and Patera 1989). No work has appeared in the hyperthermia context in this area to date.

However, it would seem urgent that investigations begin, given that ultrasound is gaining in popularity for use in treating a variety of tumor sites and heterogeneous tissue effects can no longer be avoided as this modality continues to gain momentum.

18.3.2 Applicator Modeling

18.3.2.1 Electromagnetic

Significant efforts have been made to model hyperthermia applicators. For the most part, the motivation has been to characterize applicator behavior in idealized homogeneous, or perhaps layered models of tissues. The techniques utilized to make these kinds of calculations are typically different than the finite difference, finite element, and integral equation methods employed in anatomical modeling. They can be viewed as analytical or quasi-analytical approaches and a variety of possibilities exist.

One common approach is to view the field away from the applicator as a superposition of the field due to point or line sources, the composite of which approximates the applicator itself. By integrating over the collection of elemental sources, each with a different weighting depending on the location within the applicator, the field distribution can be obtained (HAND et al. 1986). Usually the strength of the elemental sources is dictated by an assumed current and/or charge density distribution or through an equivalent field representation (JORDAN and BALMAIN 1968). In these situations the integrations that need to be performed are done so numerically, but the integrand itself is completely specified; hence, the integral equation that results is different than those arising in classical integral equation methods, where the integrand is also unknown.

Other techniques include the use of Fourier transforms (GUY 1971) and Gaussian beams (LUMORI et al. 1990a,b) to represent fields at depths across planar interfaces in terms of known aperture distributions. While these types of methods remain popular there has also been an increased use of numerical methods such as finite difference and finite element techniques to model the details of EM sources as they radiate into simple homogeneous and layered phantoms (e.g., SAITHIASEELAN et al. 1992; SHAW et al. 1992; JAMES and ANDRAASIC 1992; FURSE and ISKANDER 1989; ZHU and GANDHI 1988). Figure 18.7 shows a sample calculation of the SAR distribution produced by a two-antenna array where the antenna on the left has been designed to produce a directional heating pattern. The application being investigated is invasive heating of the prostate (YEH 1992) and the finite element method has been used to model the character of various array configurations such as the one shown in this figure. Calculations of this type have often been used to make comparisons with experimental data in order to validate various numerical models (e.g., LAU et al. 1986; RINE et al. 1990; SULLIVAN et al. 1992), but some work has appeared where heterogeneous body models have been part of the simulations (e.g., CHEN and GANDHI 1992). This has been a positive step for power deposition modeling and has brought applicator and anatomical modeling approaches closer together. Further work along this dimension is warranted and the merging of anatomical and applicator models should become a thrust area for future power deposition modeling efforts.

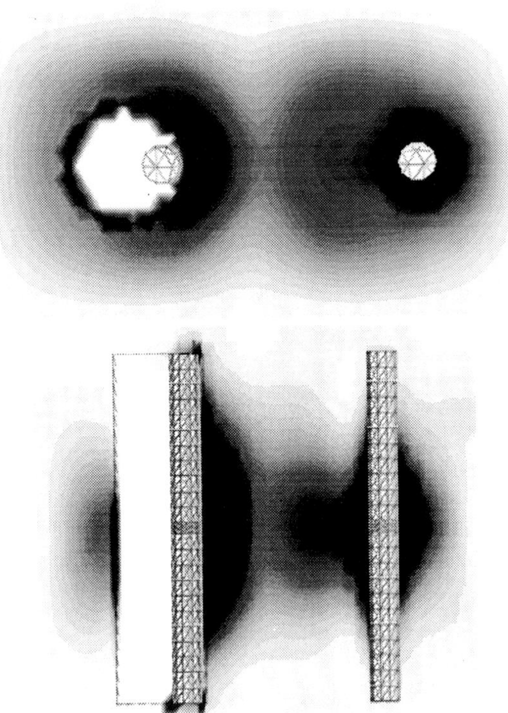

Fig. 18.7. Cross-sectional (*top*) and longitudinal (*bottom*) SAR distributions computed for a two-antenna array where one antenna (*on the left*) has been designed to produce directional power deposition

18.3.2.2 Ultrasonic

Applicator modeling has dominated the US simulations that have appeared. As indicated earlier, geometric modeling for ultrasound has been nonexistent to date (e.g., OCHELTREE and FRIZZELL 1989). The major assumption has been that ultrasound propagation is essentially unperturbed by variations in soft tissue and except for extreme cases of bone and air, computation of ultrasound fields in homogeneous medium is sufficient for accurate simulations. As a result, the primary techniques that have been utilized are analogous to those used in EM simulations (HUNT 1990). The most popular results in an integral equation over the ultrasound source where the field away from the source is described as an integral of known quantities over the source surface (HUNT 1990). Figure 18.8 conceptually illustrates this approach. These calculations, while straightforward, can nonetheless be lengthy because of the rapid spatial variation of the field to be computed, and efforts to speed up the computations have been reported (e.g., MADSEN et al. 1981; SWINDELL et al. 1982; HARTOV et al. 1990). As a result, many closely spaced samples of the field must be computed in order to capture the true distribution. For the most part, calculations of this type have appeared in homogeneous tissues, although models incorporating layered medium have also appeared (e.g., FAN and HYNYNEN 1992).

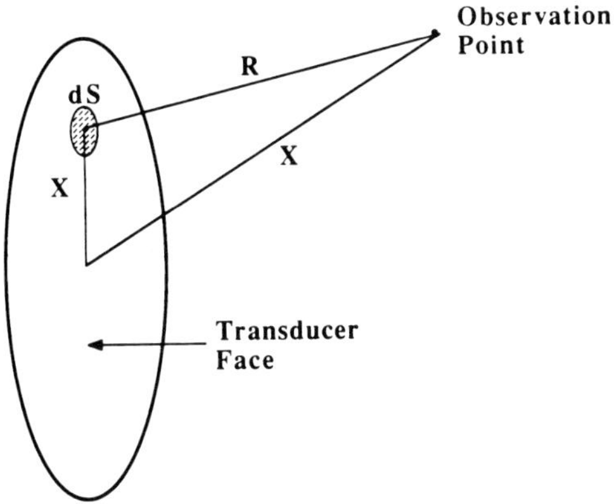

Fig. 18.8. Schematic of US field calculation at a point distant from a transducer face. The process involves integration of known quantities over the applicator. (From PAULSEN et al. 1990)

18.4 Current Status

This section discusses the current capabilities in power deposition modeling with particular attention to recent advances in numerical computation. The emphasis is on patient modeling techniques rather than device-specific applicator models since the patient models have realized a more significant level of fundamental growth over the last several years. Further, a merging of patient and applicator models is essential for continued advancement. Some evidence exists that this is already occurring (e.g., TAYLOR and LAU 1992; PIKET-MAY et al. 1992). If applicator models are to be extended beyond the analysis of homogeneous or ideally layered tissues [they currently serve this purpose well and important work continues to emerge that will be useful in advancing the design and use of present and future hyperthermia delivery systems (e.g., ZHANG et al. 1993)], ability to account for geometrically irregular tissue heterogeneities is necessary. Hence, numerical methods such as finite differences, finite elements, and integral equations will be required and advances will hinge on embedding models of the applicators within these techniques. As a result, clear understanding of current capabilities and certain future trends can be extracted from a discussion of the state of the art of these methods as applied to hyperthermia power deposition modeling.

18.4.1 Finite Difference Methods

While traditional finite difference approaches have been used in SAR calculations (e.g., SOWINSKI and VAN DEN BERG 1990, 1992), it is the finite difference time domain (FDTD) method (TAFLOVE and UMASHANKAR 1990) that has made major inroads in 3D heterogeneous models of power deposition. As indicated earlier, geometric modeling of ultrasound fields over tissue regions of interest has rarely been attempted to date with any of the numerical techniques described here, primarily due to the very small wavelengths of ultrasound in tissue. This results in problem domains that are tens to hundreds of wavelengths in size which are beyond the available computer resources when these techniques are used. Thus, finite difference power deposition modeling has concentrated on EM field simulation.

The FDTD method is an explicit time-stepping approach where the primitive Maxwell curl equations relating the magnetic and electric fields are solved alternately in time and space. The basic algorithm has been known for some time (YEE 1966) and it has continued to evolve since its inception. The most significant recent advances with respect to the hyperthermia power deposition problem include the emergence of the FD^{2}TD algorithm (SULLIVAN 1992) and the modeling of the details of specific hyperthermia applicators (PIKET-MAY et al. 1992; SAITHIASEELAN et al. 1992). The FD^{2}TD approach is to excite the body with a time-limited signal which contains a spectrum of frequencies within the zone of operating interest. By Fourier transforming the time history at each node, the frequency response of the body can be obtained. Hence, in a single execution of the algorithm, the solution for a band of frequencies can be extracted. This approach is very useful when simulating devices where operating frequency is a variable which can dramatically change the performance of the system (SULLIVAN 1992). The method has been used successfully in this mode and has made patient-specific pretreatment planning a practical reality (BEN-YOSEF et al. 1992). In fact, some of the most impressive patient-specific results have recently been reported using FDTD. Investigators have been able to correlate hot spots occurring during treatment with predicted hot spots with FDTD models (BEN-YOSEF et al. 1992; TAYLOR and LAU 1992). This is perhaps the first real evidence that SAR modeling alone can be a useful tool in delivering more effective and pain-free hyperthermia. Figure 18.9 highlights a representative result where FDTD calculations have been performed on a specific patient anatomy. The computed power deposition pattern shows high SAR levels in the left gluteal muscle and has been correlated with posthyperthermia treatment CT scans which revealed a low-density area in this region (BEN-YOSEF et al. 1992).

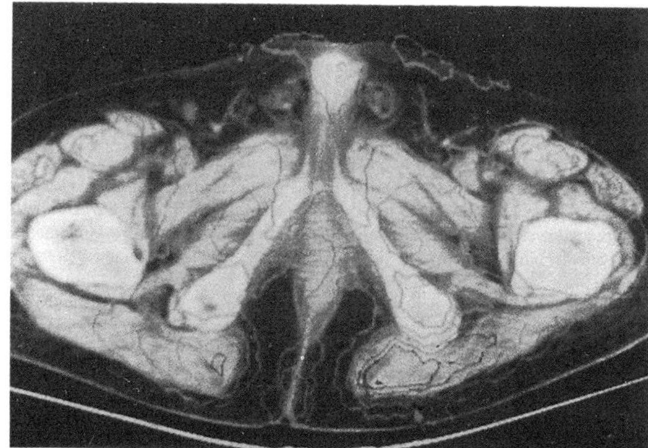

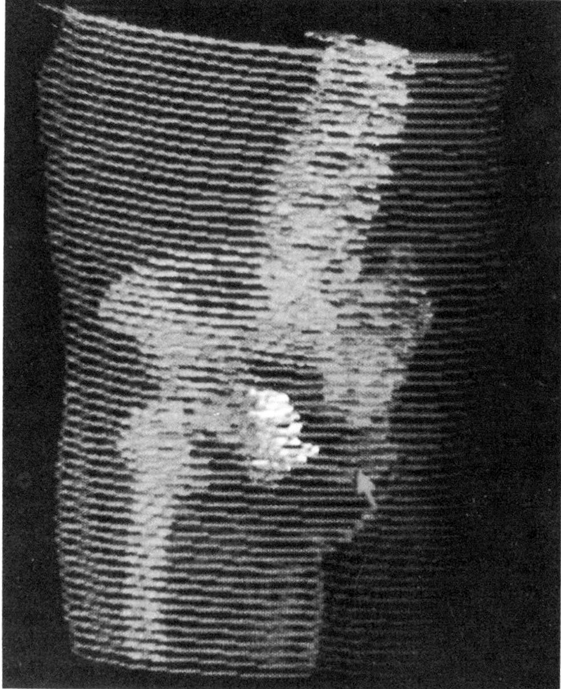

Fig. 18.9. Computed SAR distribution in a patient-specific model of prostate heating by an external annular array device. Correlations with post-treatment CT scans reveal tissue damage in the left gluteal muscle, where the calculations show a localized SAR peak. (From BEN-YOSEF et al. 1992)

The other area where recent FDTD use is important is in applicator models. Successful renderings of both noninvasive and implantable EM radiators have been reported (FURSE and ISKANDER 1989; ZHU and GANDHI 1988; PIKET-MAY et al. 1992; SAITHESEELAN et al. 1992). If it continues to be possible to incorporate the details of the hyperthermia device within the overall scheme of the FDTD algorithm, the merging of geometry and applicator models will begin to advance at an accelerated rate. Early results have focused on relatively simple radiators and verifications have been performed by comparing computed results with measurements in homogeneous phantoms, but some heterogeneous phantom results have also appeared (e.g., SULLIVAN et al. 1992; JIA et al. 1993). How effectively these models can be incorporated into heterogeneous tissue models remains to be seen. Part of the problem lies in the fact that if the tissue geometry is well resolved, the mesh spacing becomes small ($\approx$ 1 cm) and the cost associated with meshing the 3D volume outside the body which includes the external radiators becomes expensive computationally.

The future of FDTD modeling of power deposition appears to be in applicator model realization and general use of the existing method as a treatment planning and analysis tool. Advances in the algorithm itself do not appear to be overly likely in the near term. Improvements could center on algorithms for nonuniform (e.g., GAO and GANDHI 1992) and conformal meshes (e.g., JURGENS et al. 1992) and more rigorous treatment of interface and boundary conditions. While some work has appeared in these areas in other contexts, implementation typically hinders the simplicity of the basic FDTD structure and hence its practical utility in power deposition modeling.

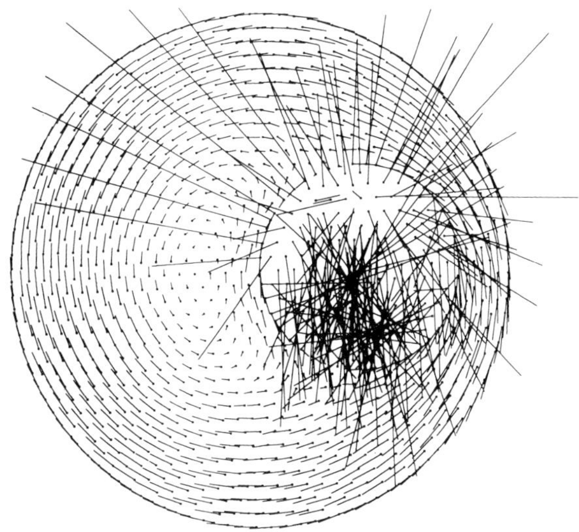

Fig. 18.10. An example of an FEM vector field calculation which is severely contaminated with parasitic solution components. For details of other similar calculations, see PAULSEN and LYNCH (1991)

18.4.2 Finite Element Methods

SAR calculations in 3D heterogeneous tissue models using finite element techniques have generally lagged the progress seen with FDTD until very recently. Although some 2D work has appeared (KAGAWA et al. 1986), 3D anatomically based models of ultrasound fields using the finite element method (FEM) have not been reported to date for the same reasons cited above for finite differences; hence, the advances that have been achieved have occurred in electromagnetic simulations of power deposition. The difficulties that have been encountered with the FEM have stemmed from three sources: (a) the occurrence of spurious solutions which corrupt the numerical computations, (b) poor convergence performance of iterative solvers for the large system of equations generated by the FEM, and (c) mesh generation problems associated with the creation of unstructured grids which conform to anatomical boundaries of the body.

The spurious solution problem is one which has perplexed FEM users for many years. It occurs in vector problems where multiple components of the field exist at each computational point. Scalar calculations such as those that appeared in 2D finite element simulations of power deposition (e.g., PAULSEN et al. 1984b, 1985) were unaffected. As a result the problem first appeared in the hyperthermia context when 2D algorithms were being extended to 3D. Spurious solutions are nonphysical solutions which satisfy the discretized form of the Maxwell equations, but which have no basis in physical reality, that is, the continuum form of these equations. Figure 18.10 shows a sample FEM calculation which is plagued by the presence of a parasitic solution which dominates the computed result as evidenced by the nonphysical character of the field displayed. After several years of analysis a new discrete form referred to as a Helmholtz form was proposed for eliminating spurious solutions with the FEM (PAULSEN and LYNCH 1991; LYNCH and PAULSEN 1991). For comparison the physically correct solution computed with this parasite-free approach for the case shown in Fig. 18.10 is provided in Fig. 18.11. This approach, if utilized with proper boundary conditions, was shown to be derivable from first principles and to possess important numerical properties for the elimination of spurious solutions (BOYSE et al. 1992; LYNCH et al. 1993). It also contained a computational economy that made its realization in 3D all the more possible (PAULSEN et al. 1992a; PAULSEN and LYNCH 1991). The Helmholtz form has been studied in both 2D and 3D and appears to offer a simple but robust method of eliminating spurious solutions in FEM EM calculations. Other approaches are also possible, but they have not been explored in the hyperthermia context (e.g., CENDES 1991).

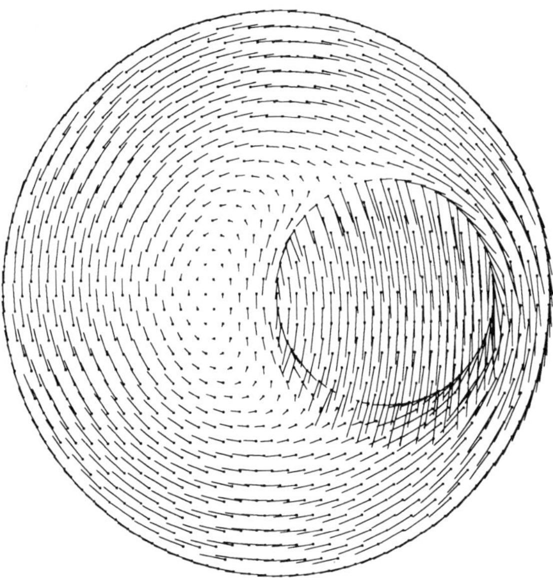

Fig. 18.11. The parasite-free (physically correct) solution for the vector field shown in Fig. 18.11

Because the FEM leads to very sparse sets of algebraic relations, iterative solvers where only the nonzero coefficients are stored become natural methods of choice for solving these relations. Unfortunately, the FEM formulation in the frequency domain leads to indefinite system matrices whose iterative solution is difficult (PAULSEN et al. 1992b). Early experience with various preconditioned forms of the conjugate gradient method revealed a major slowdown in convergence rates to the point of stalling when problem sizes reached more than 200K degrees of freedom. More recently these difficulties have been overcome with a newer algorithm with better performance on complex symmetric indefinite system matrices (JIA 1993). Recovering symmetry in the system matrix when interface relations were applied has been achieved through rotation of appropriate rows and columns into a local normal/tangential coordinate system (BOYSE et al. 1992; PAULSEN et al. 1993). Symmetric preconditioning and preconditioning based on retention of factored matrix coefficient size (rather than sparsity pattern) have been realized (JIA 1993). These advances have made iterative solution of the Helmholtz form generated by the FEM much more reliable. Present model sizes in excess of 250K degrees of freedom are showing no signs of iterative solution breakdown (JIA 1993).

Another possible avenue for defeating slowdown in iterative solver performance should it again become a factor as problem size grows by the next order of magnitude, is to use implicit time stepping. An explicit time-stepping scheme with similar efficiencies to FDTD has been realized (LYNCH and PAULSEN 1990); however, on unstructured meshes of the type of interest in power deposition modeling, stability limitations restrict the practical utility of such approaches. Implicit time integration, on the other hand, can be unconditionally stable; thus time step sizes only need be sufficiently small to resolve the period of the harmonic excitation. A matrix solution is required at each time step in order to advance the field evolution; however, this matrix is definite and well suited to fast, reliable iterative solution. Experience with implicit time integration is only now emerging, but conceptually would appear to offer important advantages (YAN 1993).

Unstructured, conforming mesh generation has been and remains the most difficult problem facing 3D heterogeneous modeling of the body with the FEM. Automatic 3D construction of meshes has made progress in recent years (e.g., JOHNSON and SULLIVAN 1993; SEEBASS et al. 1992; DAS et al. 1994) and has reached the level where models comparable in resolution and detail to those of FDTD are now possible. The mesh shown in Fig. 18.12 is an FEM rendering of the data displayed earlier in Fig. 18.4 which has been generated using some of the latest software advances. Field and SAR results have been computed based on this type of model and Fig. 18.13 illustrates a representative calculation of SAR produced by an external annular array type device in orthogonal planes through the body. Significant superficial heating, especially in the inner thighs, is evident in the computed distribution. Two advantages with computing on models such as Fig. 18.12 are readily apparent. First, the mesh conforms to the boundaries identifiable at the level of CT or MRI imaging, which allows the impact of the EM jump conditions to be felt on an accurate rendering of the body geometry. The importance of tissue interfaces in terms of creating localized peaks and valleys in SAR is well known and modeling thereof is critical. The second advantage of unstructured meshing is the ability to have variable spacing between nodes in the grid. In large-scale 3D rendering of anatomy, this allows high resolution in the treatment field with diminishing discretization elsewhere. For

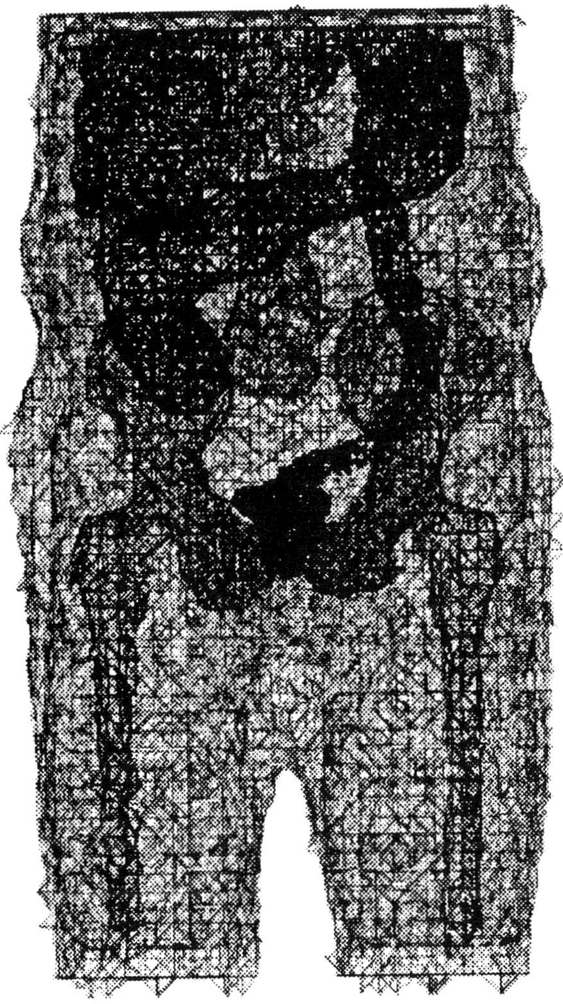

Fig. 18.12. Conforming and unstructured finite element mesh automatically generated from the patient data displayed in Fig. 18.4

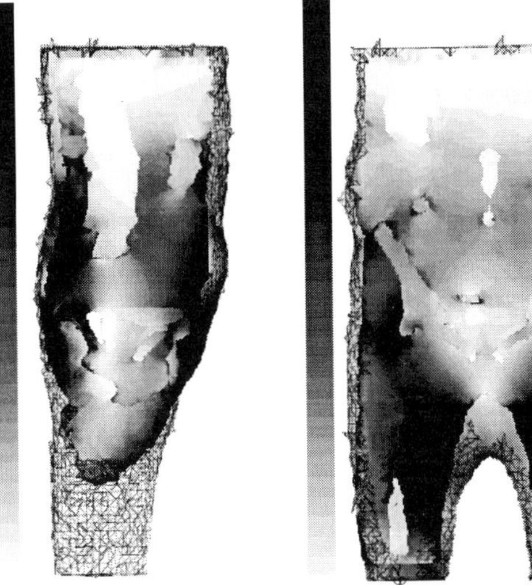

Fig. 18.13. SAR distributions computed on orthogonal planes through the body model displayed in Fig. 18.12. The impact of tissue interfaces on local peaks and valleys of SAR are readily apparent

example, it is not unusual for node spacings to vary by more than a factor of 10 inside versus outside the body, where the EM wavelengths are dramatically different. For the most part, deployment of nodes inside the body in the region of interest in higher density than elsewhere is a significant advantage. However, in terms of source modeling there is the detriment that the applicator details become submesh scale if the nodes outside the body get too far apart.

In fact, creating grid generation capabilities with smooth transitions between high and low node density is one of the major problems still facing mesh generation of anatomical geometries (PAULSEN et al. 1993). Without improvements in the future, merging of applicator and body discretizations will continue to be difficult and will slow progress. A popular refinement strategy is to cut the spacing between nodes in half and to do this selectively and repeatedly in order to attain differences in mesh scales throughout the region. Experience suggests that a smoother transition spacing of nodes is desired. Further, ability to mesh multiply-connected regions of three or more at a single point is an area where mesh generation needs improvement.

Future work on FEM-based models of power deposition can be expected to focus on applications of existing capability, merging of geometry and applicator models, model verification, and mesh generation. Because FEM modeling in 3D of size and resolution comparable to FDTD is only now available, steady application of this technology is expected over the next few years (e.g., CLEGG et al. 1994a; PAULSEN et al. 1993). Improved efforts in embedding applicator models and in more automatic and robust mesh generation must also be forthcoming if the FEM work is to keep pace with FDTD modeling. Model verification is needed as well. Some initial work has appeared (CLEGG et al. 1994b; JIA et al. 1994), but further experience is warranted. This is generally true in the FDTD arena, although effort towards model verification has been emphasized more consistently among FDTD investigators as a result of the technique having been successful in large-scale 3D computations for a longer period of time than the FEM.

18.4.3 Integral Equation Methods

In 3D computations for heterogeneous anatomies, integral equation methods have generally lagged both FDTD and FEM. Interestingly, integral equations were favorites in 2D (e.g., ISKANDER et al. 1982; VAN DEN BERG et al. 1983), but their severe computational costs have restricted their use in 3D. The primary difficulty is that the algebraic equations that result from discretization of the continuum are very dense relative to FDTD and FEM. Specifically, the strategy of integral equations is to replace the heterogeneous body by a collection of volume scatterers in free space that produce the identical field as the body. While conceptually appealing, the approach necessarily requires that the interactions between each and every scatterer be accounted for. In effect, every node in the mesh interacts with (receives a contribution from) every other node, leading to a full matrix equation (i.e., every entry in the matrix is nonzero) that needs to be solved. Under these conditions, computer memory requirements scale as the square and run time as the cube of the number of unknown field components to be computed. As a result, classical integral equation approaches have not been able to achieve the high-resolution models computed with FDTD and FEM.

Recent advances, however, have allowed this to happen (e.g., ZWAMBORN et al. 1992). In particular, the convolutional form of the resulting integral equation has allowed the use of the fast Fourier transform (FFT) to achieve matrix multiplications as part of an overall iterative solution method that scales linearly in the number of unknowns. Memory also scales in this linear way, making the overall technique very competitive in 3D models. Efficient, three-dimensional, heterogeneous calculations of SAR have been obtained on the JAAP phantom, which is a muscle–fat–air segmentation of a full-body MRI scan (ZWAMBORN et al. 1992). This model contained more than 100K degrees of freedom and had cross-sectional resolution of approximately 1.5 cm and longitudinal resolution of 3 cm. Memory consumption was modest, at 25 Mbytes. These results are comparable to the FDTD and FEM models that have also appeared recently. This FFT approach does require that the computational domain be realized on a uniform lattice; otherwise, the convolutional nature of the integral expressions is lost and so is its computational economy. The necessity of a uniform mesh places similar restrictions to the FDTD method in terms of the type of 3D heterogeneous models that can be constructed. Nonetheless, it makes a previously intractable mathematical formulation computable in a workstation environment. A sample calculation is shown in Fig. 18.14.

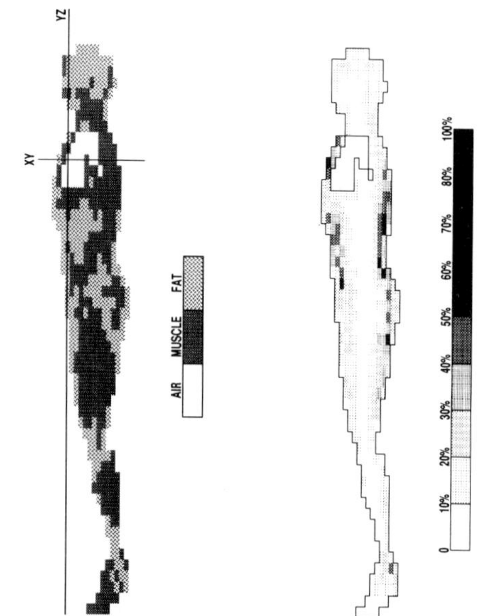

Fig. 18.14. Sagittal cut through the Jaap phantom (*left*) and absorbed power distribution (*right*) from an incident plane wave propagating from the head to the feet. (From ZWAMBORN et al. 1992)

In addition to the ability to make efficient SAR calculations using integral equations, details concerning the enforcement of interface conditions at boundaries of dielectric contrast have received attention (e.g., WUST et al. 1993). This has been important work and has highlighted some of the discrepancies that can occur between methods which enforce interface conditions strongly and those which only do so in some asymptotic way. Specifically, comparisons between finite volume integration methods (similar to FDTD) and integral equation results indicate that the finite volume approach tends to smooth out the effect of the EM jump conditions across media interfaces. Figure 18.15 shows one comparison of the different effects when the field polarization is parallel versus perpendicular to a material interface. The sharp jump in the normal component of

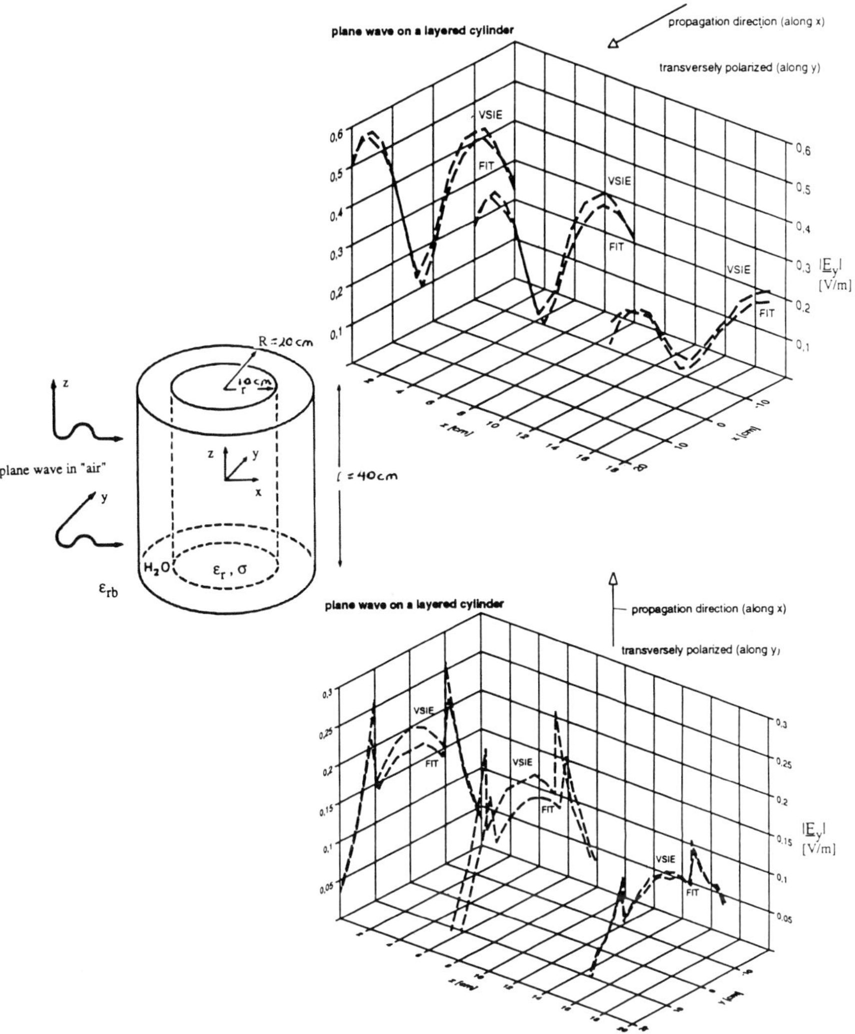

Fig. 18.15. Field computations by an improved volume scattering integral equation approach and a finite integration theory method for a layered cylinder illuminated by an incident plane wave. Tangential component agreement between the two methods is generally better than normal component agreement, where the EM jump conditions dominate. The volume scattering method takes special care to satisfy explicitly the EM jump conditions. (From WUST et al. 1993)

the solution at this interface which is evident in the integral equation calculation has been diminished in the finite volume computation. Unfortunately, implementation of the interface conditions within this integral equation framework has not allowed the efficient convolutional integral equation approach to be incorporated. It has utilized unstructured meshing, so with the interface condition satisfaction, it rivals the FEM in this regard; however, computational overhead has forced mesh sizes to remain relatively small (approximately 10% of those achievable with the FEM).

The integral equation approach has the appeal that external radiators can be incorporated relatively simply and far-field conditions are satisfied a priori. However, a move away from the typical incident and scattered field formulation is necessary when the body is in close proximity to the source. Future efforts are needed along this dimension. Further, if the attention to interface detail found in some integral equation approaches can be implemented in the fast efficient versions of other integral equation methodologies with the restrictions of structured meshing also eliminated, the integral equation technique would become difficult to outperform. Advances in these areas will be needed if integral equation technologies are to remain competitive with FDTD and FEM.

18.5 Future Trends

Based on the discussions of the previous sections, several observations and themes can be identified which provide clues to the future directions for SAR modeling. The foremost observation is very clear: 3D SAR models of anatomically complex tissue geometries are possible with several computational techniques, which has only been true for the last few years. Thus, while a certain amount of knowledge has already been gained from 3D SAR simulation, a great deal more information has yet to be extracted. Even without any additional enhancements to present modeling capabilities, the utilization of current modeling technology should be very fruitful over the coming years. In effect, the application of the software realized from the intensive 3D model development phase which has been ongoing over the last 5 years is now ready to be utilized at full force and should pay handsomely in terms of improved understanding of power deposition in tissue.

A second observation that seems clear is that patient modeling and applicator modeling, while historically distinct, are beginning to merge. Each of these modeling emphases will continue as separate entities and will continue to contribute important findings within their respective domains. However, the clinical setting under which hyperthermia is delivered consists of real devices delivering power into real patients with complex anatomies. Thus, simulations which treat both the realism of the device and the patient simultaneously are unavoidable. In many respects it seems perfectly straightforward how to implement detailed source descriptions within the numerical methods addressed in this chapter, and some work is emerging on this front. On the other hand, the level of source detail that is needed, the treatment of the feedpoint, and what can be legitimately guaranteed about the "driving" of a given device are all unknowns that must be considered; hence, it seems likely that a significant amount of effort will be needed before models with predictive capability are realized.

A third observation is that US power deposition models involving heterogeneous and geometrically complex domains are needed. A reasonable starting point from a mathematical perspective already exists; however, new approaches to solving this mathematical framework on such geometries is required. Conventional approaches suffer severe computational efficiency limitations due to the very large (in terms of wavelength) domain over which the ultrasound propagation takes place. Some of the techniques making advances in the fluid dynamics arenas appear to offer possible answers to these computational difficulties. The evolution of patient-based US power deposition models seems to be only getting more pressing, given that this modality is being explored for its potential in an increasing number of anatomical sites.

With the exception of patient-based US power deposition where computational efficiency is a major concern, the emerging theme for 3D SAR modeling will be one of computational accuracy. Over the last 5 years 3D modeling choices have largely been governed by computational efficiency considerations, with computational accuracy being secondary. Computer resources have continued to escalate and many of the computational efficiency issues have been either resolved or eliminated as a result. Hence, for 3D modeling computational efficiency is no longer the driving force that it once was. Naturally, attention is now shifting to computational accuracy.

Computational accuracy takes two forms and both will become major foci for future SAR modeling efforts. The first is the degree to which specific model implementations alter the clinical implications of the computed results. Several examples of this form of computational accuracy have been cited in earlier sections of the chapter. Two important ones are (a) the degree to which conforming meshes and strong enforcement of interface relations are essential for predicting SAR extremes and (b) the degree to which incomplete anatomical data resulting in artificial domain termination influence locally computed SAR distributions. A significant amount of insight can be expected in these areas as the use of 3D SAR models becomes more widespread. In fact, it is very possible that other unanticipated issues will arise as these newly developed models of 3D SAR get exercised under a variety of circumstances which will undoubtedly occur in the coming years.

The second form of computational accuracy

that will receive considerably more attention in the future will be one of model verification or validation against measured results. Some important work has certainly appeared in this respect, but much more is needed. A definitive approach to model validation in this context is not as obvious as it may first appear. A large amount of the motivation for developing computational models is the fact that the quantities to be computed are extremely difficult to measure in the environment under which it is desired that they be known. Two strategies seem clear, but their relative advantages are not known at the present time, nor is it apparent whether other alternatives may exist.

One appealing strategy is to develop experimental protocols that allow the quantities of interest to be measured under complex and realistic circumstances. These experiments would likely commence in anatomically based phantoms and proceed towards in vivo animal models where extensive measurements could be made. The primary difficulty with this approach is the repeatability of the experiment and the integrity of the measured values. Many confounding factors can be present in such experiments and sorting out the causes of discrepancies between measured and computed results may be impossible, especially if reliable reproducibility of measured data is problematic. A potential outcome from this type of experimental approach could well be that qualitative or semiquantitative agreement is attainable, but quantitative confirmation is less convincing. Results of this nature would have to be deemed more or less as failures given that semiquantitative levels of agreement have already been established in fairly complex phantoms.

A second general strategy for model validations is to design experiments which are relatively simple, but are aimed at testing a certain aspect of the computational model where integrity of the numerical implementation is of concern. An example of this model validation approach would be an evaluation of interface conditions and their computational accuracy. A two-region geometry could be constructed where the field polarization with respect to the interface is controllable and repeatable. Measurements could be made and compared with calculations. Sources of discrepancies would likely be resolvable given the reproducibility of the measurements as a result of the relatively simple experimental setup. While validations of this type would always retain an element of uncertainty since clinical conditions would always be more complex, they are potentially more revealing of model strengths and weaknesses given their quantitative nature. If carefully designed, these types of controlled experimental studies are likely to be able to significantly "stress" various aspects of presently available SAR models and to provide sufficient evidence to convincingly establish the ranges of their validity. The realization of such experiments will require that some new energy be devoted to enhancing the experimental techniques that are presently in widespread use in hyperthermia research.

18.6 Summary

The main points discussed can be summarized as the following:

- Power deposition models have been rapidly evolving since the early 1980s and have reached the point where realistic three dimensional computations are now possible.
- To date, power deposition models have largely fallen into two categories: (1) those which address the anatomical heterogeneity and geometrical complexity of the body and (2) those which accommodate a detailed description of the hyperthermia applicator.
- The merging of patient and applicator modeling techniques is needed in the future.
- Finite difference, finite element and integral equation methodologies are all showing some promise in power deposition modeling.
- Patient based 3D electromagnetic modeling is beginning to be used in a prospective treatment planning mode.
- Ultrasonic power deposition models involving heterogeneous and geometrically complex domains are needed.
- A major thrust in evaluating the computational accuracy of patient modeling techniques can be expected to occur over the next few years.
- Computational accuracy assessments should include evaluations of data input assumptions and comparisons with measured results obtained during repeatable experimental procedures.
- Applicator modeling efforts should be directed more heavily towards influencing the design and prototyping stages of applicator development.

References

Ben-Yosef R, Sullivan DM, Kapp DS (1992) Peripheral neuropathy and myonecrosis following hyperthermia and radiation therapy for recurrent prostatic cancer: correlation of damage with predicted SAR pattern. Int J Hyperthermia 8: 173–186

Boyse WE, Lynch DR, Paulsen KD, Minerbo GN (1992) Nodal-based finite element modeling of Maxwell's equations in three dimensions. IEEE Trans Antennas Propagat 40: 642–651

Brezovich IA, Meredith RF, Henderson RA, Brawner WR, Wepplemann B, Salter MM (1989) Hyperthermia with water-perfused catheters. In: Sugahara T, Sacto M (eds) Hyperthermic oncology 1988, vol 1. Taylor and Franscis, London, pp 809–810

Cain CA, Umemura SA (1986) Concentric ring and sector vortex phased array applicators for ultrasound hyperthermia therapy. IEEE Trans Microwave Theory Tech 34: 542–551

Cangellaris AC, Wright DB (1992) Analysis of the numerical error caused by the stair-stepped approximation of a conducting boundary in FDTD simulations of electromagnetic phenomena. IEEE Trans Antennas Propagat 39: 1518–1525

Cangellaris AC, Lee R (1992) On the accuracy of numerical wave simulations based on finite methods. J, Electromage Waves Appl 6: 1635–1653

Cendes ZJ (1991) Vector finite elements for electromagnetic field computation. IEEE Trans Magn 27: 3958–3966

Chan AK, Sigelmann RA, Guy AW (1974) Calculations of therapeutic heat generated by ultrasound in fat-muscle-bone layers. IEEE Trans Biomed Eng 21: 280–284

Chen JY, Gandhi OP (1992) Numerical simulation of annular phased arrays of dipoles for hyperthermia of deep-seated tumors. IEEE Trans Biomed Eng 39: 209–216

Clegg ST, Murphy K, Joines WT, Rine G, Samulski TV (1994a) Finite element computation of electromagnetic fields. IEEE Trans Microwave Theory Tech 42: 1984–1991

Clegg ST, Das SK, Zhang Y, McFall Y, Fullar E, Samulski TV (1994b) Verification of a hyperthermic model using MR Thermometry. Int J Hyperthermia (in press)

Curran WJ, Goodman RL (1992) Hyperthermia 1991: a critical review. In: Dewey WC, et al. (eds) Radiation Research a Twentieth-Century Perspective, vol 2: 883–888

Das SK, Clegg ST, Samulski TV (1994) Simulation of electromagnetically induced hyperthermia: a finite element gridding method. Int J Hyperthermia (in press)

Deford JA, Babbs CF, Patel UH, Bleyer MW, Marchosky JA, Moran CY (1991) Effective estimation and computer control of minimum tumor temperature during conductive interstitial hyperthermia. Int J Hyperthermia 7: 441–453

Dewhirst MW, Winget JM, Edelstein-Keshet L et al. (1987) Clinical application of thermal isoeffect dose. Int J Hyperthermia 3: 307–318

Ebbini ES, Cain CA (1991) A spherical-section ultrasound phased array applicator for deep localized hyperthermia. IEEE Trans Biomed Eng 38: 634–643

Emani B, Myerson RJ, Scott C, Gibbs F, Lee C, Perez CA (1991) Phase I/II Study, Combination of radiotherapy and hyperthermia in patients with deep-seated malignant tumors: report of a pilot study by the RTOG. Int J Radiat Oncol Biol Phys 20: 73–79

Fan X, Hynynen K (1992) The effect of wave reflection and refraction at soft tissue interfaces during ultrasound hyperthermia treatments. J Acoust Soc Am 91: 1727–1736

Feldmann HJ, Molls M, Adler S, Meyer-Schwickerath Sack H (1991) Hyperthermia in eccentrically located pelvic tumors: excessive heating of perineal fat and normal tissue temperatures. Int J Radiat Oncol Biol Phys 20: 1017–1022

Fessenden P, Lee E, Anderson TL, Strohbehn JW, Meyer JL, Samulski T, Marmor J (1984) Experience with a multitransducer ultrasound system for localized hyperthermia of deep tissues. IEEE Trans Biomed Eng 31: 126–135

Furse CM, Iskander MF (1989) Three-dimensional electromagnetic power deposition in the tumors using interstitial antenna arrays. IEEE Trans Biomed Eng 36: 977–986

Cao B, Gandhi OP (1992) An expanding grid algorithm for the finite difference time-domain method. IEEE Trans Electromagn Compat 34: 277–282

George PL (1991) Automatic mesh generation. John Wiley, New York

Gibbs FA Jr, Sapozink MD, Gates KS, Stewart JR (1984) Regional hyperthermia with an annular phased array in experimental treatment of cancer: report of work in progress with a technical emphasis. IEEE Trans Biomed Eng 31: 115–119

Gopal MK, Hand JW, Lumori MLD, Alkhairi S, Paulsen KD, Cetas TC (1992) Current sheet applicator arrays for superficial hyperthermia of chest wall lesions. Int J Hyperthermia 8: 227–240

Guy AW (1971) Electromagnetic fields and relative heating patterns due to a rectangular aperture source in direct contact with bilayered biological tissue. IEEE Trans Microwave Theory Tech 19: 214–223

Hagmann MJ (1987) Difficulty in using two-dimensional models for calculating the energy deposition in tissues during hyperthermia. Int J Hyperthermia 3: 475–476

Hagmann MJ, Levin RL (1986) Aberrant heating: a problem in regional hyperthermia. IEEE Trans Biomed Eng 33: 405–411

Hagmann MJ, Gandhi OP, Durney CH (1979) Numerical calculations of electromagnetic energy deposition for a realistic model of man. IEEE Trans Microwave Theory Tech 27: 804–809

Halac S, Roemer RB, Oleson JR, Cetas TC (1983) Magnetic induction heating of tissue: numerical evaluation of tumor temperature distributions. Int J Radiat Oncol Biol Phys 9: 881–891

Hand JW, Cheetham JL, Hind AJ (1986) Absorbed power distributions from coherent microwave arrays for localized hyperthermia. IEEE Trans Microwave Theory Tech 34: 484–489

Hartov A, Strohbehn JW, Colacchio TA (1990) A new efficient method to compute ultrasound fields on a personal computer. Proceedings of the 12th Annual International Conference of the IEEE Engineering in Medicine and Biology Society. IEEE Press, New York NY, vol 1, pp 356–358

Hill SC, Christensen DA, Durney CH (1983a) Power deposition patterns in magnetically-induced hyperthermia: a two-dimensional low-frequency numerical analysis. Int J Radiat Oncol Biol Phys 9: 893–904

Hill SC, Durney CH, Christensen DA (1983b) Numerical calculations of low-frequency TE fields in arbitrarily shaped inhomogeneous lossy dielectric cylinders. Radio Science 18: 328–336

Hunt JW (1990) Principles of ultrasound use for generating localized hyperthermia. In: Field SB, Hand JW (eds) An introduction to the practical aspects of clinical hyperthermia. Taylor and Francis, London, pp 371–422

Hynynen K (1990) Biophysics and technology of ultrasound hyperthermia. In: Gautherie M (ed) Methods of external hyperthermic heating. Springer, Berlin Heidelberg New York, pp 61–115

Hynynen K, Roemer RB, Anhalt D, Johnson C, Xu ZX, Swindell W, Cetas TC (1987) A scanned focused multiple transducer ultrasonic system for localized hyperthermia treatments. Int J Hyperthermia 3: 21–25

Iskander MF (1982) Physical aspects and methods of hyperthermia production by RF currents and microwaves. In: Nussbaum GH (ed) Physical aspects of hyperthermia. American Institute of Physics, New York, pp 151–191

Iskander MF, Turner PF, JB DuBow JB, Kao J (1982) Two-dimensional technique to calculate the EM power deposition pattern in the human body. J Microw Power 17: 175–185

James BJ, Sullivan DM (1992) Creation of three-dimensional patient models for hyperthermia treatment planning. IEEE Trans Biomed Eng 39: 238–242

James JR, Andrasic G (1992) Analysis and computation of leaky wave hyperthermia applicator. In: Fleming AHJ, Joyner KH (eds) ACES Special Issue on Bioelectromagnetic Computation, ACES journal, vol. 7, pp 72–84

Jia X (1993) Three dimensional finite element simulations for regional electromagnetic hyperthermia treatment of cancer. PhD Thesis, Thayer School of Engineering, Dartmouth College, Hanover, NH

Jia X, Paulsen KD, Buechler DN, Gibbs FA Jr, Meaney PM (1994) Finite element simulation of Sigma 60 heating in the Utah phantom: computed and measured data compared. Int J Hyperthermia (in press)

Johnston BP, Sullivan JM Jr (1993) A normal offsetting technique for automatic mesh generation in three dimensions. Int J Numer Meth Eng 36: 1717–1734

Joines WT (1984) Frequency-dependent absorption of electromagnetic energy in biological tissue. IEEE Trans Biomed Eng 31: 17–20

Jordan EC, Balmain KG (1968) Electromagnetic waves and radiating systems, 2nd edn. Prentice Hall, Englewood Cliffs, NJ

Jurgens TG, Taflove A, Umashankar K, Moore TG (1992) Finite difference time-domain modeling of curved surfaces. IEEE Trans Antennas Propagat 40: 357–366

Kagawa Y, Takeuchi K, Yamabuchi T (1986) A simulation of ultrasonic hyperthermia using a finite element model. IEEE Trans Ultrason Ferroelectrics Frequency Control 33: 765–777

King RWP, Trembly BS, Strohbehn JW (1983) The electromagnetic field of an insulated antenna in a conducting or dielectric medium. IEEE Trans Microwave Theory Tech 31: 574–583

Lau RWM, Sheppard RJ (1986) The modeling of biological systems in three dimensions using the time-domain finite-difference method. I. The implementation of the model. Phys Med Biol 31: 1247–1256

Lau RWM, Sheppard RJ, Howard G, Bleehen NM (1986) The modeling of biological systems in three dimensions using the time-domain finite-difference method. II. The application and experimental valuation of the method in hyperthermia applicator design. Phys Med Biol 31: 1257–1266

Livesay DE, Chen KM (1974) Electromagnetic fields induced inside arbitrarily shaped biological bodies. IEEE Trans Biomed Eng 22: 1273–1280

Lumori MLO, Andersen JB, Gopal MK, Cetas TC (1990a) Gaussian beam representation of aperture fields in layered lossy media: simulation and experiment. IEEE Trans Microwave Theory Tech 38: 1623–1630

Lumori MLD, Hand JW, Gopal MK, Cetas TC (1990b) Use of Gaussian beam model in prediction SAR distributions from current sheet applications. Phys Med Bio 35: 387–397

Lynch DR, Paulsen KD (1990) Time domain integration of the Maxwell equations on finite elements. IEEE Trans Antennas Propagat 38: 1933–1942

Lynch DR, Paulsen KD (1991) Origins of vector parasites in numerical Maxwell solutions. IEEE Trans Microwave Theory Tech 39: 383–394

Lynch DR, Paulsen KD, Strohbehn JW (1985) Finite element solution of Maxwell's equations for hyperthermia treatment planning. J Comp Physiol 58: 246–269

Lynch DR, Paulsen KD, Strohbehn JW (1986) Hybrid element method for unbounded electromagnetic problems in hyperthermia. Int J Numer Methods Eng 23: 1915–1937

Lynch DR, Paulsen KD, Boyse WE (1993) Synthesis of vector parasites in finite element Maxwell solutions. IEEE Trans Microwave Theory Tech 141: 1439–1448

Maday Y, Patera AT (1989) Spectral element methods for the incompressible Navier-Stokes quations. In: Noor AK, Oden JT (eds) State-of-the-art surveys on computational mechanics. American Society of Mechanical Enjineers (ASME), NY, pp 71–143

Maday Y, Ronquist EM (1990) Optimal error analysis of spectral methods with emphasis on nonconstant coefficients and deformed geometries. Comp Meth Appl Mech Eng 80: 91–115

Madsen EL, Goodsit MM, Zagzebski JA (1981) Continuous wave generated by focused radiators. J Acoust Soc Am 70: 1508–1517

Matloubieh AY, Roemer RB, Cetas TC (1984) Numerical simulation of magnetic induction heating of tumors with ferromagnetic seed implants. IEEE Trans Biomed Eng 31: 227–234

Mechling JA, Strohbehn JW (1986) A theoretical comparison of the temperature distributions produced by three interstitial hyperthermia systems. Int J Radiat Oncol Biol Phys 12: 2137–2149

Mittra R, Ramahi O (1990) Absorbing boundary conditions. for the direct solution of partial differential equations arising in electromagnetic scattering problems. In: Morgan MA (ed) Finite element and finite difference methods in electromagnetic scattering. Elsevier, London, pp 133–173

Ocheltree K, Frizzell L (1989) Sound field calculations for rectangular sources. IEEE Trans Ultrasonics Ferroelectrics Frequency Control 36: 242–248

Patera AT (1984) A spectral element flow in a channel expansion. J Computat Phys 54: 263–292

Paulsen KD (1990a) Calculation of power deposition patterns in hyperthermia. In: Gautherie M (ed)

Thermal dosimetry and treatment planning. Springer, Berlin Heidelberg New York, pp 57–117
Paulsen KD (1990b) Power deposition models for hyperthermia applicators. In: Field SB, Hand JW (eds) An introduction to the practical aspects of clinical hyperthermia. Taylor and Francis, London, pp 305–343
Paulsen KD, Lynch DR (1991) Elimination of vector parasites in finite element Maxwell solutions. IEEE Trans Microwave Theory Tech 39: 395–404
Paulen KD, Ross MP (1990) Comparison of numerical calculations with phantom experiments and clinical measurements. Int J Hyperthermia 6: 330–350
Paulsen KD, Strohbehn JW, Hill SC, Lynch DR, Kennedy FE (1984a) Theoretical temperature profiles for concentric coil induction heating devices in a two-dimensional axi-asymmetric inhomogeneous patient model. Int J Radiat Oncol Biol Phys 10: 1095–1107
Paulsen KD, Strohbehn JW, Lynch DR (1984b) Theoretical temperature distributions produced by an annular phased array type system in CT-based patient models. Radiat Res 100: 536–552
Paulsen KD, Strohbehn JW, Lynch DR (1985) Comparative theoretical performance of two types of regional hyperthermia systems. Int J Radiat Oncol Biol Phys 11: 1659–1671
Paulsen KD, Strohbehn JW, Lynch DR (1988a) Theoretical electric field distributions produced by three types of regional hyperthermia devices in a three-dimensional homogeneous model of man. IEEE Trans Biomed Eng 35: 36–45
Paulsen KD, Lynch DR, Strohbehn JW (1988b) Three-dimensional finite boundary and hybrid element solutions of the Maxwell equations for lossy dielectric media. IEEE Trans Microwave Theory Tech 36: 682–693
Paulsen KD, Jia X, Lynch DR (1992a) 3D bioelectromagnetic computation on finite elements. In: Fleming AHJ, Joyner KH (eds) ACES Special issue on bioelectromagnetic computations, vol 7, no 2. ACES Journal, pp 9–25
Paulsen KD, Lynch DR, Liu W (1982b) Conjugate direction methods for Helmholtz problems with complex-valued wavenumber. Int J Numer Methods Eng 35: 601–622
Paulsen KD, Jia X, Sullivan JM (1993) Finite element computations of specific absorption rates in anatomically conforming full-body models for hyperthermia treatment analysis. IEEE Trans Biomed Eng 40: 933–945
Perez CA, Pajak T, Emami B, Hornbeck NB, Tupchong L, Rubin P (1991) Randomized phase III study comparing irradiation and hyperthermia with irradiation alone in superficial measurable tumors. Am J Clin Oncol (CCT) 14: 133–141
Phillips TL (1993) Clinical trials of hyperthermia, presented at the 13th Annual Meeting of the North American Hyperthermia Society, Dallas, TX, March.
Piket-May MJ, Taflove A, Lin WC, Katz DS, Sathiaseelan V, Mittal BB (1992) Computational modeling of EM hyperthermia: 3D and patient specific. IEEE Trans Biomed Eng 39: 226–236
Rine GP, Samulski TV, Grant W, Wallen CA (1990) Comparison of two-dimensional numerical approximation and measurement of SAR in a muscle equivalent phantom exposed to a 915 MHz slab-loaded waveguide. Int J Hyperthermia 5: 213–226
Saithiaseelan V, Taflove A, Piket-May MJ, Reuter C, Mittal BB (1992) Application of numerical modeling techniques in electromagnetic hyperthermia. In: Fleming AHJ, Joyner KH (eds) ACES Special issue on bioelectromagnetic computations, vol 7. ACES Journal, pp 61–71
Samulski TV, Grant WJ, Oleson JR, Leopold KA, Dewhirst MW, Vallario P, Blivin J (1990) Clinical experience with multi-element ultrasonic hyperthermia system: analysis of treatment temperatures. Int J Hyperthermia 6: 909–922
Sapozink MD, Joszef G, Astrahan MA, Gibbs FA, Petrovich Z, Stewart JR (1990) Adjuvant pelvic hyperthermia in advanced cervical carcinoma. I. Feasibility, thermometry and device comparison. Int J Hyperthermia 6: 985–996
Sapozink MD, Corry PM, Kapp DS (1991) RTOG quality assurance guidelines for clinical trails using hyperthermia for deep-seated malignancy. Int J Radiat Oncol Biol Phys 20: 1109–1115
Seebass M, Nadobny J, Wust P, Felix R (1992) 2D and 3D finite element mesh generator for hyperthermia simulations. In: Geener EW (ed) Hyperthermic oncology 1992. Proceedings of the 6th International Congress on Hyperthermic Oncology. Arizona Board of Regents, Tucson, AZ, p 229
Shaw JA, Durney CH, Christensen DA (1991) Computer aided design of two-dimensional electric type hyperthermia applicators using the finite difference time-domain method. IEEE Trans Biomed Eng 38: 861–870
Shepard MJ, Weatherill P (eds) (1991) Special issue on adaptive meshing. Int J Numer Meth Eng 32: 651–937
Sowinski MJ, Van Den Berg PM (1990) A three dimensional iterative scheme for an electromagnetic capacitive applicator. IEEE Trans Biomed Eng 37: 975–986
Sowinski MJ, Van Den Berg PM (1992) A three dimensional iteratve scheme for an electromagnetic inductive applicator. IEEE Trans Biomed Eng 39: 1255–1264
Strohbehn JW (1983) Temperature distributions from interstitial RF electrode hyperthermia systems: theoretical predictions. Int J Radiat Oncol Biol Phys 9: 1655–1667
Strohbehn JW, Roemer RB (1984) A survey of computer simulations of hyperthermia treatment. IEEE Trans Biomed Eng 31: 136–149
Strohbehn JW, Trembly BS, Douple EB (1982) Blood flow effects on the temperature distributions from an invasive microwave antenna array used in cancer therapy. IEEE Trans Biomed Eng 29: 649–661
Strohbehn JW, Paulsen KD, Lynch DR (1986) Use of finite element methods in computerized thermal dosimetry. In: Hand JW, James JR (eds) Physical techniques in clinical hyperthermia. Research Studies Press, Letchworth, Herts, England, pp 383–451
Sullivan D (1990) Three-dimensional computer simulation in deep regional hyperthermia using the finite difference time-domain method. IEEE Trans Microwave Theory Tech 38: 204–211
Sullivan DM (1992) A frequency dependent FDTD method for biological applications. IEEE Trans Microwave Theory Tech 40: 532–539
Sullivan DM, Gandhi OP, Taflove A (1988) Use of the finite difference time-domain method in calculating EM absorption in man models. IEEE Trans Biomed Eng 35: 179–185
Sullivan DM, Buechler D, Gibbs FA (1992) Comparison of measured and simulated data in an annular phased array using an inhomogeneous phantom. IEEE Trans Microwave Theory Tech 40: 600–604

Swindell W, Roemer RB, Clegg ST (1982) Temperature distributions caused by dynamic scanning of focused ultrasound transducers. Proceedings of IEEE Ultrasonic Symposium, IEEE Press, New York, NY, pp 750–753

Taflove A, Umashankar KR (1990) The finite difference time-domain method for numerical modeling of electromagnetic wave interactions with arbitrary structures. In: Morgan MA (ed) Finite element and finite difference methods in electromagnetic scattering. Elsevier, London, pp 287–373

Taylor HC, Lau RWM (1992) Evaluation of clinical hyperthermia treatment using time-domain finite difference modeling technique. In: Fleming AHJ, Joyner KH (eds) ACES Special issue on bioelectromagnetic computations, ACES Journal, vol 7, pp 85–96

Turner PF (1984) Regional hyperthermia with an annular phased array. IEEE Trans Biomed Eng 31: 106–114

Turner PF, Schaefermeyer T (1989) BSD-2000 approach for deep local and regional hyperthermia: clinical utility. Strahlenther Onkol 165: 700–704

Van Den Berg PM, DeHoop AT, Segal A, Praagman N (1983) A computational model of electromagnetic heating of biological tissue with application to hyperthermic cancer therapy. IEEE Trans Biomed Eng 30: 797–805

Wang C, Gandhi OP (1989) Numerical simulation of annular phased arrays for anatomical based models using the FDTD method. IEEE Trans Microwave Theory Tech 37: 118–126

Wust P, Nadobny J, Felix R, Deuflhard P, Louis A, John W (1991) Strategies for optimized application of annular-phased array systems in clinical hyperthermia. Int J Hyperthermia 7: 157–174

Wust P, Nadobny J, Dohlus M, John W, Felix R (1993) 3D computation of E-fields by the volume-surface integral equation (VSIE) method in comparison to the finite-integration theory (FIT) method. IEEE Trans Biomed Eng 40: 745–759

Yan Z (1993) Implicit time-stepping solution of Maxwell's equations on finite elements. MS Thesis, Thayer School of Engineering, Dartmouth College, Hanover, NH

Yee KS (1966) Numerical solutions of initial boundary value problems involving Maxwell's equations in isotropic media. IEEE Trans Antennas Propagat 14: 302–207

Yeh MM (1992) An intracavitary microwave antenna array system for hyperthermia of the prostate. MS Thesis, Thayer School of Engineering, Dartmouth College, Hanover, NH

Young JH, Wang MT, Brezovich IA (1980) Frequency/depth-penetration considerations in hyperthermia by magnetically induced currents. Electron Lett 16: 358–359

Yuan X, Lynch DR, Paulsen KD (1991) Importance of normal field continuity in inhomogeneous scattering calculations. IEEE Trans Microwave Theory Tech 39: 638–642

Zhang Y, Samulski TV, Clegg ST, Joines W (1993) Theoretical and measured electromagnetic fields radiated by a spiral microstrip antenna. 13th Annual Meeting of the North American Hyperthermia Society, Dallas, TX, March.

Zhu X, Gandhi OP (1988) Design of RF needle applicators for optimum SAR distributions in irregularly shaped tumors. IEEE Trans Biomed Eng 35: 382–388

Ziolkowski RW, Madsen NK, Carpenter RC (1983) Three-dimensional computer modeling of electromagnetic fields; a global lookback lattice truncation scheme. J Comput Phys 50: 360–408

Zwamborn APM, van den Berg PM, Mooibroek J, Koenis FTC (1992) Computation of three dimensional electromagnetic field distributions in a human body using the weak form of the CGFFT method. In: Fleming AHJ, Joyner KH (eds) ACES special issue on bioelectromagnetic computation 5, ACES Journal, vol 7, no. 2, pp 22–42

19 Basics of Thermal Models

J. MOOIBROEK, J. CREZEE, and J.J.W. LAGENDIJK

CONTENTS

19.1 Introduction

An aspect of clinical hyperthermia which is still in the midst of its developmental stage is the determination of three-dimensional (3D) temperature distributions for treatment planning purposes (COMAC BME/ESHO 1990, 1992). As long as noninvasive 3D temperature measurement techniques cannot be applied routinely in clinics, we must rely for temperature information on thermal probes inserted in tumor mass and healthy tissues. However, these invasive techniques cannot provide sufficient spatial information on the actual 3D temperature field and therefore thermal models are the method of choice to bridge the gap (CLEGG et al. 1985; CLEGG and ROEMER 1989, 1993; LIAUH et al. 1991; see also Chap. 20).

Even if the energy deposition in living tissues were to be known accurately (see Chap. 18), the prediction of the resulting temperature response would not be a trivial task. The largest bottleneck in thermal modeling is the fact that a general thermal theory, i.e., one that is applicable to any body site, has not been completed for the description of convective heat transport by moving blood, which comprises about 10% of the total body volume (GUYTON 1986) and may contribute up to 90% of all heat transport (LAGENDIJK et al. 1988).

The first problem encountered in the formulation of such a theory is the identification of those vessel structures responsible for major heat exchange (PENNES 1948; CHEN and HOLMES 1980; CHATO 1980; WEINBAUM et al. 1984, 1992; JIJI et al. 1984; WEINBAUM and LEMONS 1992). The next problem is to judge, on the basis of vessel architecture (e.g., number density) and rheological factors (e.g., flow), whether these structures are accessible for a continuum formulation. By this we mean that control volumes can be discerned in the tissue which are large with respect to the microscopic dimensions of the identified vessel structure, thus permitting volume averaging of their combined effect, but small compared to the macroscopic dimensions of the temperature field. If certain classes of vessels cannot be described in this way, they have to be treated on an individual basis as discrete vessels (TORELL and NILSSON 1978; LAGENDIJK 1982; MOOIBROEK and LAGENDIJK 1991; CREZEE and LAGENDIJK 1990, 1992; CHEN and ROEMER 1992; ROEMER 1990). A third complicating factor is that a general clinically applicable theory should also provide tools to cope with the dynamic behavior of tissue–blood heat exchange, i.e., the physiological response at elevated tissue temperatures. Note that, for example, skeletal muscle tissue perfusion can vary 20- to 25-fold from resting conditions to

J. MOOIBROEK, MSc, Department of Radiotherapy, University Hospital Utrecht, Heidelberglaan 100, NL-3584 CX Utrecht, The Netherlands

J. CREZEE, PhD, Department of Radiotherapy, University Hospital Utrecht, Heidelberglaan 100, NL-3584 CX Utrecht, The Netherlands

J.J.W. LAGENDIJK, PhD, Department of Radiotherapy, University Hospital Utrecht, Heidelberglaan 100, NL-3584 CX Utrecht, The Netherlands

heavy exercise (GUYTON 1986). Although the literature is not equivocal about the fact that tumor blood flow is always increased (LAGENDIJK et al. 1988; REINHOLD and VAN DEN BERG 1990; FELDMAN et al. 1992), because it may be a tumor type-specific phenomenon, acute local and global (nervous and humoral) induced blood flow changes in normal or tumor tissue are significant. Some indications exist that this will lead to a nonlinear theory for local thermoregulatory responses (CHATO 1990; LEMONS and WEINBAUM 1992; WEINBAUM and LEMONS 1992).

The relevance of a reliable theory is obvious as it would have immediate consequences for dosimetry, system design and optimization, and treatment planning.

19.2 Review of Progress in Thermal Modeling

19.2.1 Introduction

A comprehensive survey of the existing literature is not possible in the allotted space; therefore we will limit ourselves to the presentation of those contributions on which today's thermal models are based. General introductions to thermal models and their clinical applications are given by LAGENDIJK (1987, 1990), CHATO (1990), and ROEMER (1988, 1990) and in the COMAC BME/ESHO Task Group report on treatment planning and modelling in hyperthermia (COMAC BME/ESHO 1992).

Two major approaches have been followed to clarify which vessel structures are responsible for blood–tissue heat exchange. Several authors (CHEN and HOLMES 1980; CHATO 1980; BAISH et al. 1986a,b; WEINBAUM et al. 1984; JIJI et al. 1984) have tackled the lowest end of the vessel bed and tried to formulate a continuum theory for microvascular heat transfer, while other, more clinically involved groups (LAGENDIJK 1982; MOOIBROEK and LAGENDIJK 1991; CREZEE and LAGENDIJK 1990, 1992; CHEN and ROEMER 1992) have started with a discrete description of the largest vessels of the vascular tree. The latter, more pragmatic approach was adopted for the following clinical reasons: Cold tracks along large vessels cause underdosage of tumor areas, which makes knowledge of their spatial trajectory indispensible. As vessel imaging methods like magnetic resonance angiography (MRA) have evolved enormously, e.g., 0.5-mm-diameter vessels in the brain can be resolved presently (DUMOULIN et al. 1993), a top-down strategy can be followed in the discrete vessel formulation until the constraints of the imaging systems and computational resources have been reached. As both aforementioned methods are based on the same hydrodynamic notions, i.e., thermal equilibration length and countercurrent heat exchange, these will be outlined first.

19.2.1.1 Thermal Equilibration Length of Single Vessels

Vessels transporting blood at a different temperature than the surrounding tissue will lose or gain thermal energy across the vessel–tissue interface. The rate at which this happens is described by the Nusselt number N_u, a dimensionless hydrodynamic parameter. The Nusselt number depends on the flow pattern in the vessels and may vary from large values for turbulent vessel flow to a constant value for well-developed, e.g., laminar, flow. ZHU et al. (1990) recently established a value of 4.36 under more general conditions than have previously been used to define this quantity. Using this parameter an estimate can be made of the characteristic length of a vessel over which an initial temperature difference has relaxed to e^{-1} of this value. This length is called the thermal equilibration length (L_{eq}) of a vessel. Applying the simplified representation of a thin-walled, centrally located, flow pipe in a cylindrical medium for a vessel in a tissue cylinder and assuming a constant heat flux across the pipe wall, several authors have calculated L_{eq} for different branches of the vascular tree. Together with some structural and flow dynamic parameters, values for L_{eq} are listed in Table 19.1 (CREZEE 1993). A sensitivity analysis shows that L_{eq} strongly depends on flow and vessel diameter and to a lesser extent on the tissue parameters (MOOIBROEK 1992).

19.2.1.2 Countercurrent Heat Exchange

A structural feature which is very abundant in the human body is countercurrent flow. By this we mean that a supplying artery and a draining vein are closely juxtaposed, thus following the same spatial course but with opposite flow directions. This principle is already manifest from the third generation of the vessel bed and proceeds until the terminal arteries and veins of the microcircuitry. The description of heat transfer in such

Table 19.1. Vessel parameters for a 13-kg dog. Diameter, length, flow, and number from MALL (1888) and GREEN (1995), L_{eq} computed with $\rho_b = 10^3\,\mathrm{kg\,m^{-3}}$, $c_b = 4.10^3\,\mathrm{J\,kg^{-1}\,°C^{-1}}$, $k_b = 0.6\,\mathrm{W\,°C^{-1}\,m^{-1}}$ and $\Lambda = 1.5$

Vessel type	Diameter (mm)	Length l_v (cm)	Flow (cm/s)	Nusselt number	L_{eq} (cm)	L_{eq}/l_v
Aorta	10	40	50	1	12 500	310
Large arteries	3	20	13	40	290	15
Main branches	1	10	8	600	20	2.0
Secondary branches	0.6	4	8	1800	7.2	1.8
Tertiary branches	0.14	1.4	3.4	7.6×10^4	0.17	0.1
Terminal branches	0.05	0.1	2	10^6	0.013	0.1
Terminal arteries	0.03	0.15	0.4	1.3×10^7	0.0009	0.006
Arterioles	0.02	0.2	0.3	4×10^7	0.0003	0.002
Capillaries	0.008	0.1	0.07	1.2×10^9	0.00001	0.0001
Venules	0.03	0.2	0.07	8×10^7	0.00016	0.001
Terminal branches	0.07	0.15	0.07	1.3×10^7	0.0009	0.006
Terminal veins	0.13	0.1	0.3	10^6	0.013	0.1
Tertiary veins	0.28	1.4	0.8	7.6×10^4	0.16	0.1
Secondary veins	1.5	4	1.3	1800	7.3	1.8
Main veins	2.4	10	1.5	600	22	2.2
Large veins	6	20	3.6	40	320	16
Vena cava	12.5	40	33	1	12 900	320

structures is more complicated than for the single vessel case because heat exchange also occurs between the countercurrent vessel pair. A relaxation parameter similar to L_{eq} has been defined, i.e., L_{eqcc}, and quantified using techniques from hydrodynamics. A fundamental contribution originates from BAISH et al. (1986a), using two heat conduction coupling parameters: the first reflects the combined contribution of both vessels to the surrounding tissue while the second accounts for the heat exchange between the vessel pair. This approach has been used extensively (WEINBAUM and JIJI 1987; WISSLER 1987a,b) and was recently extended by ZHU et al. (1990) for the more clinically relevant situation of eccentrically located, unequally sized artery–vein pairs.

Although different analytical expressions have been derived (MOOIBROEK 1992) to quantify L_{eqcc}, the general conclusion which can be drawn from all studies is that L_{eqcc} is smaller than L_{eq} for the single vessel case and therefore the values listed in Table 19.1 can be used as a conservative estimate for the thermal significance of individual and countercurrent vessels.

19.2.2 Continuum Formulations

19.2.2.1 Heat Sink/Source Description

Capillaries were originally thought to be the vascular site for blood–tissue heat exchange. Based on their distributive nature, i.e., large contact surface area with tissue, high number density, and close proximity to the living cells, and in analogy with other transport processes such as O_2 diffusion and CO_2 removal, PENNES (1948) postulated his bioheat equation. He hypothesized that arterial blood traversing all generations of the vessel bed does not have any heat exchange with tissue until it reaches the capillaries, where it equilibrates instantaneously with the local tissue temperature and is subsequently removed via the venous route, again without any tissue interaction. In terms of L_{eq} this means that all vessels of the vascular tree are characterized by an L_{eq} approaching infinity while the capillaries have an L_{eq} approaching zero. Assuming an isotropic arrangement of the capillaries, he equated what is referred to in the hyperthermic literature as the Pennes heat sink/source term: $w_b c_b(T_{art} - T_{tis})$, with w_b the volumetric tissue perfusion and T_{art} mostly defined as the body core temperature (37°C). Although the underlying hypothesis was never confirmed experimentally, this formulation has been used extensively. Its power lies in its mathematical simplicity and the ability to adjust the perfusion term such that a good match can be obtained between measured and calculated data. CHEN and HOLMES (1980) derived a perfusion-related heat sink/source term by evaluating the vascular contribution to tissue heat transfer in a generalized vessel network consisting of serveral generations of bifurcations and confluences. Because of the continuous branching towards vessels with smaller thermal equilibration lengths, the blood in the arterial branch is inevitably forced to reach to local tissue temperature. In the confluencing venous vessel tree, blood collects in sections with a larger equilibration length. Chen and Holmes showed that if the thermal equilibration length is longer than the actual length of the vessels in each section, heat can escape the system, resulting in the Pennes heat sink term. The contribution of the first generations of major arteries and branches with diameters larger than 0.6 mm must be described individually. Unlike Pennes, CHEN and HOLMES based their heat sink/source term on the local arterial temperature T_a^* and the perfusion rate w_a^* of the last individually treated bifurcation. The amount of heat which escapes the control volume via the venous route is equated in their bioheat formulation by: $Q = w^* \rho_b c_b (T_a^* - T_{tis})$.

Recently CHARNY et al. (1989, 1990) and WEINBAUM et al. (1992), assuming countercurrency, demonstrated that the heat perfusion term has to be associated with the small countercurrent vessel bleed-off circuitry connecting the walls of the countercurrent vessels larger than 250–300 μm in diameter. It was shown that, depending on the physiological conditions, blood leaving the arterial wall at temperature T_a could arrive at the venous wall at a temperature T_v, which could vary between T_a and the local tissue temperature. In the latter case a Pennes term arises. With the different structural basis in mind and the recognition that T_a is the local arterial temperature and not the body core temperature, this term is now phrased as the modified heat/sink source term of Pennes.

19.2.2.2 Effective Thermal Conductivity (k_{eff}) Description

The recognition that vessels larger in diameter than the arterioles (40 μm), capillaries (10–20 μm), and venules (50 μm) had equilibration lengths comparable to their physical lengths provided the impetus to formulate a new thermal theory for blood–tissue heat exchange. CHEN and HOLMES (1980) convincingly showed that terminal arteries and veins with diameters in the range of 200–500 μm are the primary sites for blood–tissue heat equilibration. Note that the physical length of those vessels (Table 19.1) is in the mm to cm range, which roughly coincides with the extension of thermal gradients under hyperthermic conditions. Blood in these vessels will be in a continuous process of heat exchange along their length and thus will retain during passage some memory of the thermal history, e.g., blood in the proximal part of a vessel may gain a certain amount of thermal energy which partly may be released at its distal portion. This type of thermal energy transport resembles the common conductive heat transport where thermal energy is transported from locations at a higher temperature towards locations at a lower temperature via molecular collisions. The theoretical basis of the k_{eff} concept was firmly established by the fundamental work of CHEN and HOLMES (1980) and was later refined by WEINBAUM and JIJI (1985) (see next section), who showed that the countercurrent arrangement of these vessels results in a tensorial heat transfer coefficient which, under specific conditions, i.e., isotropically arranged vessel pairs, results in a scalar k_{eff} term. The k_{eff} concept has been verified experimentally (WEINBAUM et al. 1984; JIJI et al. 1984; CREZEE and LAGENDIJK 1990, 1991) and by simulations using the discrete vessel models (LAGENDIJK and MOOIBROEK 1986).

19.2.2.3 Further Refinements of Continuum Formulations

The foregoing continuum formulations on local vascular architecture and hydrodynamic parameters (L_{eq} and L_{eqcc}) represented a major leap forwards in thermal modeling. However, it should be kept in mind that their basic notions were derived mostly under idealized conditions not met in practice. For example, the equilibration lengths of single or countercurrent vessels were equated under the simplifying assumptions of a constant temperature at the tissue perimeter and definite ratios between vessel and tissue cylinder diameter. Although such assumptions may be justified at specific body sites, it is not expected that they will be generally applicable. This implies that a general theory will be more complex than the presented ones. WEINBAUM and JIJI (1985) presented a more refined bioheat equation than the one previously formulated by CHEN and HOLMES (1980) in that they used the notion of a local *average* tissue temperature, i.e., the mean of the local arterial and venous temperature. Additionally they noted that the gradient in this local *average* tissue temperature equals the gradient in the local mean vessel temperature (closure condition). As a consequence of these observations their final formulation does not contain a direct reference to vessel temperatures, but their presence is accounted for implicitly by use of this local *average* tissue temperature and the locally defined enhanced tensorial thermal conductivity. For the more subtle details of Weinbaum and Jiji's formulation and the subsequent discussion (WISSLER 1987a,b; WEINBAUM and JIJI 1987) of the validity of the closure condition, the reader is referred to the original papers. It is important to note here that their final formulation contains mutually dependent heat sink/source and k_{eff} contributions. They stressed that the countercurrent heat exchange mechanism is dominant under the restriction that the ratio $e = L_{eqcc}/L < 0.3$, with L the extension of the macroscopic tissue temperature gradient, and that for increasing values of e the heat sink/source term will become increasingly important. The significance of this ratio was also recognized by BAISH et al. (1986b) and later by CHARNY et al. (1990) in a comparative study between their three equation model, the Pennes model, and the Weinbaum and Jiji formulation. These considerations show the necessity of introducing further refinements into the thermal theory as the parameter e may vary spatially as well as temporally during hyperthermia.

19.2.3 Discrete Vessel Formulation

So far the efforts to formulate a thermal theory have been restricted to the collective contribution of vessels ranging in diameter from 50 to 500 μm. Other significant contributions to the development of an all-encompassing thermal theory for hyperthermic applications have been made by authors describing the impact of the largest vessels of the vascular tree on the final temperature distribution. LAGENDIJK et al. (1984) devised a numerical method to describe the influence of large thermally significant vessels and pointed to the occurrence of underdosed areas when such vessels traverse or closely pass tumor volumes. This method was extended by MOOIBROEK and LAGENDIJK (1991) to allow for the computation of true 3D bending and branching vascular structures, which was subsequently optimized for computational speed through implementation of a multitime level scheme as proposed by DuFort and Frankle (MITCHELL and GRIFFITHS 1980). Using these numerical models as an investigational tool, these authors also confirmed the concept of a countercurrent-related increase in the tissue thermal conductivity k_{eff} (LAGENDIJK and MOOIBROEK 1986). Based on calculations of the thermal equilibration length of vessels, L_{eq}, they arrived at a tripartition of the vessel bed with respect to heat transfer, similar to CHATO (1980). Large individual arterial vessels will remain predominantly at core temperature so their presence can be accounted for by defining additional boundary conditions ($T_{art} = T_{core}$) along their trajectory. Insofar as the number density of branches of these vessels is small and their equilibration length is comparable with their physical length, they must be described individually. The local number density of further generations of thermally significant vessels, i.e., the intermediate size vessels, is such that these vessels are in a transition region of an individual versus a collective description and thus presently pose the largest problem for a thermal theory. The smallest branches were found to be described best by an enhanced effective tissue thermal conductivity k_{eff}. It was further stressed on the basis of theoretical considerations (CREZEE and LAGENDIJK 1992) that due to the heat resistance in the vessel and the vessel wall the underdosed areas along the vessels could turn out to be smaller than originally anticipated and therefore these areas could be heated to therapeutic levels if local specific absorption rate (SAR) control were sufficient (see Chap. 20). The use of discrete vessel models has advantages but also clear limitations. The former follow from the observation that no inherent simplifying assumptions need to be made about the vessel and surrounding tissue temperatures and gradients. Blood and tissue temperatures thus relax freely to their final values according to the defined initial and boundary conditions without applying simplifying assumptions not generally met in clinical applications. By scaling down to the correct dimensions this method is an ideal research tool to verify underlying hypotheses as used in the continuum formulation. Two major limitations can be discerned in existing discrete vessel models: The first is related to the spatial resolution (0.5 mm) needed to derive both the arterial and the venous network. This resolution is becoming achievable with MRA at body locations, such as the brain, where organ movement does not play a critical role, as is the case in the pelvic or abdominal region (DUMOULIN et al.

1993). However, the initial problems related to loading the enormous amount of vascular data into discrete models are now diminishing due to the progress made in devising reconstruction algorithms (KOTTE 1993) of the imaging data. The second limitation is related to the computing resources: A $10 \times 10 \times 10\,\mathrm{cm}^3$ volume with a 0.5-mm resolution requires 32 Mbytes just for storage of the temperature distribution. As computing time is directly related to this matrix size it is also important to keep the number of nodes limited. Depending on the volumes heated, this inevitably leads to grid sizes in which not all the significant vessels can be resolved individually. Strategies are now being developed to extend the discrete vessel model with continuum formulations for the unresolved thermally significant vessels (VAN LEEUWEN 1993).

19.3 Validation of Thermal Models

The present stage of experimental verification of thermal models will be illustrated by some examples from the literature. We will discuss two types of experiments: in vivo or ex vivo, using isolated perfused organs. The latter require special perfusion techniques (HOLMES et al. 1984; ZAERR et al. 1990; BOS et al. 1991). A disadvantage of most in vivo tests is the absence of perfusion control; this frustrates attempts to separate convective and conductive heat transport because the absolute blood flow level is (a) difficult to determine and (b) will probably display time- and temperature-dependent behavior. However, it is possible to retain (some) control over blood flow.

19.3.1 Ex Vivo Tests

Several thermal model tests comparing the conventional bioheat equation and the effective thermal conductivity model were carried out at our department using isolated perfused bovine organs like kidney and tongue. In the first series an artificial vessel was introduced into the kidney cortex, which also served as a heat source. The stationary temperature profiles around this vessel were determined at different flow rates within the cortex tissue, ranging between 0 and $3\,\mathrm{kg\,m^{-3}\,s^{-1}}$. Both the amplitude and the shape of the resulting temperature profiles agreed with the effective conductivity model prediction.

There are several methods for determination of the effective thermal conductivity, k_{eff}. ANDERSON et al. (1992) describe a method using a thermal diffusion probe, a self-heated thermistor where the ambient conductivity is derived from the temperature elevation caused by a fixed power level. Measurements in isolated perfused canine kidney show that k_{eff} increases approximately linearly with perfusion.

A more global method is measurement of the propagation velocity of heat diffusion in the tissue, which is proportional to the conductivity. A method for the determination of heat diffusion that is suitable for interstitial hyperthermia, provided power deposition is concentrated near the needles, uses the time delay τ_w before the temperature starts to rise at a distance x from a needle after the heating has been switched on: $k_{\mathrm{eff}} = \rho_t c_t x^2/(4\tau_w)$. A threefold increase in k_{eff} was observed under specific experimental conditions using hot water tube heating (CREZEE et al. 1991).

19.3.2 In Vivo Tests

WEINBAUM et al. (1984) examined the importance of countercurrent heat exchange by evaluating the radial temperature profile in rabbit thigh, measured in vivo with a thin thermocouple wire. Vessel data and the location of the thermocouple with respect to the vessels were obtained by producing a corrosion cast of the thigh afterwards. No external heating was used. The radial temperature gradient between the cutaneous plexus in the skin and the central artery and vein was almost linear, increasing from 27°C to 33.5°C. The arterial temperature was nearly equal to the venous temperature for any countercurrent pair encountered along the track; even for the main artery and vein of the hind leg the difference was just 0.3°C. According to the Pennes heat sink model, the arterial and venous temperatures should have been equal to the core temperature and the local tissue temperature, respectively, causing arteriovenous temperature differences of up to 6.5°C. The absence of significant arteriovenous temperature differences indicates that countercurrent heat exchange is a dominant mode of heat transfer. However, this conclusion may not apply to humans as these data were obtained in a much smaller species. In similar experiments LEMONS et al. (1987) made a detailed registration of the arteriovenous temperature differences for rabbit thigh in vivo and found, under normothermic conditions, both with and without surface cooling, that the lower limit for thermal nonequilibration was 100 μm for arteries versus 400 μm for veins. This asymmetry was ascribed to the difference in radius of the artery and vein in a countercurrent pair. ROEMER et al. (1989) measured steady state temperature profiles in canine thighs heated by scanned focused ultrasound, both in vivo at some uncontrolled perfusion level and at zero blood flow after death. A comparison was made with both limited k_{eff} and heat sink model predictions; a better qualitative agreement was found with the latter, especially regarding the presence of a depression in the temperature profile at the center of the scan. Similar experiments were described in more detail by MOROS et al. (1993). HYNYNEN et al. (1989) used a setup designed by DEYONG et al. (1986), consisting of a flow transducer and a cuff around the renal artery of dogs. Feedback of the flow data enabled controlled renal perfusion at levels between 0 and 240 ml min^{-1} in vivo. The kidney was heated with scanned focused ultrasound, and the resulting steady state temperature profiles were compared with the heat sink model prediction. Agreement was reasonably good.

Summarizing, these experiments support the validity of k_{eff} in the description of small vessel heat transfer and of the heat sink term for larger vessels, but only regarding the gross temperature distribution. A more accurate description of the temperature distribution will require the inclusion of discrete vessels in the thermal model.

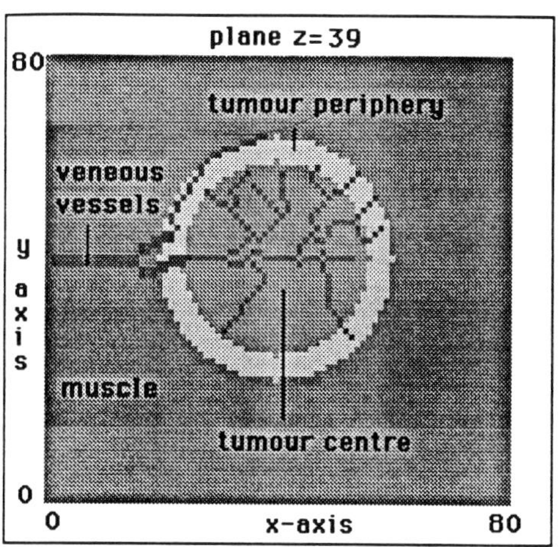

Fig. 19.1. Cross-sectional view of model geometry consisting of 80 × 80 × 80 (x, y, z) cubical nodes spaced 1 mm apart showing the plane (z = 39) containing the venous part of a countercurrent vessel network (arteries: z = 41). Thermal parameters for muscle and tumor are: k = 0.6 W m^{-1} °C^{-1}, ρ = 10^3 kg m^{-3}, c_p = 3600 J kg^{-1} °C^{-1}. Isotemperature values (T = 37°C) are assumed on all boundary planes

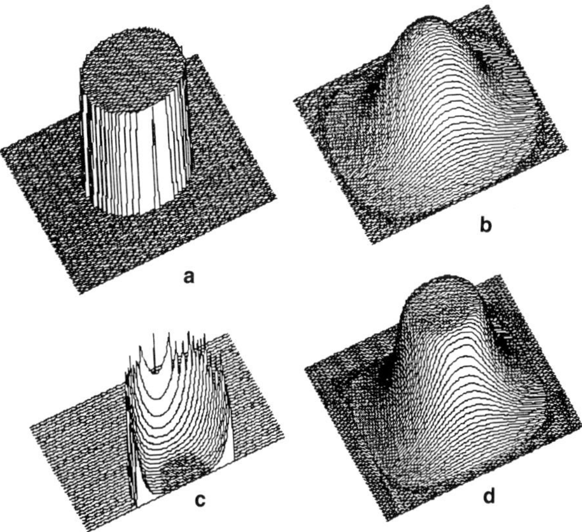

Fig. 19.2. Normalized landscape plots of uniform power deposition in tumor (**a**) and resulting temperature distribution (**b**) in model midplane (z = 40). Power distribution (**c**) needed to derive a uniform temperature distribution in the tumor (**d**)

19.4 Basic Differences Between Frequently Used Thermal Models

In the following the basic differences between some frequently applied thermal models will be highlighted. No attempt will be made to correlate the different models or to dispute the correctness of these models. The only purpose here is to show how the resulting temperature distribution will depend on the model used. In order to have a common basis we used our 3D thermal program for inhomogeneous media, which also permits the simultaneous definition of branching vessel networks, volumetric perfusion, and/or enhanced tissue thermal conductivity. An overview of the model parameters is presented in Fig. 19.1, where we used an idealized tumor geometry with central countercurrent vascularization (z = 39 and z = 41 plane) and a spherical SAR distribution enclosing the tumor volume. This SAR distribution (Fig. 19.2c) was constructed such that in the unperfused situation the resulting tumor temperature was nearly uniform and rapidly decayed in healthy tissue (see Fig. 19.2d). As the literature is not equivocal about the perfusional status of tumors under hyperthermic conditions, we investigated three extreme cases, i.e., low muscle perfusion with high tumor perfusion, the opposite case, and finally equal muscle and tumor perfusion. In some cases we will indicate how the SAR distribution has to be tailored in order to retrieve the original uniform tumor temperature.

The following expression for conductive and convective heat transport will serve as a common basis:

$$\rho \times C_p \times dT/dt = \Delta(k \cdot \Delta T) + B + P + Q_{\text{met}} \quad [\text{W m}^{-3}], \tag{19.1}$$

where ρ is the density (kg m^{-3}), C_p the specific heat capacity ($\text{J kg}^{-1}\,°\text{C}^{-1}$), k the intrinsic thermal conductivity ($\text{W m}^{-1}\,°\text{C}^{-1}$), and T the local tissue temperature (°C).

In Eq. 19.1 the left-hand term denotes the net rate of accumulated heat in an infinitesimal control volume. P and Q_{met} are the local volumetric power depositions related to external and internal (metabolic) heat sources, respectively. The first term on the right-hand side is the Fourier conduction term related to molecular collisions. The second term symbolizes the crucial convective heat transport contribution, to be discussed next.

In order to emphasize the differences we first establish the stationary distribution in the midplane of the model when no convective heat transport is present, i.e., we assume $B = 0$ and $k = 0.6$ ($\text{W m}^{-1}\,°\text{C}^{-1}$), while the SAR distribution is uniform. It is clear (Fig. 19.2a) that a uniform SAR distribution cannot heat the inner region (tumor) uniformly because the external region (muscle) acts as thermal load. The heat loss at the outer region of the tumor thus has to be compensated for by a locally increased power deposition (Fig. 19.2c).

19.4.1 Heat Sink/Source Description

In the Pennes formulation the convective term B has the following shape:

$$B = -W_b C_b (T - T_{\text{art}}), \tag{19.2}$$

where w_b is the volumetric perfusion rate ($\text{kg m}^{-3}\,\text{s}^{-1}$), c_b is the specific heat capacity of blood ($\text{J kg}^{-1}\,°\text{C}^{-1}$), T is the local tissue temperature (°C), and T_{art} is usually taken to be equal to the core temperature, i.e., $T_{\text{art}} = 37°\text{C}$. The leading minus sign accounts for the fact that heat can be withdrawn (sink) from the control volume if $T_{\text{art}} < T$, which is the case under hyperthermic conditions, or released (source) if $T_{\text{art}} > T$, as under normo- or hypothermic conditions.

In Fig. 19.3 landscape plots are presented for the three different perfusional cases following the SAR distribution which in the unperfused case revealed a nearly uniform temperature distribution of 44°C. If only the tumor is perfused ($4\,\text{kg m}^{-3}\,\text{s}^{-1}$), two characteristic features are observed: the tumor temperature drops to a maximum value of 40.3°C and the shape of the distribution becomes bimodal. To restore the original uniform tumor temperature we have to raise the central tumor power density, which involves a reshaping of the power distribution according to Fig. 19.3d. If only muscle perfusion is increased ($4\,\text{kg m}^{-3}\,\text{s}^{-1}$), an overall temperature drop of 1.2°C is observed, but the shape of the distribution remains nearly the same. This is explained by the fact that the power distribution only encloses the tumor volume and the muscle temperatures are already so low that the heat sink term will not contribute much in this region. Minor reshaping of the power distribution is needed; only its absolute value has to be increased to compensate for the 1.2°C drop. A similar bimodal temperature distribution and an additional 0.7°C decrease is obtained when tumor and muscle are perfused equally. The original uniform tumor temperature is obtained by using the reshaped power distribution of Fig. 19.3f. The main characteristic of this type of model is that the description of convective heat transport remains

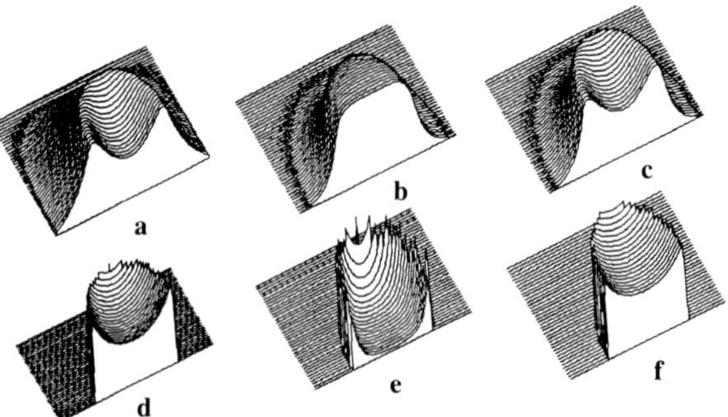

Fig. 19.3. Normalized landscape plots (**a–c**) of temperature distribution in plane $z = 40$ under different perfusion conditions (see text), applying the heat sink/source model. Normalized landscape plots (**d–f**) of power distributions needed to change **a,b** and **c** into uniform tumor temperature distribution

limited to the tissue volume enclosed by the power distribution. If a uniform tumor temperature distribution is the final goal, a perfusion-dependent readjustment of the power distribution and power level is needed.

19.4.2 Effective Thermal Conductivity (k_{eff}) Description

In this formulation the term B obtains the form:

$$B = \Delta(k_{conv} \cdot \Delta T), \qquad (19.3)$$

in which k_{conv} is a scalar quantity and therefore has the same shape as the first term in Eq. 19.1. In practice they are always combined and referred to as $k_{eff} = k_{tis}(1 + k_{conv}/k_{tis})$. Note that in Eq. 19.3 no reference is made to any locally defined arterial or venous temperature.

When the power distribution of Fig. 19.2c was used to calculate the temperature distribution in the model midplane ($z = 40$) for different values of k_{eff} for muscle and tissue, typical results as presented in Fig. 19.4 were obtained. In Fig. 19.4a a $k_{eff} = 4$ ($\mathrm{W\,m^{-1}\,°C^{-1}}$) was used for the tumor and a $k_{eff} = 1$ ($\mathrm{W\,m^{-1}\,°C^{-1}}$) for muscle. The maximum value decreased from 44°C to 41.2°C and could be restored to 44°C by increasing the power level, without the need for reshaping. In the opposite case (Fig. 19.4b), with $k_{eff} = 4$ ($\mathrm{W\,m^{-1}\,°C^{-1}}$) for muscle, the tumor temperature remained nearly uniform ($T = 43.1$°C) and only a small adjustment of power level was needed. If for both muscle and tissue a $k_{eff} = 4$ ($\mathrm{W\,m^{-1}\,°C^{-1}}$) value was taken, the maximum temperature fell to 39.7°C but the distribution remained nearly the same as in Fig. 19.4a. Characteristic features of this type of thermal model are that predicted temperature distributions have a smoother appearance and that there is no need to reshape the power deposition pattern when k_{eff} changes occur during heating.

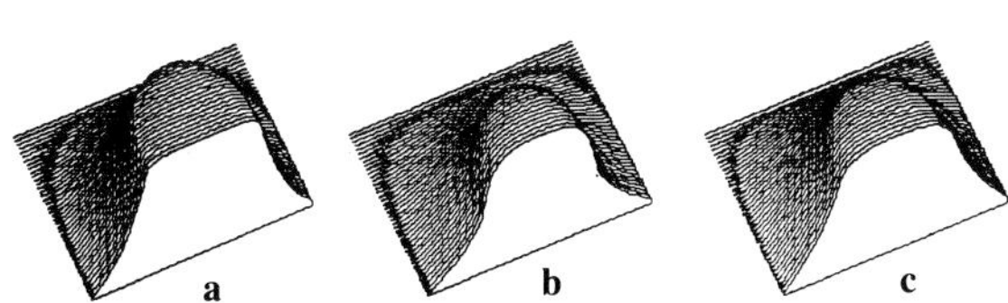

Fig. 19.4a–c. Normalized landscape plots of temperature distribution in plane $z = 40$ for different k_{eff} values for muscle and tumor (see text)

19.4.3 Discrete Vessel Heat Transport

In this formulation the term B is decomposed into contributions related to the presence of those vessels (B_{discr}) which are still tractable by vessel imaging methods such as MRA (Kotte 1993) and a k_{conv} term to describe the remaining nonresolved vessel structures, i.e.:

$$B = B_{discr} + \Delta(k_{conv} \cdot \Delta T). \qquad (19.4)$$

Vessels characterized by an equilibration length much longer than their physical length, L_{ves}, are treated as locally defined isothermal boundary conditions, i.e., $T_{ves} = T_{core}$, and in principle this strategy is prolonged until a class of vessel segments is encountered for which L_{ves} becomes comparable with L_{eq}. This type of vessel is treated on an individual basis as described by Mooibroek and Lagendijk (1991).

As an example we defined a co-planar countercurrent vessel network with veins located in plane $z = 39$ and arteries in plane $z = 41$. Similar to the foregoing cases, the power distribution of Fig. 19.2c is used to calculate the temperture distribution in plane $z = 37$ (Fig. 19.5a), the model midplane (Fig. 19.5b), and at $z = 43$, i.e., at a distance 2 mm from the plane containing the arterial network (Fig. 19.5c).

A characteristic feature of this method is that the predicted temperature distributions show steep gradients normal to predominantly the arterial vessel trajectories. It should be noted that in the foregoing calculations we assumed $k_{eff} = 1$ ($\mathrm{W\,m^{-1}\,°C^{-1}}$) for muscle and tumor to focus on the impact of individual vessel segments. Temperature distributions in these planes improve

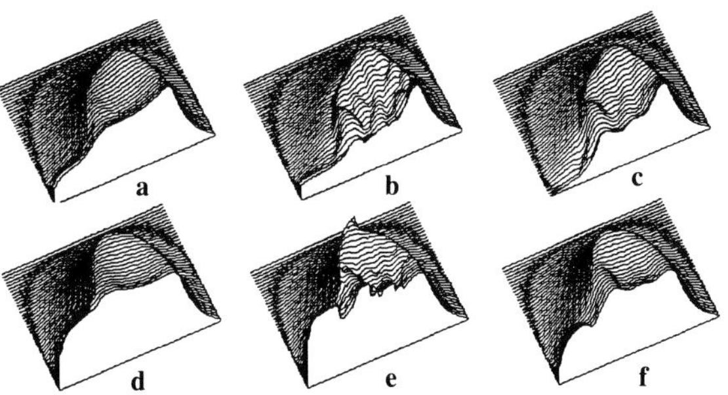

Fig. 19.5. Normalized landscape plots (**a–c**) of temperature distribution in plane $z = 37$ (**a**), $z = 40$ (**b**), and $z = 43$ (**c**) applying the discrete vessel model. Improved temperature distributions result in these planes when a locally increased power density in a tissue cylinder ($d_{cyl} = 3 \times d_{ves}$) around each vessel is assumed (**d–f**)

when a locally increased power density is applied in a tissue cylinder ($d_{cyl} = 3 \times d_{ves}$) around each vessel (Fig. 19.5d–f). At higher k_{eff} values the distribution will obtain a smoother appearance (not shown).

19.5 Discussion

The past decade has been very fruitful with respect to thermal modeling because important issues have been clarified at a basic level. Several authors have shown the inconsistency of the Pennes heat sink/source term when it is related to the isotropically arranged capillaries making up the terminal part of microvascularity. Due to the extremely short thermal equilibration lengths, blood in these vessels will be in complete thermodynamic equilibrium with their surrounding tissue and thus the driving potential for blood–tissue heat exchange is lacking. According to present insights, however, vascularized tissues can exhibit a Pennes-like behavior, which is now associated with the bleed-off circulation of the thermally significant countercurrent vessels ($D \simeq 300\,\mu$m) or with the larger vessels themselves ($D > 500\,\mu$m). This raises a question mark as to its use in today's clinical applications. It does not seem justified to use the perfusion-based heat sink values because these significant countercurrent vessels follow definite spatial trajectories, while their volumetric densities may be three orders of magnitude lower than the isotropic capillaries, meaning that volumetric averaging must be performed with some caution.

It has further been established that the countercurrent terminal arteries and veins ($D > 150\,\mu$m) are the dominant sites where blood–tissue heat exchange takes place. Depending on their number densities and spatial organization, this implies that the heat exchange can be described in terms of a scalar or tensorial effective thermal conductivity.

The recognition that the various parts of connected vascular entities can lead to different formulations of blood–tissue heat exchange has far-reaching consequences: First, it justifies the use of fully hybrid models in thermal modeling; these models will describe the thermally significant vasculature discretely as far as these vascular data are available from 3D MRA. The small vessel heat transfer will be decribed by the continuum effective thermal conductivity, while small heat sinks, related to the discretely described vessels, will fill in the gap, describing (a) those vessels too small to be imaged but too large to be described by the effective thermal conductivity and describing (b) the countercurrency bleed off. Second it also forces us to establish the conditions where the contribution of either type is dominant in heat transfer. In general this will be organ specific as the vascular organization will differ from organ to organ and/or tumor to tumor. It will also depend on the physiological response of the heated tissues. Increased blood flow rates will lead to larger thermal equilibration lengths; however, this effect will be counteracted by the increased effective thermal conductivity in the tissue around the vessel, leading to a reduction in the equilibration length.

The presented computational examples provide valuable information for system designers, and point to the need for an SAR tailoring concept (Zhou and Fessenden 1993), i.e., local control of the 3D SAR pattern to compensate for the local heat losses during hyperthermia treatments. Modern systems and techniques based on this concept are now being developed; the scanning focused ultrasound techniques as well as new 3D controlled interstitial techniques are ideal methods for local 3D SAR control (see Chap. 20). An immediate consequence of this approach is that such a refined spatial power control must be backed by either extensive invasive thermometry or reliable thermal models (see Chap. 10, Sect. 10.6).

19.6 Summary

- Thermal models are methods to bridge the gap in information between scarce spatial thermometry data obtained with invasive thermometry and the actual 3D temperature distribution.
- So far no general thermal theory has been developed which is applicable to any body site; especially the description of convective heat transfer is incomplete, i.e., the identification of vessel structures responsible for major heat exchange and the description of continuous or discrete vessel models and the dynamic behavior of the tissue-blood heat exchange hyperthermia.
- Vessels transporting blood at a different temperature than the surrounding tissue lose or gain thermal energy across the vessel–tissue

interface. This is described by the characteristic thermal equilibrium length of vessels, which strongly depends on flow and vessel diameter. Another structural feature of importance is the countercurrent flow and heat exchange. For countercurrent vessels the characteristic equilibrium length is smaller than for the single-vessel case.

- Continuum formulations address small vessels (50–500 μm) using the heat sink/source description, the effective thermal conductivity description and further refinements of continuum formulations. Discrete vessel formulations address the impact of the largest vessels on the thermal distribution.
- Ex vivo and in vivo studies have been designed to test and validate different thermal models. They support the validity of k_{eff} in the heat transfer description of small vessels and of the heat sink term for large vessels. More accurate descriptions need to include discrete vessels in the thermal model.
- The different formulations of blood-tissue heat exchange have far-reaching consequences: they justify the use of fully hybrid models in thermal modeling and require an organ- or tumor-specific description of the vascular pattern. They also depend on the physiological response of the tissues.
- As a consequence, all modern heating techniques must be backed by either extensive invasive thermometry or reliable thermal models to provide useful data on the heating characteristics.

References

Anderson GT, Valvano JW, Santos RR (1992) Self-heated thermistor measurements of perfusion. IEEE Trans Biomed Eng 39: 877–885

Baish JW, Ayyaswamy PS, Foster KR (1986a) Small-scale temperature fluctuations in perfused tissue during local hyperthermia. J Biomech Eng 108: 246–250

Baish JW, Ayyaswamy PS, Foster KR (1986b) Heat transport mechanisms in vascular tissues: a model comparison. J Biomech Eng 108: 324–331

Bos CK, Crezee J, Mooibroek J, Lagendijk JJW (1991) A perfusion technique for tongues to be used in bioheat transfer studies. Phys Med Biol 36: 843–846

Charny CK, Weinbaum S, Levin RL (1989) An evaluation of the Weinbaum-Jiji bioheat transfer model for simulations of hyperthermia. Adv Bioeng ASME WAM 126: 1–10

Charny CK, Weinbaum S, Levin RL (1990) An evaluation of the Weinbaum-Jiji bioheat equation for normal and hyperthermic conditions. Biomech Eng-T ASHE 112: 80–87

Chato JC (1980) Heat transfer to blood vessels. J Biomech Eng 102: 110–118

Chato JC (1990) Fundamentals of bioheat transfer. In: Crautherie M (ed) Thermal dosimetry and treatment planning. Springer, Berlin Heidelberg New York, pp 1–56

Chen MM, Holmes KR (1980) Microvascular contributions in tissue heat transfer. Ann NY Acad Sci 335: 137–151

Chen ZP, Roemer RB (1992) The effects of large blood vessels on temperature distributions during simulated hyperthermia. J Biomech Eng 114: 473–481

Clegg ST, Roemer RB (1989) Estimation of three-dimensional temperature fields from noisy data during hyperthermia. Int J Hyperthermia 5: 967–989

Clegg ST, Roemer RB (1993) Reconstruction of experimental hyperthermia temperature distributions: application of state and parameter estimation. Trans ASME 115: 380–388

Clegg ST, Roemer RB, Cetas TC (1985) Estimation of complete temperature fields from measured transient temperatures. Int J Hyperthermia 1: 265–286

COMAC-BME/ESHO (1990) Workshop on modelling and planning in hyperthermia (Lagonissi 1990). Conclusions, subgroup Thermal Modelling (by Lagendijk JJW). COMAC-BME Hyperthermia Bulletin 4: 47–49

COMAC BME/ESHO Task Group Report (1992) Treatment planning and modelling in hyperthermia (Task Group committee chairman: Lagendijk JJW). Tor Vergata Medical Physics Monograph Series

Crezee J (1993) Experimental verification of thermal models. PhD Thesis. Addix, Wijk bij Duurstede

Crezee J, Lagendijk JJW (1990) Measurement of temperature profiles around large artificial vessels in perfused tissue. Phys Med Biol 35: 905–923

Crezee, J, Lagendijk, JJW (1992) Temperature uniformity during hyperthermia: the impact of large vessels. Phys Med Biol 37: 1321–1337

Crezee J, Mooibroek J, Bos CK, Lagendijk JJW (1991) Interstitial heating: experiments in artificially perfused bovine tongues. Phys Med Biol 36: 823–833

Crezee J, Mooibroek J, Lagendijk JJW (1993) Thermal model verification in interstitial hyperthermia. In: Seegenschmiedt MH, Sauer R (eds) Interstitial and intracavitary thermoradiotherapy. Springer, Berlin Heidelberg New York, pp 147–153

DeYoung DW, Kundrat MA, Cetas TC (1986) In vivo kidneys as preclinical thermal models for hyperthermia. Proc IEEE 9th Ann Conf Med Biol Soc (Boston: IEEE No. 87CH2513-0): 994–996

Dumoulin CL, Souza SP, Pele NJ (1993) Phase-sensitive flow imaging. In: Potchen EJ, Haacke EM, Siebert JE, Gottschalk A (eds) Magnetic resonance angiography. Mosby, St. Louis, pp 173–188

Feldmann HJ, Molls M, Hoederath A, Krümpelmann S, Sack H (1992) Blood flow and steady state temperatures in deep-seated tumors and normal tissues. Int J Radiat Oncol Biol Phys 23: 1003–1008

Guyton AC (1986) Textbook of medical physiology. Saunders, Philadelphia, pp 206–336

Green HD (1950) Circulatory system: physical principles. In Medical Physics II, edited by O. Glasser (Chicago, Year Book Publishers), pp 228–251

Holmes KR, Ryan W, Weinstein P, Chen MM (1984) A fixation technique for organs to be used as perfused tissue phantoms in bioheat transfer studies. In: Spiker RLS (ed) 1984 Advances in bioengineering. NY ASME WAM: 9–10

Hynynen K, DeYoung D, Kundrat M, Moros E (1989) The effect of blood perfusion rate on the temperature distributions induced by multiple, scanned and focussed ultrasonic beams in dogs' kidneys in vivo. Int J Hyperthermia 5: 485–498

Jiji LM, Weinbaum S, Lemons DE (1984) Theory and experiment for the effect of vascular microstructure on surface tissue heat transfer II. Model formulation and solution. J Biomech Eng 106: 331–341

Lagendijk JJW (1982) The influence of blood flow in large vessels on the temperature distribution in hyperthermia. Phys Med Biol 27: 17–23

Lagendijk JJW (1984) A new theory to calculate temperature distributions in tissues, or why the "bioheat transfer" equation does not work. In: overgaard J (ed) Hyperthermic oncology 1984, vol 1, Taylor&Francis, London, pp 507–510

Lagendijk JJW (1987) Heat transfer in tissues. In: Field SB, Franconi S (eds) Physics and technology of hyperthermia. Martinus Nihjof, Amsterdom, pp 517–561

Lagendijk JJW (1990) Thermal models: principles and implementation. In: Field SB, Hand JW (eds) An introduction to the practical aspects of clinical hyperthermia. Taylor and Francis, London, pp 478–512

Lagendijk JJW, Mooibroek J (1986) Hyperthermia treatment planning. Recent Results Cancer Res 101: 119–131

Lagendijk JJW, Schellekens M, Schipper J, Van der Linden PM (1984) A three-dimensional description of heating patterns in vascularised tissues during hyperthermic treatment. Phys Med Biol 29: 495–507

Lagendijk JJW, Hofman P, Schipper J (1988) Perfusion analyses in advanced breast carcinoma during hyperthermia. Int J Hyperthermia 4: 479–495

Lagendijk JJW, Crezee J, Mooibroek J (1992) Progress in thermal modelling development. In: Gerner Eq, Cetas TC (eds) Hyperthermic Oncology 1992, vol 2. Arizona Board of Regents, Tucson, AZ, pp 257–260

Lemons DE, Weinbaum S (1992) Heat transfer and local thermal control of the microcirculation. Adv Biol Heat Mass Transfer 231: 129–134

Lemons DE, Chien S, Crawshaw LI, Weinbaum S, Jiji LM (1987) Significance of vessel size and type in vascular heat transfer. Am J Physiol 253: R128–R135

Liauh CT, Clegg ST, Roemer RB (1991) Estimating three-dimensional temperature fields during hyperthermia: studies of the optimal regularization parameter and time sampling period. Trans ASME 113: 230–238

Mall F (1888) Die Blut- und Lymphwege im Dünndarm des hundes. Abhandlungen der Königlich Sächsische Gesellschaft der Wissenschaften, Mathematisch-Physischen Classe 14, pp 151–200

Mitchell AR, Griffiths DF (1980) The finite difference method in partial differential equations. Wiley, New York, pp 89–91

Mooibroek J (1992) In: COMAC BME/ESHO taskgroup report. Treatment planning and modelling in hyperthermia Task Group committee chairman: Lagendijk JJW). Tor Vergata Medical Physics Monograph Series, pp 89–99

Mooibroek J, Lagendijk JJW (1991) A fast and simple algorithm for the calculation of convective heat transfer by large vessels in three dimensional inhomogeneous tissues. IEEE Trans Biomed Eng 38: 490–501

Mooibroek J, Crezee J, Lagendijk JJW (1993) Thermal modelling of vascular patterns and their impact on interstitial heating technology and temperature monitoring. In: Seegenschmiedt MH, Sauer R (eds) Interstitial and intracavitary thermo-radiotherapie. Springer, Berlin Heidelberg New York, pp 131–137

Moros EG, Dutton AW, Roemer RB, Burton M, Hynynen K (1993) Experimental evaluation of two simple thermal models using hyperthermia in muscle in vivo. Int J Hyperthermia 9: 581–598

Pennes HH (1948) Analysis of tissue and arterial blood tempertures in the resting human forearm. J Appl Physiol 1: 93–122

Reinhold HS, van den Berg AP (1990) In: Field SB, Hand JW (eds) An introduction to the practical aspects of clinical hyperthermia. Taylor and Francis, London, pp 77–107

Roemer RB (1988) Heat transfer in hyperthermia treatments: basic principles and applications. In: Paliwal BR, Hetzel FW (eds) Biological, physical and clinical aspects of hyperthermia. American Institute of Physics, New York, pp 210–242

Roemer RB (1990) Thermal dosimetry. In: Gautherie M (ed) Thermal dosimetry and treatment planning. Springer, Berlin Heidelberg New York, pp 119–214

Roemer RB, Moros EG, Hynynen K (1989) A comparison of bioheat transfer and effective conductivity equation predictions to experimental hyperthermia data. Adv Bioeng ASME WAM, HTD 126: 11–15.

Torell LM, Nilsson SK (1978) Temperature gradients in low-flow vessels. Phys Med Biol 23: 106–117

Weinbaum S, Jiji LM (1985) A new simplified bioheat equation for the effect of blood flow on local average tissue temperature. Biomech Eng -T ASME 107: 131–139

Weinbaum S, Jiji LM (1987) Discussion of papers by Wissler and Baish et al. concerning the Weinbaum-Jiji bioheat equation. J Biomech Eng -T ASME 109: 234–237

Weinbaum S, Lemons DE (1992) Heat transfer in living tissue: the search for a blood-tissue energy equation and the local thermal microvascular control mechanism. BMES Bull 16: 38–43

Weinbaum S, Jiji LM, Lemons DE (1984) Theory and experiment for the effect of vascular microstructure on surface tissue heat transfer. Anatomical foundation and model conceptualization. J Biomech Eng-T ASME 106: 321–330

Weinbaum S, Jiji LM, Lemons DE (1992) The bleed off perfusion term in the Weinbaum-Jiji bioheat equation. J Biomech Eng-T ASME 114: 376–380

Wissler EH (1987a) Comments on the new bioheat transfer equation proposed by Weinbaum and Jiji. J Biomech Eng 109: 226–233

Wissler EH (1987b) Comments on Weinbaum and Jiji's discussion of their proposed bioheat equation. J Biomech Eng 109: 355–356

Wulff W (1974) The energy conservation equation for living tissue. IEEE Trans Biomed Eng 21: 494–495

Wust P, Nadobny J, Felix R, Deuflhard P, Louis A, John W (1991) Strategies for optimized application of

annular-phased-array systems in clinical hyperthermia. Int J Hyperthermiz 7: 157–173
Zaerr J, Roemer RB, Hynynen K (1990) Computer-controlled dynamic phantom for ultrasound hyperthermia studies. IEEE Trans Biomed Eng 37: 1115–1118
Zhou L, Fessenden P (1993) Automation of temperature control for large-array microwave surface applicators. Int J Hyperthermia 9: 479–490
Zhu M, Weinbaum S, Jiji LM (1990) Heat exchange between unequal countercurrent vessels asymmetrically embedded in a cylinder with surface convection. Int J Heat Mass Transfer 33: 2275–2284

20 Principles of Treatment Planning

J.J.W. LAGENDIJK, J. CREZEE, and J. MOOIBROEK

CONTENTS

20.1 Introduction

In treatment planning three aspects can be considered in general: tumor localization, treatment strategy, and treatment simulation. In tumor localization the exact location of the tumor is defined in relation to critical organs and patient coordinates. All information about available equipment and equipment behavior in relation to tumor location defines the treatment strategy. Finally, the complete treatment has to be simulated on the planning computer; furthermore, when using radiotherapy a treatment simulator is often employed, and when using hyperthermia "dry runs" with the actual heating equipment are sometimes conducted to complete the simulation procedure (MYERSON et al. 1991). In radiotherapy, patient treatment position verification using the laser alignment system, the light field, and the optical distance indicator in relation to skin markers and megavolt imaging (MEERTENS et al. 1990; VISSER et al. 1990) completes the treatment planning and guarantees an overall accuracy of about 5% (BRAHME et al. 1988). In hyperthermia, because of the influence of physiology where 80%–90% of all heat transfer is directly related to blood flow (LAGENDIJK et al. 1988), it is impossible to predict the final temperature distribution with reasonable accuracy. It is an absolute necessity to have a feedback system during the actual treatment. ROEMER and CETAS (1984) called this concurrent dosimetry; it entails the use of (invasive) thermometry and E-field probes to measure the temperature, the absorbed power (SAR) distributions, tissue cooling rates (ROEMER 1990; DE LEEUW et al. 1993), and effective thermal conductivities (CREZEE and LAGENDIJK 1990). After treatment all these treatment data can be used to optimize the treatment planning computations. ROEMER and CETAS (1984) called this retrospective thermal dosimetry, i.e., the use of all treatment data to calculate the final temperature/thermal dose distribution given. However, in must be stated that, except for simple temperature control feedback, no clinical (treatment planning) systems have been described in the literature which use these concurrent and retrospective thermal dosimetry aspects systematically to optimize treatment. As a first step, in vivo SAR measurements for optimizing regional RF hyperthermia are entering clinical use (DE LEEUW et al. 1993; WUST et al. 1992).

The final goal of hyperthermia treatment planning is to design the optimal treatment and to calculate the thermal dose given by this treatment. One problem is the definition of thermal dose (DEWHIRST 1992). For simplicity and practicability the treatment is normally described using the time-dependent temperature at the sensor sites

J.J.W. LAGENDIJK, PhD, Department of Radiotherapy, University Hospital Utrecht, Heidelberglaan 100 NL-3584 CX Utrecht, The Netherlands
J. CREZEE, PhD, Department of Radiotherapy, University Hospital Utrecht, Heidelberglaan 100, NL-3584 CX Utrecht, The Netherlands
J. MOOIBROEK, MSc, Department of Radiotherapy, University Hospital Utrecht, Heidelberglaan 100, NL-3584 CX Utrecht, The Netherlands

(HAND et al. 1989). This results in a spatial and temporal sampling of the actual temperature distribution (ROMANOWSKI et al. 1991) and a treatment description using parameters like T_{10}, T_{50} and T_{90} (the temperature that 10%, 50%, and 90% of all measured temperatures were at or above, respectively) as indicators of the actual temperature distribution and the thermal dose delivered. The temperature distribution depends on the SAR distribution generated by the heating system, the 3D distribution of the thermal properties (thermal property anatomy), the blood flow (perfusion) distribution, the discrete blood vessel network (thermally significant vessels) and the boundary conditions. Because of (a) changes in physiology, (b) changes in the actual treatment due to on-line interpretation of temperature data and (c) uncertainty/instability of system settings all these parameters will/may change during treatment. As described above, this renders obsolete the conventional treatment planning procedures. In hyperthermia treatment planning the concurrent dosimetry aspect is mandatory; conventional treatment planning will only provide guidelines to set up treatment and to design heating equipment. This physiology dependency and additional time-dependent parameter changes make hyperthermia treatment planning extremely difficult and necessitate the use of a wide variety of measurements during treatment.

In the currently available hyperthermia literature "treatment planning" is mostly limited to computation of SAR distributions. However, there is no straightforward relation between SAR and the thermal dose/temperature, as will be outlined in Sect. 20.2 on treatment strategy.

Great progress has been made in SAR planning for regional RF hyperthermia (see Chap. 18). First SAR planning systems are entering the clinic, for both radiofrequency systems (JAMES and SULLIVAN 1992; WUST et al. 1993; ZWAMBORN and VAN DEN BERG 1992) and ultrasound systems (McGOUGH et al. 1992). Present research on radiofrequency modeling is focused on techniques to perform 3D anatomy/dielectric imaging of individual patients (JAMES and SULLIVAN 1992; VAN DER KOIJK et al. 1993), the description of antennas and boundary conditions (HORNSLETH 1992; MOOIBROEK et al. 1993), and computer requirements and code optimization. Special attention is being given to the experimental and theoretical verification of the different models developed (COMAC BME/ESHO 1992). For regional and interstitial hyperthermia using low-frequency RF techniques, high-resolution quasi-static models have been developed (SOWINSKI and VAN DEN BERG 1990; VAN DER KOIJK et al. 1993). In ultrasound hyperthermia treatment planning the effort is focused on the 3D imaging of bony structures, soft tissue, and air and the alignment of the treatment beams in these structures, including looking for optimal entrance windows in order to prevent bone heating (McGOUGH et al. 1992). The short wavelengths using ultrasound allow easy steering but complicate the accurate SAR computation in complex anatomies due to the limited resolution of the computer models (HAND 1993).

At present SAR models find their major use in the understanding of heating systems, system optimization, and system design. The clinical application is still limited, mainly due to the computer and 3D imaging requirements, but first applications, especially to check for local hot spots/overdosage, have been published (BEN-YOSEF et al. 1993). The clinical application of hyperthermia treatment planning is mainly restricted by the need for further progress in thermal modeling (see Chap. 19) and especially in the anatomical/vascular input of the models.

In this chapter we will consider treatment strategy, tumor localization, i.e., the 3D imaging techniques and image processing techniques of interest for hyperthermia planning, and some clinical applications.

A thorough description of the requirements for hyperthermia treatment planning is given in the COMAC BME/ESHO task group report, *Treatment Planning and Modelling in Hyperthermia* (COMAC BME/ESHO 1992).

20.2 Treatment Strategy

The fundamental question in defining the treatment strategy is: what type of temperature distribution do we want and what type of SAR distribution and boundary conditions do we need to achieve this temperature distribution. No clear definition exists, taking into account all biological parameters, as to what type of temperature distribution is optimal. For reasons of simplicity we take as the optimal temperature distribution a distribution as uniform as possible in the tumor area, at the desired level, without any unwanted hot spots. To achieve this type of distribution, taking into account the important insight gained from thermal modeling theory that the major temperature inhomogeneities are caused by the thermally significant vessels (CHEN and HOLMES 1980; LAGENDIJK 1982) and especially their spatial density (the amount of vessels entering per cm^2) (LAGENDIJK et al. 1992), three basic strategies can be employed, as detailed below.

20.2.1 Strategy 1: Blood Preheating

This strategy is based on the idea that if the blood in the incoming vessels is preheated, a uniform temperature distribution will result. An essential parameter is the thermal equilibration length L_{eq} of the incoming vessels (TORELL and NILSSON 1978; CHEN and HOLMES 1980; CHATO 1980; LAGENDIJK 1982), i.e., the length it will take for the blood to become heated to within e^{-1} of the surrounding tissue temperature. This L_{eq} is of such a size, e.g., 10–20 cm for a typical 1-mm-diameter vessel, that large areas of normal tissue have to be heated to ensure that the blood enters the tumor at the desired temperature. The situation is even worse if we go further back along an arterial tree: we move towards larger vessels with a longer L_{eq}. However, we can state in general that the larger the normal tissue area heated, the better the temperature distribution will be, with the ultimate limit of a systemic temperature rise. Especially in regional radiofrequency hyperthermia, systemic temperature rise is normal and will directly improve the local temperature uniformity. The definition of L_{eq} considers with single vessels in a tissue cylinder with a uniform high boundary temperature, which implies that when there is a more or less uniform SAR the vessel density must be uniform to result in uniform temperature. Normally the vessel density will not be uniform: locations with a low vessel density and thus little cooling will reach a high temperature while locations with a high vessel density will stay at a generally low temperature. This implies that parallel entrance of more vessels or, directly related, vessel branching, will cool down the area and thus lengthen the thermal equilibration length and worsen the temperature situation. On the other hand, countercurrent heat exchange with venous blood vessels leaving a heated area will reduce the L_{eq} of incoming arteries and improve the temperature uniformity pleading for heating the whole organ containing the tumor. In general, the strategy of blood preheating calls for deposition of SAR outside the tumor target volume, mainly along the paths of the incoming vessels, and/or systemic temperature rise.

20.2.2 Strategy 2: Blood Cooling Compensation

This strategy is based on the idea that, if by having 3D small-scale SAR control the cooling towards the blood vessels in the tumor area is compensated, a relatively useful uniform temperature distribution results (LAGENDIJK et al. 1992, 1994). CREZEE and LAGENDIJK (1992) calculated the temperature distribution around a vessel with emphasis on the minimum temperature at the vessel wall (Fig. 20.1). They showed that because of the heat resistance of the blood in laminar flow vessels, acceptable temperatures at the vessel wall/tumor boundary can be achieved even with a worst case central blood temperature as low as 37°C provided that the k_{eff} is high enough and the local SAR is sufficient to compensate for the heat loss towards the vessel. The power needed and the resulting vessel wall tem-

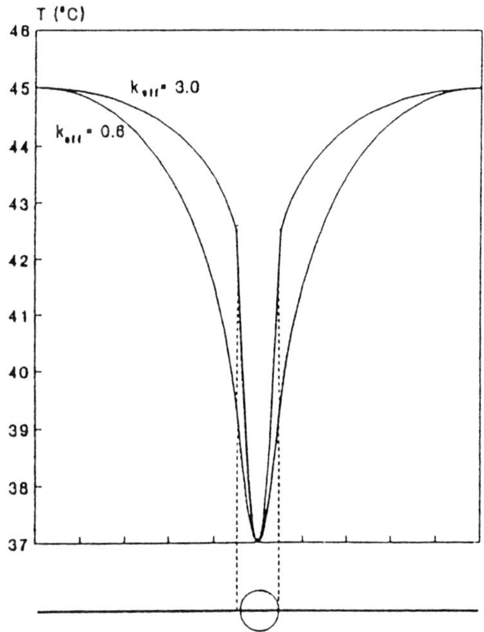

Fig. 20.1. Worst case radial temperature profile around a thermally developed vessel (vessel diameter 2 mm, tissue diameter 2 cm) with central temperature at body core temperature for an effective thermal conductivity of 0.6 and 3.0 $W m^{-1} °C^{-1}$. (From CREZEE and LAGENDIJK 1992)

perature depend on the local effective thermal conductivity (Fig. 20.2); higher wall temperatures are achieved in tissues with a high effective thermal conductivity (high perfusion), because the high effective thermal conductivity is associated with a low heat resistance in the tissue surrounding the vessel, while the vessel heat resistance in series with this tissue heat resistance is fixed. If this spatial SAR control can be realized the temperature boundary conditions for obtaining a minimal L_{eq} are being achieved (see strategy 1), which improves the situation even further due to optimal blood preheating. It must be realized that due to the three-dimensional vessel network the SAR steering must be fundamentally 3D; 2D steering will be of not great value. At present only interstitial hyperthermia (IHT) (potentially) and scanned focused ultrasound (SFUS) techniques can provide this smallscale SAR control. Using blood cooling compensation, two effects play an important role:

1. Vessel density: each vessel withdraws a certain amount of heat from the tissue. Without spatially controlled SAR, differences in vessel density cause differences in gross tissue cooling and thus large underdosed areas (LAGENDIJK et al. 1992, 1994) (Fig. 20.3a,b); 3D local SAR steering with about 1 cm resolution can compensate for this and cause a relatively uniform temperature distribution (Fig. 20.3c,d).
2. Single vessel: the underdosed area around a single vessel is diminished, its wall temperature is increased, and its L_{eq} is shortened by a high SAR at the vessel location (CREZEE and LAGENDIJK 1992).

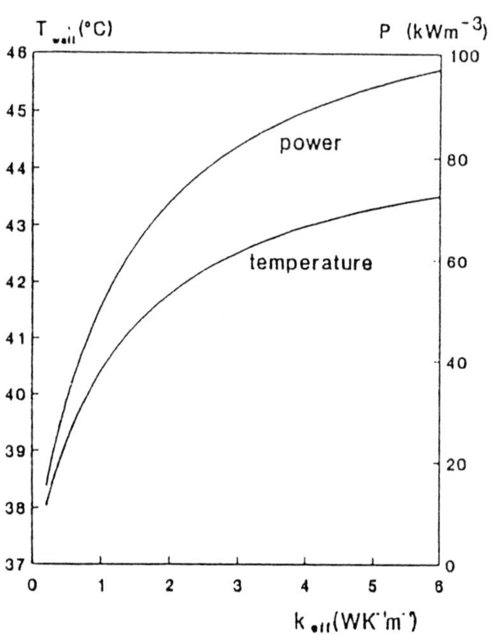

Fig. 20.2. Minimal vessel wall temperature and the power needed to raise the maximum temperature to 45°C versus k_{eff}. (From CREZEE and LAGENDIJK 1992)

20.2.3 *Strategy 3: High-Temperature Short-Duration (HTSD) Hyperthermia*

The principle behind HTSD hyperthermia is that the total thermal dose is given in such a short time that heat transfer towards vessels is too slow to cause any significant underdosage; the cooling influence of the vessels is limited to their immediate surroundings. This technique only works with very short heating times (5–20 s) and consequently requires high temperatures (47°–53°C; BORELLI et al. 1990). Studies concerning the development of HTSD are all based on scanned focused ultrasound techniques (HUNT et al. 1991; DORR and HYNYNEN 1992; LAGENDIJK et al. 1994). It is expected that this technique will enable a relatively uniform dose to be given without the need to have any knowledge of perfusion or location of and blood flow velocity within large vessels.

In Sect. 20.4 we will investigate how the above-described strategies impact on the design and application of heating techniques.

20.3 Imaging

20.3.1 *Specific Absorption Rate*

We shall first consider the calculation of the absorbed power distribution. As in radiotherapy treatment planning, computed tomography (CT) and magnetic resonance imaging (MRI) will supply the basic data for the planning in general. It is essential to realize that in contrast with much radiotherapy treatment planning, no simple 2D solution is satisfactory. In radiofrequency hyperthermia the influence of the 3D boundaries/anatomy is so strong that only 3D modeling will provide relevant data (WUST et al. 1992). In ultrasound hyperthermia 3D imaging is essential to guide the positioning of the beams relative to the air cavities and bony structures (McGOUGH et al. 1992).

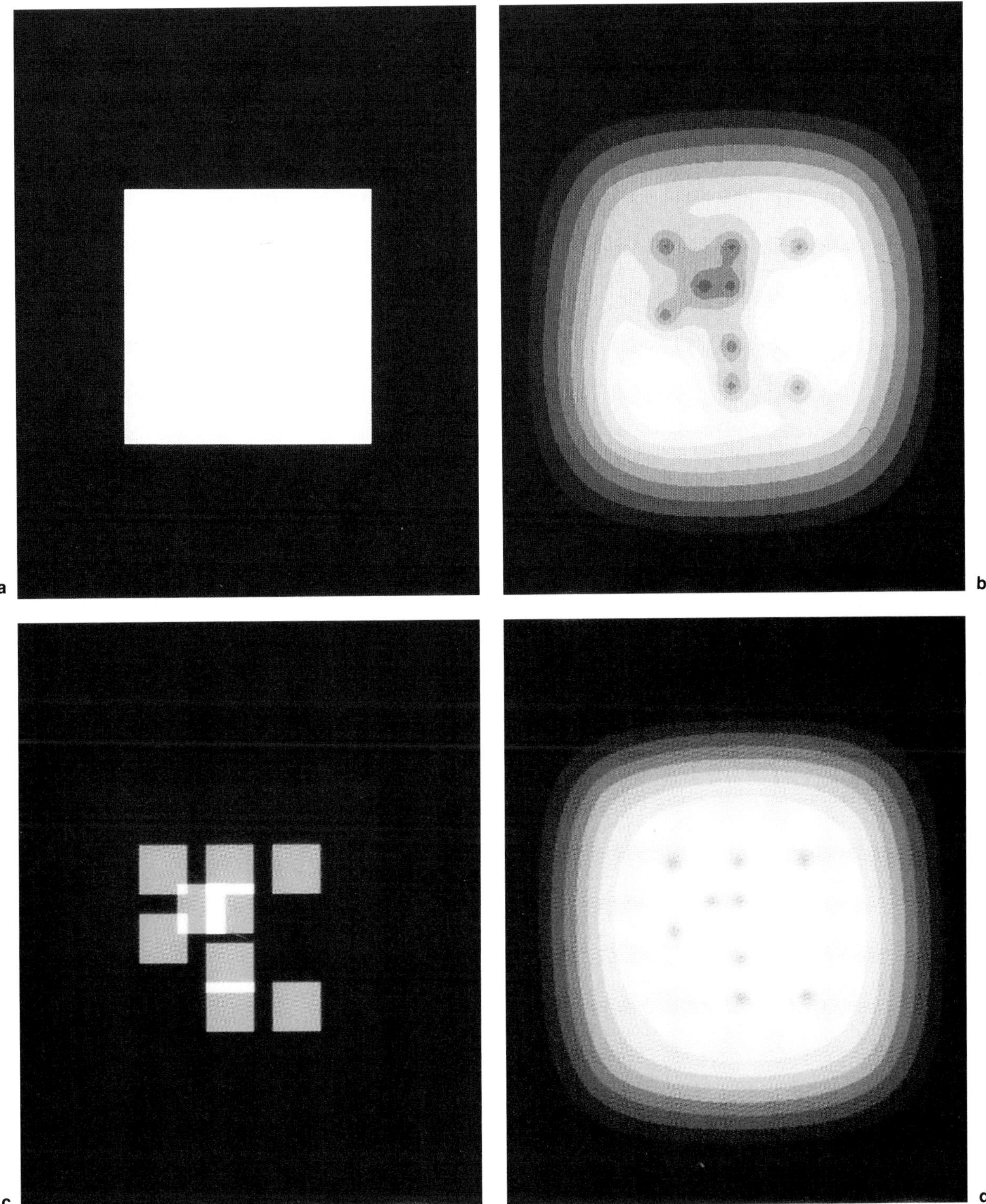

Fig. 20.3. The application of a uniform SAR (**a**: 5 × 5 cm area) to the volume containing a variable density of discrete vessels (nine vessels, blood temperature 37°C, k_{eff} = 1.8 W m^{-1}°C^{-1}) results in a highly nonuniform thermal dose distribution (**b**). Spatial control over SAR (**c**) results in the greatest temperature uniformity (**d**)

For both 3D CT and 3D MRI the present spatial small volume resolution is better than 1 mm and sufficient for the determination of the 3D anatomy. Geometrical accuracy for CT is perfect, while for MRI some care must be taken (a) in using external markers for positioning due to marker shifts caused by patient-induced susceptibility artifacts (BHAGWANDIEN et al. 1992) and (b) due to geometrical distortion caused by machine- and patient-related magnetic field nonuniformity and nonlinearity of the gradients (BAKKER et al. 1992).

Demands concerning patient positioning, repositioning, and position verification will vary greatly depending on the type of heating technology used. In SFUS the imaging position must be exactly the treatment position, as with radiotherapy; in regional radiofrequency (RF) hyperthermia no studies are yet available to define the positioning accuracy needed. In addition, the extension of the water bolus cannot be imaged at all and must be added later. The anatomy input requirements differ greatly for the two basic heating technologies, ultrasound (US) and RF.

20.3.1.1 RF: Dielectric Imaging

All RF and microwave techniques require the dielectric anatomy for accurate SAR computation. Segmentation according to gray scales is possible with CT. JAMES and SULLIVAN (1992) have provided a first study on the relation between Hounsfield units and dielectric properties. By gray-scale segmentation they can differentiate between low water content tissues like fat and bone and high water content tissues; lung will show values between air and soft tissue, dependent on the lung density. Because no physical relation exists between Hounsfield units and dielectric constants, James and Sullivan's method cannot differentiate between (high water content) soft tissues like gray and white brain matter. Physically the dielectric properties are related to the water content of tissues (GUY 1971; SCHEPPS and FOSTER 1980), which can relatively easily and automatically be defined in MRI by proton density imaging. VAN DER KOIJK et al. (1993) tested a multiple echo/multiple repetition time imaging procedure for acquiring the water content in different phantoms. A 5% accuracy was obtained with varying T_1 and T_2.

For small-scale hyperthermia applications like IHT, no major problems exist. However, for regional RF applications large volumes must be imaged which, depending on the model resolution desired, may result in long imaging times (and, using CT, considerable radiation doses). Data reduction techniques like replacing the legs and trunk with standard anatomies in the computation of pelvic SAR distributions using regional RF techniques must be evaluated.

Different segmentation techniques can be used:

1. Working at the voxel level, each voxel may be assigned specific dielectric properties allowing an accurate 3D computation with maximum detail. Care must be taken in choosing the resolution; too large a voxel may homogenize the anatomy due to partial volume effects. Working at the voxel level hinders easy 3D display of anatomy and SAR; normally 2D slices will be displayed with isodoses.
2. Working with volumes demands a volume segmentation guided by the clinician; this is time consuming but allows easy 3D display of organs and their spatial relations. Each volume is assigned a single set of dielectric properties, diminishing the detail in the computation. Clearly easy volume display, not allowing too much structure, is in conflict with detailed SAR computations.

20.3.1.2 US: Bone/Soft Tissues/Air

As stated above, in SFUS the imaging position must be the treatment position; this may represent a severe restriction in the development of SFUS heating techniques. The major interest lies in the 3D imaging of bony (and air) structures; the differences in soft tissues are only of minor importance and are not taken into account in the computations (HYNYNEN 1990). Because bone can easily be defined using CT imaging, the data acquisition for SFUS SAR planning will usually not be a problem. The major problem lies in the treatment position, which must be imageable. Relative positioning using on-line ultrasound imaging (LIZZI et al. 1988), small heating pulses to locate the focus related to the spatially known temperature sensors (HYNYNEN and LULU 1990), and/or an invasively positioned small ultrasound probe to calibrate the focus position (CAIN 1993) may diminish the positioning demands.

20.3.2 Thermal Modeling

For thermal modeling the imaging demands are much harder to fulfill. For thermal modeling we need:

1. Location, diameter, and flow velocity of all thermally significant vessels
2. Tissue perfusion (effective thermal conductivity)
3. The 3D anatomy (intrinsic thermal conductivity, specific heat)
4. Transient effects

For strategy 1, blood preheating, gross scale solutions may be sufficient to guide the treatment. Within the COMAC/ESHO task group report (1992) there was agreement to use the modified bioheat transfer equation as given Eq. 19.1 in Chap. 19. The heat transfer in the smaller vessels is described in this equation by the effective thermal conductivity (Chen and Holmes 1980; Crezee and Lagendijk 1990). This effective thermal conductivity includes the intrinsic thermal conductivity of the tissue, which is, however, of minor importance in the total heat transfer in tissue (Lagendijk et al. 1988). This implies that the anatomy is mainly of importance insofar as the tissue type defines the local physiological data/blood flow. Both CT and MRI are expected to be able to supply these data. The intrinsic perfusion distribution can be obtained from dynamic contrast imaging using both CT and MRI (Le Bihan and Turner 1993). A major problem, however, is the physiological reaction to the hyperthermia treatment, which makes on-line measurement techniques a necessity. Techniques to measure on-line blood flow-related parameters, such as the tissue cooling coefficient (Roemer 1990; Roemer et al. 1985; Lagendijk et al. 1988) and effective thermal conductivity (Crezee and Lagendijk 1992), have been described in the literature.

It will be clear that strategy 2, blood cooling compensation, requires that discrete large vessels (diameter $> \approx 0.5$ mm) be incorporated into the numerical thermal model. Recent developments in digital subtraction angiography (DSA) and especially magnetic resonance angiography (MRA) can be used to supply the vascular data. DSA is characterized by a good spatial resolution; however, it supplies only data on arterial vessels. Also, 3D reconstruction of the vessel locations from multiple 2D data is a major effort (Sun 1989). During the last few years, MRA has entered the clinical routine and evolved as a noninvasive technique which, at specific body sites, e.g., cerebral vessel anatomy, can compete with other standard angiographic methods (Potchen et al. 1993). It is expected that optimization of the hardware and software and use of special pulse sequences and/or contrast agents (Gd-DTPA), will further improve the resolution, and that other body sites such as the abdomen, pelvis, and extremities will become accessible (Potchen et al. 1993). A major advantage of MRA over other methods is its ability to image not only the 3D arterial architecture but also the venous vessel anatomy. Because in hyperthermia treatment planning the interest lies in the 3D path of the vessel, and not in, for example, the localization of stenoses, special pulse sequences are required. 3D low flow velocity and phase contrast techniques look promising: they supply the 3D tissue anatomy and the vessel tracks and give an indication of the flow velocity (Dumoulin et al. 1993).

The quantification of blood flow by MRA shows the same evolutionary trend as vessel imaging, although with some phase lag. The state of art in respect of this technique is reviewed by Firmin et al. (1993). Indirect quantification of large vessel blood flow via tissue perfusion and vessel network flow theory has to be evaluated.

One of the problems with respect to thermal modeling is how to represent both the vessel architecture and the flow in such a way that they can be loaded in a hyperthermia treatment planning system. For DSA several techniques have been developed to reconstruct vessel architecture from 2D or 3D vessel imaging data (Sun 1989). MRA-based work has been presented by Smets (1990), Vandermeulen (1991), and Kotte (1993). Kotte (1993) developed a special region growing algorithm to extract individual vessel segments from phase contrast MRA data which matches the segmental approach of vessels in the discrete vessel model (Mooibroek and Lagendijk 1991) (Fig. 20.4).

Image processing activities like stacking the 2D images into a 3D data set, contouring, voxel segmentation, 3D anatomy visualization, CT and MRI image correlation, and dose display fall outside the scope of this chapter but are discussed extensively in several handbooks, e.g., for 3D radiotherapy planning. General visualization software packages like AVS are being used to develop modules for hyperthermia and radiotherapy treatment planning (McGough et al. 1992; Buhle 1993).

20.4 Some Applications of (3D) Hyperthermia Treatment Planning

20.4.1 Scanned Focused Ultrasound

Scanned focused ultrasound is unique among noninvasive methods of inducing hyperthermia in that the SAR distribution may be controlled at a scale of 0.5 cm or better. This implies that, theoretically, extremely uniform temperature distributions can be obtained (Lagendijk et al. 1992, 1994). However, as discussed, the complete 3D discrete vessel network must be known and a 3D discrete vessel thermal model must be available to compute the temperature distribution to guide the steering of the focal volume. Research towards the minimum number of invasive thermometry sensors needed to guide the steering in the absence of such a model must be performed.

Tools to guide SAR steering in a 3D bony/air/soft tissue anatomy are being developed. These include aperture optimization or geometrical planning techniques (Hynynen 1990) to guide beam positioning, including optimizing entrance windows and tumor coverage without overheating bony structures (McGough et al. 1992). Intensity pattern optimization may be used to prevent too high focal intensities (Ebbini and Cain 1991).

Several studies on the development of SFUS-based HTSD techniques have been reported (Hunt et al. 1991; Dorr and Hynynen 1992; Lagendijk et al. 1994). HTSD SFUS techniques will diminish the extreme thermal modeling treatment planning demands; however, HTSD heating is sensitive to the effective thermal conductivity. In particular, heterogeneity in small vessel blood flow/perfusion and thus effective thermal conductivity can result in heterogeneity in the thermal dose distribution (Billard et al. 1990). Because every volume is irradiated once using a small focus without use of temperature distribution smearing due to heat transfer, the required positioning accuracy is extremely high. Relative positioning within the tumor volume on the order of the focus dimension, usually a few mm, is needed. To prevent background heating the focus must step slowly and preferably via a semirandom pattern through the volume (Lagendijk et al. 1994).

20.4.2 Interstitial Hyperthermia

In IHT, thermometry can be performed from within the brachytherapy catheters/needles already present; in theory this means that a good impression of the 3D temperature distribution can be obtained. This fact, the well-defined heating techniques, and the relatively small volumes heated make IHT an ideal test site for hyperthermia treatment planning.

Many authors have computed the temperature distribution in IHT using the conventional bioheat transfer equation (Chap. 19 in this volume; Strohbehn et al. 1982; Strohbehn 1983; Brezovich and Atkinson 1984; Babbs et al. 1990; Schreier et al. 1990). The common pattern in these predictions is an underdosage between the interstitial needles which increases with increasing perfusion, with temperatures remaining high near the needles. The predictions made by the effective thermal conductivity model and experimental verifications do not show these unfavorable perfusion effects (Crezee and Lagendijk 1990; Crezee and Lagendijk 1992). Schreier et al. (1990), heating porcine thighs, also found more favorable temperatures than predicted with the conventional bioheat equation. As discussed in Chap. 19 by Mooibroek et al., these results can be expected since the main temperature nonuniformity is caused by the discrete vessels, while small vessel blood flow homogenizes the temperature distribution. As described in Sect. 20.2, to achieve optimal uniform temperature distributions, 3D spatial SAR control with about 1 cm resolution is needed to compensate for discrete vessel cooling. It can easily be shown that the interstitial techniques which provide just 2D control in an anatomy containing 3D vessel structures are only able to obtain a useful temperature distribution if this volume is small and the electrodes/antennas are short. Present-day systems are often characterized by uncontrolled inhomogeneities in the temperature distributions obtained (Goffinet et al. 1990). This dose nonuniformity limits the clinical acceptance despite some good preliminary clinical results (Cosset 1990; Salcman and Samaras 1983; Roberts et al. 1986; Silberman et al. 1985). Sneed et al. (1992) showed in the treatment of gliomas that a more uniform dose (higher T_{90}) directly resulted in a higher local response. Volumes larger that a few cubic centimeters can only be heated uniformly with IHT systems which provide sufficient longitudinal *and* transversal SAR control.

In Utrecht we are developing, in collaboration with the Dr. Daniel den Hoed Cancer Center in Rotterdam and Nucletron International, a multielectrode current source IHT system and an IHT hyperthermia treatment planning system (LAGENDIJK et al. 1995). We incorporate the 3D anatomy (10 × 10 × 10 cm) at a 1 mm spatial resolution. By the use of local analytical solutions, discrete vessels and catheters/needles down to about 0.5 mm diameter can be inserted in the model (DE BREE 1994; KOTTE 1993). Modern Unix workstations can easily handle this amount of data while both the Dufort Frankle algorithm and multigrid methods speed up computation. Speed and interactivity are important because predicted areas of underdosage may require direct insertion of extra catheters during implant in IHT, or direct control of focus intensity and location in SFUS. Present applications are limited by the 3D angiography input, not by computer power. As an example of the 3D IHT treatment planning computations, Fig. 20.4 gives the temperature distribution predicted in a seven-catheter implant in brain, using a segmented anatomy and realistic vessel network. The temperature distribution has been calculated for both 4-cm-long LCF electrodes and segmented "current source electrodes." Figure 20.5 gives the temperature volume histogram for both situations.

20.4.3 Regional RF Hyperthermia

With respect to treatment strategy, deep regional heating comes closest to the strategy of blood preheating, as relatively large tissue volumes containing normal tissue are raised to temperatures in the range of 40°–43°C (VAN ES et al. 1992; ANSCHER et al. 1992; LEOPOLD et al. 1992; FELDMANN et al. 1993). This feature leads to a gradual increase in systemic temperature with concomitant changes in heart rate and blood pressure. Reported figures on systemic temperatures reached during regional hyperthermia range from 37.5° to 40.0°C. (FELDMANN et al. 1993; VAN Es et al. 1992). Large vessel blood entering the tumor volume will therefore not only have higher basal temperatures but also gain an additional temperature increase through heat exchange in the heated healthy tissues around the tumor. Inasmuch as such an intentionally applied strategy is not treatment limiting through unacceptable systemic stress, local pain complaints, or enhanced tissue toxicity, this contributes to higher T_{90} temperatures (local data).

Efforts in clinical treatment planning have mostly been limited to the computation of the 2D SAR distribution with the aim of optimization of system settings, i.e., phase and amplitude of individual applicators (STROHBEHN et al. 1989; WUST et al. 1991) or by patient shift (DE LEEUW et al. 1993). Despite some critical remarks on the dimensionality of SAR models with respect to the computing demands (PAULSEN and ROSS 1990), the general opinion is that 3D SAR modeling is a necessity because of the influence of the 3D boundaries/anatomy (PAULSEN 1990; Chap. 18 in this volume). 2D models tend to overestimate the power penetration depth while important features like aberrant heating (HAGMANN and LEVIN 1986) and influence of bolus extension (MOOIBROEK et al. 1993) are missed completely. Moreover, the 3D SAR models are indispensable for system optimization (WUST et al. 1993; MOOIBOEK et al. 1993) or new system design. Recently SULLIVAN et al. (1993) reported on the clinical use of a fully 3D computer program based on individual patient anatomical CT data (JAMES and SULLIVAN 1992).

20.5 Summary

- A major problem in hyperthermia is the still limited capacity of the present heating systems in providing the thermal dose and dose uniformity clinically wanted.
- The temperature uniformity problems can be solved following the three different strategies each with its own treatment planning demands. In our opinion strategy 2, namely blood cooling compensation by spatial SAR control at a centimetre scale, has the best prospects.
- Spatial SAR control can be obtained with 3D controlled interstitial (IHT) systems and scanned focused ultrasound systems (SFUS).
- SFUS has to rely fully on the knowledge provided by treatment planning, the IHT systems may rely too on extensive in vivo thermometry in the catheters already present; the latter may first enter the clinic.
- To exploit the full potential of 3D spatial SAR control a multi-electrode (64 channels) current

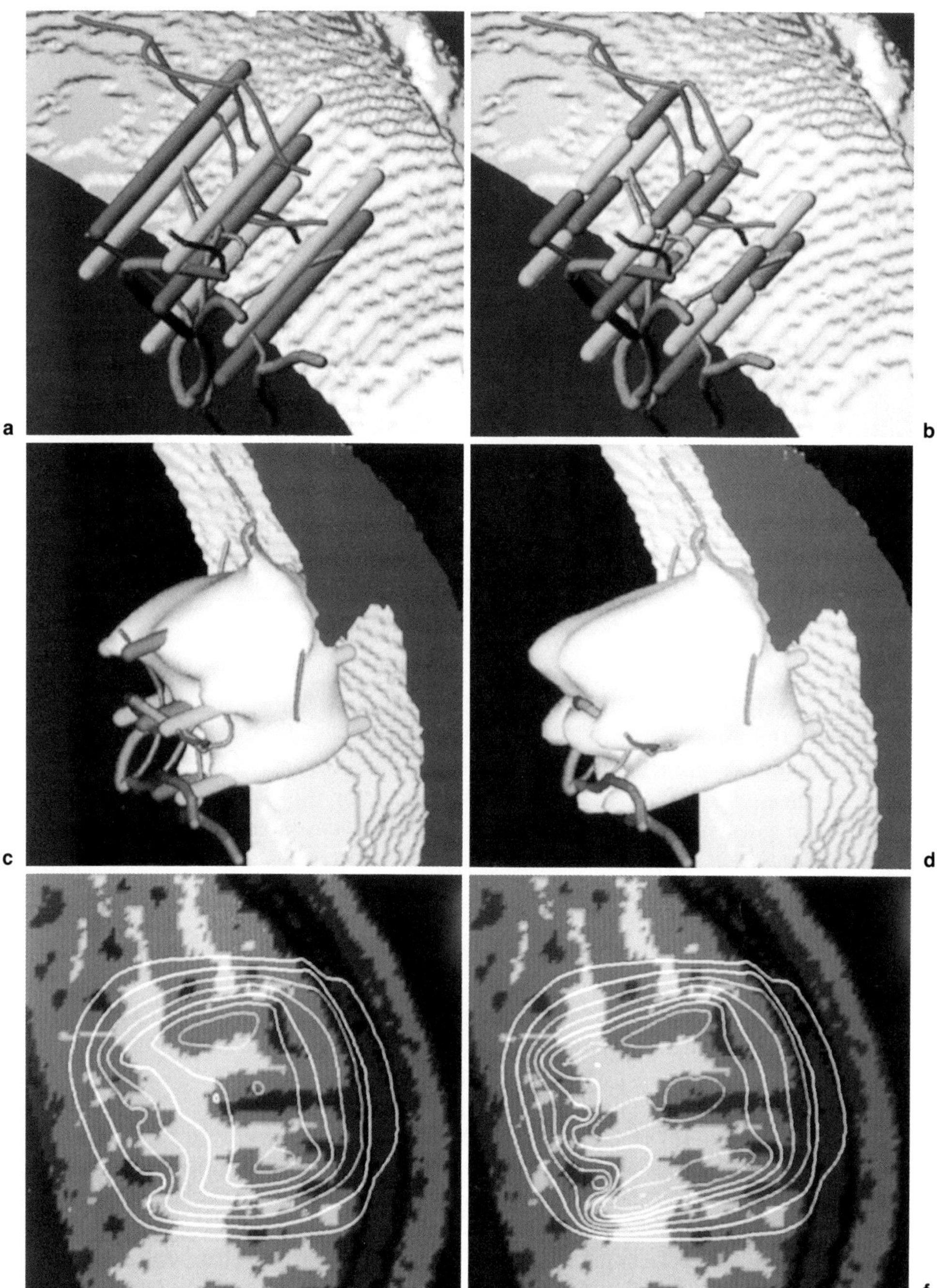

Fig. 20.4a–f. Seven-catheter implant and vascular anatomy, 6 × 6 × 6 cm volume of the upper right part of the brain. **a** Mono electrodes; **b** segmented electrodes (three segments 1.3 cm along one catheter, spacing 0.5 cm). **c,d** Simulated temperature distribution; 3D 42°C isosurface display. **c** Mono electrodes; **d** segmented electrodes. **e,f** Simulated temperature distribution; 2D isotherm display through central electrodes. **e** Mono electrodes; **f** segmented electrodes

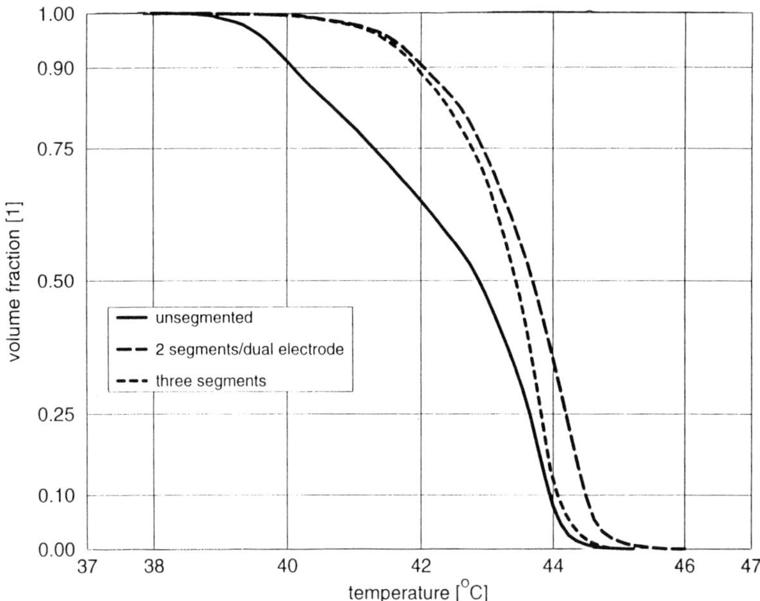

Fig. 20.5. Temperature volume histograms for the stationary distributions of Fig. 20.4

source (MECS) interstitial hyperthermia system and a complete on-line interstitial hyperthermia treatment planning system is being developed to be used for simultaneous hyperthermia and external radiation.

References

Anscher MS, Samulski TV, Leopold KA, Oleson JR (1992) Phase I/II study of external radio frequency phased array hyperthermia and external beam radiotherapy in the treatment of prostate cancer: technique and results of intraprostatic temperature measurements. Int J Radiat Oncol Biol Phys 24: 489–495

Babbs CF, Fearnot NE, Marchosky JA, Moran CJ, Jones JT, Plantenga TD (1990) Theoretical basis for controlling minimal tumor temperature during interstitial conductive heat therapy. IEEE Trans Biomed Eng 37: 662–672

Bakker CJG, Moerland MA, Bhagwandien R, Beersma R (1992) Analysis of machine-dependent and object-induced geometric distortion in 2DFT MR imaging. Magn Reson Imaging 10: 597–608

Ben-Yosef R, Sullivan DM, Kapp DS (1993) Peripheral neuropathy and myonecrosis following hyperthermia and radiation therapy for recurrent prostatic cancer: correlation of damage with predicted SAR pattern. Int J Hyperthermia 8: 173–185

Bhagwandien R., van Ee R., Beersma R., Bakker CJG, Moerland MA, Lagendijk JJW (1992) Numerical analysis of the magnetic field for arbitrary magnetic susceptibility distributions in 2D. Magn Reson Imaging 10: 299–313

Billard BE, Hynynen K, Roemer RB (1990) Effect of physical parameters on high temperature ultrasound hyperthermia. Ultrasound Med Biol 16: 409–420

Borelli J, Thompson LL, Cain CA, Dewey WC (1990) Time-temperature analysis of cell killing of BHK cells heated at temperatures in the range of 43.5°C to 57.0°C. Int J Radiat Oncol Biol Phys 19: 389–399

Brahme A, Chavaudra J, Landberg T et al. (1988) Accuracy requirements and quality assurance of external beam radiotherapy with photons and electrons. Acta Oncol 27: Suppl. 1

Brezovich IA, Atkinson WJ (1984) Temperature distributions in tumor models heated by self-regulating nickel-copper alloy thermoseeds. Med Phys 11: 145–152

Buhle EL Jr (1993) Use of AVS in radiotherapy treatment planning. AVS Network News 2: 46–48

Chato JC (1980) Heat transfer to blood vessels. J Biomech Eng 102: 110–118

Chen MM, Holmes KR (1980) Microvascular contributions in tissue heat transfer. Ann NY Acad Sci 335: 137–151

COMAC BME/ESHO Task Group Report (1992) Treatment planning and modelling in hyperthermia (Task Group committee chairman: Lagendijk JJW). Tor Vergata Medical Physics Monograph Series

Cosset JM (1990) Interstitial hyperthermia. In: Goutherie M (ed) Interstitial, endocavitary and perfusional hyperthermia. Springer, Berlin Heidelberg New York, pp 1–41

Crezee J, Lagendijk JJW (1990) Measurement of temperature profiles around large artificial vessels in perfused tissue. Phys Med Biol 35: 905–923

Crezee J, Lagendijk JJW (1992) Temperature uniformity during hyperthermia: the impact of large vessels. Phys Med Biol 37: 1321–1337

De Leeuw AAC, Mooibroek J, Lagendijk JJW (1991) SAR-steering by patient positioning in the "Coaxial TEM" system: phanton investigation. Int J Hyperthermia 7: 605–611

De Leeuw AAC, Crezee H, Lagendijk JJW (1993) Temperature and SAR measurements in deep-body hyperthermia with thermocouple thermometry. Int J Hyperthermia 9: 685–697

Dewhirst MW (1992) Thermal dosimetry. In: Gerner EG, Cetas TC (eds) Hyperthermic oncology 1992, vol 2. Arizona Board of Regents, pp 39–43

Dorr LN, Hynynen K (1992) The effects of tissue heterogeneities and large blood vessels on the thermal exposure induced by short high-power ultrasound pulses. Int J Hyperthermia 8: 45–60

Dumoulin CL, Souza SP, Pele NJ (1993) Phase-sensitive flow imaging. In: Potchen EJ, Haacke EM, Siebert JE, Gottschalk A (eds) Magnetic resonance angiography. Mosby, St. Louis, pp 173–188

Ebbini ES, Cain CA (1991) Optimization of the intensity gain of multiple-focus phased-array heating pattern. Int J Hyperthermia 7: 953–973

Feldmann HJ, Molls M, Heinemann H-G, Romanowski R, Stuschke M, Sack H (1993) Thermoradiotherapy in locally advanced deep seated tumours- thermal parameters and treatment results. Radiother Oncol 26: 38–44

Firmin DN, Dumoulin CL, Mohiaddin RH (1993) Quantitative flow imaging. In: Potchen EJ, Haacke EM, Siebert JE, Gottschalk A (eds) Magnetic resonance angiography. Mosby, St. Louis, pp 187–219

Goffinet DR, Prionas SD, Kapp DS et al. (1990) Interstitial 192 Ir flexible catheter radiofrequency hyperthermia treatments of head and neck and recurrent pelvic carcinomas. Int J Radiat Oncol Biol Phys 18: 199–210

Guy AW (1971) Analysis of electromagnetic fields induced in biological tissues by thermographic studies on equivalent phantom models. IEEE Trans Biomed Eng 31: 115–119

Hagmann MJ, Levin RL (1986) Aberrant heating: a problem in regional hyperthermia. IEEE Trans Biomed Eng 33: 405–411

Hand JW, Lagendijk JJW, Andersen, JB, Bolomey JC (1989) Quality assurance quidelines for ESHO protocols. Int J Hyperthermia 5: 421–428

Hornsleth SN (1992) The finite difference time domain method and its application to hyperthermia simulations. In: Gerner EG, Cetas TC (eds) Hyperthermic oncology, vol 2. Arizona Board of Regents, pp 271–273

Hunt JW, Lalonde R, Ginsberg H, Urchuk S, Worthington A (1991) Rapid heating: critical theoretical assessment of thermal gradients found in hyperthermia treatments. Int J Hyperthermia 7: 703–718

Hynynen K (1990) Biophysics and technology of ultrasound hyperthermia. In: Gautherie M (ed) Methods of external hyperthermic heating. Springer, Berlin Heidelberg New York, pp 61–115

Hynynen K, Lulu BA (1990) State of art in medicine: hyperthermia in cancer treatment. Invest Radiol 25: 824–834

James BJ, Sullivan DM (1992) Creation of three-dimensional patient models for hyperthermia treatment planning. IEEE Trans Biomed Eng 39: 238–242

Lagendijk JJW (1982) The influence of blood flow in large vessels on the temperature distribution in hyperthermia. Phys Med Biol 27: 17–23

Lagendijk JJW, Hofman P, Schipper J (1988) Perfusion analyses in advanced breast carcinoma during hyperthermia. Int J Hyperthermia 4: 479–495

Lagendijk JJW, Crezee J, Mooibroek J (1992) Progress in thermal modelling development. In: Gerner EG, Cetas TC (eds) Hyperthermic Oncology 1992, vol 2. Arizona Board of Regents, pp 257–260

Lagendijk JJW, Hand JW, Crezee J (1994) Dose uniformity in scanned focused ultrasound hypethermia. Int J Hyperthermia 10/6: 775–784

Lagendijk JJW, Visser AG, Kaatee RSJP et al. (1995) The multi-electrode current source interstitial hyperthermia method. Activity Special Report 6: 83–90

Le Bihan D, Turner R (1993) Diffusion and perfusion nuclear magnetic resonance imaging. In: Potchen EJ, Haacke EM, Siebert JE, Gottschalk A (eds) Magnetic resonance angiography. Mosby, St. Louis, pp 323–342

Leopold KA, Dewhirst M, Samulski T et al. (1992) Relationships among tumor temperature treatment time, and histopathological outcome using preoperative hyperthermia with radiation in soft tissue sarcomas. Int J Radiat Oncol Biol Phys 22: 989–998

Lizzi F, Ostromogilski M, Dumke A, Lunzer B, Driller J, Loleman D (1988) A computer imaging and graphics system for planning ultrasound therapy in the eye. J Ultrasound in Medicine 7(Suppl): 556

McGough RJ, Ebbini ES, Cain CA (1992) Optimization of apertures and intensity patterns for hyperthermia with ultrasound pased array systems. In: Gerner EG, Cetas TC (eds) Hyperthermic oncology 1992, vol 2. Arizona Board of Regents, pp 205–209

Meertens H, Bijhold J, Stackee J (1990) A method for the measurement of field placement errors in digital portal imaging. Phys Med Biol 35: 299–323

Mooibroek J, Lagendijk JJW (1991) A fast and simple algorithm for the calculation of convective heat transfer by large vessels in three dimensional inhomogeneous tissues. IEEE Trans Biomed Eng 38: 490–501

Mooibroek J, De Leeuw AAC, Lagendijk JJW (1993) Theoretical and experimental investigation of 3-D SAR distribution in elliptical phantoms irradiated by the "Coaxial TEM" applicator. Proc 2nd Int Sc Meeting: Microwaves in Medicine, Rome, pp 105–108

Myerson RJ, Leybovich L, Emami B, Grigsby PW, Straube W, Von Gerichten D (1991) Phantom studies and preliminary clinical experience with the BSD 2000. Int J Hyperthermia 7: 937–951

Paulsen KD (1990) Calculation of power deposition patterns in hyperthermia. In: Gautherie M (ed) Thermal dosimetry and treatment planning. Clinical thermology, subseries thermotherapy. Springer, Berlin Heidelberg New York, pp 57–117

Paulsen KD, Ross MP (1990) Comparison of numerical calculations with phantom experiments and clinical measurements. Int J Hyperthermia 6: 333–349

Potchen EJ, Haacke EM, Siebert JE, Gottschalk A (eds) (1993) Magnetic resonance angiography, Mosby, St. Louis

Roberts DW, Coughlin CT, Wong TZ, Fratkin JD, Douple EB, Strohbehn JW (1986) Interstitial hyperthermia and iridium brachytherapy in treatment of malignant glioma. J Neurosurg 64: 581–587

Roemer RB (1990) The local tissue cooling coefficient: a unified approach to thermal washout and steady-state "perfusion" calculations. Int J Hyperthermia 6: 421–430

Roemer RB, Cetas TC (1984) Applications of bioheat transfer simulations in hyperthermia. Cancer Res 44: 4788s–4798s

Roemer RB, Fletcher AM, Cetas TC (1985) Obtaining

local SAR and blood perfusion data from temperature measurements: steady-state and transient techniques compared. Int J Radiat Oncol Biol Phys 11: 1539–1550

Romanowski R, Schott C, Feldmann HJ, Molls M (1991) Numeric description of thermometry quality in regional hyperthermia: the S-quotient. Strahlenther Onkol 167: 337

Salcman M, Samaras GM (1983) Interstitial hyperthermia for brain tumors. J Neurooncol 1: 225–236

Schepps JL, Foster KR (1980) The UHF and microwave dielectric properties of normal and tumor tissues: variation in dielectric properties with tissue water content. Phys Med Biol 25, pp 1149–1159

Schreier K, Budihna M, Lesnicar H et al. (1990) Preliminary studies of interstitial hyperthermia using hot water. Int J Hyperthermia 6: 431–444

Silberman AW, Rand RW, Storm FK, Drury B, Benz ML, Morton DL (1985) Phase I trial of thermochemotherapy for brain malignancy. Cancer 56: 48–56

Smets C (1990) A knowledge-based system for the automatic interpretation of blood vessels on angiograms. PhD Thesis. Katholieke Universiteit Leuven

Sneed PK, Gutin PH, Stauffer PR et al. (1992) Thermoradiotherapy of recurrent malignant brain tumors. Int J Radiat Oncol Biol Phys 23: 853–861

Sowinski MJ, van den Berg PM (1990) A three-dimensional iterative scheme for an electromagnetic capacitive applicator. IEEE Trans Biomed Eng 37: 975–986

Strohbehn JW (1983) Temperature distributions from interstitial rf electrode hyperthermia systems: theoretical predictions. Int J Radiat Oncol Biol Phys 9: 1655–1667

Strohbehn JW, Trembly BS, Douple EB (1982) Blood flow effects on the temperature distributions from an invasive microwave antenna array used in cancer therapy. IEEE Trans Biomed Eng 29: 649–661

Strohbehn JW, Curtis EH, Paulsen KD, Yuan X, Lynch DR (1989) Optimization of the absorbed power distribution for an annular phased array hyperthermia system. Int J Radiat Oncol Biol Phys 16: 589–599

Sullivan DM, Ben-Yosef R, Kapp DS (1993) Stanford 3D hyperthermia treatment planning system. Technical review and clinical summary. Int J Hyperthermia 9: 627–643

Sun Y (1989) Automated identification of vessel contours in coranary arteriograms by an adaptive tracking algorithm. IEEE Trans Med Imaging 8: 78–88

Torell LM, Nilsson SK (1978) Temperature gradients in low-flow vessels. Phys Med Biol 23: 106–117

Van der Koijk JF, Bakker CJG, de Bree J et al. (1993) Development of an interstitial hyperthermia treatment planning system. Proc 2nd Int Sc Meeting: Microwaves in Medicine, Rome, pp 109–112

Van der Meulen D (1991) Methods for registration, interpolation of three dimensional medical image data for use in 3D display, 3D modelling and therapy planning. PhD Thesis, Katholieke Universiteit Leuven

Van Es CA, Wijrdeman HK, De Leeuw AAC, Lagendijk JJW, Battermann JJ (1992) Pilot study. Regional hyperthermia with the "Coaxial TEM" system in advanced pelvic disease. In: Gerner EW (ed) Hyperthermic oncology 1992, vol 1. Summary papers. Arizona Board of Regents, p 415

Visser AG, Huizenga H, Althof VG, Swanenburg BN (1990) Performance of a prototype fluoroscopic radiotherapy imaging system. Int J Radiat Oncol Biol Phys 18: 43–50

Wust P, Nadobny J, Felix R, Deuflhard P, Louis A, John W (1991) Strategies for optimized application of annular-phased-array systems in clinical hyperthermia. Int J Hyperthermia 7: 157–173

Wust P, Nadobny J, Seebass M, Fahling H, Felix R (1992) Potential of radiofrequency hyperthermia: planning, optimization, technological development. In: Gerner EG, Cetas TC (eds) Hyperthermic oncology 1992, vol 2. Arizona Board of Regents, pp 65–72

Wust P, Nadobny J, Seebass M, Dohlus M, John W, Felix R (1993) 3D computation of E fields by the volume surface integral equation (VSIE) method in comparison with the finite integration theory (FIT) method. IEEE Trans Biomed Eng vol. 40 (8): 745–759

Zwamborn APM, van den Berg PM (1992) The three-dimensional weak form of the conjugate gradient FFT method for solving scattering problems. IEEE Trans Microwave Theory Tech 40: 1757–1766

21 Technical and Clinical Quality Assurance

A.G. VISSER and G.C. VAN RHOON

CONTENTS

21.1 Introduction

Several documents have recently been published that are generally related to technical and clinical aspects of quality assurance (QA) in hyperthermic oncology, and these documents can now serve as a baseline for all institutions involved in clinical HT applications and multicenter trials. In Table 21.1 the main area of interest for each of these documents is given. Furthermore, QA guidelines for hyperthermic treatments have been discussed within the framework of the European COMAC-BME Hyperthermia project which ran between 1989 and 1992, and specifically during a workhop on "Quality Assurance in Hyperthermia" held in Sabaudia, Italy (COMAC Hyperthermia Bulletin 5, 1991).

Besides the aim of maximizing clinical outcome, an equally important goal of QA is the provision of a basic set of objective physical parameters to enable evaluation and comparison of the performance of the available heating systems at specific tumor sites. In this chapter we give an overview of available QA *methods* for different types of hyperthermia treatments (i.e., external heating of both superficial and deep-seated tumors and interstitial methods), rather than a complete summary of existing QA guidelines. It should be mentioned that we have refrained from discussing the QA aspects of hyperthermia treatments using ultrasound (see Chap. 15 regarding ultrasound thermometry QA).

After discussing the need for QA in hyperthermic oncology, emphasis will be put on the background of techniques to characterize the performance for electromagnetic applicators. Furthermore, for superficial hyperthermia of chest wall recurrences and locoregional hyperthermia of deep-seated malignancies in the pelvis, the thermometry requirements are discussed in some depth as these tumor sites are the most frequently heated in the clinical situation. Additionally, minimal requirements are proposed for the hyperthermia staff needed to provide good-quality hyperthermia treatments. Finally, a discussion is presented on current trends in applicator research which aim to improve the quality of the electromagnetic heating techniques.

21.2 The Need for Quality Assurance

During the last two decades many clinical studies on superficially located tumors have demonstrated that local hyperthermia given in combination with

A.G. VISSER, PhD, Department of Clinical Physics, Dr. Daniel den Hoed Cancer Center, P.O. Box 5201, Groene Hilledijk 301, NL-3008 AE Rotterdam, The Netherlands G.C. VAN RHOON PhD, Department of Hyperthermia, Dr. Daniel den Hoed Cancer Center, P.O. Box 5201, Groene Hilledijk 301, NL-3008 AE Rotterdam, The Netherlands

Table 21.1. Overview of recently published QA guidelines for hyperthermic oncology

Authors	Reference	Main area of interest
AAPM (1989)	Am Assoc Phys Med.	Performance evaluation of equipment
HAND et al. (1989)	Int J Hyperthermia 5: 421–428	ESHO QA guidelines: superficial HT
SHRIVASTAVA et al. (1989)	IJROBP 16: 571–587	General QA guidelines
DEWHIRST et al. (1990)	IJROBP 18: 1249–1259	QA for multi-institutional trials, emphasis on microwave heating
SAPOZINK et al. (1991)	IJROBP 20: 1109–1115	Deep-seated tumors (>3 cm depth)
WATERMAN et al. (1991)	IJROBP 20: 1099–1107	Ultrasound heating
EMAMI et al. (1991)	IJROBP 20: 1117–1124	Interstitial heating

IJROBP, International Journal of Radiation Oncology, Biology, Physics

radiotherapy has a great potential to improve the local control rate. For chest wall recurrences of metastatic breast cancer the local control rates with conventional therapy are poor: the administration of low-dose radiotherapy alone at doses of about 30–35 Gy results in complete response (CR) rates ranging from 20% to 27%. With the same range of radiotherapy doses in combination with local hyperthermia a much better local control rate is commonly obtained, with CR rates from 58% to 88% (GONZALEZ GONZALEZ et al. 1988; HOFMAN et al. 1984; JO et al. 1987; KAPP et al. 1988a; KJELLEN et al. 1989; PEREZ et al. 1986; PEREZ and EMAMI 1989; SEEGENSCHMIEDT et al. 1988; VAN DER ZEE et al. 1988; MASUNAGA et al. 1990).

Although these results are impressive, several studies indicate that the clinical outcome can still be improved substantially by improving the quality of the hyperthermic treatment. Correlations between minimum or average intratumoral temperature and patient treatment outcome, response rate, and duration of response have been found (OLESON et al. 1984, 1989; LUK et al. 1984; HIRAOKA et al. 1984; ARCANGELI et al. 1985; VAN DER ZEE et al. 1985, 1986; DEWHIRST et al. 1986). More recently the impact of QA on the therapeutic outcome of the RTOG 81-04 study has been reported by PEREZ et al. (1989). These authors hypothesized that the CR rate for patients with smaller chest wall tumors (diameter < 3 cm) was higher than that for larger tumors (diameter > 3 cm), 55% versus 24%, because the smaller tumors were easier to heat adequately. Other clinical data illustrating the impact of QA on clinical outcome are provided by MYERSON et al. (1990), who showed a significant correlation between local control and tumor coverage by at least the 25% iso-SAR contour [65% (22/34) vs 21% (4/19)] and by VAN DER ZEE et al. (1992b). In the latter, DDHCC, study we demonstrated that in our patient group with large superficial breast cancer recurrences (diameter > 3 cm), a significant ($P = 0.006$) increase occurred in the CR rate from 31% (4/13) to 75% (30/40) for which no other explanation could be found than the use of a better heating technique in the more recently treated patients (27-MHz capacitive heating, 433-MHz single applicator ("patchwork") heating, and 2450-MHz multiapplicator heating versus the present 433-MHz multiapplicator multigenerator hyperthermia system). At the same time the CR achieved in small superficial breast cancer recurrences (diameter ≥ 3 cm) was 92% (12/13) with the older heating techniques versus 91% (42/46) for the present 433-MHz heating system. For our patient group the influence of the quality of the heat treatment on the therapeutic outcome may be demonstrated quantitatively in the following formula:

$$P_{(cr)} = 0.6 \times P_{(ht)} + 0.3,$$

where: $P_{(cr)}$ is the *net* probability of a CR; $P_{(ht)}$ is the probability of adequate heating; the probability of CR when treated with radiotherapy alone (RT; 8 × 4 Gy) is taken to be 0.3; and the term 0.6 stems from the difference between the probability of CR (0.9; small tumors) for RT given with an assumed 100% adequate heating and the CR (0.3) for RT alone. In multi-institutional trials the quality of the hyperthermia treatment can be expected to show variations and this will be reflected in a decreased response rate and thus in the need for a larger patient population within multi-institutional phase III studies. Using this linear relation between the probabilities of adequate heating and CR, the effect of variations in the quality of the

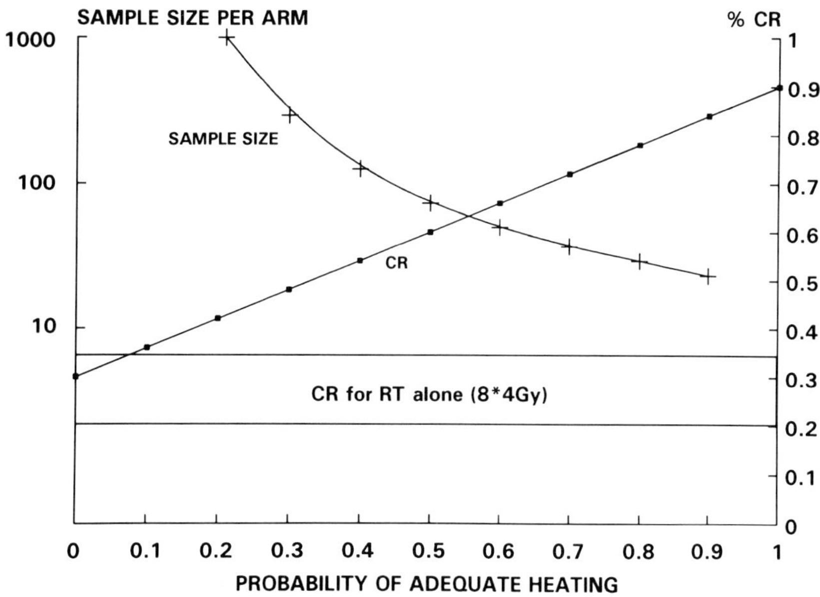

Fig. 21.1. The impact of adequate heating on the complete response rate (CR) for chest wall tumors and the sample size per treatment arm for a randomized phase III trial

hyperthermia treatment on CR and the sample size needed for phase III trials is illustrated in Fig. 21.1.

Hence, there is sufficient clinical evidence to support the view that a large group of patients could benefit substantially from improved quality standards. Although these clinical data concern only combined radiotherapy plus hyperthermia for superficially located tumors, there is no reason to suppose that the same would not apply to the treatment of deep-seated tumors.

21.3 Procedures for Quality Assurance

The existing QA guidelines as listed in Table 21.1 describe in detail which QA performance checks have to performed to characterize the performance of a hyperthermia system. It must be realized, however, that these QA checks are performed under laboratory conditions. During clinical treatments conditions will be less than ideal and each hyperthermia group should include a number of specific QA checks to investigate how the performance of their hyperthermia system (applicator, thermometry, software, etc.) will be affected under more realistic conditions.

Generally, QA for the clinical application of hyperthermia treatments can be regarded as consisting of a number of successive steps. Prior to any clinical activities the first step is to verify whether the hyperthermia system performs as specified by the manufacturer, i.e., an acceptance test needs to be performed. The next step is to implement a service protocol with a schedule of periodic reviews of the equipment performance. Depending upon the vulnerability of the various parts of the hyperthermia system, the interval between inspection and performance checks can vary from 1 day (e.g., for thermometry) to 1 year (e.g., for applicators).

After the hyperthermia system has been fully characterized, it has to be decided which tumors, i.e., location, size, and depth, can be heated. Such a protocol with standard criteria will be a helpful guide in making a fast and consistent (pre)selection of tumors which potentially can be heated by the hyperthermia system. At this stage the size of the required treatment volume of the tumors proposed for hyperthermia treatment must be defined accurately in three dimensions. Naturally, a treatment protocol for a specific tumor should prescribe the dimensions of the treatment volume.

The next step will be to select the hyperthermia applicator setup, which can consist of a single or multiple applicator in an array setting. At present no universal guidelines for applicator selection exist. For superficial tumor locations a commonly used recommendation (RTOG) for applicator selection is that at least the margins of the treatment volume at the skin surface should be covered by the 25% iso-SAR contour measured in a flat muscle equivalent phantom. The 50% iso-SAR contour is recommended by the ESHO QA guidelines. However, since in the ESHO guidelines normalization of the SAR distribution is carried out at a depth of 10 mm, the two approaches are similar. For deep-seated tumors no recommendations on applicator selection were found in the QA guidelines available. Although applicator selection for deep-seated tumors is very complex task and the SAR distribution within the body will strongly depend upon the anatomy, it seems evident that acceptance of a minimum requirement regarding enclosure of the macroscopic tumor volume by a specific iso-SAR contour would improve clinical outcome. Within our group in the DDHCC the starting values for frequency, phase, and amplitude settings of the Sigma-60 applicator are selected on the basis that the macroscopic tumor volume should be enclosed by the 80% iso-SAR contour as predicted by the 2D treatment planning program (supplied by BSD) in a homogeneous elliptical model of similar size. Of course, as soon as the presently emerging 3D planning programs for electromagnetic heating are available, they should be applied for clinical treatments of deep-seated tumors. It should then be investigated whether the additional effort in 3D hyperthermia treatment planning does indeed contribute to the achievement of better temperature distributions and, ultimately, higher clinical response rates.

After applicator selection the optimum positions of the thermometry catheters have to be selected in accordance with the recommendations given in existing QA guidelines. The next step in the QA procedure is the accurate and extensive documentation of the treatment setup followed by the documentation of all relevant changes made during treatment, e.g., in response to complaints of the patient or to improve patient tolerance and/or measured temperatures. In an optimum setting all data will be recorded according to the Hyperthermia Data Standard (HDS) file format as proposed by SAPARETO and CORRY (1989).

In our experience the final (essential) step in guaranteeing QA will be the discussion of the hyperthermia treatment performance within the complete hyperthermia team before the next hyperthermia treatment is given. On the basis of the thermal dose delivered and the experience of the hyperthermia staff regarding patient tolerance, changes in the system setup can be considered in order to improve the treatment performance.

21.4 Instrumentation for Quality Assurance

The requirements regarding the instrumentation to perform the checks as prescribed by the QA guidelines have been excellently described by SHRIVASTAVA et al. (1989). For a hyperthermia department only applying hyperthermia treatments to superficial tumor locations, the demand for instrumentation will include at least a standard thermometer, a standard power meter, a calibrated leakage radiation survey meter, a reliable precision waterbath, and a number of standard tissue-equivalent phantoms (muscle and fat) of different sizes and shapes. If hyperthermia treatments are also applied to deep-seated tumors, there is a clear need for more advanced instrumentation to perform additional QA tests. For these departments and departments which are active in the field of applicator development, it is recommended that the minimum set of instrumentation is expanded by a network-analyzer or a vector-voltmeter in the required frequency range, bidirectional couplers, a high-power dummy load, a frequency meter, calibrated RF power sensors and meters, radiation survey meters to monitor both the magnetic and electric field, and phantoms to test the performance of applicators. As will be explained below, this additional instrumentation is required to ensure that the actual phase and amplitude settings of the deep hyperthermia system are indeed the values needed for optimum performance.

Furthermore, with the growing ability to perform SAR steering it will be necessary to implement SAR measuring systems which are able to measure the SAR distribution quantitatively and not only qualitatively. This means, for example, that for the phantoms using a matrix of light-emitting diodes (LEDs), methods will have to be developed to quantify the light output of each LED (see Chap. 17).

21.5 Characterization of the Performance of Electromagnetic Applicators

The energy distribution induced by an electromagnetic (EM) applicator will be dependent on amplitude, frequency, and polarization of the applied electric field together with the dielectric properties, size, and anatomy of the patient. To limit the hyperthermia treatment to a localized region of the body it is required that the applicator be in close proximity to the skin. This means that the body is almost always exposed to the near field of the applicator. In this area it is difficult to predict the complex electric field distribution of the applicator accurately, and experimental assessment of the applicator characteristics to evaluate the feasibility of heating a specific tumor location is very important. It will be clear that, if the information obtained from phantom studies can be supplemented with theoretical modeling, it will be possible to make a more appropriate choice of heating technique.

The ESHO guidelines concentrate on the use of radiative applicators for the hyperthermic treatment. However, within Europe and especially in France a large number of institutes are using RF capacitive hyperthermia systems. The ESHO guidelines do not provide precise requirements for this type of applicator. The penetration depth *must* be measured in a direction containing the maximum SAR value, and this is not necessarily located at the center of the aperture of the applicator. For radiative applicators the size of the phantom should be expressed as multiples of the plane wave penetration depth (phantom tickness 3 times penetration depth; surface area = bolus surface dimension plus 1–2 times penetration depth). For capacitive devices the phantom thickness must be as thick as the tissue thickness between the electrodes in the clinical setup.

To perform phantom studies materials are needed to simulate human tissue. There are several extensive reviews (e.g., CHOU 1987; HAND 1990) which describe in detail the many recipes available to construct liquid or solid phantoms.

21.5.1 Phantom Studies

The objective of phantom studies is usually to obtain a precise characterization of the complete vector field of an electromagnetic applicator, that is the experiment must provide information on the the amplitude, phase, and polarization of the electric field with sufficient spatial resolution in the lossy media of the phantom. In practice, the information is only obtained partially. There are two methods available, which can be characterized as the power-pulse and split-phantom techniques, respectively.

The first and most commonly used method of measuring the electric field is to determine the rate of change of temperature (dT/dt) after a short period of heating at high power, e.g., such that the temperature increase is determined only by the amount of absorbed energy. Under this condition, the SAR at any point in the phantom can be calculated from the temperature rise through:

$$\mathrm{SAR} = c\frac{dT}{dt} = \frac{1}{2\rho}\sigma|E|^2, \tag{21.1}$$

where c is the specific heat of the phantom material.

For this method it is essential that the experiments be performed within a short time interval to minimize artifacts due to thermal conduction. A good estimate of the scale of the thermal conduction effects on the temperature distribution can be obtained from the heat penetration depth into a uniform infinite half space:

$$x = \sqrt{\frac{\pi k t}{\rho c}},$$

where k = thermal conductivity (W/m/°C), t = time, c = specific heat capacity (J/kg/°C), ρ = the mass density (kg/m^3), and x = the penetration depth (m). Clearly, the demands on the heating time will vary with the required spatial resolution for the measurement of the SAR distribution. For loco-regional deep heating a spatial resolution of 5 mm is often sufficient and heating times from 1 to 5 min can be used. In contrast, for interstitial hyperthermia devices, where a spatial resolution of 1–2 mm is needed, the duration of the experiment (heating + measurement) should be less than 20 s.

The second method is an established and accurate technique, namely measurement of the temperature distribution by infrared thermography using the split-phantom technique (GUY 1971). This method requires the use of a solid (or gelled) phantom which can be split into two parts at the plane of interest. The exposed, two-dimensional temperature distribution can be measured quickly by an infrared-thermographic camera. Over the years several other methods have been introduced to replace the costly infrared-thermographic camera. As an alternative, the use of liquid crystal sheets in combination with a color photographic camera also quickly provides two-dimensional information about the temperature distribution over a chosen plane.

The temperature distribution can also be measured by temperature sensors which are scanned through the phantom. The clear disadvantage of this method is that after each power-pulse the temperature distribution in the phantom should be allowed to return to steady-state values. Consequently, the measurement of the SAR distribution over the whole plane of interest will be a time-consuming procedure. An important advantage of the power-pulse technique using temperature probes is that it can also be applied during the clinical treatment and thus provides a way to correlate measured SAR with predicted SAR at selected sites in the body. Whether the temperature distribution is measured by infrared thermography, liquid crystal, or temperature sensors, caution should be exercised to ensure that the measuring technique does not disturb the SAR distribution (HAND 1990; SCHAUBERT 1984). The SAR distribution measured by temperature rise only provides information about the local magnitude of the electromagnetic field and not about the polarization of the electric field. By introducing layers of different phantom material in front of the applicator some information can be obtained about the relative strength of the tangential and perpendicular components of the electric field.

21.5.2 E-Field Probes

A different method to obtain information about the SAR distribution is to use miniature probes which measure the electric field directly. Typically, an electric field sensor can be divided into three sections: (a) the receiving antenna, (b) the cables to transport the measured signal, and (c) the instrument to analyze and present the information. Although many different antenna types (BASSEN and SMITH 1983) are available, a miniature dipole antenna is most commonly used to measure the electric field. If the proper conditions for the phantom setup are met (coaxial cable perpendicular to the electric field to minimize perturbation), information can be obtained about the amplitude and phase of the electric field. In this case the signal of the dipole antenna should be transmitted by a "balanced coaxial" cable to a vector-voltmeter or a network analyzer. In other situations the coaxial cable arrangement may cause significant disturbance of the electric field distribution. If information about the phase of the electric field is not needed, it is a common procedure to place a diode at the base of the dipole and to measure the resultant DC-voltage. Normally, carbon-loaded Teflon leads are used to transport the DC-signal to the measuring unit (BASSEN et al. 1975; RASKMARK and GROSS 1987). Alternatively, one may use an LED and fiberoptic techniques to measure the signal (BASSEN et al. 1977). Both carbon-loaded Teflon leads and optical fibers have the advantage that they do not disturb the electric field distribution.

As the dipole antenna is predominantly sensitive to one polarization of the electric field, all three (x, y, and z) polarizations must be measured to obtain the entire electric field. For this purpose the dipole needs to be placed parallel to the direction of the electric field polarization of interest, which may not always be easy to achieve. If, however, the dipole is placed at an angle of $\text{arctg}(\sqrt{2}) = 54.7°$ to the axis of the probe [corresponding to the angle of a line from the origin to the point (1, 1, 1) with any of the three axes (x, y, z)], three simple rotations of the probe over 120° can resolve the entire electric field (RASKMARK and GROSS 1987).

Until now only the BSD Medical Corporation (TURNER 1988) has been successful in developing an electric field probe with a diameter smaller than 1 mm, i.e., small enough to fit in standard thermometry catheters. In order to reduce the diameter of the electric field probe, insulation of the probe to the surrounding tissue is realized through a thin layer of shrinking tube material. Disadvantages of a thin insulation layer are that the sensitivity of the electric field probe is dependent upon the dielectric permittivity of the tissue surrounding the probe and that interaction errors due to the proximity of tissue boundaries (BASSEN and SMITH 1983) are increased. More recently the use of a miniaturized electric field dipole probe to characterize the SAR pattern of interstitial and intracavitary applicators has been reported by ENGELBRECHT et al. (1993). Their miniature electric field sensor is constructed on a ceramic substrate and is capable of measuring two perpendicular components of the electric field simultaneously (ERB et al. 1993). GOPAL et al. (1993) have developed an electric field probe capable of measuring both the amplitude and the phase of the electric field at frequencies of 434 and 915 MHz. They incorporated a thick insulating layer of low dielectric permittivity around the probe, resulting in a response error due to the surrounding media of less than 5%.

All electric field probe techniques mentioned thus far provide information only about a single site in the phantom. Automated scanning techniques have been introduced to measure the SAR pattern of a whole plane but even then the experiment requires long measurement periods. To overcome this problem SCHNEIDER and VAN DIJK (1991) have developed a matrix of 137 LEDs to visualize the electric field distribution over a whole cross-section of an elliptical phantom. The leads of the LEDs form the dipole of the electric field probes as described above. The advantage of the LED matrix is the fact that the effect of changing phase relation, amplitudes, or position of the applicators can be observed instantaneously (see Chap. 17 for further discussion of phantom measurements).

21.6 Thermometry Requirements

21.6.1 Developments in Thermometry

Invasive thermometry is an essential part of each hyperthermia treatment. It provides the clinical data necessary to control SAR steering during treatment, to perform "thermal dose" response studies, and to evaluate and compare the performance of heating systems. Under clinical circumstances the quality of the measured temperature distributions is critically dependent on the accuracy of the thermometry system and the distribution of the temperature measuring points over the treatment volume.

During the last decade good progress has been made with regard to thermometry. Unfortunately, all noninvasive thermometry methods, such as electric impedance imaging, active microwave imaging, and microwave radiography are still at an experimental stage and applied only by a few research groups. With currently available techniques, relying only on noninvasive thermometry is not considered good and safe practice and would not be in accordance with requirements for clinical trials. Therefore, invasive thermometry using electric or optical temperature probes is still a necessity in hyperthermia. Currently there is a tendency to use more complex hyperthermia systems to heat larger tumor volumes, therefore the thermometry requirements need to be extended. One way to improve the information on the temperature distribution is to increase the density of temperature measuring points along the invasive catheter track by thermal mapping. This raises the question of whether the sampling sites in the tumor tissue are sufficiently representative for the whole of the tumor volume. This problem has not yet been resolved. The number of thermometry probes within the treatment area is limited by the number of thermometry catheters which can be inserted in the treatment volume. If the invasive catheters are left in place during a treatment series, the anatomy or patient movements may restrict the placement of catheters. The QA criteria as formulated by the RTOG (DEWHIRST et al. 1990) and ESHO (HAND et al. 1989) cannot always be met. Furthermore, tumors often have a chaotic vessel network and the blood flow over the tumor volume will be far from uniform. If multiple sensor sites are used to sample the temperature distribution, the probability that one or more probes will indicate the normal-tissue temperature of the inflowing blood rather than that of the heated tumor tissue increases with the number of sensors. It has been demonstrated from clinical data that the minimum temperature correlates with the number of temperature probes (CORRY et al. 1988; PEREZ and EMAMI 1989). Attempts to characterize the mostly highly nonuniform temperature distributions by a single parameter for the "thermal dose" are thus rather problematic. In practice this requires a method that uses various weighting factors to integrate the large amount of temperature data and probe distributions into a single thermal dose parameter (EDELSTEIN et al. 1989; ENGLER et al. 1989; CLEGG and ROEMER 1989; CORRY et al. 1988; DEWHIRST et al. 1987; FIELD 1988; OLESON et al. 1989; SIM et al. 1984).

21.6.2 Criteria for Thermometry

21.6.2.1 Calibration and Source of Errors

The fundamental aspects of calibration of temperature probes, electric or optical, are well understood. Recently two extensive reviews concerning the practical aspects of thermometry during clinical hyperthermia have been published (CETAS 1990; SAMULSKI and FESSENDEN 1990). Generally, in a good clinical verification procedure a two-point temperature calibration should be made prior to each treatment (or less frequently, depending upon the nature of the thermometer) to cope with the nonlinear relationship between measured signal and temperature. This calibration can be performed against traceable calibration standards such as mercury glass thermometers, stable thermistor thermometers, or constant temperature cells (gallium, succinonitrile). A summary of the recommendations made by the ESHO guidelines (HAND et al. 1989) and SHRIVASTAVA et al. (1989) regarding thermometry QA is given in Table 21.2.

Regarding interference effects (electromagnetic and ultrasound) and thermal conduction effects, the principal errors are again well understood. These sources of error are discussed in detail in both thermometry reviews mentioned above. Errors in the temperature readings due to electromagnetic interference are the main disadvantage of systems using thermocouples. Under normal conditions the time constant of a temperature probe is approximately 1 s. However, due to EM interference a small tissue cylinder surrounding the thermometry catheter might be preferentially heated. If this is the case it takes more time before the measured temperature in the thermometry catheter approaches the actual tissue temperature sufficiently after the EM power has been switched off. Especially in deep hyperthermia, where it is difficult to place the probes perpendicular to the direction of the electric field, the increase in the time constant of the probes can be substantial. Several groups are working on procedures to improve the power-pulse technique with regard to this type of error. The use of biphasic temperature–time curves or two successive measurements at the start of the treatment have been suggested to separate the "EM thermometry artifact" from the actual temperature increase. In this respect the following recommendations were arrived at during the COMAC QA workshop in Sabaudia:

1. If the artifact is ⩾1°C then do *not* use the temperature data in the analysis of trials
2. If the artifact is <1°C then correct the temperature data until the residual error is ⩽0.2°C
3. When the power-pulse technique is used the temperature representing the tissue temperature should be measured: for superficial hyperthermia after ⩾3 s; for deep hyperthermia after ⩾5 s.

Table 21.2. Recommendations on the QA for thermometry systems according to guidelines of the EHSO (HAND et al. 1989) and SHRIVASTAVA et al. (1989)

Test/procedure	Acceptability criteria	Frequency of testing
Standard calibration thermometer accuracy over 20°–50°C range	0.05°C	A,Y
Clinical thermometry systems		
Accuracy over 37°–46°C	0.2°C	A,Q
Precision for 10 successive readings (1 SD)	⩽0.1°C	A,Q
Stability	⩽10.11°C	A,Q
Response time	<10 s	A,Y
Accuracy of sensor position	2 mm	A,Q
Perturbation/artifacts	<0.1°C	A,C,Y
Electromagnetic interference	<0.1°C	A,C,Y,
Pretreatment accuracy check at ⩽37°C and ⩾43°C or a single calibration check at 43°C	0.2°C	T or R
Inspection for probe damage	Qualitatively	A,T

A, Acceptance testing and equipment installation; Y, yearly; Q, quarterly; T, each treatment; R, recommended by manufacturer; C, when components of the standard setup are changed

21.6.2.2 Recommended Probe Positions and Position Recording

Clearly, it is generally recognized that the number of invasive thermometry catheters which can be placed in the patient is limited. There are many constraints in planning the placement of thermometry catheters, and these have been described in detail in the RTOG QA guidelines (DEWHIRST et al. 1990; SAPOZINK et al. 1991). An important aspect of the thermometry placement procedure, and one which can usually be met, is to choose the catheter track within the radiation portal. In this way seeding of tumor cells along the catheter track can be avoided (Van der Zee et al. 1992a).

As mentioned above, thermal mapping or the use of multisensor temperature probes is mandatory to increase the number of temperature measuring points and to improve the description of the temperature field within the treatment volume. Regarding the desired spatial resolution of the temperature measuring points along the thermometry catheters, the recommendations of the different guidelines are summarized in Table 21.3. A thermal mapping probe should not be used as a control probe in a computer-controlled feedback system.

With regard to recording probe positions for tumors extending to depths greater than 1.5 cm, the demands put forward by the RTOG QA guidelines are often viewed as too strict by the European hyperthermia community. For most European hyperthermia groups the high degree of occupation of CT or MRI equipment limits the access to these sophisticated imaging systems for the purposes of localization or verification of the thermometry probes. Therefore any practical guideline for position recording using CT or MRI systems will be difficult to comply within multi-institutional trials. Nevertheless, it is strongly recommended that CT, MRI, or US imaging techniques be used whenever possible to localize probe positions and to follow the RTOG guidelines (Dewhirst et al. 1990).

Table 21.3. QA guidelines for temperature data acquisition

Spatial resolution
1. If the tumor size is ≤5 cm then the temperature should be measured with a spatial resolution of 5 mm within the tumor
2. For large tumors a spatial resolution of 10 mm is acceptable
3. Normal tissue temperatures should be measured along the catheter track and at the surface

Frequency of measurement
1. Thermal mapping must be done on a routine base with a maximum interval between the mappings of 10 min
2. If stationary multisensor probes are used, the frequency of temperature measurement should be increased to preferably once per minute

A higher number of temperature probes, and thus better spatial resolution, is to be preferred to more frequent read-outs of a small number of temperature sensors.

Minimum requirements for probe position documentation as formulated at the COMAC-BME QA in Sabaudia (1991) are as follows:

1. Use the best available position description with a goal of 2 mm resolution in all coordinates.
2. Use transparencies (scale 1:1) to outline tumor, catheters (including angle of insertion), applicators, scars, etc.

21.6.2.2.1 Superficial Tumors. For superficial hyperthermia the number of invasive thermometry catheters acceptable to the patient will vary between 3 and 6. In general the guidelines on probe positioning in the RTOG protocol (Dewhirst et al. 1990) are more favorable for noninterfering probes and less applicable when thermocouples are used. For the institutes using conventional (thermocouple) thermometry systems it seems easier to follow the ESHO guidelines (Hand et al. 1989) for probe positioning.

The RTOG guidelines specify in detail how many temperature sensors should be used and where to place them for superficial locations. The approach of the ESHO QA committee is to provide an absolute minimum requirement in respect of thermometry and to design more detailed thermometry requirements on a protocol-specific basis.

In general, thermometry catheters should be placed so that there will be a good distribution of temperature probes over the whole treatment volume. The QA guidelines of the RTOG and ESHO on invasive thermometry are summarized in Table 21.4. Skin surface temperature measurements must be performed at sites at risk for the development of burns, such as protruding bones or tumor areas or other areas with an expected high SAR. Scar tissues and burns of previous treatment must also be monitored carefully.

As mentioned above, within Europe probe position recording for superficial hyperthermia is only rarely performed by means of CT or MRI. A procedure for treatment documentation using transparent sheets has been described in detail by Broekmeyer-Reurink et al. (1992) for superficial hyperthermia of chest wall recurrences of breast cancer. On a transparent sheet a life-size drawing (Fig. 21.2) is made which includes information on:

Table 21.4. QA guidelines of RTOG and ESHO for invasive thermometry

	RTOG[a] (Dewhirst et al. 1990)	ESHO[b] (Hand et al. 1989)
Superficial bulky malignancies, isolated single nodules	2 catheters parallel to midplane or 2 catheters cross through midplane *plus* 1 tangential at base 2 catheters parallel to midplane and 1 orthogonal, extending through deep base along the midaxis	A minimum of three sensors within 1 cm of the periphery of the tumor. One must be at depth and two at diametrically opposed locations. (Requirement for ESHO protocol 1–85)
Diffuse erythematous infiltration	Invasive thermometry catheters should be placed at a depth of 0.5–1.0 cm along with a large number of skin surface measurements. $25\,cm^2$: 1 invasive catheter $25–100\,cm^2$: 2 invasive catheters $>100\,cm^2$: $\geq$3 invasive catheters	
Multiple small nodules	Invasive thermometry catheters placed at the bases of the nodules such that a maximum number of nodules are intersected. Multiple skin surface sites must be monitored. $25\,cm^2$: 1 invasive catheter $25–100\,cm^2$: 2 invasive catheters $>100\,cm^2$: $\geq$3 invasive catheters	

[a] Only optimal strategies are given
[b] The ESHO QA guidelines state that the minimum number of temperature probes and the exact positioning is a protocol-specific requirement

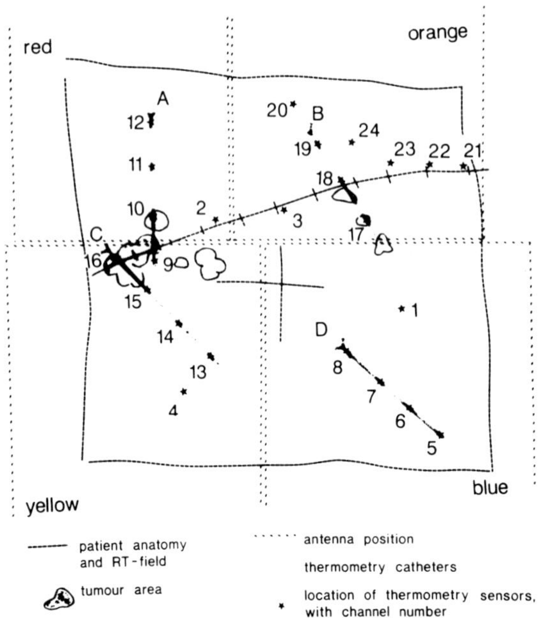

Fig. 21.2. Transparency with life-size drawing. The numbers in the drawing correspond with the channel numbers of the thermometry system. Colors listed represent the color codes used for the various applicator – amplifier combinations

1. Edges of the radiation field, in relation to some reference mark on the patient
2. Location of tumor and scar tissues
3. Margins of the apertures of the selected applicator(s)
4. Site of insertion and direction of the thermometry catheters

The location of each thermometry catheter is further documented by measurements of the total length, the external length, the insertion depth, and the parts of each thermometry catheter running through palpable tumor tissue (Fig. 21.3).

21.6.2.2.2 Deep-Seated Tumors. For deep-seated tumors the situation is much more complicated and in general the physician in charge will be pleased if he/she is able (and allowed) to insert one deep-seated thermometry catheter. Without exception, placement of a 15-cm-long thermometry catheter in the pelvis, abdomen, or thorax must be performed under CT or MRI guidance. The CT or MRI image obtained from this catheter placement procedure can be used to document the anatomical location of the catheter and to identify the tissue type along the catheter track. Catheter placement will be restricted

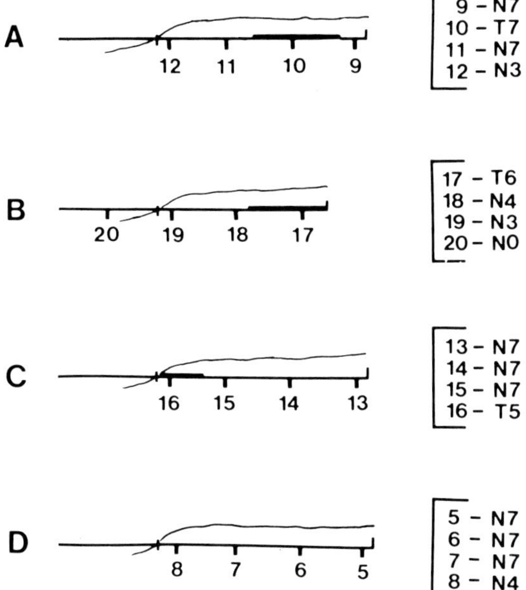

Fig. 21.3. Catheter drawings; schematic representation of catheter trajectories and thermometry probes in the tissue

by the risk of causing physical trauma, e.g., perforation of intestinal lumen, major blood vessels, or organs with high blood flow. Bone is also an effective barrier for many tumor locations. Furthermore, the risk of kinking of the thermometry catheter due to pressure of the water bolus or shearing forces on the catheter due to patient movement will restrict catheter placement. For catheters which stay in place during the whole treatment series the risk of kinking can be reduced somewhat by inserting a nylon wire into the catheter.

As loco-regional hyperthermia is presently mainly concentrated on the treatment of deep-seated tumors in the pelvis using radiative electromagnetic applicators, only the guidelines for placement of thermometry catheters at these locations are mentioned here. For other sites of deep-seated malignancies we refer to the RTOG QA guidelines (SAPOZINK et al. 1991). For deep-seated tumors in the pelvic region, thermometry should be performed in the intracavitary locations if feasible, as this will provide important additional information on the temperature distribution. Although it seems relatively easy to perform thermometry at these sites, it should be realized that side-effects of the radiation treatment may cause thermometry at these sites to become a painful procedure. Skin surface temperature measurements should be performed in areas with only limited (Chap. 15, Sect. 15.6.1) contact with the water bolus and at locations where a high SAR can be expected, such as the perineum and the anal cleft. If indicated, additional cooling should be applied at these areas. With regard to the invasive thermometry catheters the optimal strategy would include: one temperature map extending from a deep tumor margin to the surface along the longitudinal axis; a second temperature map extending from a deep tumor margin to the surface along a radius perpendicular to the longitudinal axis; and a third catheter to monitor temperatures along a tumor margin. In Fig. 21.4 the various strategies (optimal, less optimal, and minimum acceptable) as defined by the RTOG QA guidelines (SAPOZINK et al. 1991) are illustrated.

21.6.3 Thermometry Requirements in Interstitial Hyperthermia

In the RTOG QA guidelines for interstitial hyperthermia a number of different recommended locations for thermometry probe placement have been defined. It seems useful to summarize these definitions and the recommendations regarding the number of thermometry probes required as a function of implant geometry. In a given implant, for example a rectangular implant area treated with 16 applicators, i.e., antennas or electrodes (arranged in four parallel planes of four applicators each), the following probe locations can be distinguished:

1. The center of the implant
2. The centers of subarrays [in general a subarray can consist of three applicators (triangle), four applicators (square), or more]
3. The tumor periphery
4. The surrounding normal tissue

The preferred number of thermometry probes applied depends on the total number of heating applicators and the specific implant geometry. Global recommendations for the number of thermometry catheters as given in the RTOG guidelines (EMAMI et al. 1991) are summarized in Table 21.5. Either thermometry catheters should be loaded with multipoint thermometry probes or thermal mapping with single probes along the catheter tracks should be performed.

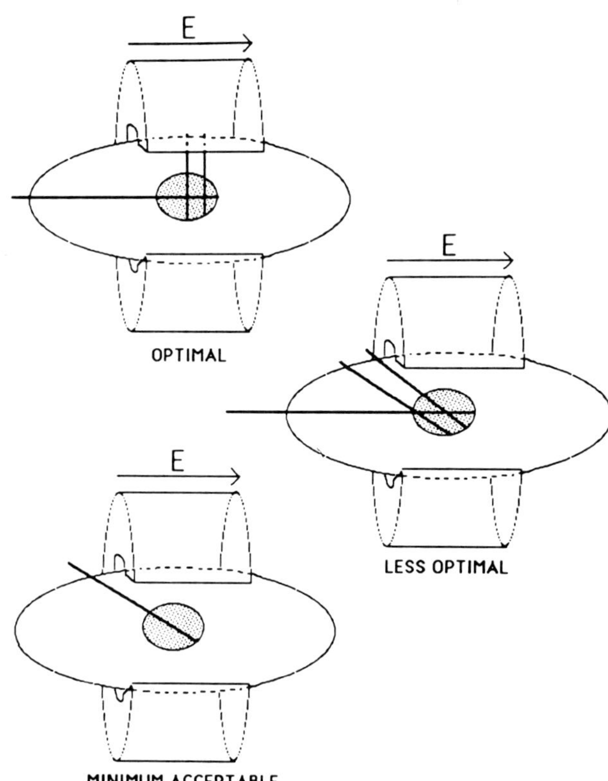

Fig. 21.4. Strategies for thermometry catheter placement in association with annular MW or RF array devices. (From DEWHIRST et al. 1990)

Table 21.5. Summary of the recommended number of thermometry probes as a function of the number of heating applicators and the implant geometry (after EMAMI et al. 1991)

No. of heating applicators	Position A: center of implant	Position B: centers of subarrays	Position C: periphery
3–8	1	0	1
9–16	1	1	1
17–32	1	2	1
>32	1	3	2

Regarding the temperature monitoring during treatment the RTOG recommends the following:

1. Multisensor probes or thermal mapping
2. Each sensor location measured at least every 15 min
3. Spacing between probe locations or map points:
   a) 5 mm for tumors less than 5 cm
   b) 10 mm for larger tumors

Regarding the recommended minimum time interval between measurements at each probe location one may note that the requirement of measuring each location at least every 15 min is less strict than, for example, the QA guidelines for ESHO protocols (HAND et al. 1989) dealing with (external) superficial hyperthermia. For reporting a summary of the treatment the latter guidelines recommend that the temperature at each sensor location must be recorded at 5-min intervals during the treatment; the data acquisition system should be able to scan all temperature sensors at 10- to 20-s intervals, while the data should be printed at 1-min intervals. Because there is no obvious reason to suppose that temperature distributions obtained with interstitial hyperthermia will be more uniform and stable compared with external heating methods, it seems prudent to set similar (strict) requirements for the frequency of temperature measurements.

21.6.4 Problems of Measuring Inside Interstitial/Intracavitary Applicators

Typical examples of thermometry inside heating applicators are thermal measurements within RF needles, within or directly adjacent to MW antennas or RF-capacitive-coupling applicators. Generally this type of measurement is used to represent the temperatures obtained in tissue regions close to the applicators, often the maximum temperature regions within the implanted volume. Advantages of this mode of thermometry are (a) the possibility of individual power control of all applicators, and (b) the indication of maximum temperature, possibly allowing prevention of treatment side-effects and toxicity.

An important drawback of this type of thermometry is the possible presence of thermometry artifacts, e.g., due to self-heating in the case of microwave (MW) antennas or radiofrequency (capacitive-coupling) applicators and/or due to thermal resistance between the probe and the surrounding tissue. The accuracy of thermometry inside MW antennas has been discussed by ASTRAHAN et al. (1988). Measured temperatures were found to differ from the estimated local tissue temperature by up to 8°C. In their discussion, self-heating distal to the antenna junction appeared to be the primary source of this error.

For capacitive-coupling (27-MHz) applicators the dielectric properties of the catheter material can be of importance: material with a relatively high loss factor can be expected to show significant heating of the catheter.

The magnitude of any possible thermometry artifact has to be known in order to be able to obtain meaningful data representing the actual local tissue temperatures. If either self-heating or electromagnetic interference is found to have an influence, measurements during power-off periods should be performed. If reliable temperatures can be obtained, these thermometry concerns refer only to the regions close to the applicators, where generally significantly higher temperatures are obtained in comparison to the tissue regions between the applicators. It is therefore recommended that thermometry inside heating applicators should always be supplemented by measurements with probes in nonheated catheters.

Advantages of thermometry in nonheated catheters are: (a) assessment of actual tissue temperatures between the applicators, where temperature levels are generally lower; (b) minimal or no artifacts from the heating applicators, and therefore (c) reliable data for thermal dose-response evaluation. A drawback might be the possible underestimation of the high temperatures close to the heating applicators, which might be relevant for treatment toxicity, especially when patients are treated under general anesthesia.

In order to obtain a full perception of the temperature distribution over the target volume, the application of thermal modeling using measured temperatures as input data is an interesting possibility. The principal advantage of interstitial hyperthermia is the large number of invasive catheters and their small separation relative to the size of the target volume. By using power-pulse measurement techniques with multipoint temperature probes in all catheters it should be possible to obtain small-scale data on the heat transport through blood flow over the whole target volume. In this respect interstitial hyperthermia may serve as a useful test case for thermal models (LAGENDIJK et al. 1992). In combination with small-scale and sufficiently fast thermometry data, it should then be possible to obtain detailed information on the temperature distribution as a whole and to utilize this information for optimization.

Additional discussion of thermometry-related quality assurance may be found in Chap. 15.

21.7 Hyperthermia Staff Requirements

With respect to clinical treatments it seems prudent to realize that good hyperthermia equipment does not guarantee a good hyperthermic treatment. A motivated and experienced group from various disciplines is a requirement if reliable and consistent clinical results are to be obtained. For hyperthermia treatments of good quality the staff of a hyperthermia department should consist of a physician, a physicist, and hyperthermia technologists. A description of the qualifications needed for each discipline was given by LUK (1988).

1. *The physician* who prescribes and supervises hyperthermia should be a licensed clinician with special training in oncology and the basic biological and physical principles of hyperthermia, as well as adequate experience in clinical applications of hyperthermia. A minimum of 6 months of additional training in hyperthermia should be required to achieve the necessary knowledge and clinical proficiency.

2. *The physicist*, who is responsible for all the physical and quality aspects of the hyperthermia

equipment, must be trained at the level of a radiation physicist. Additional training in thermometry, electromagnetic, and thermal treatment modeling and in the physics of ultrasound, radiofrequency, and microwaves is required, as well as a thorough knowledge of the biological and physiological responses of tumor and normal tissues to heat. Furthermore, an excellent knowledge of the operation, maintenance, and QA procedures of hyperthermia equipment and the clinical application of the hyperthermia treatment is required.

3. *The hyperthermic technologist* should have a training in basic health and physical sciences such as would normally be given to a radiation therapy technician. Supplementary, special training in the operation, maintenance, and QA procedures of hyperthermia equipment and in the clinical application of the hyperthermia treatment is required.

The requirements regarding the presence of the hyperthermia team are quite different for hyperthermia treatments of superficial and deep-seated tumors. For superficial hyperthermia the presence of three disciplines is required in the preparation of the first hyperthermia treatment, i.e., the physician is responsible for the insertion of the thermometry catheters and documentation of the condition of the patient and the treatment area; the technologist assists the physician and prepares the hyperthermia system; and the attendance of the physicist will be required for selection of the applicators and sites where thermometry is indicated. In general the subsequent superficial hyperthermia treatments are administered by a technologist. Although the physicist is responsible for the quality of the hyperthermia treatment, he/she is only actively involved with the application of the first hyperthermia treatment. For all successive treatments the physicist will be available on demand of the technologist to solve specific problems.

For deep hyperthermia the involvement of the physician and the physicist is much more labor-intensive. The impact of deep heating on the physiological condition of the patient, i.e., core temperature, pulse rate, blood pressure, and pain, is such that it requires continuous supervision of the physician to ensure patient safety. The state of the art of current deep hyperthermia systems requires that the hyperthermia treatment is administered by a physicist or under his/her direct supervision (which requires that the physicist stays in the control room). The tasks of the technologists (generally 2) are to prepare the hyperthermia system and the patient, i.e., perform the pretreatment thermometry checks, introduce intracavitary thermometry catheters, etc., and to take care of the comfort of the patient during the whole treatment, i.e., supply drinks, cool the patient with wet towels, etc.

For interstitial hyperthermia the staff requirement will depend strongly on the interstitial hyperthermia system used. Of course, the clinician always needs to introduce the catheters necessary for the interstitial treatments, both for brachytherapy and for hyperthermia. The demands regarding the involvement of a physicist to administer the hyperthermia treatment will depend strongly on the interstitial hyperthermia technique used. With the hot water perfusion techniques the treatment can be administered by a technologist with a physicist as supervisor, while with the more complex RF or MW techniques the treatment needs to be administered by a physicist.

21.8 Current Trends in Research Towards Higher Quality in Hyperthermia

21.8.1 Superficial Hyperthermia

Superficial hyperthermia is the most frequently used modality in the clinical situation and over the years superficial heating methods have become well elucidated. Nevertheless, the equipment still presents severe limitations in terms of effective field size, spatial power control, the underheating of certain tumor areas but overheating of critical regions (scars, bone, and fat), and accessibility. In spite of these limitations and problems the clinical results obtained are encouraging and warrant further investigations. Recent developments in electromagnetic applicators, e.g., current sheet applicators, microwave blankets, and open-sided horn applicators, have advanced the state of art, but the clinical evaluation of these innovations is still pending.

Conventionally, superficial hyperthermia is defined as the heating of tumors penetrating less that 3 cm, e.g., chest wall recurrences and some head and neck and limb tumors. In this summary the heating of tumors penetrating more than 3 cm, e.g., axillary tumors and tumors of other larger head and neck sites, is designated as "deep superficial hyperthermia." Obviously, the two groups demand different approaches.

For chest wall tumors and other malignancies penetrating less than 3 cm both microwave and ultrasound systems should be considered, but at the present time microwave applicators are primarily in clinical use. A limitation of the presently available applicators is their small effective treatment area compared to the aperture size. Especially in the hyperthermic treatment of chest wall recurrences, which generally extend over large areas (>200 cm^2), the small effective treatment area is a severe disadvantage. Therefore, there is a growing interest in the development of applicators capable of treating large areas. Recent and promising applicator research is concentrating on the development of applicator arrays (FESSENDEN et al. 1988; LEE et al. 1992; JOHNSON et al. 1988; HAND 1990; MAGIN and PETERSON 1989). The rationale for this approach is that the ability to adjust the output of each individual array element provides a better spatial control of the SAR distribution than can be obtained with a single element.

Array elements under clinical investigation are those composed of current sheet applicators (LUMORI et al. 1990; GOPAL et al. 1992) and microstrip spiral applicators (FESSENDEN et al. 1988; SAMULSKI et al. 1990). The Lucite Cone waveguide applicator (RIETVELD and VAN RHOON 1991) is still at the experimental phase. Differences between these arrays are field polarization (circular or linear) and energy coupling (***E*** or ***H*** field): spiral applicator: circular and ***E*** field; current sheet applicator: linear and ***H*** field; Lucite Cone applicator: linear and *E* field. There appears to be no benefit of coherent use of EM arrays in chest wall tumors compared to incoherent use. Therefore power steering to the array can be obtained by both one generator per element or by power scanning over several elements using time modulation. Characterization of usefulness in the clinic is presently studied only for the spiral microstrip applicator array and it is too early to decide whether one applicator type is to be preferred.

Small elements will provide high spatial resolution of power control and are capable of conforming to body contour; however, they will have less penetration depth. Under clinical conditions the size of the aperture will be a compromise between a small aperture size to improve spatial resolution of SAR control and a large aperture size for sufficient penetration depth. Note that it is not yet completely understood which degree of penetration depth and spatial resolution of SAR control will be needed to obtain a good therapeutic outcome for all tumors of the chest wall, such as breast recurrences, which generally extend over large areas and have variable thickness. This needs further investigation and it may well turn out that within a hyperthermia department several systems with different specifications, large penetration depth with less spatial control and small penetration depth with high spatial control, will be needed. Furthermore, with the increasing complexity of array configurations, the requirements regarding thermometry and control algorithms become more demanding. For this purpose the contribution of surface temperature probes must be investigated.

For the "deep superficial tumors" penetrating more than 3 cm there are, at present, very few applicators capable of heating large volumes adequately at depth. Ultrasound appears to be the most promising system available. Further technical development of both EM and US devices is essential in this field and the clinical assessment of techniques like focused ultrasound, evanescent mode, and lens applicators is needed. For head and neck tumors an additional problem is accessibility and here the development of slim, conformal applicators is vital.

Important aspects for quality control are patient positioning and bolus characteristics. Reproducibility is still a major problem and depends strongly on the local situation and anatomical problems. The comfort of the patient is a critical factor regarding reproducibility and the overall quality of the treatment. Discomfort or pain suffered by the patient should be distinguished according to whether it is related to heat or to the positioning of the applicator(s) on the treatment field: especially in patients with ulcerating tumors just the pressure of the water bolus and the applicator(s) can cause irritating pain.

21.8.2 Deep Hyperthermia

To obtain a sufficient penetration depth the electromagnetic heating systems have to operate at low frequencies, in the range 10–120 MHz. A physical consequence of this restriction is that the wavelength will be very large. Therefore in contrast to ultrasound systems, selective tumor heating with electromagnetic deep heating systems can only be obtained if the tumor blood flow is low compared to that of the surrounding normal tissue (STROHBEHN et al. 1989; WUST et al. 1991). To optimize the SAR – and the temperature distribution for different patient dimensions and tumor locations – most of the radiative hyperthermia systems for locoregional deep heating provide SAR steering by phase and amplitude and frequency variation. Depending on the electromagnetic applicator type used, the transition between tissues with low and high permittivity may cause significant changes in the local SAR. This in turn may result in localized hot spots in normal tissue which are often power limiting and thus result in a lower thermal dose within the tumor.

In clinical treatments high-quality hyperthermic treatments are still difficult to obtain and to maintain for a reasonable duration (KAPP et al. 1988; SAPOZINK et al. 1988; SHIMM et al. 1988). In approximately 90% of the clinical treatments with the old annular phased array system (BSD-1000 system), local pain, general discomfort, and rise in normal tissue temperature were power limiting while the tumor temperature remained too low (HOWARD et al. 1986; KAPP et al. 1988; PILEPICH et al. 1987; SAPOZINK et al. 1988; SHIMM et al. 1988, 1989). These disadvantages reduce the clinical application and the efficacy of the treatment.

Only limited data are available on clinical experience with the new BSD-2000 Sigma-60 system. MYERSON et al. (1991) reported preliminary data with seven patients treated in 26 sessions with the Sigma-60 applicator. They were able to obtain a minimum temperature of 42°C in 85% of all tumor temperature measuring points. Other important observations were: (a) improved patient tolerance demonstrated by the fact that the tumor temperature could be maintained above 42°C for more than 30 min in 65% of the treatments; (b) the RF powers necessary to reach therapeutic temperatures were much lower than with the old APA system. As similar results have been reported by others (FELDMANN et al. 1991; WUST et al. 1990), there are indications that the approach of the BSD-2000 Sigma-60 system may indeed lead to an improved quality of the hyperthermic treatment of deep-seated tumors. However, old problems might be replaced by new problems when using the new BSD-2000 system. FELDMANN et al. (1991) found during his patient treaments (eight patients, 57 treatments) that preferential heating of the perineal fat can be treatment limiting. OLESON (1991) reported that hot spots are produced in bony prominences of the pelvis, particularly over the sacrum, the hip joint, the superior iliac crest, and the pubic bone. Additionally, fringing fields from the area where the water bolus bag contacts the skin result in hot spots in the anterolateral thighs.

The above findings emphasize the need for continuous applicator development with the aim of improving the flexibility and adaptability of the SAR distribution to the patient's anatomy. Present research in loco-regional hyperthermia is concentrating on:

1. The use of advanced and sophisticated three-dimensional electromagnetic planning procedures to provide information on the optimum settings of frequency, amplitude, and phase for radiative array systems.
2. Implementation of specific QA procedures to ensure that the actual delivered treatment will match the optimized treatment plan. A method for the accurate measurement of the amplitude and phase setting of the BSD-2000 system has been described by HORNSLETH (1993). Phase deviations of 20° have been found between phase measured at the low power side (before pre-amp) and at the high power side just before the Sigma-60 applicator.
3. Better control of the location of the "focal spot" by introducing a possibility to adapt the phase offset for the four channels of the Sigma-60 applicator.
4. Longitudinal control of the SAR distribution by dividing the present 45-cm-long biconal dipole antenna in the Sigma-60 applicator into three segments of 15 cm with separate phase and amplitude control. This will, of course, increase the complexity of the control algorithm.

Besides the improvements presently being investigated for the Sigma-60 applicators, several groups are working on deep heating systems using a different electromagnetic applicator. The open water bolus system of the coaxial TEM applicator as developed and investigated in Utrecht is markedly distinct from all other applicators. In the future, comparisons of the thermal dose obtained with the TEM applicator with that obtained with radiative systems using a closed water bolus for similar patient categories are needed to evaluate the benefit of this approach.

In contrast to the electromagnetic approach, the use of ultrasound to induce deep heating has important physical advantages (HUNT 1990; HYNYNEN et al. 1992) such as the low absorption coefficient and the short wavelength in human tissues, which enable highly focused energy deposition at depth. Of all the noninvasive hyperthermia systems developed for locoregional deep heating, only ultrasound has the potential to deposit the energy at selective locations within the tumor volume. The clinical use of ultrasound is, however, cumbersome due to two distinct physical disadvantages: reflection at interfaces between soft tissue and air or bone, and high absorption in bone. Especially with the early single, stationary, and planar ultrasound transducer designs these problems resulted in limiting normal tissue heating or pain in many of the clinical treatments (CORRY et al. 1988; HYNYNEN et al. 1989; KAPP et al. 1988; SHIMM et al. 1988).

Presently, the use of a well-focused ultrasound beam which is scanned rapidly by mechanical or electronic means across the tumor to generate an improved temperature distribution is being actively investigated (IBBINI and CAIN 1990; MOROS et al. 1990; HAND et al. 1992).

21.8.3 Interstitial Hyperthermia

The motivation for applying interstitial or intracavitary hyperthermia is usually based on one or more of the following considerations:

1. The brachytherapy technique used may enable use of this hyperthermia technique when localized heating might otherwise not be possible.
2. These techniques allow better sparing of normal surrounding tissues.
3. A higher level of treatment control can be attained because a greater number of applicators and temperature sensors are used in comparison to external methods.

Research aimed at improving quality is focused on exploiting the latter advantage to a greater degree: better localized heating combined with better treatment control.

The following techniques for interstitial heating are being used and improved upon:

1. *Radiative*, using microwave (MW) antennas operating in the range of about 300–2450 MHz. Microwave antennas have the capability to deposit power at a distance from the applicator, allowing (at least in theory) somewhat larger separations between applicators; constructive interference between coherently driven antennas can be used to improve the power deposition at depth. Problem areas with microwave antennas are the difficulty in varying the length to be heated, the dependence on the insertion depth, and, depending on antenna design, the presence of a "cold tip," i.e., insufficient power deposition at the tip of the antenna. Research activities include design variations to improve longitudinal heating (along the applicator), helical coil designs, and coherent vs noncoherent arrays of applicators.

2. *Radiofrequency* (RF), using frequencies in the range between 500 kHz and about 27 MHz. The use of frequencies at the lower end of this range, to drive electrodes (e.g., implanted needles) which are in galvanic contact with the tissue volume to be heated, is conceptually the simplest technique for interstitial heating, often indicated as local current field (LCF) heating. The use of higher frequencies (27 MHz) for interstitial heating is mainly motivated by utilizing capacitive coupling of electrodes inside nonconductive catheters instead of direct galvanic contact with the surrounding tissue. This technique is therefore designated as capacitive-coupling (CC) interstitial hyperthermia. Research activities include the use of segmented applicators to improve spatial SAR control, for both the LCF and CC methods, and improved treatment control through computer steering. As pointed out by LAGENDIJK et al. (1992), interstitial hyperthermia seems an interesting test case for the test of thermal modeling.

3. *Conductive* techniques, which are quite different from the electromagnetic heating methods in the sense that they rely only on thermal conduction to reach hyperthermic temperatures and no power is deposited in the tissue. Both the technique using inductively heated ferromagnetic seeds (FMS) and hot-source methods (i.e., hot-water circulation systems or hot-wire systems) belong to this category. Hot-water systems have the important advantage of simplicity. Research activities for FMS are focused on the development of seeds of new materials with a chosen well-controlled Curie temperature and a steep susceptibility versus temperature behavior.

Recent developments in these three areas have been summarized in a Task Group Report published by ESHO (Visser et al. 1993), as well as in Chap. 13 of this volume.

21.9 Summary

- There is conclusive evidence from superficial hyperthermia applications that the outcome of treatments can be improved substantially by improving the quality of the hyperthermic treatments. There is no reason to suppose that the same would not apply to all hyperthermia applications.
- Emphasis has been put on the background of techniques to characterize – and thus to improve- the performance of electromagnetic applicators.
- In clinical hyperthermia practice two tumor sites are freqently heated: chest wall recurrences and deep seated tumors in the pelvis. For these common indications the thermometry requirements and practical clinical experience have been discussed in some depth.
- The staff of a hyperthermia department should consist of a physician, a physicist and hyperthermia technologists. The level of involvement of each discipline depends on the technique of hyperthermia applied. Hyperthermia of deep seated tumors seems most labour intensive for all disciplines.
- A summary has been given of current trends in applicator research which are likely to result in higher quality of hyperthermic treatments. In all areas discussed – i.e., superficial, deep and interstitial heating – distinct possibilities can be indicated for improving the localization of the absorbed power distribution, in combination with better treatment control.

References

AAPM Report 26 (1989) Performance evaluation of hyperthermia equipment (Report of AAPM Task Group no 1. Hyperthermia Committee). American Association of Physicists in Medicine

Arcangeli G, Arcangeli G, Guerra A, Lovisolo G, Cividalli A, Marino G, Mauro F (1985) Tumour response to heat and radiation: prognostic variables in the treatment of neck node metastases from head and neck cancer. Int J Hyperthermia 1: 207–217

Astrahan MA, Luxton G, Sapozink MD, Petrovich Z (1988) The accuracy of temperature measurements from within an interstitial microwave antenna. Int J Hyperthermia 4: 593–607

Bassen H, Smith GS (1983) Electric field probes – a review. IEEE Trans Antennas Propagation 31: 710–718

Bassen H, Swicord M, Abita J (1975) A miniature broadband electric field probe. Ann NY Acad Sci 247: 481–493

Bassen H, Herchenroeder P, Cheung A, Neuder S (1977) Evaluation of an implantable electric field probe within finite simulated tissues. Radio Science 12: 15–25

Broekmeyer-Reurink MP, Rietveld P JM, Van Rhoon GC, Van der Zee J (1992) Some practical notes on documentation of superficial hyperthermia treatment. Int J Hyperthermia 8: 401–406

Cetas TC (1990) Thermometry. In: Field SB, Hand JW (eds) An introduction to the practical aspects of clinical hyperthermia. Taylor & Francis, London, pp 423–477

Chou CK (1987) Phantoms for electromagnetic studies. In: Field SB, Franconi C (eds) Physics and technology of hyperthermia. Martinus Nijhoff, Dordrecht, pp 294–318

Clegg ST, Roemer RB (1989) Towards the estimation of three-dimensional temperature fields from noisy temperative measurements during hyperthermia. Int J Hyperthermia 5: 467–484

COMAC Hyperthermia Bulletin COMAC-BME workshop on quality assurance in hyperthermia 5: 78–99

Corry PM, Jabboury K, Kong JS, Armour EP, McCraw FJ, LeDuc T (1988) Evaluation of equipment for hyperthermia treatment of cancer, Int J Hyperthermia 4: 53–74

Dewhirst MW, Sim DA (1986) Estimation of therapeutic gain in clinical trials involving hyperthermia and radiotherapy. Int J Hyperthermia 2: 165–178

Dewhirst MW, Winget JM, Edelstein-Keshet L et al. (1987) Clinical application of thermal isoeffect dose. Int J Hyperthermia 3: 307–318

Dewhirst MW, Phillips TL, Samulski TV et al. (1990) RTOG quality assurance guidelines for clinical trials using hyperthermia. Int J Radiat Oncol Biol Phys 18: 1249–1259

Edelstein-Keshet L, Dewhirst NW, Oleson JR, Samulski TV (1989) Characterization of tumour temperature distributions in hyperthermia based on assumed mathematical forms. Int J Hyperthermia 5: 757–777

Egawa S, Tsukiyama I, Akine Y, Kajiura Y, Ogino T, Yamashita K (1988) Hyperthermic therapy of deep seated tumors: comparison of the heating efficiencies of an APA and a capacitively coupled RF system. Int J Radiat Oncol Biol Phys 14: 521–528

Emami B, Stauffer P, Dewhirst MW et al. (1991) RTOG quality assurance guidelines for interstitial hyperthermia. Int J Radiat Oncol Biol Phys 20: 1117–1124

Engelbrecht R, Erb J, Schaller G (1993) Entwicklung von miniaturisierten E-feldsonden zur Vermessung von Hyperthermie-Applikatoren. In: Müller RG, Erb J (eds) Medizinische Physik 1993 (24 Wissenschiftliche Tagung der Deutschen Gesellschaft für Medizinische Physik), Erangen, pp 88–89

Engler MJ, Dewhirst MW, Oleson JR (1989) Stability of temperatures during hyperthermia treatments. Int J Hyperthermia 5: 59–67

Erb J, Engelbrecht R, Schaller G, Seegenschmiedt HM, Müller RG, Sauer R, Roos D (1993) Charakterisierung und Qualitätssicherung von interstitiellen koaxialen Mikrowellen-Dipolantennen. In: Müller RG, Erb J (eds) Medizinische Physik 1993 (24 Wissenschiftliche Tagung der Deutschen Gesellschaft für Medizinische Physik), Erlangen, pp 86–87

Feldmann HJ, Molls M, Adler S, Meyer-Schwickerath M, Sack H (1991) Hyperthermia in eccentrically located pelvic tumours: excessive heating of the perineal fat and normal tissue temperatures. Int J Radiat Oncol Biol Phys 20: 1017–1022

Fessenden P, Lee ER, Kapp DS, Tarczy-Hornoch P, Prionas SD, Sullivan DM (1988) Improved microwave (MW) applicators for surface hyperthermia. 5th International Symposium on Hyperthermic Oncology, Kyoto, Vol. 1, Sugaharu T, Saito M (eds) Taylor & Froncis, London, New York, Philadelphia, pp 773–774

Field SB (1988) The concept of thermal dose. Recent Results Cancer Res 107: 1–6

Gonzalez Gonzalez D, van Dijk JDP, Blank LECM (1988) Chest wall recurrences of breast cancer: results of combined treatment with radiation and hyperthermia. Radiother Oncol 12: 95–103

Gopal MK, Hand JW, Lumori MLD, Alkhair S, Paulsen KD, Cetas TC (1992) Current sheet applicator arrays for superficial hyperthermia of chest wall lesions. Int J Hyperthermia 8: 227–240

Guy, AW (1971) Analysis of electromagnetic fields induced in biological tissues by thermographic studies on equivalent phantom models. IEEE Trans Microwave Theory Tech 19: 189–214

Hand JW (1990) Biophysics and technology of electromagnetic hyperthermia. In: Goutherie M (ed) Methods of external hyperthermic heating. Springer, Berlin Heidelberg New York, pp 1–59

Hand JW, Lagendijk JJW, Andersen JB, Bolomy JC (1989) Quality assurance guidelines for ESHO protocols. Int J Hyperthermia 5: 421–428

Hand JW, Vernon CC, Prior MV (1992) Early experience of a commercial scanned focused ultrasound hyperthermia system. Int J Hyperthermia 8: 587–607

Hiraoka M, Jo S, Dodo Y, Ono K, Takahashi M, Nishida H, Abe M (1984) Clinical results of radiofrequency hyperthermia combined with radiation in the treatment of radioresistant cancers. Cancer 54: 2898–2904

Hofman P, Lagendijk JJW, Schipper J (1984) The combination of radiotherapy with hyperthermia in protocolized clinical studies. In: Overgaard J (ed) Hyperthermic oncology 1984, vol 1. Summary papers. Taylor and Francis, London, pp 379–382

Hornsleth SN (1993) Quality assurance procedures for the BSD-2000. Abstract at "Hyperthermia in Clinical Oncology", 7th BSD users meeting, Munich

Howard GCW, Sathiaseelan V, King GA, Dixon AK, Anderson A, Bleehen NM (1986) Regional hyperthermia for extensive pelvic tumours using an APA applicator: a feasibility study. Br J Radiol 59: 1195–1201

Hunt JW (1990) Principles of ultrasound used for generating localized hyperthermia. In: Field SB, Hand JW (eds) An introduction to the practical aspects of clinical hyperthermia. Taylor & Francis, London, pp 371–422

Hynynen KH, Anhalt DP, Shimm DS, Roeemer RB, Cassady JR (1989) Scanned, multiple focussed beam system with real time imaging, 5th. Int Symposium of Hyperthermic Oncology, Kyoto, Japan, (see fursther kieller et al.), pp 666–669

Hynynen KH, Frederiksen F, Gautherie M (1992) Ultrasound hyperthermia: Task Group Report of the European Society for Hyperthermic Oncology. Tor Vergata Medical Physics Monograph Series, University of Rome Tor Vergata, Rome

Ibinni MS, Cain CA (1990) The concentric-ring array for ultrasound hyperthermia: combined mechanical and electrical scanning. Int J Hyperthermia 6: 401–419

Johnson RH, Preece AW, Murfin JL (1988) Flexible electromagnetic hyperthermia applicators, Abstracts of the 5th International Symposium on Hyperthermic Oncology, Kyoto, P44-a-6, 317

Jo S, Hiraoka M, Akuta K, Nishimiura Y, Nagata Y, Takahashi M, Abe M (1987) Clinical results of thermoradiotherapy for breast cancer. In: Onoyama Y (ed) Proceedings of the 3rd annual meeting of the Japanese Society of Hyperthermic oncology, Mag Bros. Inc., Tokyo, 339–340

Kapp DS, Fessenden P, Samulski TV et al. (1988b) Stanford University institutional report. Phase I evaluation of equipment for hyperthermic treatment of cancer, Int J Hyperthermia 4: 75–115

Kjellen E, Lindholm CE, Nilsson P (1989) Radiotherapy in combination with hyperthermia in recurrent or metastatic mammary carcinomas. 5th International Symposium on Hyperthermic oncology, Kyoto, Japan, Vol 2, Sugaharu T, Saito M, (eds) Taylor & Francis, London, New York, Philodelphia

Lagendijk JJW, Crezee J, Mooibroek J (1992) Progress in thermal modeling development. In: Gerner EW (ed) Hyperthermic oncology 1992, vol 1. Proceedings of the 6th Int Congress on Hyperthermic Oncology, Tucson, Avizona Board of Regents, p 456

Lee ER, Wilsey TR, Tanczy-Hornoch P, Kapp DS, Fessenden P, Lohnbach A, Prionas SD (1992) Body conformable 915 MHz microstrip array applicators for large surface area hyperthermia. IEEE Trans Biomed Eng 39: 470–483

Luk KH (1988) Training and certification issues in hyperthermia. In: Paliwal BR, Hetzel FW, Dewhirst MW (eds) Biological, physical and clinical aspects of hyperthermia. Medical Physics Monograph 16. American Inst of Physics, New York, pp 476–483

Luk KH, Pajak TF, Perez CA, Johnson RJ, Conner N, Dobbins T (1984) Prognostic factors for tumor response after hyperthermia and radiation In: Overgaard J (ed) Hyperthermic oncology, vol 1. Summary papers. Taylor & Francis, London, pp 353–356

Lumori MLD, Hand JW, Gopal MK, Cetas TC (1990) Use of Gaussian beam model in predicting SAR distributions from current sheet applicators. Phys Med Biol 35: 387–397

Magin RL, Peterson AF (1989) Noninvasive microwave arrays for local hyperthermia: a review. Int J Hyperthermia 5: 429–450

Masunaga S, Hiraoka M, Takahashi M et al. (1990) Clinical results of thermotherapy for locally advanced and/or recurrent breast cancer – comparison of results with radiotherapy alone. Int J Hyperthermia 6: 487–497

Moros EG, Roemer RB, Hynynen KH (1990) Pre-focal plane high-temperature regions induced by scanning focused ultrasound beams. Int J Hyperthermia 6: 351–366

Myerson RJ, Perez CA, Emami B, Straube W, Kuske RR, Leybovich L, Von Gerichten D (1990) Tumor control in long-term survivors following superficial hyperthermia. Int J Radiat Oncol Biol Phys 18: 1123–1129

Myerson RJ, Leybovich L, Emami B, Staube W, Von Gerichten D (1991) Phantom studies and preliminary clinical experience with the BSD-2000. Strahlenther Onkol 167, p 54

Oleson JR, Sim DA, Manning MR (1984) Analysis of prognostic variables in hyperthermia treatment of 161 patients. Int J Radiat Oncol Biol Phys 10: 2231–2239

Oleson JR, Dewhirst MW, Harrelson JM, Leopold KA, Samulski TV, Tso CY (1989) Tumor temperature distributions predict hyperthermia effect. Int J Radiat Oncol Biol Phys 16: 559–570

Perez CA, Emami B (1989) Clinical trials with local (external and interstitial) irradiation and hyperthermia. Radiol Clin North Am 27: 525–542

Perez CA, Kuske RR, Emami B, Fineberg B (1986) Irradiation alone or combined with hyperthermia in the treatment of recurrent carcinoma of the breast in the chest wall. A non-randomized comparison. Int J Hyperthermia 2: 179–187

Perez CA, Gillespie B, Pajak T, Hornback NB, Emami B, Rubin P (1989) Quality assurance problems in clinical hyperthermia and their impact on therapeutic outcome: a report by the Radiation Therapy Oncology Group. Int J Radiat Oncol Biol Phys 16: 551–558

Pilepich MV, Myerson RJ, Emami BN, Perez CA, Leybovich L, Von Gerichten D (1987) Regional hyperthermia: a feasibility analysis. Int J Hyperthermia 3: 247–351

Raskmark P, Gross E (1987) Balanced applicator tests. Internal report, Institute for Electronic Systems, University of Aalborg, Aalborg, Denmark

Rietveld PJM, Van Rhoon GC (1991) Preliminary results of the improved 433 MHz water filled waveguide applicator in an array application. Strahlenther Onkol 167: 335–336

Samulski TV, Fessenden P (1990) Thermometry in therapeutic hyperthermia. In: Gautherie M (ed) Methods of hyperthermia control. Springer, Berlin Heidelberg New York, pp 1–34

Samulski TV, Fessenden P, Lee ER, Kapp DS, Tanabe E, McEuen A (1990) Spiral microstrip hyperthermia applicators: technical design and clinical performance. Int J Radiat Oncol Biol Phys 18: 233–242

Sapareto SA, Corry PM (1989) A proposed standard data file format for hyperthermia treatments. Int J Radiat Oncol Biol Phys 16: 613–627

Sapozink MD, Gibbs F, Thomson JW, Eltringham JR, Stewart JR (1986) A comparison of deep regional hyperthermia from an annular array and a concentric coil in the same patients. Int J Radiat Oncol Biol Phys 11: 179–190

Sapozink MD, Gibbs FA, Gibbs P, Stewart JR (1988) Phase I evaluation of hyperthermia equipment – University of Utah Institutional Report. Int J Hyperthermia 4: 117–132

Sapozink MD, Corry PM, Kapp DS et al. (1991) RTOG quality assurance guidelines for clinical trials using hyperthermia for deep-seated malignancy. Int J Radiat Oncol Biol Phys 20: 1109–1115

Schaubert DH (1984) Electromagnetic heating of tissue-equivalent phantoms with thin, insulating partitions. Bioelectromagnetics 5: 221–232

Schneider CJ, Van Dijk JDP (1991) Visualisation by a matrix of light-emitting diodes of interference effects from a radiative four-applicator hyperthermia system. Int J Hyperthermia 7: 355–366

Schneider CJ, Van Dijk JDP, De Leeuw AAC, Wust P, Baumhoer W (1993) Quality assurance in various radiative hyperthermia systems applying a phantom with LED-matrix. Int J Hyperthermia, vol. 10, 5: 733–747

Seegenschmiedt MH, Brady LW, Sauer R, Karlsson UL, Herbst M, Tobin R (1988) Radiation therapy for superficial chest wall recurrences. Presented at the 8th meeting of the NAHG

Shimm DS, Cetas TC, Oleson JR, Cassady JR, Sim DA (1988) Clinical evaluation of hyperthermia equipment: the University of Arizona institutional report for the NCI hyperthermia equipment evaluation contract. Int J Hyperthermia 4: 39–51

Shimm DS, Cetas TC, Hynynen KH, Beuchler DN, Anhalt DP, Sykes HF, Cassady JR (1989) The CDRH helix, a phase I clinical trial. Am J Clin Oncol Cancer Clin Trials 12: 110–113

Shrivastava P, Luk K, Oleson JR et al. (1989) Hyperthermia quality assurance guidelines. Int J Radiat Oncol Biol Phys 16: 571–587

Sim DA, Dewhirst MW, Oleson JR, Grochowski JK (1984) Estimating the therapeutic advantage of adequate heat. In: Overgaard J (ed) Hyperthermic oncology 1984, vol I. Taylor & Francis, London, pp 359–362

Strohbehn JW, Curtis EH, Paulsen KD, Yuan X, Lynch DR (1989) Optimization of the absorbed power distribution for an annular phased array hyperthermia system. Int J Radiat Oncol Biol Phys 16: 589–599

Turner PF (1988) BSD-2000 operators manual

Van der Zee J, Van Rhoon GC, Wike-Hooley JL, Reinhold HS (1985) Clinically derived dose effect relationship for hyperthermia given in combination with low dose radiotherapy. Br J Radiol 58: 243–250

Van der Zee J, Van Putten WLJ, Van den Berg AP, Van Rhoon GC, Wike-Hooley JL, Broekmeyer-Reurink MP, Reinhold HS (1986) Retrospective analysis of the response of tumours is patients treated with a combination of radiotherapy and hyperthermia. Int J Hyperthermia 2: 337–345

Van der Zee J, Treurniet-Donker AD, The SK et al. (1988) Low dose reirradiation in combination with hyperthermia: a palliative treatment in combination with breast cancer recurring in previously irradiated areas. Int J Radiat Oncol Biol Phys 15: 1407–1413

Van der Zee J, Veeze-Kuijpers B, Wiggers T, Treurniet-Donker AD (1992a) Risk of tumour growth along thermometry catheter tract. A case report. Int J Hyperthermia 8: 621–624

Van der Zee J, Van Rhoon GC, Verloop-van't Hof EM, Van der Ploeg SK, Rietveld PJM, Van den Berg AP (1992b) The importance of adequate heating techniques for therapeutic outcome. In: Gerner EW, Cetas TC (eds) Hyperthermic oncology, vol 2. Arizona Board of Regents, Arizona, pp 349–352

Visser AG, Chive M, Hand JW, Lagendijk JJW, Marchal C, Roos D, Seegenschmiedt MH, Van Dijk JDP (1993) COMAC BME/EHSO Task Group Report. Interstitial and intracavitary hyperthermia. Tor Vergata Medical Physics Monograph Series, vol 4. University of Rome

Waterman FM, Dewhirst MW, Samulski TV et al. (1991) RTOG quality assurance guidelines for clinical trials using hyperthermia administered by ultrasound. Int J Radiat Oncol Biol Phys 20: 1099–1107

Wust P, Nadobny J, Fahling H, Felix R (1990) First clinical experiences with the BSD-2000: experimental and theoretical evaluation. Strahlenther Onkol 167: 55

Wust P, Nadobny J, Felix R, Deuflhard P, Louis A, John W (1991) Strategies for optimized application of annular-phased-array systems in clinical hyperthermia. Int J Hyperthermia 7: 157–173

Subject Index

List of Contributors

JEAN-CHARLES BOLOMEY, PhD
Professor, Electromagnetics Department
SUPELEC
University of Paris XI
Plateau du Moulon
91190 Gif-sur-Yvette
France

PAUL BURGMAN, PhD
Department of Medical Physics
and Radiation Oncology
Memorial Sloan-Kettering Cancer Center
1275 York Avenue
New York, NY 10021
USA

I.B. CHOI, MD
Radiation Biology Section
Department of Therapeutic Radiology
University of Minnesota
Box 494 UMHC
Minneapolis, MN 55455
USA

J. CREZEE, PhD
Department of Radiotherapy
University Hospital Utrecht
Heidelberglaan 100
3584 CX Utrecht
The Netherlands

OLAV DAHL, MD
Department of Oncology
University of Bergen
Haukeland Hospital
5021 Bergen
Norway

MARK W. DEWHIRST, DVM, PhD
Tumor Microcirculation Laboratory
Department of Radiation Oncology
Duke University Medical Center
P.O. Box 3455
Durham, NC 27710
USA

C.J. DIEDERICH, PhD
Department of Radiation Oncology
University of California
P.O. Box 0226
San Francisco, CA 94143
USA

ROLAND FELIX, MD
Department of Radiation Oncology
Universitätsklinikum Rudolf Virchow
Standort Wedding
Freie Universität Berlin
Augustenburger Platz 1
13353 Berlin
Germany

KULLERVO HYNYNEN, PhD
Department of Radiology
Brigham and Women's Hospital
Harvard Medical School
75 Francis Street
Boston, MA 02115
USA

DEBRA K. KELLEHER, PhD
Institute of Physiology and Pathophysiology
University of Mainz
Duesbergweg 6
55099 Mainz
Germany

A.W.T. KONINGS, PhD
Department of Radiobiology
University of Groningen
Bloemsingel 1
9713 BZ Groningen
The Netherlands

JAN J.W. LAGENDIJK, PhD
Department of Radiotherapy
University Hospital Utrecht
Heidelberglaan 100
3584 CX Utrecht
The Netherlands

D. le Bihan, MD
Department of Health & Human Services
National Institutes of Health
The Warren G. Clinical Center
Building 10, Room 1C660
Bethesda, MD 20892
USA

Eric R. Lee, BSEE
Physical Science Research
SLAC-Mail Stop 61
Stanford, CA 94305
USA

Gloria C. Li, PhD
Departments of Medical Physics
and Radiation Oncology
Memorial Sloan-Kettering Cancer Center
1275 York Avenue
New York, NY 10021
USA

S. Mizushina, PhD
Professor, Research Institute of Electronics
Shizuoka University
3-5-1 Johoku
Hammamatsu 432
Japan

Jaap Mooibroek, MSc
Department of Radiotherapy
University Hospital Utrecht
Heidelberglaan 100
3584 CX Utrecht
The Netherlands

Jacek Nadobny, PhD
Abteilung Radiologie mit Poliklinik
Universitätsklinikum Rudolf Virchow
Standort Wedding
Freie Universität Berlin
Augustenburger Platz 1
13353 Berlin
Germany

B.S. Nah, MD
Radiation Biology Section
Department of Therapeutic Radiology
University of Minnesota
Box 494 UMHC
Minneapolis, MN 55455
USA

Andre Nussenzweig, PhD
Department of Medical Physics
and Radiation Oncology
Memorial Sloan-Kettering Cancer Center
1275 York Avenue
New York, NY 10021
USA

R. Olmi, PhD
IROE – National Research Council
Via Panciachiti 64
50127 Firenze
Italy

J.L. Osborn, BS
Radiation Biology Section
Department of Therapeutic Radiology
University of Minnesota
Box 494 UMHC
Minneapolis, MN 55455
USA

Keith D. Paulsen, PhD
Thayer School of Engineering
Dartmouth College
Hinman Box 8000
Hanover, NH 03755
USA

Deborah M. Prescott, DVM, PhD
Assistant Professor
Department of Radiation Oncology
Duke University Medical Center
P.O. Box 3455
Durham, NC 27710
USA

Dan I. Roos, PhD
Department of Gynecological Oncology
Örebro Medical Center Hospital
70185 Örebro
Sweden

S.K. Sahu, PhD
Radiation Biology Section
Department of Therapeutic Radiology
University of Minnesota
P.O. Box 494 UMHC
Minneapolis, MN 55455
USA

C.J. SCHNEIDER, PhD
Department of Radiotherapy
Amsterdam University Hospital
Academisch Medisch Centrum
Meibergdreef 9
1105 AZ Amsterdam
The Netherlands

MARTIN SEEBASS, PhD
Konrad Zuse Zentrum
for Information Technology
Heibronner Straße 10
10711 Berlin
Germany

M. HEINRICH SEEGENSCHMIEDT, MD
Department of Radiation Oncology
University of Erlangen-Nürnberg
Universitätsstraße 27
91054 Erlangen
Germany

Chang W. Song, PhD
Radiation Biology Section
Department of Therapeutic Radiology
University of Minnesota
Box 494 UMHC
Minneapolis, MN 55455
USA

BENGT SORBE, MD
Department of Gynecological Oncology
Örebro Medical Center Hospital
70185 Örebro
Sweden

PAUL R. STAUFFER, MSEE
Department of Radiation Oncology
University of California
P.O. Box 0226
San Francisco, CA 94143
USA

CHRISTIAN STREFFER, PhD, MD h.c.
Professor, Department of Medical Radiobiology
Universitätsklinikum Essen
45122 Essen
Germany

JAN D.P. VAN DIJK, PhD
Department of Radiotherapy
Amsterdam University Hospital
Academisch Medisch Centrum
Meibergdreef 9
1105 AZ Amsterdam
The Netherlands

GERARD C. VAN RHOON, PhD
Department of Hyperthermia
Dr. Daniel den Hoed Cancer Center
P.O. Box 5201
Groene Hilledijk 301
3008 AE Rotterdam
The Netherlands

PETER W. VAUPEL, MD
Professor, Institute of Physiology
and Pathophysiology
University of Mainz
Duesbergweg 6
55099 Mainz
Germany

CLARE C. VERNON, MA, FRCR
Department of Clinical Oncology
Hammersmith Hospital
Ducane Road
London, W12 OHS
England

ANDRIES G. VISSER, PhD
Department of Clinical Physics
Dr. Daniel den Hoed Cancer Center
P.O. Box 5201
Groene Hilledijk 301
3008 AE Rotterdam
The Netherlands

FRANK M. WATERMAN, PhD
Professor of Medical Physics
Department of Radiation Oncology
Thomas Jefferson University Hospital
111 South 11th Street
Philadelphia, PA 19107-5097
USA

PETER WUST, MD
Department of Radiation Oncology
Universitätsklinikum Rudolf Virchow
Standort Wedding
Freie Universität Berlin
Augustenburger Platz 1
13353 Berlin
Germany